Craniofacial Microsomia and Treacher Collins Syndrome

David M. Yates • Michael R. Markiewicz
Editors

Craniofacial Microsomia and Treacher Collins Syndrome

Comprehensive Treatment of Associated Facial Deformities

Springer

Editors
David M. Yates
Division of Cranial and Facial Surgery
El Paso Children's Hospital
El Paso, TX
USA

Michael R. Markiewicz
Department of Oral and
Maxillofacial Surgery
University at Buffalo
Buffalo, NY
USA

ISBN 978-3-030-84732-6 ISBN 978-3-030-84733-3 (eBook)
https://doi.org/10.1007/978-3-030-84733-3

This Springer imprint is published by the registered company Springer Nature Switzerland AG
The registered company address is: Gewerbestrasse 11, 6330 Cham, Switzerland

This book is dedicated to the following individuals:

Soli Deo Gloria

Most importantly this book is dedicated to my wife, Mariana, who has tirelessly supported and loved me. She is my sounding board, my advisor, my co life-adventurer, and my best friend. Thanks for living life with me.

My children – Ana, Luke, Liliana, Noah – YOU are my GREATEST inspirations. You bring me great joy everyday, and love me unconditionally. You give me hope for the future and I love you all very much!

My parents – Jess and Bertie – Thank you for loving me, molding me, and shaping me into the father, man, and surgeon I am today.

My Mentors – Dr Ghali Ghali, Richard Finn, Douglas Sinn, John Zuniga, John Stella, Paul Tiwana, Robert V. Walker, and Kenny Gambrell – thank you for all your efforts with me, your patience, your time, and commitment to train and make me the surgeon that I am today

My Partners – Drs Vernon Burke, Reo Pugao, Natasha Fürchtgott, and Hans Brockhoff – You make work fun! I could not imagine a better group of individuals to work and grow with! Thank you for your commitment to training our fellow, and for your loyalty, kindness, and friendship.

David M. Yates

To those family, friends, colleagues, mentors, students, and patients, who have enriched my life, professionally and personally by supporting and making me better. Thank you.

Michael R. Markiewicz

Foreword

The "foreword" to a book or other works of literature, in contrast to the "preface," is usually written by someone other than the authors or editors. An expert, a prominent figure in the field, or someone who because of previous experience or publications on the subject is chosen to review the book. I am flattered that Drs. Markiewicz and Yates asked me to write this foreword as I have been interested in first and second pharyngeal arch deformities for almost 50 years. The role of the foreword writer is to provide a short (hence fore***word***) objective assessment and overall summary of the work to help the potential audience decide whether to buy and read the book. Presumably, the foreword will be laudatory, give the book credibility, and recommend it to the readers. In contrast, a preface is usually written by the authors to explain why they chose the subject, the aims of the book, the learning goals, and a summary. In the craniomaxillofacial surgery literature, a preface is attached to works more commonly than a foreword. It should be noted that the correct spelling is "foreword," not "forward," and this has been called the most frequently misspelled word in the English language.

Often, the authors or editors of a book are experts in the particular subject(s). Searching the literature using the terms hemifacial microsomia (HFM), craniofacial microsomia, first and second pharyngeal arch deformities, branchial arch deformities, Treacher Collins syndrome (TCS), Nager syndrome, facioauriculovertebral syndrome, ocular-auriculo-vertebral spectrum, and lateral-facial dysplasia, among others. does not produce significant contributions by the editors of this book. Exploring how these two editors became interested in craniomaxillofacial deformities is informative for department chairs, program directors, and oral and maxillofacial surgery (OMS)faculty. It demonstrates how exposure during the early phases of dental education can have a profound effect on students and their career choices.

I first met Michael Markiewicz as a 2nd or 3rd year dental student during his observational visits to the craniofacial clinic at Boston Children's Hospital, where he often witnessed the interactions between myself and Dr. John Mulliken on children with complicated deformities. He had an interest in research and he participated in projects with Dr. Tom Dodson at Massachusetts General Hospital (MGH). Markiewicz was then accepted to the Harvard School of Public Health for an MPH under the tutelage of Dr. Dodson who was the director of the MGH OMS Center for Advanced Clinical Investigation. These two experiences started him on his path to an academic career in OMS with a special interest in craniomaxillofacial deformities. Similarly, David Yates, as a student on a 2-month mission trip in Mexico, was exposed to patients with craniofacial deformities, many of whom had cleft lip and palate. Oral and maxillofacial surgeons were performing reconstructive operations for underserved children in poverty. In addition, he was inspired by the book *Ships of Mercy* which describes the work of Dr. Gary Parker, an OMS who has treated many children with congenital facial deformities and who served as the chief medical officer on these floating "ships of mercy." These experiences motivated Yates to become an OMS. He applied and was accepted in dental school and completed his residency in OMS at the University of Texas Southwestern, Parkland Hospital. He recalled: "One of my first weeks there, Dr. Sinn did two craniosynostosis patients… I was hooked!" He completed the residency and then a fellowship in cleft-craniofacial surgery.

Dr. Markiewicz and Dr. Yates are now well trained, board certified surgeons concentrating on craniomaxillofacial and cleft deformities with a career commitment to treating these patients. As young surgeons looking for guidance in the literature, they found that there is no central repository to be used as a resource for diagnosis and management of children and adults with first and second pharyngeal arch deformities. Hence, they decided to recruit a group of experts in this field to produce an authoritative text for clinicians. The result is: *Comprehensive Management of Craniofacial Microsomia and Treacher Collins Syndrome* by Michael Markiewicz and David Yates (editors).

When I began my career in the early 1970s, there was no unified concept of the asymmetric and symmetric first and second pharyngeal arch deformities. The patients were often treated in isolation by various specialists: otolaryngologists worked on hearing issues, plastic surgeons on soft tissue deficiencies, both on the problem of microtia, orthodontists on the teeth, oral and maxillofacial surgeons on the jaws and skeletal contour asymmetries, and speech pathologists on speech. Many patients also had cleft lip and palate. Hemifacial microsomia was considered a unilateral deformity without consideration of the effects of the primary defect on the adjacent and contralateral facial skeleton. There was very little coordination of care and no road map for the timing and sequence of treatment. Much progress has been made over the past 50 years. There is a better, although not complete, understanding of the etiopathogenesis, epidemiology, sequence of growth, and effects on the adjacent and contralateral facial skeleton. In addition, the majority of patients are now treated in specialized multidisciplinary craniofacial centers with input from all the relevant specialists. There have been considerable advances in imaging for diagnosis, individualized virtual treatment planning, and corrective surgery using personalized cutting guides and fixation hardware. However, because these are rare conditions and there are few large series from single institutions, many challenges remain. The optimal timing and sequence for surgical procedures, the role of growth-modifying dental orthopedics, the management of facial nerve, hearing, and soft tissue deficits, to mention a few, are yet to be determined using prospective controlled studies with high-quality data. As a practical matter, a comprehensive evidenced-based text serving as a resource to help students, residents, fellows, and practicing clinicians caring for these patients would be a significant contribution. This is the goal of *Comprehensive Management of Craniofacial Microsomia and Treacher Collins Syndrome.*

It is a tribute to their credibility in craniomaxillofacial surgery and their dedication to this subject that Drs. Markiewicz and Yates have been able to assemble a large group of credible experts to accomplish this comprehensive text. There are 26 chapters; the first 12 are devoted primarily to craniofacial microsomia/hemifacial microsomia (HFM) with some material also on TCS (Chaps. 9 and 10) as it relates to hearing and external ear deformities that occur in both syndromes. Chapters 13, 14, 15, 16, 17, 18, 19, 21, 22, 23, 24, 25, and 26 are primarily dedicated to TCS, and Chap. 20 reviews the use of alloplastic temporomandibular joint placement (TMJR) in both HFM and TCS. There are 70 listed contributors representing multiple specialties, geographic locations, and a broad range of ages and years of experience. Perusing the list of contributors one can infer that the book does not represent a specific or consistent conceptual philosophy or point of view. Rather, it is a general encyclopedic treatise on multiple aspects concerning HFM and TCS. In addition, there is a good deal of repetition and overlap of general information in the chapters. Recognizing these inherent issues with multi authored textbooks covering a broad subject area, the editors bring both parts of the book to closure in Chaps. 12 and 26, the overviews for HFM and TCS. A chapter worth mentioning, "Etiology and Anatomical Variation in Treacher Collins," by FJ Smith, begins with an enlightening and inspirational personal perspective on this condition, as the author has Treacher Collins syndrome.

The variety of authors and specialties involved in this book provide a real-life template on how to think and work collegially on these complicated patients, appreciating the contributions of each area of expertise. This is an example of interdisciplinary collaboration, the model for how these patients should be managed. In addition, the book brings to the reader a comprehensive resource under one cover with background, historic perspective, and multiple points of view with references. It will help students, residents, fellows, and young and older surgeons understand the complexity of these deformities and provide high-quality patient care.

Leonard B. Kaban
Walter C. Guralnick
Department of Oral & Maxillofacial Surgery
Harvard School of Dental Medicine
Massachusetts General Hospital
Boston, MA, USA

Preface

The premise of this book is simple. When searching for a comprehensive resource on the management of patients with craniofacial microsomia and Treacher Collins syndrome, we found that this text did not exist. In fact, we were surprised when we realized that there were no definitive texts, on either subject. Given the common management and procedures utilized to manage patients with both Craniofacial Microsomia and Treacher Collins Syndrome, we felt that both entities would be best addressed in the form of a sequential two volume text.

As two early career cleft and craniofacial surgeons, we were immediately confronted with patients suffering from these difficult and rare conditions. The majority of which had undergone multiple procedures – most of which did little to improve their cosmetic appearance, functional outcomes, or quality of life. This was certainly not due to the honorable intentions by the previous treating surgeons. In fact, most patients had been operated on by multiple surgeons from various specialties in an attempt to improve the life of these patients. These patients suffer significant functional limitations related to speech, mastication, breathing, hearing, and vision. In addition, they have cosmetic concerns including facial deformities and microtia, resulting in a significant psychological burden. When we turned to the literature on these topics, we found an abundance of information, but it appeared to be disjointed and incomplete. Most importantly, there was no definitive text that delivered a comprehensive approach for managing patients with these challenging conditions.

We wanted to compose a book which addressed the diagnosis and management of all aspects of these two entities, a manual by which a practitioner could open the first page, read through the chapters, and upon completion be provided with a roadmap on how to treat these rare conditions. Therefore, we compiled a list of necessary and pertinent subject matter, and engaged expert level authors to address these topics in a comprehensive evidence based manner. This book is multidisciplinary in nature and takes a comprehensive look at craniofacial microsomia and Treacher Collins syndrome, specifically with regards to surgical management.

This book has been a labor of love and its content has already changed the way in which we manage our own patients. We are very grateful to the authors who have contributed and the content they have offered. Our hope is that this text will provide guidance to young and experienced surgeons alike so that we may optimize the management of these patients who entrust us with their lives and care.

El Paso, TX, USA David M. Yates
Buffalo, NY, USA Michael R. Markiewicz

Contents

Contributors

Shelly Abramowicz, DMD, MPH, FACS Division of Oral and Maxillofacial Surgery, Department of Surgery, Emory University School of Medicine, Chief of Oral and Maxillofacial Surgery, Children's Healthcare of Atlanta, Atlanta, GA, USA

Imran Ahson, DMD, MD New Hampshire Oral and Maxillofacial Surgery, Nashua, NH, USA

Kristan P. Alfonso, MD Department of Otolaryngology- Head and Neck Surgery, Emory University, Atlanta, GA, USA

Division of Pediatric Otolaryngology, Children's Healthcare of Atlanta, Center for Advanced Pediatrics, Atlanta, GA, USA

Veerasathpurush Allareddy, BDS, PhD Department of Orthodontics, Department of Orthodontics, College of Dentistry, University of Illinois at Chicago, Chicago, IL, USA

Malena M. Amato, MD, FACS Department of Ophthalmology, The University of Texas at Austin Dell Medical School, Austin, TX, USA

Shika Andhole, BSA, MS The University of Texas at Austin, Austin, TX, USA

Sharon Aronovich, DMD, FRCD(C), FACS University of Michigan, Oral and Maxillofacial Surgery, Ann Arbor, MI, USA

Kevin E. Bright, MD, FACS Department of Surgery, Texas Tech School of Medicine, Lubbock, TX, USA

El Paso Cleft Palate and Craniofacial Team, El Paso, PA, USA

Valerie Bright, BS Biochemistry El Paso, TX, USA

Laura Brooks, M.Ed. CCC-SLP BCS-S Children's Healthcare of Atlanta, Atlanta, GA, USA

Zachary Brown, DDS, MD University of Texas Health Sciences Center San Antonio, Department of Oral and Maxillofacial Surgery, San Antonio, TX, USA

Partner at Facial Surgery Group, Kansas City, MO, USA

Sediqua Bufford, MSBT Morehouse School of Medicine, Atlanta, GA, USA

Vernon Burke, DMD, MD High Desert Oral and Facial Surgery, El Paso Children's Hospital, El Paso, TX, USA

Kevin Chow, BA McGovern Medical School, University of Texas Health Science Center at Houston, Houston, TX, USA

Maura Cosetti, MD Ear Institute, New York Eye and Ear of Mount Sinai, New York, NY, USA

Department of Otolaryngology-Head and Neck Surgery and Neurosurgery, Icahn School of Medicine at Mount Sinai, New York, NY, USA

Evan C. Cumpston, MD Department of Otolaryngology-Head & Neck Surgery, Resident at UT Health San Antonio, San Antonio, TX, USA

Adriana da Silveira, DDS, Ms, PhD Dell Children's Medical Center of Central Texas, Dell Seton Medical Center at The University of Texas, Private Practice, Austin, TX, USA

Karin De La Fuente, M.S., CCC-SLP EL PASO SPEECH AND LANGUAGE SERVICE EXCELLENCE INC, El Paso, PA, USA

Pollyana Marques de Moura, DDS, Ms, PhD Private Practice, Dallas, TX, USA

Sean Peter Edwards, MD, DDS, FRCD(C), FACS University of Michigan, Oral and Maxillofacial Surgery, Ann Arbor, MI, USA

Mark A. Egbert, DDS Department of Surgery, Division of Plastic Surgery, University of Washington School of Medicine, Seattle, WA, USA

Department of Oral and Maxillofacial Surgery, University of Washington School of Dentistry, Seattle, WA, USA

Craniofacial Center, Seattle Children's Hospital, Seattle, WA, USA

Mohammed H. Elnagar, DDS, PhD Department of Orthodontics, College of Dentistry - University of Illinois at Chicago, Chicago, IL, USA

Ashish Francis, MD Department of Surgery and Perioperative Care, The University of Texas at Austin Dell Medical School, Austin, TX, USA

Division of Craniofacial and Pediatric Plastic Surgery, Dell Children's Medical Center of Central Texas, Austin, TX, USA

Division of Craniofacial and Pediatric Plastic and Reconstructive Surgery, Akron Children's Hospital, Akron, OH, USA

Jaymee Franknecht, AuD Department of Otolaryngology-Head and Neck Surgery, Columbia University Medical Center, New York, NY, USA

Natasha Fürchtgott, DDS, MS Partner, Private Practice, High Desert Oral and Facial Surgery, El Paso, TX, USA

Vice Chair Department of Oral and Maxillofacial Surgery El Paso Children's Hospital, El Paso, TX, USA

Assistant Clinical Professor, Texas Tech University Health Sciences Center El Paso, WLH School of Dental Medicine, El Paso, TX, USA

Adjunct Faculty, University of Texas Health Sciences Center San Antonio, Department of Oral and Maxillofacial Surgery, San Antonio, TX, USA

Danielle Gill, DMD Carolinas Center for Oral and Facial Surgery, Charlotte, NC, USA

Paulo Zupelari Goncalves, DDS, PhD University of Michigan, Oral and Maxillofacial Surgery, Ann Arbor, MI, USA

University Center of Ourinhos, São Paulo, Brazil

Steven Goudy, MD Children's Healthcare of Atlanta, Atlanta, GA, USA

Department of Otolaryngology-Head and Neck Surgery, Emory University School of Medicine, Atlanta, GA, USA

Raymond Harshbarger, MD, FACS, FAAP Department of Surgery and Perioperative Care, The University of Texas at Austin Dell Medical School, Austin, TX, USA

Division of Craniofacial and Pediatric Plastic Surgery, Dell Children's Medical Center of Central Texas, Austin, TX, USA

Richard A. Hopper, MD, MS Department of Surgery, Division of Plastic Surgery, University of Washington School of Medicine, Seattle, WA, USA

Craniofacial Center, Seattle Children's Hospital, Seattle, WA, USA

Hitesh Kapadia, DDS, PhD Craniofacial Center, Division of Craniofacial Orthodontics, Seattle Children's Hospital, Seattle, WA, USA

University of Washington School of Dentistry, Seattle, WA, USA

Lauren Kaplan, AuD Ear Institute, New York Eye and Ear of Mount Sinai, New York, NY, USA

Patrick Kelley, MD Department of Surgery and Perioperative Care, The University of Texas at Austin Dell Medical School, Austin, TX, USA

Division of Craniofacial and Pediatric Plastic Surgery, Dell Children's Medical Center of Central Texas, Austin, TX, USA

Paul W. Kloostra, DDS, MD Cleft and Craniofacial Surgery, CAMC Cleft and Craniofacial Center, Charleston Area Medical Center Women & Children's Hospital, Charleston, WV, USA

Tania Kraai, MD University of New Mexico Health Science Centers, Department of Surgery, Albuquerque, NM, USA

Jessica S. Lee, DDS, MD, MA Northeast Facial and Oral Surgery Specialists, Florham Park, NJ, USA

Former Pediatric Cleft and Craniofacial Surgery Fellow, Cleft and Craniofacial Center, Charleston Area Medical Center, Women & Children's Hospital, Charleston, WV, USA

Sheryl Lewin, MD Lewin Ear Reconstruction, Torrance, CA, USA

Aaron Liddell, MD, DMD, FACS Private Practice. Colorado Oral and Maxillofacial Surgery, Denver, CO, USA

Yi-Chun Carol Liu, MD Department of Otolaryngology-Head and Neck Surgery, Baylor College of Medicine, Houston, TX, USA

Division of Pediatric Otolaryngology, Texas Children's Hospital, Houston, TX, USA

James Maclaine, BDS Clinical Instructor, Department of Developmental Biology, Boston Children's Hospital and Harvard School of Dental Medicine, Boston, MA, USA

Ashley Manlove, DMD, MD, FACS Carle Illinois College of Medicine, Department of Oral and Maxillofacial Surgery, Carle Foundation Hospital, Director Cleft and Craniofacial Team, Urbana, IL, USA

Michael R. Markiewicz, DDS, MD, MPH, FACS, FAAP Department of Oral and Maxillofacial Surgery, University at Buffalo, Buffalo, NY, USA

Alexander P. Marston, MD Tufts University School of Medicine, Department of Otolaryngology – Head and Neck Surgery, Division of Pediatric Otolaryngology, Division of Facial Plastic and Reconstructive Surgery, Boston, MA, USA

Michael Miloro, MD, DMD, FACS Department of Oral and Maxillofacial Surgery, University of Illinois, Chicago, IL, USA

Brian Mitchell, DDS Department of Oral and Maxillofacial Surgery, Carle Foundation Hospital, Urbana, IL, USA

Alexis Olsson, DDS, FACS Oral and Maxillofacial Surgery, Northwestern University Feinberg School of Medicine, Northwestern Memorial Hospital, Chicago, IL, USA

Paul W. Orjuela, DDS Department of Oral & Maxillofacial Surgery, The University of Oklahoma Health Sciences Center, Oklahoma City, OK, USA

Bonnie L. Padwa, DMD, MD, FACS Harvard School of Dental Medicine and Harvard Medical School, Boston, MA, USA

Department of Plastic and Oral Surgery, Boston Children's Hospital, Boston, MA, USA

Daniel Perez, DDS Oral and Maxillofacial Surgery Department, UT Health San Antonio, San Antonio, TX, USA

Brian Perry, MD Department of Otolaryngology-Head & Neck Surgery, University of Texas-Rio Grande Valley, Edinburg, TX, USA

Cory M. Resnick, DMD, MD, FACS Harvard School of Dental Medicine and Harvard Medical School, Boston, MA, USA

Department of Plastic and Oral Surgery, Boston Children's Hospital, Boston, MA, USA

Pat Ricalde, DDS, MD, FACS Florida Craniofacial Institute, University of South Florida, St. Joseph's Cleft & Craniofacial Center, Tampa, FL, USA

Fabio G. Ritto, DDS, MD, MS, PhD Department of Oral & Maxillofacial Surgery, The University of Oklahoma Health Sciences Center, Oklahoma City, OK, USA

E. Weston Santee, DDS, MD High Desert Oral and Facial Surgery and El Paso Children's Hospital 2019-2020, El Paso, TX, USA

Andrew R. Scott, MD Tufts University School of Medicine, Department of Otolaryngology – Head and Neck Surgery, Division of Pediatric Otolaryngology, Division of Facial Plastic and Reconstructive Surgery, Boston, MA, USA

Rosemary Seelaus, BS, MAMS, CCA The Craniofacial Center, Department of Surgery, University of Illinois at Chicago, Chicago, IL, USA

Farooq Shahzad, MBBS, MS, FACS, FAAP Division of Plastic & Reconstructive Surgery, Memorial Sloan-Kettering Cancer Center, Weill Medical College of Cornell University, New York, NY, USA

Rodrigo C. Silva, MD Department of Otolaryngology-Head and Neck Surgery, Baylor College of Medicine, Houston, TX, USA

Division of Pediatric Otolaryngology, Texas Children's Hospital, Houston, TX, USA

Douglas P. Sinn, DDS, FACS University of Texas Southwestern Medical Center/ Parkland Hospital, Mansfield, TX, USA

Francis Joel Smith, PhD Department of Cell & Developmental Biology, Modern Human Anatomy Program, University of Colorado Anschutz Medical Campus, School of Medicine, Aurora, CO, USA

Kevin S. Smith, DDS, FACS, FACD Department of Oral & Maxillofacial Surgery, The University of Oklahoma Health Sciences Center, Oklahoma City, OK, USA

Srinivas M. Susarla, DMD, MD, MPH Department of Surgery, Division of Plastic Surgery, University of Washington School of Medicine, Seattle, WA, USA

Department of Oral and Maxillofacial Surgery, University of Washington School of Dentistry, Seattle, WA, USA

Craniofacial Center, Seattle Children's Hospital, Seattle, WA, USA

Andrea Sweetnam, M.S., CCC/A Pediatric and Cochlear Implant Audiologist at Southwest Ear, Nose, and Throat Consultants, El Paso, TX, USA

Randi Tepper, AuD Ear Institute, New York Eye and Ear of Mount Sinai, New York, NY, USA

Paul S. Tiwana, DDS, MD, MS, FACS, FACD Department of Oral & Maxillofacial Surgery, The University of Oklahoma Health Sciences Center, Oklahoma City, OK, USA

Katherine Vandenberg, MD University of New Mexico Health Science Centers, Department of Surgery, Albuquerque, NM, USA

Adam Wandell, DDS Oral and Maxillofacial Surgery Department, UT Health San Antonio, San Antonio, TX, USA

Larry M. Wolford, DMD Clinical Professor of Oral and Maxillofacial Srugery and Orthodontics, Texas A&M University College of Dentistry, Private Practice; Baylor University Medical Center, Dallas, TX, USA

David M. Yates, MD, DMD, FACS Division of Cranial and Facial Surgery, El Paso Children's Hospital, El Paso, TX, USA

Paul Foster School of Medicine El Paso, El Paso, TX, USA

Oral and Maxillofacial Surgery, University of Texas Health Sciences Center, San Antonio, TX, USA

Part I
Craniofacial Microsomia CFM

Chapter 1
Etiology and Anatomical Variance in Craniofacial Microsomia

Ashley Manlove, Brian Mitchell, and Shelly Abramowicz

Introduction

Craniofacial microsomia (CFM) is a condition that includes a spectrum of phenotypic craniofacial anomalies that result from abnormal development of the first and second branchial arches. The term CFM is often used interchangeably with other names, most commonly hemifacial microsomia (HFM). Historically there has been a variety of nomenclature used to describe the different phenotypical anomalies associated with CFM including HFM, Goldenhar syndrome, oculoauriculovertebral dysplasia, oromandibular dysostosis, as well as others. The degree of overlap (or lack thereof) of phenotypic characteristics has led some experts to believe CFM is a spectrum. The term oculoauriculovertebral spectrum has been used as an encompassing term for these variable phenotypes and has also been used interchangeably with CFM or HFM [1].

CFM occurs in 1:3000 to 1:5000 live births [2, 3]. Most cases are sporadic, but there are rare familial cases [4]. CFM does not have definitive diagnostic criteria, such as a genetic test, but consists of a spectrum of phenotypic presentations with underdevelopment of the various parts of facial skeleton and underlying soft tissues.

A. Manlove
Carle Illinois College of Medicine, Department of Oral and Maxillofacial Surgery, Carle Foundation Hospital, Director Cleft and Craniofacial Team, Urbana, IL, USA
e-mail: Ashley.Manlove@carle.com

B. Mitchell
Department of Oral and Maxillofacial Surgery, Carle Foundation Hospital, Urbana, IL, USA
e-mail: Brian.Mitchell@Carle.com

S. Abramowicz (✉)
Division of Oral and Maxillofacial Surgery, Department of Surgery, Emory University School of Medicine, Chief of Oral and Maxillofacial Surgery, Children's Healthcare of Atlanta, Atlanta, GA, USA
e-mail: sabram5@emory.edu

D. M. Yates, M. R. Markiewicz (eds.), *Craniofacial Microsomia and Treacher Collins Syndrome*, https://doi.org/10.1007/978-3-030-84733-3_1

The orbits, zygomatic arch, maxilla, mandible, ears, facial nerves, and facial muscles may be affected. These anomalies can cause airway compromise, feeding issues, facial paralysis, hearing challenges, and malocclusion. Therefore, a child with CFM is best treated by a multidisciplinary team and followed from birth to adulthood. This chapter will discuss pathogenesis, classification, and clinical presentation of CFM.

Pathogenesis

The first and second pharyngeal arches form around the 4th week of embryologic development when the migration of neural crest cells from the neural tube begins the development of branchial arch ectomesenchyme [5, 6]. Each branchial arch has three layers (endoderm, mesenchyme, and ectoderm) which produce the four primordial components – muscle, artery, nerve, and cartilage [6]. These arches give rise to the structures of the face innervated by cranial nerves V and VII. The first branchial arch gives rise to the maxilla, mandible, zygoma, trigeminal nerve, muscles of mastication, and the anterior portion of the ear (tragus, root, and superior helix) as well as the malleolus and incus. The second branchial arch gives rise to the hyoid bone, the styloid process and facial nerve, the facial muscles and most of the ear (helix, antihelix, antitragus, and lobule), as well as the stapes [7]. For these structures to fully form, the mesenchymal cells of the arches must maintain continuous tissue-to-tissue communication to support the development of the skeletal, muscular, and neural components [8]. Disruption of this communication can result in hypoplasia or aplasia of the affected structure [2].

The pathogenesis of CFM has not been definitively proven; however, etiology is presumed to be due to abnormalities in the development of the first and second branchial arches [9]. There are two prevailing theories in which the disruption of branchial arch development causes subsequent malformation of craniofacial structures and, thus, CFM forms (1) vascular abnormalities and hemorrhage and (2) abnormal cranial neural crest cell migration.

Vascular Abnormalities and Hemorrhage

In 1948 Braithwaite and Watson initially suggested that abnormal development or the absence of the stapedial artery in utero could lead to ischemia and necrosis of developing tissue, thus resulting in the phenotype of CFM [2]. The stapedial artery is a transient structure within normal fetal development that arises around the 33rd day in utero. It provides the vascular distribution to supply the primordia of the first and second branchial arches and is the dominant blood supply to the face. It later connects the future external carotid artery to the internal carotid artery. The stapedial artery regresses by the 45th day of development [10]. Poswillo led a well-known study in 1973 consisting of mice and *M. irus* monkey models with the first and second branchial arch anomalies. The animals had similar findings to CFM. He evaluated the embryos throughout their development and identified small areas of hemorrhage and hematoma formation shortly following the anastomosis of vessels that form the stapedial arterial stem. The bleeding affected the first and second branchial arches [2]. This theory also explains the variable nature of CFM, as a varying amount of hemorrhage would produce different sizes and shapes of hematomas, thus resulting in damage to local developing tissues in differing ways. This could result in a wide spectrum of phenotypic variability [10].

Abnormal Cranial Neural Crest Cells

Anomalies or deficiencies in migration, proliferation, and differentiation of neural crest cells (NCCs) have also been proposed as a possible mechanism for CFM [11, 12]. The neural crest cells are a migratory cell population specific to vertebrates that originate from the developing neural tube. The cells delaminate and migrate to different regions of the embryo where they differentiate into a broad range of cell types, stimulating local tissue growth during development [5, 12]. The migration of neural crest cells also gives rise to the branchial arch ectomesenchyme around the 4th week in utero. In the cranial region, NCCs generate odontoblasts, cartilage, bone, connective tissue, and smooth muscle, playing a key role in the development of a large portion of the structures of the face and anterior neck [12, 13]. Given that most craniofacial structures involved in CFM are derivatives of cranial NCCs, direct disturbances of the migration, proliferation, and differentiation of cranial NCCs have been suggested to be the origin of the developmental deformities found in CFM. Giving support to this idea, NCCs have been shown to form the basis of craniofacial, vertebral, CNS, cardiovascular, and urogenital anomalies, which have all been frequently observed in the CFM population [14, 15]. The abundance of extra-craniofacial anomalies in CFM patients suggests that the NCCs could be the source of the anomalies. Phenotypic variability in CFM could be explained by the extent of the neural crest cell loss, leading to varying degrees of severity of the facial malformations [11]. There have been several transgenic mouse models described in the literature in which neural crest problems appeared to cause the first and second branchial arch anomalies, although these models have not perfectly mirrored the constellation of findings in CFM [16].

There are extrinsic and intrinsic pathogenic factors that can cause vascular abnormalities and hemorrhage as well as lead to abnormal neural crest cell migration. Teratogenic drugs such as thalidomide, alcohol, and retinoic acid have shown CFM-like phenotype in animal models [11]. And intrinsic factors such as diabetes and second-trimester bleeding are also correlated as major risk factors for CFM (Table 1.1) [17, 18].

Table 1.1 Pathogenic factors [2, 17, 18, 30–33]

Extrinsic factors	Intrinsic factors
Thalidomide	Diabetes
Pseudoephedrine	Multiple gestation
Retinoic acid	Bleeding during the second trimester
Triazene	Autosomal dominance
Alcohol consumption	

Classification

The wide variance in presentation of patients with CFM has led to many different classification systems as well as different names. The term CFM is often used interchangeably with hemifacial microsomia (HFM), first and second branchial arch syndrome, and otomandibular dysostosis. Goldenhar syndrome, or oculoauriculovertebral syndrome, may be used interchangeably but is more commonly discussed as being on the CFM "spectrum" [9]. Goldenhar syndrome and oculoauriculovertebral syndrome are variants of CFM that include extracranial anomalies in addition to those found in CFM including epibulbar dermoids (benign congenital eye tumors) as well as vertebral and rib anomalies such as incomplete formation, fusion, or missing ribs [1]. The classification systems attempt to make it easier to communicate among providers, predict future growth, and plan surgical interventions. The two most commonly used classification systems are Kaban-Pruzansky and OMENS/OMENS Plus. Most agree that the mandibular deformity is the foundation of the classification system and best determines the overall deformity and treatment.

Kaban-Pruzansky Classification

In 1969 Pruzansky described three mandibular deformities associated with hemifacial microsomia patients. However, Pruzanksy did not consider the position of the condyle relative to the glenoid fossa. Kaban et al. analyzed patients with HFM three-dimensionally and classified them by the mandibular deformity [19]. Kaban et al. modified the classification system in their article in 1988 breaking down *Type II* into *Type IIA* and *Type IIB* to clarify the degree of condylar deformity and position of the condyle with relation to the glenoid fossa. These observations were important since the surgical treatment differs greatly between patients with *Type IIA* and *Type IIB*. Kaban et al. report that neither the soft tissue ear deformity nor the cranial nerve involvement correlates with the severity of the mandibular skeletal deformity [20, 22]. In contrast, Vento et al. found a positive association between mandibular hypoplasia and the severity of associated facial deformity [21]. These observations resulted in Kaban-Pruzansky classification (Table 1.2).

Table 1.2 Kaban-Pruzanksy classification

Type 1	All structures are present but all are hypoplastic/short
Type II	Small mandibles with an abnormally shaped ramus and underdeveloped TMJ that is abnormally positioned – usually displaced anteriorly and medially
Type IIA	TMJ that is deformed but functions normally (Fig. 1.1a, b)
Type IIB	The TMJ is malpositioned inferiorly, medially, and anteriorly [19]
Type III	The mandible has an absent ramus and glenoid fossa (i.e., TMJ is missing)

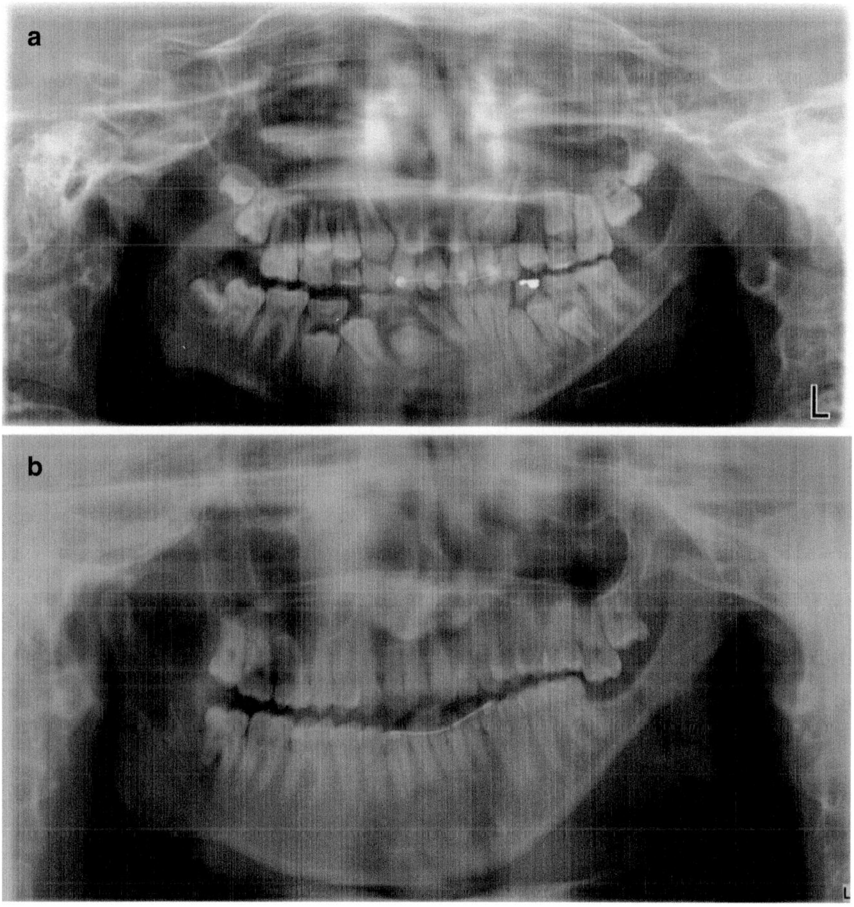

Fig. 1.1 Kaban-Pruzansky class IIA CFM. (**a**) An 11-year-old: note hypoplastic and short ramus-condyle unit on the left that is malpositioned but functions normally. (**b**) Same patient at 20 years old denied treatment. Note mandibular and maxillary hypoplasia and asymmetry

OMENS Classification

The OMENS classification system was developed to include the major manifestations of HFM in a comprehensive and succinct fashion. Veneto et al. developed the classification system to be comprehensive and allow for evaluation and analysis of each deformity independently [21]. This classification system evaluates the patient for (O) orbital distortion, (M) mandibular hypoplasia, (E) ear deformity, (N) nerve involvement, and (S) soft tissue deficiency [21]. Within each subgroup, each manifestation is numerically classified by the level of deformity from zero (normal) to three (most severe) (Table 1.3).

Table 1.3 OMENS classification [21]

Orbit
O0: Normal size and position
O1: Abnormal size
O2: Abnormal orbital position (arrow depicts whether superior or inferior)
O3: Abnormal size and position
Mandible
M0: Normal mandible
M1: Mandible and glenoid fossa are small with shortened ramus
M2: Mandibular ramus is short and abnormally shaped
M2A: Glenoid fossa is in relatively normal position compared with contralateral side
M2B: Temporomandibular joint is inferior, medial, and anteriorly displaced with hypoplastic condyle
M3: Complete absence of ramus, glenoid fossa, temporomandibular joint
Ear
E0: Normal ear
E1: Mild hypoplasia and cupping with all structures present
E2: Absence of external auditory canal with variable hypoplasia of concha
E3: Malpositioned lobule (usually inferior and anterior) with absent auricle
Facial nerve
N0: No facial nerve involvement
N1: Upper facial nerve involvement; temporal and zygomatic branches
N2: Lower facial nerve involvement; buccal, mandibular, and cervical branches
N3: All branches of facial nerve affected
(Other nerves such as trigeminal and hypoglossal may be denoted with superscript, i.e., $N^{5}0$ or $N^{12}0$)
Soft tissue
S0: No soft tissue or muscle deficiency
S1: Minimal soft tissue or muscle deficiency
S2: Moderate soft tissue or muscle deficiency
S3: Severe soft tissue or muscle deficiency

OMENS Plus Classification

The OMENS Plus classification system was developed and published in 1995 after an editorial critique of the OMENS system. The suggestions were that the classification should include non-craniofacial anomalies to strengthen the system [23, 24]. OMENS Plus includes anomalies such as cardiovascular, renal, central nervous system, skeletal, GI, and pulmonary [15]. When extracranial findings are present, it is reported as OMENS+ X system, where X is the number of anomalies in that system. If more than one system is involved, it is reported at OMENS+ X system, Y system. For example, if only one system is affected but multiple anomalies occur within that system, it is documented at OMENS+ 2 skeletal (1 = C2–C3 fusion, 2 = scoliosis). If two systems are affected, it would be documented as OMENS+ 1 cardiac (1 = VSD) and 2 CNS (1 = hydrocephalus, 2 = Chiari malformation).

Clinical Features

CFM has a variable phenotype. Variability involves the bone (e.g., hypoplasia/malformation of mandible, maxilla, zygoma, temporal bone, external, and middle ear), soft tissues and neural and muscles [9, 25] (Table 1.4). The phenotypic expression

Table 1.4 Affected systems in CFM [6, 9, 25]

Affected system	Possible clinical features	
Mandibular deficiency (89–100%)	Malformed glenoid fossa	
Midface	Maxillary hypoplasia Zygomatic hypoplasia	Occlusal cant
Ocular and orbital anomalies	Orbital dystopia Coloboma upper eyelid	Epibulbar dermoids Lacrimal duct atresia or stenosis
Ear anomalies (65–99%)	Microtia or anotia Preauricular skin tags Conductive hearing loss Preauricular sinus	Middle ear (ossicle) defects Pinna abnormalities External auditory canal atresia Sensorineural hearing loss
Soft tissue defects (17–95%)	Masticatory or facial muscle hypoplasia Parotid gland hypoplasia	Deficiency of subcutaneous tissue Macrostomia or oral clefting
Associated craniofacial	Velopharyngeal insufficiency Palatal deviation Hypodontia	Frontal plagiocephaly Cranial skull base abnormality
Cranial nerve involvement (10–45%)	CN VII nerve palsy	
Extracranial abnormalies	Vertebral or rib defects Cervical spine anomalies Scoliosis Cardiac anomalies	Pigmentation Limb anomalies Pulmonary disease Renal or GU defects CNS anomalies

can range from subtle facial asymmetry with a small skin tag in front of an otherwise normal-appearing ear to bilateral involvement with microtia or anotia and atresia of the ear canals, microphthalmia, and severe mandibular hypoplasia [6, 19]. Typical presentation, about 70–95% of cases, is unilateral. However, even in cases that present as bilateral, asymmetry and variable expression of each side is typically observed [7, 25] (Fig. 1.2a, b). At birth, the defect often appears mild; however the

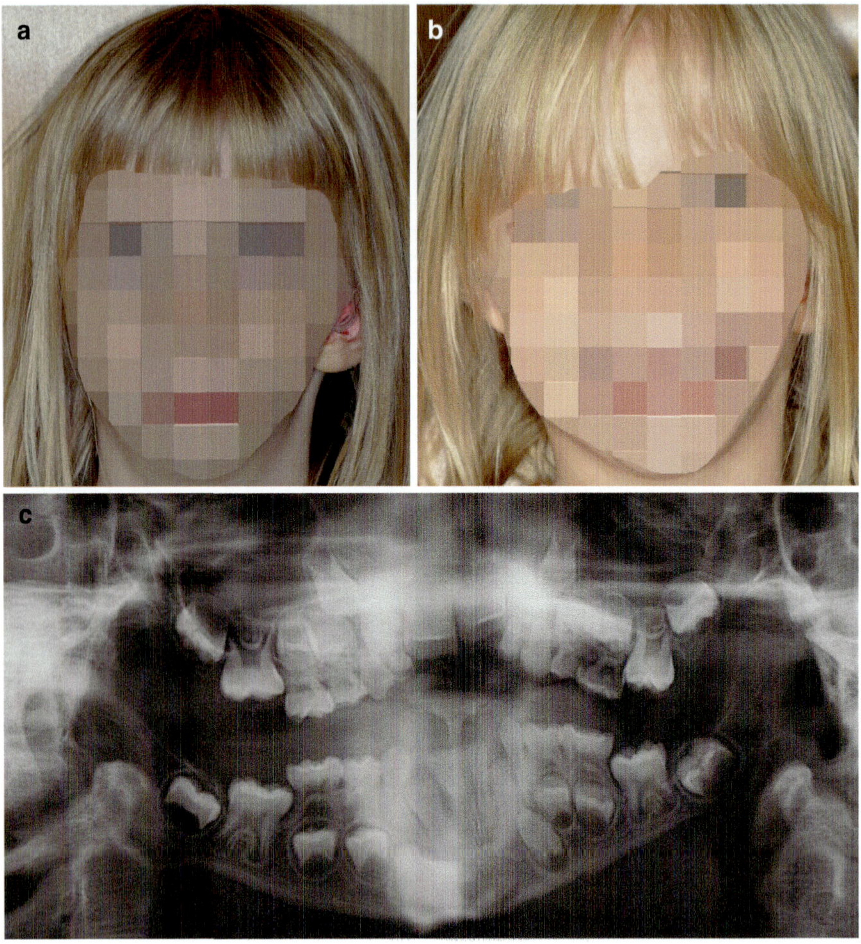

Fig. 1.2 Bilateral CFM with variable expression on the right side versus left side. (**a**) Clinical photograph at 6 years old showing facial and mandibular asymmetry with deficient soft tissue on the left. The presence of hearing aid on the left. (**b**) Clinical photograph at 8 years old showing mixed dentition, soft tissue, and mandibular asymmetry with deficiency on the left. Malformed right ear. (**c**) Panorex radiograph at 6 years old showing early mixed dentition, bilateral CFM with absent coronoid on the right, and Kaban-Pruzansky IIA on the left. (**d**) Panorex radiograph at 8 years old showing mixed dentition, maxillary expander in place, and minimal change in mandibular asymmetry

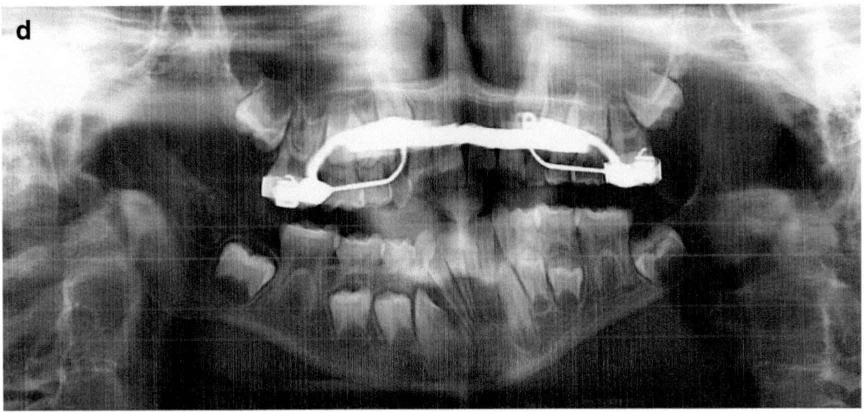

Fig. 1.2 (continued)

asymmetry becomes more distinct with growth of the child and progressive development of the normal side [3].

While there are no official diagnostic criteria, most craniofacial experts agree that mandibular and soft tissue deficiencies are necessary features for diagnosis of CFM [20, 25]. Mandibular hypoplasia has been described as the cornerstone of CFM, with a correlation demonstrated between the severity of mandibular hypoplasia and other defects [21]. Mandibular deficiency can vary from minimal underdevelopment of the condyle to the absence of the ascending ramus and condyle with underdevelopment of the horizontal ramus. The entire temporomandibular joint (TMJ) can be involved, including the glenoid fossa of the temporal bone [3].

Macrostomia, a transverse facial cleft, is a rare defect believed to be causes by failure of mesodermal migration and merging within the maxillary and mandibular prominences of the first branchial arch [26]. Macrostomia presents as a 1- to 2-cm extension lateral to the normal position of the oral commissure [3]. It can occur alone but is frequently associated with deformities of the structures developing from the first and second branchial arches [27–29].

Auricular defects can range from mild to severe (Fig. 1.3). A mild deformity would present as preauricular skin tags with or without cartilage or a preauricular sinus with a normal inner ear [3]. Anomalies of the auricle and middle ear ossicles can be present [25]. The most severe deformity consists of underdevelopment of all parts of the external ear (auricle and external auditory canal) and middle ear (tympanic membrane, tympanic cavity, auditory ossicles, mastoid antrum, mastoid cells, and Eustachian tube).

The maxilla, zygoma, temporal bone, and orbit may also be affected in CFM [9]. Maxillary underdevelopment is evidenced by decreased width from the midline palatal raphe to the lingual surface of the teeth on the affected side [3]. An underdeveloped zygoma consists of flat malar eminence and shortened span of the zygomatic arch, contributing to the decrease in length of the canthal-tragal line on the

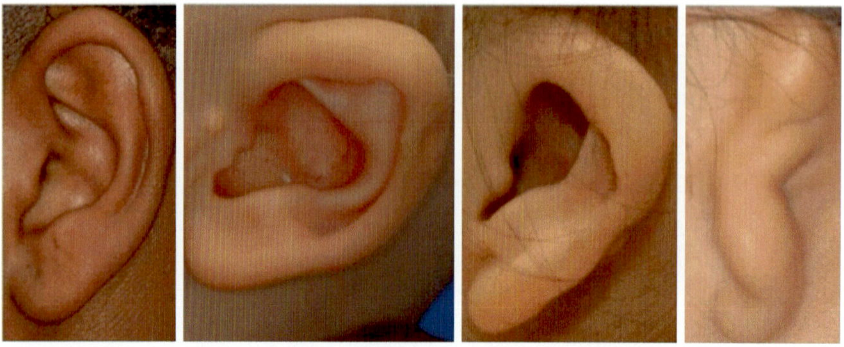

Normal ear

Grade I. Slightly smaller auricle; mild deformity, but each part can be clearly distinguished.

Grade II. Auricle is ½ to 2/3s of predicted size; its structure is only partially retained.

Grade III. Severely malformed auricle; often "peanut-shaped"

Fig. 1.3 Spectrum of auricular deformities that may present in HFM

affected side (Fig. 1.4) [3]. The temporal bone does not have its origin in the first and second branchial arches, but its development is intimately related to these visceral arches. Potential temporal bone abnormalities include underdevelopment or the absence of the zygomatic and mastoid processes. Dissections of the temporal bone in autopsy have shown that any part of the temporal bone other than the petrous portion which houses the inner ear might be underdeveloped [3]. The orbit may demonstrate vertical displacement (Fig. 1.5: 18 mos. with left vertical orbital dystopia). Coloboma of the upper eyelid and/or iris may be found. Microphthalmia or anophthalmia is rare but has been observed [6].

The muscles innervated by the fifth and seventh cranial nerves may be underdeveloped, with possible paresis. Patients may have sensorineural hearing loss and impairment of extraocular movements [3].

Extracraniofacial anomalies may be present in 55% of patients with CFM [29]. Patients with bilateral CFM are more likely to develop extracraniofacial anomalies [14, 29]. These anomalies most often present in the vertebrae, ribs, circulatory system, CNS, urogenital tract, and gastrointestinal (GI) tract. Vertebral anomalies may be found in cervical/lumbar/thoracic spine and/or ribs as hemivertebrae, block vertebrae, and/or scoliosis. These anomalies can range from asymptomatic to severe, some causing significant health consequences [29]. CNS anomalies in CFM can include hydrocephaly, ventriculomegaly, intracranial cysts, Arnold-Chiari malformations, or spinal cord anomalies. Circulatory system anomalies include ventricular or atrial septal defects, patent ductus arteriosus, and valve malformations. GI tract anomalies consist of inguinal/umbilical hernia, imperforate anus, or esophageal atresia. Urogenital anomalies may include renal aplasia, undescended testis, or hydronephrosis. Respiratory tract anomalies are possible but rare, such as laryngomalacia, tracheomalacia, or lung hypoplasia [14, 29].

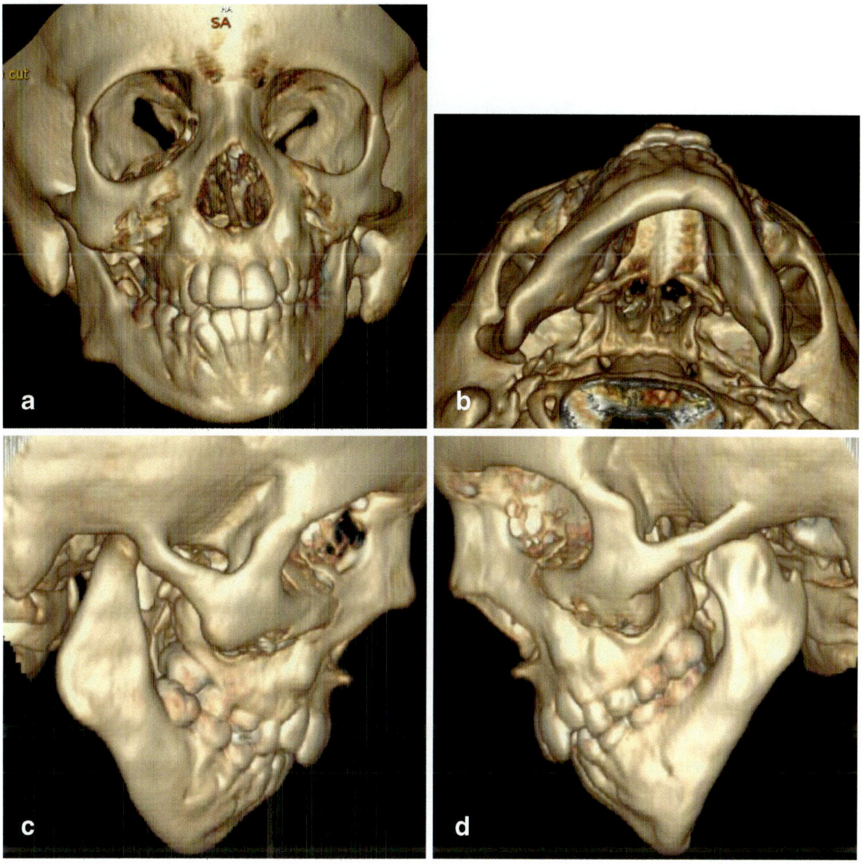

Fig. 1.4 Facial asymmetry including zygomatic, maxillary, and mandibular hypoplasia in 3D facial CT of patient with bilateral CFM. (**a**) Frontal view showing mandibular asymmetry. (**b**) Base view showing mandibular hypoplasia on the left with Kaban-Pruzansky IIA deformity as well as hypoplasia of the zygoma on the left when compared to the right. (**c**) Right lateral view showing the absence of coronoid. (**d**) Left lateral view showing deformity of ramus-condyle unit

Conclusions

CFM has a variable presentation that can range from mild ear deformity and asymmetry to near-absent auricle and agenesis of the ramus and condyle. The two prevailing pathogenic models of CFM include vascular abnormalities in the developing embryo and abnormalities with cranial NCC migration. Given the extreme phenotypic variation, numerous classification systems have been proposed with the two most common being Kaban-Pruzansky and OMENS Plus. Careful analysis and diagnosis by a multidisciplinary team is important to be able to provide appropriate care to patients with CFM from infancy to adulthood. The multidisciplinary team is

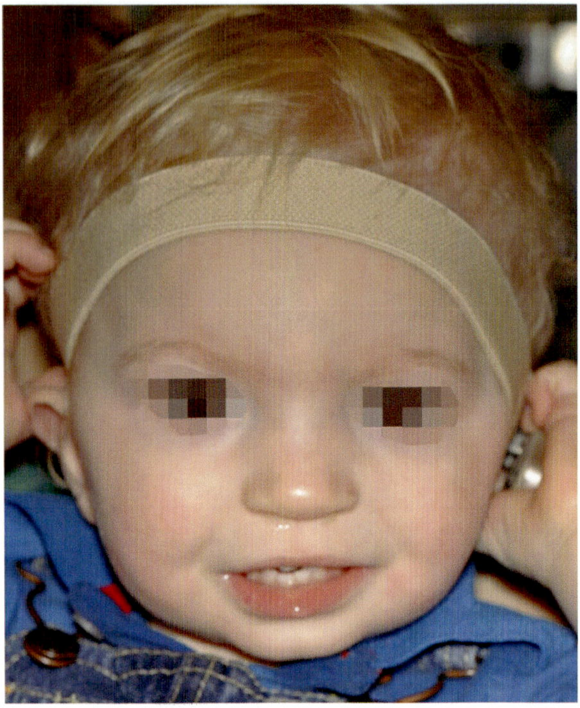

Fig. 1.5 Clinical photograph of 18-month-old with left vertical orbital dystopia

especially important in childhood (i.e., skeletal immaturity), where the potential for future growth after surgical reconstruction exists. The remainder of this book will provide additional information and examples regarding treatment of children with CFM.

References

1. Cohen MM, Rollnick BR, Kaye CI. Oculo-auriculo-vertebral spectrum: an updated critique. Cleft Palate J. 1989;26:276–86.
2. Poswillo D. The pathogenesis of the first and second branchial arch syndrome. Oral Surg Oral Med Oral Pathol. 1973;35(3):302–28.
3. Grabb WC. The first and second branchial arch syndrome. Plast Reconstr Surg. 1965;36(5):485–508.
4. Singer SI, Haan E, Slee J, Goldblatt J. Familial hemifacial microsomia due to autosomal dominant inheritance. Case Reports. Aust Dent J. 1994;39(5):287–91.
5. Monahan R, Seder K, Patel P, Alder M, Grud S, O'Gara M. Hemifacial microsomia: etiology, diagnosis, and treatment. J Am Dent Assoc. 2001;132:1402–8.
6. Heike CL, Luquetti DV, Hing AV. Craniofacial microsomia overview. 2009 Mar 19 [Updated 2014 Oct 9]. In: Adam MP, Ardinger HH, Pagon RA, et al., editors. GeneReviews® [Internet]. Seattle: University of Washington, Seattle; 1993–2020. Available from: https://www.ncbi.nlm.nih.gov/books/NBK5199/.

7. Birgfeld CB, Luquetti DV, Gougoutas AJ, Bartlett SP, Low DW, Sie KC, et al. A phenotypic assessment tool for craniofacial microsomia. Plast Reconstr Surg. 2011;127:313–20.
8. Stark RB, Saunders DE. The first branchial syndrome. The oral-mandibular-auricular syndrome. Plast Reconstr Surg Transplant Bull. 1962;29:229–39.
9. Brandstetter KA, Patel KG. Craniofacial microsomia. Facial Plast Surg Clin North Am. 2016;24(4):495–515.
10. Robinson LK, Hoyme HE, Edwards DK, Jones KL. Vascular pathogenesis of unilateral craniofacial defects. J Pediatr. 1987;111(2):236–9.
11. Chen Q, Zhao Y, Shen G, Dai J. Etiology and pathogenesis of hemifacial microsomia. J Dent Res. 2018;97(12):1297–305.
12. Minoux M, Rijli FM. Molecular mechanisms of cranial neural crest cell migration and patterning in craniofacial development. Development. 2010;137(16):2605–21.
13. Johnston MC, Bronsky PT. Animal models for human craniofacial malformations. J Craniofac Genet Dev Biol. 1991;11:277–91.
14. Renkema RW, Caron CM, Pauws E, Wolvius EB, Schipper JM, Rooijers W, Dunaway DJ, Forrest CR, Padwa BL, Koudstaal MJ. Extracraniofacial anomalies in craniofacial microsomia: retrospective analysis of 991 patients. Int J Oral Maxillofac Surg. 2019;48(9):1169–76.
15. Horgan JE, Padwa BL, LaBrie RA, Mulliken JB. OMENS-Plus: analysis of craniofacial and extracraniofacial anomalies in hemifacial microsomia. Cleft Palate Craniofac J. 1995;32(5):405–12.
16. Cousley R, Naora H, Yokoyama M, Kimura M, Otani H. Validity of the Hfm transgenic mouse as a model for hemifacial microsomia. Cleft Palate Craniofac J. 2002;39(1):81–92.
17. Werler MM, Starr JR, Cloonan YK, Speltz ML. Hemifacial microsomia: from gestation to childhood. J Craniofac Surg. 2009;20(1):664–9.
18. Wang R, Graham JM. Infants of diabetic mothers are at increased risk for the oculo-auriculo-vertebral sequence: a case-based and case-control approach. J Pediatr. 2002;141(5):611–7.
19. Kaban LB, Mulliken JB, Murray JE. Three dimensional approach to analysis and treatment of hemifacial microsomia. Cleft Palate J. 1981;18(2):90–9.
20. Murray JE, Kaban LB, Mulliken JB. Analysis and treatment of hemifacial microsomia. Plast Reconstr Surg. 1984;74:186–99.
21. Vento AR, LaBrie RA, Mulliken JB. The O.M.E.N.S. classification of hemifacial microsomia. Cleft Palate Craniofac J. 1991;28(1):68–76.
22. Kaban LB, Moses MH, Mulliken JB. Surgical correction of hemifacial microsomia. Plast Reconstr Surg. 1988;82:9–19.
23. Cohen MM. A critique of the OMENS classification of hemifacial microsomia. Cleft Palate Craniofac J. 1991;28:77.
24. Cousley RRJ. A comparison of two classification systems for hemifacial microsomia. Br J Oral Maxillofac Surg. 1993;31:78–82.
25. Cousley RRJ, Calvert ML. Current concepts in the understanding and management of hemifacial microsomia. Br J Plast Surg. 1997;50:536–51.
26. Rogers GF, Mullikan JB. Repair of transverse facial cleft in hemifacial microsomia: long-term anthropometric evaluation of commissural symmetry. Plast Reconstr Surg. 2007;120(3):728–37.
27. Akinmoladun VI, Owotade FJ, Afolabi AO. Bilateral transverse facial cleft as an isolated deformity: case report. Ann Afr Med. 2007;6(1):39–40.
28. Makhija LK, Jha MK, Bhattacharya S, Rai A, Dey AB, Saha A. Transverse facial cleft: a series of 17 cases. Indian J Plast Surg. 2011;44(3):439–43.
29. Renkema RW, Caron CJJM, Mathijssen IMJ, et al. Vertebral anomalies in craniofacial microsomia: a systematic review. Int J Oral Maxillofac Surg. 2017;46(10):1319–29.
30. Vargesson N. Thalidomide-induced teratogenesis: history and mechanisms. Birth Defects Res C Embryo Today. 2015;105(2):140–56.

31. Louryan S, Heymans O, Goffard JC. Ear malformations in the mouse embryo following maternal administration of triazene, with clinical implications. Surg Radiol Anat. 1995;17(1):59–63.
32. Lammer EJ, Chen DT, Hoar RM, Agnish ND, Benke PJ, Braun JT, Curry CJ, Fernhoff PM, Grix AW Jr, Lott IT, et al. Retinoic acid embryopathy. N Engl J Med. 1985;313(14):837–41.
33. Werler MM, Sheehan JE, Hayes C, Padwa BL, Mitchell AA, Mulliken JB. Demographic and reproductive factors associated with hemifacial microsomia. Cleft Palate Craniofac J. 2004;41(5):494–50.

Chapter 2
Initial Evaluation of a Patient with Craniofacial Microsomia

Natasha Fürchtgott, Zachary Brown, and Valerie Bright

Introduction

Craniofacial microsomia (CFM, OMIM 164 210) is the term used to describe a developmental disorder with a spectrum of congenital abnormalities that affect anatomical structures derived from the first and second branchial arches. Multiple names have been used to describe this aberrant embryologic development; CFM can also be known in the literature as:

- Hemifacial microsomia [1, 2]
- First and second branchial arch syndrome [3]
- Oral-mandibular-auricular syndrome [4]
- Otomandibular dysostosis [5, 6]
- Otomandibular dysmorphogenesis [7]

N. Fürchtgott (✉)
Private Practice, High Desert Oral and Facial Surgery, El Paso, TX, USA

Department of Oral and Maxillofacial Surgery El Paso Children's Hospital, El Paso, TX, USA

Texas Tech University Health Sciences Center El Paso, WLH School of Dental Medicine, El Paso, TX, USA

University of Texas Health Sciences Center San Antonio, Department of Oral and Maxillofacial Surgery, San Antonio, TX, USA
e-mail: furchtgott@hdofs.com

Z. Brown
University of Texas Health Sciences Center San Antonio, Department of Oral and Maxillofacial Surgery, San Antonio, TX, USA

Partner at Facial Surgery Group, Kansas City, MO, USA
e-mail: drbrown@facialsurgerygroup.com

V. Bright
El Paso, TX, USA

D. M. Yates, M. R. Markiewicz (eds.), *Craniofacial Microsomia and Treacher Collins Syndrome*, https://doi.org/10.1007/978-3-030-84733-3_2

- Oculoauriculovertebral spectrum (OAVS), sequence, or dysplasia [8, 9]
- Facioauriculovertebral sequence or syndrome [10]
- Lateral facial dysplasia [11]
- Auriculobranchiogenic dysplasia [12]
- Intrauterine facial necrosis [13]
- Hemignathia and microtia syndrome [14]
- Necrotic facial dysplasia [15]
- Mandibular laterognathism [16]
- Goldenhar syndrome

Due to the significant variability in the presentation of the spectrum and the fact that bilateral involvement is observed in 5–30% of the cases [11, 17], the term craniofacial microsomia is now preferred, and these entities are accepted to exist within a continuum. From the Greek words *micros* (small) and *sōma* (body), microsomia refers to the main phenotypical characteristics of a hypoplastic and malformed unilateral affected side of the craniofacial skeleton. It most commonly affects the external ear, middle ear, mandible, temporomandibular joint, muscles of mastication, facial muscles, and other facial soft tissues of one side of the craniofacial region. Other facial structures, such as the orbit, eye, nose, cranium, or neck, may be involved [18]. When the entity is bilateral, it is usually an asymmetric presentation.

In addition to craniofacial anomalies, there may be cardiac, vertebral, central nervous system, genitourinary, and renal defects. As mentioned in the previous chapter, the phenotype is highly variable as the expression varies from microtia to a near complete agenesis of the affected side of the mandible and overlying soft tissues.

This chapter compiles the many classification schemes and patient variations in anatomic expression of craniofacial microsomia to provide a roadmap for patient evaluation at various stages of patient presentation. The initial evaluation naturally leads to further investigation of possible extracraniofacial abnormalities and guides treatment sequencing for the patient's life. Standardized evaluation of patients with craniofacial deformities leads to better communication among clinicians and inevitably better treatment outcomes for patients.

Craniofacial Microsomia Classification Systems

Several classification systems have been developed since 1969 in an attempt to better differentiate the complex and variable phenotypical expression. Auriculofacial defects are the predominant and pathognomonic features of CFM, and it is generally agreed upon that its diagnosis requires the presence of at least one hypoplastic structure derived from the first or second branchial arches. However, the presence of isolated microtia, preauricular skin tags, or macrostomia without other CFM features would be arguable to not fit criteria for establishment of a CFM diagnosis.

Because there is lack of consensus on the diagnostic criteria for this condition, its prevalence, classification, and defined treatment protocols are not fixed. The literature today presents the medical community with multiple classification systems to score the severity and guide treatment planning.

The mandible is the "keystone" to the skeletal deformities of CFM [19] and therefore the basis in which the classification systems have been developed. Cousley suggested the guidelines for minimum diagnostic criteria for CFM [20]. These criteria are not definitively accepted, despite their widely accepted use:

1. Ipsilateral mandibular *and* auricular defects (external or middle ear)
2. Asymmetric mandible *or* auricular defects (external or middle ear) *with either*:
    (a) Involvement of two or more indirectly associated anomalies
    (b) Positive family history of CFM

Skeletal Deformity Classifications

The purpose of the Pruzansky Mandibular Deformity Classification system is to organize the severity of mandibular hypoplasia (Table 2.1). Kaban's Modification to Pruzansky's Original Classification intends to include the glenoid fossa and TMJ development based on radiological findings (Table 2.2). Surgical treatment strategies will vary based on the category, and this will be further discussed in the following chapters.

Table 2.1 Pruzansky mandibular deformity classification (Pruzansky, 1969)

Grade I	Mandible of smaller than normal size but with morphologic characteristics of the ramus being clearly present
Grade II	Condyle, ramus, and sigmoid notch, while still identifiable, are grossly distorted, and the mandible is strikingly different in size and shape from normal
Grade III	Mandible is severely malformed, ranging from poorly identifiable ramal components to complete agenesis of the ramus

[7]

Table 2.2 Kaban modification of Pruzansky's classification (Kaban, 1988)

Type I	All mandibular and TMJ components are present and normal in shape but hypoplastic to a variable degree
Type IIA	The mandibular ramus, condyle, and TMJ are present but hypoplastic and abnormal in shape
Type IIB	The mandibular ramus is hypoplastic and markedly abnormal in form and location, being medial and anterior. There is no articulation with the temporal bone
Type III	The mandibular ramus, condyle, and TMJ are absent. The lateral pterygoid muscle and temporalis, if present, are not attached to the mandibular remnant

[21, 22]

Treatment of types I, IIA, and some IIB mandibular deformities can be accomplished by osteotomy (with or without bone grafting) or by distraction osteogenesis. Treatment of many type IIB and all type III deformities requires total construction of the ramus condyle unit and, in some cases, the glenoid fossa.

Auricular Deformity Classification

The Meurman grades of microtia was first described in 1957 to expand on classification systems of microtia. This system has been incorporated into more inclusive classification systems seen later in this chapter. The severity of microtia starts with hypoplasia of the auricle but with retained anatomic structures but then advances to complete aplasia of crucial components. Grade I is classified as a malformed auricle of smaller than normal size but retaining characteristic features. Grade II expands with having a lack of fundamental features that may consist of a low, oblong elevation hook formed at the cranial end corresponding to the helix. Grade III is characterized with a more defective auricle with a malformed lobule and the rest of the pinna being totally absent [23].

Soft Tissue Deformity Classifications

The Murray Grading of Severity of Soft Tissue Deformities was developed in 1984. This system evaluates primarily microtia, CN deficits, and presents of clefts (Table 2.3). The degree of soft tissue hypoplasia is directly proportional to the severity of the mandibular deformity. Muscles of mastication may be absent or reduced to fibrous tissue.

Multisystem Deformity Classifications

SAT Classification System

The SAT Classification System is an alphanumeric coding system based on the TNM classification of malignant tumors. It combines elements of the Pruzansky's mandible classification, Meurman's microtia staging, and Murray's soft tissue deformity grading (Table 2.4).

Table 2.3 Murray grading of severity of soft tissue deformities (Murray, 1984)

Mild	Minimal deficiency; no ear or cranial nerve involvement
Moderate	Between mild and severe
Severe	Major soft tissue deficiency plus ear distortion, nerve deficits, and clefts of the face or lips

[24]

Table 2.4 SAT Classification System (David, 1987)

S – Skeletal categories	
S1	Small mandible with normal shape
S2	Condyle, ramus, and sigmoid notch identifiable but grossly distorted; mandible strikingly different in size and shape from normal
S3	Mandible severely malformed, ranging from poorly identifiable ramal components to complete agenesis of ramus
S4	An S3 mandible plus orbital involvement with gross posterior recession of lateral and inferior orbital rims
S5	The S4 defects plus orbital dystopia and frequently hypoplasia and asymmetrical neurocranium with a flat temporal fossa
A – Auricle categories	
A0	Normal
A1	Small, malformed auricle retaining characteristic features
A2	Rudimentary auricle with hook at the cranial end corresponding to the helix
A3	Malformed lobule with the rest of pinna absent
T – Soft tissue categories	
T1	Minimal contour defect with no cranial nerve involvement
T2	Moderate defect
T3	Major defect with obvious facial scoliosis, possibly severe hypoplasia of cranial nerves, parotid gland, muscles of mastication, eye involvement, clefts of the face or lips

[19]

OMENS Classification (Vento, 1991)

The OMENS Classification is much more comprehensive than its predecessors, as it includes elements of the previous classifications, but it separates orbital and mandibular defects into separate categories, as well as soft tissue and CN VII function (Table 2.5) [26].

Horgan et al. described the importance of including extracraniofacial anomalies in this system, after they found that the frequency of patients with CFM and other organ system involvement was 55.4%. The classification system has been enhanced to OMENS Plus (+), where the + sign and a number are added at the end of the acronym to designate the presence and quantity of extracraniofacial findings [27]

Phenotypic Assessment Tool for Craniofacial Microsomia

The Phenotypic Assessment Tool for Craniofacial Microsomia (PAT-CFM) is a comprehensive pictorial classification system that allows for standarization of the assessment of patients with CFM (Fig. 2.1). The pictorial representation of the OMENS+ classification was developed by Gougoutas et al, and further expanded to include laterality and minor anomalies by the Craniofacial Clinic at Seattle Children's Hospital.

Table 2.5 OMENS classification (Vento, 1991)

Orbit categories	
O_0	Normal orbital size and position
O_1	Abnormal orbital size
O_2	Abnormal orbital position (O2↑ or O2↓ depending on the horizontal position of orbit relative to the less affected side)
O_3	Abnormal orbital size and position
Mandible categories	
M_0	Normal mandible
M_1	Small mandible and glenoid fossa with a short ramus
M_2	Short and abnormally shaped ramus (M_{2A}, if the glenoid fossa is in a similar position to the opposite TMJ; M_{2B} if the TMJ is inferiorly, medially, and anteriorly displaced with a severely hypoplastic condyle)
M_3	Complete absence of ramus, glenoid fossa, and TMJ
Ear categories	
E_0	Normal ear
E_1	Mild hypoplasia and cupping with all structures present
E_2	Absence of external auditory canal with variable hypoplasia of the concha
E_3	Malpositioned lobule with absent auricle
Nerve (facial nerve) categories	
N_0	Normal facial nerve
N_1	Upper facial nerve involvement (temporal and zygomatic branches)
N_2	Lower facial nerve involvement (buccal, mandibular, and cervical branches)
N_3	All branches of the facial nerve affected
Soft tissue categories	
S_0	No obvious soft tissue or muscle deficiency
S_1	Minimal subcutaneous/muscle deficiency
S_2	Moderate deficiency
S_3	Severe deficiency due to subcutaneous and muscular hypoplasia

[25]

Patient Evaluation and Diagnosis

As with any other craniofacial condition, a multidisciplinary team approach for the management of these patients is ideal. Here, qualified professionals from a myriad of health disciplines work in a coordinated effort to deliver proper and consistent medical, dental, and psychosocial care. The team should include a pediatrician, audiologist, speech-language pathologist, orthodontist, pediatric dentist, oral maxillofacial surgeon, plastic surgeon, and otolaryngologist with access to neurosurgeon, ophthalmologist, radiologist, social worker, psychologist, geneticist, orthopedic surgeon, cardiologist, cardiothoracic surgeon, and urologist.

Although CFM is the second most common craniofacial congenital disorder, its multidisciplinary team approach is not as well outlined as the management of patients with cleft lip and palate. Table 2.6 contains a comprehensive list of anomalies commonly found in craniofacial microsomia. Due to the wide breadth of physical

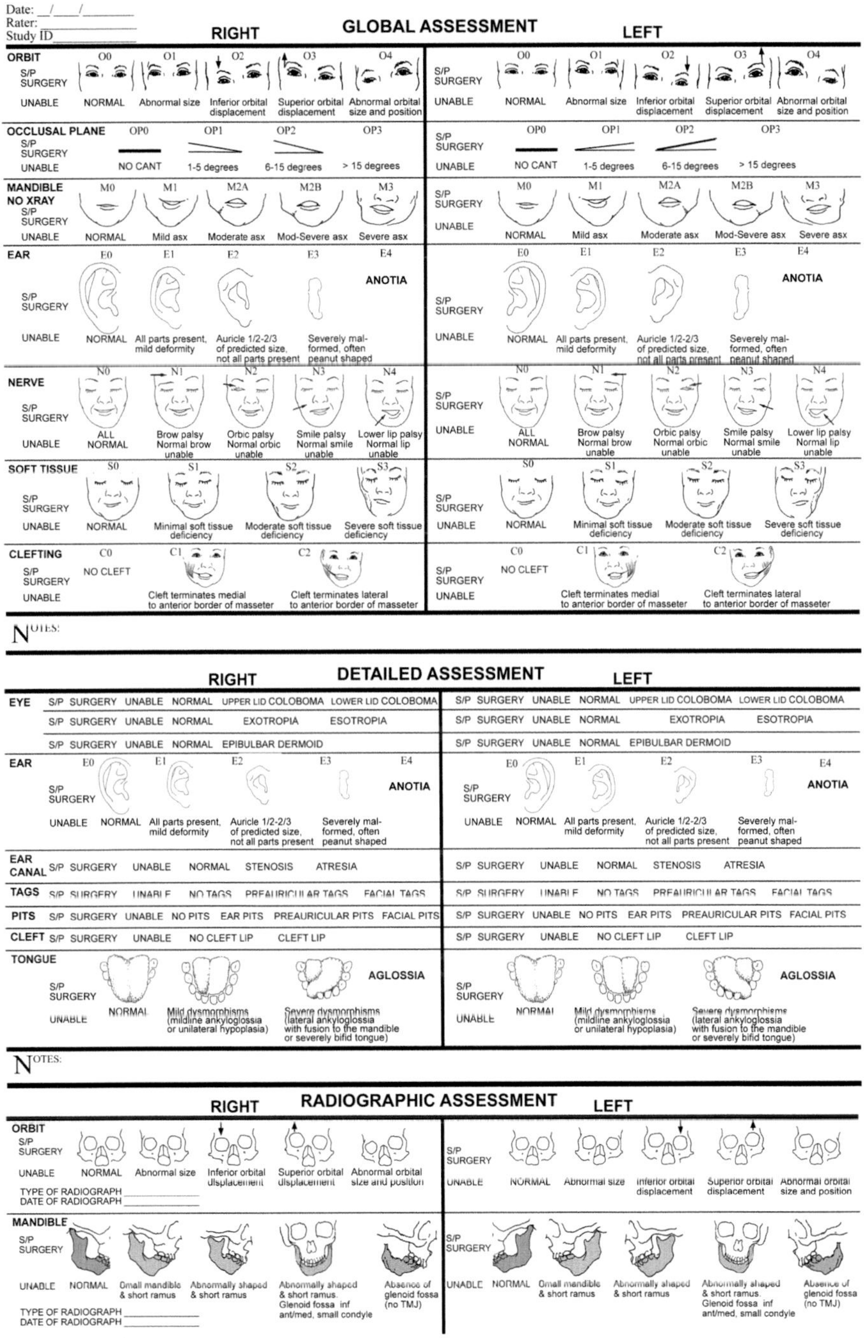

Fig. 2.1 Phenotypic assessment tool for craniofacial microsomia [37]

Table 2.6 List of anomalies commonly found in craniofacial microsomia

Facial skeleton anomalies	Mandibular hypoplasia Malformed glenoid fossa Maxillary hypoplasia Occlusal canting Zygomatic hypoplasia Palatal deviation Aplasia/hypoplasia of temporomandibular joints
Ocular anomalies	Orbital dystopia Ocular motility disorders Epibulbar dermoids Eyelid defects Lacrimal duct atresia/stenosis Microphthalmia Exophthalmia Anophthalmia Strabismus Eyes asymmetry/dysmorphy Lipodermoids Coloboma
Auricular anomalies	Microtia/anotia Preauricular appendages Conductive hearing loss Preauricular fistulae Middle ear (ossicle) defects Dacryocystitis Atresia of the external auditory canal Ear dysplasia with or without hearing loss due to ossicular chain defects Ear asymmetry
Craniofacial soft tissue anomalies (17–95%)	Masticatory/facial muscle hypoplasia Macrostomia CN VII Palsy Parotid gland hypoplasia
Other craniofacial anomalies	Bifid tongue, other tongue anomalies Velopharyngeal insufficiency Cranial base anomalies Palatal deviation Cleft lip and/or cleft palate Agenesis of the second premolars and the third molars Supernumerary teeth Malformations of enamel and dentin Delay in tooth development Microcephaly Dolichocephaly Plagiocephaly Trigeminal anesthesia

Table 2.6 (continued)

Extracraniofacial skeletal system	Vertebral defects (hemivertebrae/vertebral anomaly) and rib defects Cervical spine anomalies Cleft spine Extremities anomalies Club foot Radial hemimelia Scoliosis Congenital hip deformity Pectus excavatum and other chest wall deformities Hyposegmented sternum Short, webbed neck Radial/ulnar hypoplasia Toe syndactyly Digital polydactyly/syndactyly Pes cavus
Cardiac anomalies (4–33%)	Murmur Atrial and ventricular septal defects (the most frequent) Tetralogy of Fallot Patent ductus arteriosus Anomalous pulmonary return Conotruncal defects Aortic stenosis Pulmonic stenosis Aortic arch anomalies Transposition of the great vessels Other outflow tract abnormalities Dextrocardia
Renal and genitourinary anomalies (4–15%)	Renal size discrepancy Ectopic kidneys Renal agenesis Fused kidneys Reflux Multicystic kidneys Double ureter Hydroureter Hydronephrosis

(continued)

Table 2.6 (continued)

Central nervous system anomalies (5–18%)	Cranial nerve defects other than facial nerve (V, IX, XII) Agenesis of corpus callosum Corpus callosum lipoma Diffuse cerebral hypoplasia Seizure disorder Hydrocephalus due to aqueduct of Sylvius stenosis Dilated lateral cerebral ventricles or asymptomatic hydrocephalus Asymmetric lateral ventricles Absence of septum pellucidum Diffuse cerebral hypodensity Frontal hypodensities Encephalocele/Dandy-Walker syndrome Developmental delay Spine deformities Holoprosencephaly Arnold-Chiari malformation Hypothalamic hamartoma
Gastrointestinal tract anomalies (2–12%)	Rectal atresia Tracheoesophageal fistula Esophageal atresia Inguinal hernias Gastroesophageal reflux Imperforate anus Intestinal malrotation Displaced/absent rectum
Respiratory system anomalies (1–15%)	Choanal atresia Tracheal stenosis Obstructive sleep apnea Abnormal anatomy of larynx and pharynx Disorder of lobular anatomy of lungs

[20, 27–36]

anomalies, patients should always have a thorough physical exam at initial presentation to guide screening tests. Given the wide phenotypic diversity, creating evidence-based guidelines for screening and care is difficult in this patient population [38]

Prenatal Period

Prenatal diagnosis of sporadic cases has been reported with the use of fetal ultrasound; however, this is still very infrequent. It is more likely to detect a severe malformation with these studies, and with the evolution of 3D scanning, some milder cases of microtia, preauricular tags, and mandibular hypoplasia have been identified [29].

Prenatal and birth history should aim to determine any maternal-fetal factors. Medications and substances that have been linked to CFM due to their ability to cause vascular abnormalities and hemorrhage, damage to Meckel's cartilage, and abnormal development of neural crest cells include thalidomide, triazene, retinoic acid, pseudoephedrine, methotrexate, and heavy alcohol consumption. Environmental factors also linked to CFM include hypoxia, ionizing radiation, and hyperthermic stress [39–42].

Maternal intrinsic factors such as multiple gestations, diabetes, hypothyroidism, and bleeding in the second trimester are major risk factors [29, 43].

Neonatal Period

The main goal during this time is to assure adequate respiratory support and address any feeding difficulties. Additionally, extracraniofacial findings must be ruled out, particularly those requiring emergent cardiothoracic surgical management.

Symptoms associated with respiratory distress include tachypnea, stridor, cyanosis, retractions, and episodic upper airway obstruction with apnea. If there are respiratory concerns due to airway obstruction, a surgical consultation for airway management is necessary [44–46].

Some life-threatening congenital cardiac defects will require immediate repair. Therefore, a chest x-ray, electrocardiogram, and echocardiogram are indicated as part of the work-up in this age period.

Lactation consultants and speech-language pathologists can assess and provide parents with necessary techniques to modify nursing and feeding times. Specialized feeding bottles, nasogastric feeds, and even gastrostomy feeds might be necessary for severe cases.

Work-up testing should also include a newborn hearing screening and renal ultrasound. Strict monitoring of weight, height, and development is to be carried out by the pediatricians.

Oral and mandibular abnormalities are identified within the first few hours of life. An examination by the craniofacial surgeon should occur not only for the assessment of respiratory support adequacy but also for parent education and establishment of an initial relationship for the long-term treatment plan.

Cervical/spinal and renal abnormalities can occur in up to 15% of patients with CFM; however, routine neonatal screening is not definitively recommended. A retrospective review of 514 patients with isolated microtia or aural atresia without facial asymmetry demonstrated that initial screening was inconsistent among the cohort population. Of those screened, only 2% of the patients had renal abnormalities on ultrasound, and none of the patients had cervical or spinal abnormalities. Routine screenings for renal or cervical/spinal abnormalities lack in consistency and insurance approval and, more importantly, fail to capture true abnormality rates. Routine screens with renal ultrasounds and spinal x-rays may not be warranted at this stage unless clinically indicated [38, 47].

0–12 Months

Ideally, an appointment will be made for initial visit with the craniofacial team prior to discharge from hospital care after birth. The pediatrician can also trigger this referral, and the first appointment should happen within the first weeks of life.

At the first craniofacial team visit, reassurance and educational resources are given. This is an opportunity for the parents to meet with all members of the team and determine barriers to care as well as to obtain referrals for pending studies.

It is important to establish a complete history and physical examination. This should include a review of systems aiming to consider meeting developmental milestones, obstructive sleep apnea symptoms, difficulty with swallowing and feeding, speech development, and a psychosocial assessment. Polysomnography, audiograms, and swallow evaluations by a speech-language pathologist could be indicated based on these symptoms.

The pediatrician is key to continue the patient's close follow-up for monitoring of continued development, weight gain, and growth charting.

Photography is used to document facial appearance throughout the patient's growth, starting at the initial visit and throughout the treatment process. Traditionally, posteroanterior cephalograms have been the gold standard for assessment of facial asymmetry. Nowadays, the use of cone-beam computerized tomography and the ability to obtain three-dimensionally reconstructed images in a relatively low-dose radiation study has gained popularity.

Since CFM is most commonly a simplex case with unknown etiology, risk recurrence estimates are empiric. It is estimated that the sibling recurrence risk is estimated to be 2–3%, assuming normal chromosomes and no family history. No specific genetic testing is available, and only a few cases have demonstrated de novo chromosome abnormalities. The identification of subtle clinical manifestations in a patient's relatives is important, as well as a three-generation family history. The family history must inquire about other relatives with facial asymmetry, ear tags, ear pits, hearing loss, vertebral malformations, eye abnormalities, abnormalities of extremities, and cardiac or urogenital malformations [29, 48].

Childhood and Adolescence

During this phase, serial multidisciplinary evaluations must take into account the improvement of facial symmetry and management of malocclusion, maximize hearing and communication, and support psychosocial needs.

An important consideration that is commonly overlooked is that airway problems that appear in infancy worsen with adolescence [49, 50].

It is not the purpose of this chapter to elaborate on the details of surgical management required for these patients, as they will be discussed further. However, this excellent timeline elaborated at the Craniofacial Center at Seattle Children's Hospital can be a useful guide (Fig. 2.2).

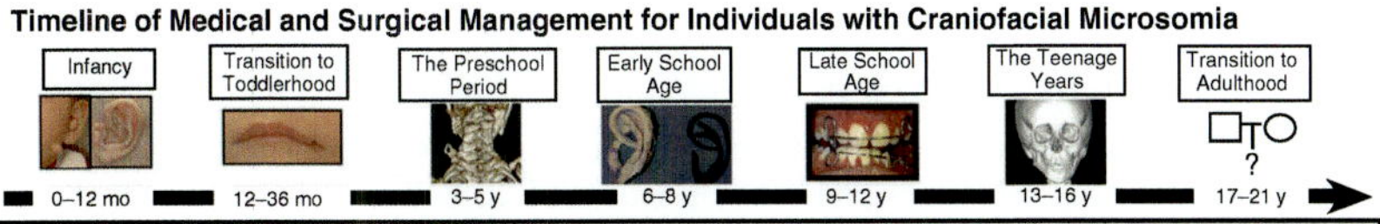

	Infancy (0–12 mo)	Transition to Toddlerhood (12–36 mo)	The Preschool Period (3–5 y)	Early School Age (6–8 y)	Late School Age (9–12 y)	The Teenage Years (13–16 y)	Transition to Adulthood (17–21 y)
Obtain:	-Hearing evaluation -Renal ultrasound	-Hearing evaluation[a]	-Hearing evaluation[a] -Cervical spine films	-Hearing evaluation[a] -CT if aural atresia -Orthodontic records	-Hearing evaluation[a] -Orthodontic records	-Hearing evaluation[a] -Orthodontic records	-Hearing evaluation
Evaluate:	-Respiratory status -Feeding & growth -Other anomalies	-Respiratory status -Feeding & growth -Other anomalies -Facial symmetry -Palatal function -Oral health	-Obstructive sleep symptoms -Nutrition -Development -Facial symmetry -Speech -Oral health	-Obstructive sleep symptoms -Growth -Development -Facial symmetry -Speech -Oral health	-Obstructive sleep symptoms -Growth -Occlusion -Psychosocial well-being -Oral health	-Obstructive sleep symptoms -Occlusion -Psychosocial well-being -Oral health	-Obstructive sleep symptoms -Occlusion -Psychosocial well-being -Oral health
Discuss:	-CFM diagnosis -Short and long-term plan -Adjustment to condition -Hearing status -Barriers to care	-Short and long-term plan -Adjustment to condition -Hearing status -Barriers to care	-Treatment options -Preparation for pre-school, kindergarten -Barriers to care -Communication -Importance of good oral hygiene	-Treatment options -Child and family's treatment goals -Self-esteem, concerns -Barriers to care -School accomodations for hearing loss[a]	-Treatment options -Child and family's treatment goals -Self-esteem, concerns -Barriers to care -School accomodations for hearing loss[a]	-Treatment options -Teens treatment goals -Self-esteem, concerns -Barriers to care -School accomodations for hearing loss[a]	-Teens treatment goals -Final treatment plan -Self-esteem, concerns -Barriers to care -Transition to adult care
Provide:	-Reassurance -Resource information -Genetics referral -Echocardiogram[a] -Ophthalmology referral[a]	-Reassurance -Support resources -Early intervention services[a]	-Information on resources & school support -Orthopedics referral[a] -Early intervention services[a]	-Information on resources & school support -Psychosocial support -Assistance with surgical decision-making	-Information on resources & school support -Psychosocial support -Assistance with surgical decision-making	-Information on resources & school support -Psychosocial support -Assistance with surgical decision-making	-Resource information -Psychosocial support -Genetics referral to discuss recurrence risks -A transfer summary of care provided -Referrals for adult care
Common surgeries[b]**:**	-Ear & facial tag removal -Oral cleft repair -Tympanostomy tubes -Airway procedures	-Tympanostomy tubes -Eyelid surgery -Oral cleft repair -Airway procedures	-Tympanostomy tubes -Eyelid surgery -Oral cleft repair -Airway procedures	-Ear reconstruction or prosthesis -Aural atresia repair -Consider early jaw surgery	-Fat grafting -Airway procedures	-Ear reconstruction or prosthesis -Jaw surgery -Fat grafting -Rhinoplasty	-Jaw surgery -Fat grafting -Microsurgery -Soft tissue augmentation
Consider:	A genetics evaluation can aid in assessment of the differential diagnoses, which may include: CHARGE, Townes-Brocks, Branchio-oto-renal Nagar, Miller, and Treacher-Collins syndromes.	A history suggestive of airway compromise (eg, sleep apnea and/or poor growth) requires an airway evaluation with an ENT and consideration of a sleep study. Obstructive symptoms vary with age and should be evaluated regularly.	Evaluations with an audiologist and ENT are critical to maximize hearing & communication. Parents may find this period challenging and may be anxious to proceed with treatments prior to the ideal.	Coordination between treatment for microtia with orthognathic surgery is critical in order to optimize long-term results for jaw and ear placement. This may require postponing ear reconstruction for children with significant jaw asymmetry.	Communication between the team and local dental & orthodontic providers is criticial for efficient orthodontic treatment with an integrated plan.	Consider final soft tissue augmentation after skeletal deficiencies have been corrected. Assurance that the teeen has realistic expectations during the pre-surgical planning phase is essential for optimization of patient satisfaction.	Final orthodontic treatments and jaw surgeries often occur at time when it interrupts social, athletic, and academic activities. Acknowledgement of this fact and communication with the patient is critical to achieving an optimal outcome.

Fig. 2.2 Timeline for care of patients with craniofacial microsomia (CFM). (a) When indicated. (b) Although these are common craniofacial surgeries in CFM, not all children will require every procedure [51].

Differential Diagnosis

Clinical findings overlap with other syndromes that have identifiable causative genes, such as Treacher Collins syndrome, Townes-Brocks syndrome, CHARGE syndrome, branchiootorenal spectrum disorders, and mutations of EFTUD2 [29]. Other entities for differential diagnosis include a traumatic postnatal deformity, Parry-Romberg syndrome, juvenile rheumatoid arthritis, unilateral condylar hyperplasia, Nager acrofacial dysostosis syndrome, and Pierre Robin sequence.

Summary

The initial evaluation of patients with craniofacial microsomia can be complex due to a wide range of potential facial and extracraniofacial deformities. A methodical, step-wise approach to patient evaluation with the help of the many classification schemes available can guide clinicians to find not only the correct diagnosis but also the corresponding steps to patient care. In evaluating these complex patients, it is always helpful to standardize the initial evaluation to maintain consistency in reporting and diagnosis.

Citations

1. Canton E. Arrest of development of the left ramus of the lower jaw, combined with malformation of the external ear. Trans Pathol Soc Lond. 1861;12:237.
2. Gorlin RJ, Cohen M, Hennekam RC. Syndromes of the head and neck. Oxford University Press; 2001.
3. Grabb WC. The first and second branchial arch syndrome. Plast Reconstr Surg. 1965;36:485–508.
4. Stark R, Saunders D. The first branchial syndrome: the oral-mandibular-auricular syndrome. Plast Reconstr Surg. 1962;29:229–39.
5. Francois J. L'hérédité en ophtalmologie [Heredity in ophthalmology]. Bull Soc Belge Ophtalmol. 1958;118(Pt 1):1-300. French. PMID: 13618716.
6. Obwegeser HL. Correction of the skeletal anomalies of otomandibular dysostosis. J Maxillofac Surg. 1974;2:73.
7. Pruzansky S. Not all dwarfed mandibles are alike. Birth Defects. 1969;4:120–9.
8. Gorlin RJ, Jue K, Jacobsen U, Goldschmidt E. Oculoauriculovertebral dysplasia.
9. Gorlin R. J., Cohen M. M., Jr., Hennekam R. C. M. (1990). Syndromes of the Head and Neck. Oxford: Oxford University Press.
10. Jongbloet PH. Goldenhar syndrome and overlapping dysplasias in vitro fertilisation and ovopathy. J Med Genet. 1987;24:616.
11. Ross RB. Lateral facial dysplasia (first and second brachial arch syndrome, hemifacial microsomia). Birth Defects. 1975;11:51.
12. Caronni EP. Embryogenesis and classification of branchial auricular dysplasia. In: Transactions of the Fifth International Congress of Plastic and Reconstructive Surgery.
13. Walker DG. Malformations of the face. Baltimore: Williams & Wilkins; 1961.
14. Stark R, Saunders D. The first brachial arch syndrome, the oral-mandibular-auricular syndrome. Plast Reconstr Surg. 1962;29:229.
15. Keith A. Three demonstrations on congenital malformations of the face, head and foot. Br J Surg. 1940;28:173.
16. Dingman RO, Grabb WC. Mandibular laterognathism. Plast Reconstr Surg. 1963;31:563.
17. Posnick JC. Craniofacial and maxillofacial surgery in children and young adults. Philadelphia: W.B. Saunders; 2000, p. 860–907.
18. McKusick VA, Hamosh A. OMIM Entry - % 164210 - HEMIFACIAL MICROSOMIA; HFM. 6/2/1986. https://www.omim.org/entry/164210.
19. David DJ, Mahatumarat C, Cooter RD. Hemifacial microsomia: a multisystem classification. Plast Reconstr Surg. 1987;80:525–35.
20. Cousley RR, Calvert ML. Current concepts in the understanding and management of hemifacial microsomia. Br J Plast Surg. 1997;50:536–51.
21. Kaban LB, Moses ML, Mulliien JB. Surgical correction of hemifacial microsomia in the growing child. Plast Reconstr Surg. 1988;9:82.
22. Kaban LB, Padwa BL, Mulliien JB. Surgical correction of mandibular hypoplasia in hemifacial microsomia: the case for treatment in early childhood. J Oral Maxillofac Surg. 1998;56:628–38.
23. Meurmany Y. Congenital microtia and meatal atresia: observations and aspects of treatment. AMA Arch Otolaryngol. 1957;663(4):443–6.
24. Murray JE, Kaban LB, Mulliken JB. Analysis and treatment of hemifacial microsomia. Plast Reconstr Plast. 1984;74:186.
25. Vento AR, LaBrie RA, Mulliken JB. The O.M.E.N.S. classification of hemifacial microsomia. Cranio. 1991;28:68–76.
26. Cousley RRJ. A comparison of two classification systems for hemifacial microsomia. Br J Oral Maxillofac Surg. 1993;31(2):78–82. https://doi.org/10.1016/0266-4356(93)90165-S.

27. Horgan JE, Padwa BL, Labrie RA, Mulliken JB. OMENS-plus: analysis of craniofacial and extracraniofacial anomalies in hemifacial microsomia. Cleft Palate Craniofac J. 1995;32(5):405–12. https://doi.org/10.1597/1545-1569_1995_032_0405_opaoca_2.3.co_2.
28. Bogusiak K, Puch A, Arkuszewski P. Goldenhar syndrome: current perspectives. World J Pediatr. 2017;13(5):405–15. https://doi.org/10.1007/s12519-017-0048-z.
29. Beleza-Meireles A, Clayton-Smith J, Oliveira R, Reis CF, Venancio M. Oculo-auriculo-vertebral spectrum: a review of the literature and genetic update. Eur J Med Genet. 2015;58:455–65.
30. Rosa RFM, Graziadio C, Lenhardt R, Alves RPM, Paskulin GA, Zen PRG. Central nervous system abnormalities in patients with oculo-auriculo-vertebral spectrum (Goldenhar syndrome). Arq Neuropsiquiatr. 2010;68(1):98–102.
31. Lima MD, Marques YM, de Melo Alves S Jr, Ortega KL, Soares MM, Magalhaes MH. Distraction osteogenesis in Goldenhar Syndrome: case report and 8-year follow-up - PubMed. Med Oral Patol Oral Cir Bucal. 2007;12:528–31. https://pubmed.ncbi.nlm.nih.gov/17978778/.
32. Wilson GN. Cranial defects in the Goldenhar syndrome. Am J Med Genet. 1983;14:435–43.
33. Roodneshin F, Agah M. Management of anesthesia in Goldenhar syndrome: case-series study. Tanaffos. 2009;8:43–50.
34. Bielicka B, Nęcka A, Andrych M. Interdisciplinary treatment of patients with Goldenhar syndrome-clinical reports. Dent Med Probl. 2006;43:458–62.
35. Wolford LM, Bourland TC, Rodrigues D, Perez DE, Limoeiro E. Successful reconstruction of nongrowing hemifacial microsomia patients with unilateral temporomandibular joint total joint prosthesis and orthognathic surgery. J Oral Maxillofac Surg. 2012;70:2835–53.
36. Tasse C, Böhringer S, Fischer S, Lüdecke HJ, Albrecht B, Horn D. Oculo-auriculo-vertebral spectrum (OAVS): clinical evaluation and severity scoring of 53 patients and proposal for a new classification. Eur J Med Genet. 2005;48:397–411.
37. Birgfeld CB, Luquetti DV, Gougoutas AJ. A phenotypic assessment tool for craniofacial microsomia. Plast Reconstr Surg. 2011;127(1):313–20.
38. Vong A, Funamura J. Multidisciplinary management of oculo-auriculo-vertebral spectrum. Curr Opin Otolaryngol Head Neck Surg. 2018;26(4):234–41.
39. Vargesson N. Thalidomide-induced teratogenesis: history and mechanisms. Birth Defects Res C Embryo Today. 2015;105(2):140–56.
40. Werler MM. Teratogen update: pseudoephedrine. Birth Defects Res A Clin Mol Teratol. 2006;76(6):445–52.
41. Lammer E, Chen D, Hoar R, et al. Retinoic acid embryopathy. N Engl J Med. 1985;313(14):837–41.
42. Sulik K, Cook C, Webster W. Teratogens and craniofacial malformations: relationships to cell death. Development. 1988;103:213–31.
43. Wang R, Graham J. Infants of diabetic mothers are at increased risk for the oculo-auriculo-vertebral sequence: a case-based and case-control approach. J Pediatr. 2002;141(5):611–7.
44. Meenan K, Kadakia S, Bernstein J. Revisiting the work of Maurice Goldenhar-an overview of Goldenhar syndrome. Eur J Plast Surg. 2014;37:575–82.
45. Luna-Paredes C, Antón-Pacheco J, García Hernández G, Martínez Gimeno A, Romance García A, García RI. Screening for symptoms of obstructive sleep apnea in children with severe craniofacial anomalies: assessment in a multidisciplinary unit. Int J Pediatr Otorhinolaryngol. 2012;76:1767–70.
46. Antón-Pacheco J, Luna-Paredes C, Martínez Gimeno A, García Hernández G, Martín de la Vega R, Romance García A. The role of bronchoscopy in the management of patients with severe craniofacial syndromes. J Pediatr Surg. 2012;47:1512–5.
47. Zim S, Lee J, Rubinstein B. Prevalence of renal and cervical vertebral anomalies in patients with isolated microtia and/or aural atresia. Cleft Palate Craniofac J. 2017;54:664–7.

48. Chen Q, Zhao Y, Shen G, Dai J. Etiology and pathogenesis of hemifacial microsomia. J Dent Res. 2018;97(12):1297–305.
49. Hoch B, Hochban W. Four-year-old girl with Goldenhar-sequence and severe obstructive sleep apnea, symptoms, diagnosis and therapy. Int J Pediatr Otorhinolaryngol. 1998;43:277–81.
50. Sahni N, Bhatia N. Successful management of difficult airway in an adult patient of Goldenhar syndrome. Saudi J Anaesth. 2014;8:98–100.
51. Birgfeld CB, Heike C. Craniofacial microsomia. Semin Plast Surg. 2012;26(2):91–104.

Chapter 3
A Look at Breathing, Feeding/Swallowing, and Speech Impairment in Patients with Craniofacial Microsomia

Laura Brooks and Steven Goudy

Introduction

Craniofacial microsomia (CFM) includes a spectrum of malformations primarily involving structures derived from the first and second branchial arches. Characteristics of this condition can include the following:

- Mandibular hypoplasia/micrognathia.
- Facial asymmetry.
- Ear malformations that can include microtia, anotia, or aural atresia.
- Preauricular or facial tags.
- Hearing loss.
- Feeding/swallowing disorders.
- Cleft lip and/or palate.
- Extra craniofacial malformations can include vertebral, renal, cardiac, and limb involvement.

The primary anomalies of CFM include the airway, oropharynx, and auditory structures [1]. The goals of treatment for CFM are to optimize breathing, feeding/swallowing, hearing, communication, facial symmetry, dental occlusion, and quality of life [1]. Intervention is age-dependent, time-sensitive, and dependent on the stage of craniofacial development.

L. Brooks
Children's Healthcare of Atlanta, Atlanta, GA, USA
e-mail: Laura.Brooks@choa.org

S. Goudy (✉)
Children's Healthcare of Atlanta, Atlanta, GA, USA

Department of Otolaryngology-Head and Neck Surgery, Emory University School of Medicine, Atlanta, GA, USA
e-mail: steven.goudy@emory.edu

D. M. Yates, M. R. Markiewicz (eds.), *Craniofacial Microsomia and Treacher Collins Syndrome*, https://doi.org/10.1007/978-3-030-84733-3_3

Breathing

Mandibular hypoplasia is one of the most common features in patients with CFM [1, 2]. This upper airway obstruction places children with CFM at a high risk for obstructive sleep apnea (OSA) with symptoms of snoring, increased work of breathing, and apnea in the neonatal period [2, 3]. Significant obstructive sleep apnea can result in failure to thrive, pulmonary hypertension, and even death [2, 4]. Sleep-disordered breathing in this population can be associated with one or more of the following sites of airway obstruction: glossoptosis, micrognathia, adenotonsillar hyperplasia, midface hypoplasia, nasoseptal deviation, and rhinitis [1]. Patients with more severe mandibular and orbital deformities seem to be at a greater risk for obstructive sleep apnea [5]. Breathing patterns in patients with OSA can include increased work of breathing, tachypnea and/or gas exchange abnormalities [6].

Obstructive sleep apnea has been defined as complete cessation of airflow for more than two breaths or 10 seconds, and hypopnea is characterized by a >50% reduction in ventilation with decrease in oxygen saturation (i.e., >3%). OSA can range from mild to severe, and the classification and severity of obstructive sleep apnea (OSA) are traditionally based on apnea-hypopnea index (AHI). Although some definitions vary, the most commonly accepted definition in pediatric OSA is as follows: ≤1 event/hour is normal, 1–5 is mild, 5–10 is moderate, and >10/hour is severe OSA [2, 5, 7, 8].

Infants with difficulty breathing due to upper airway obstruction undergo monitoring by pulse oximetry, overnight polysomnography, and potentially direct laryngoscopy and/or bronchoscopy [1]. A Pediatric Sleep Questionnaire (PSQ) could be completed by the parents and includes questions regarding sleep-disordered breathing and sleep habits [3]. Interventions can be nonsurgical or surgical. Nonsurgical treatments for upper airway obstruction include prone positioning, positive pressure (nasal, mask), nasal decongestants, and intubation. Surgical treatments for upper airway obstruction include tongue lip adhesion, adenotonsillectomy, tongue base reduction, septorhinoplasty, mandibular distraction, skeletal expansion, maxillary advancement, and tracheotomy [1, 5, 9].

If the upper airway obstruction is severe and adequate respiration is not achieved by positive pressure or surgical intervention, a tracheotomy may be performed. A tracheostomy bypasses the upper airway and is the most effective intervention for severe OSA. The goal of a tracheostomy is for eventual decannulation when a child can adequately achieve respiration through the upper airway with surgical intervention or maturation. When a patient has a tracheostomy with or without ventilator dependence, a speech/language pathologist (SLP) can evaluate the infant or child's ability to orally feed and to tolerate application of a speaking valve. A speaking valve can allow for inhalation to occur through the tracheostomy tube and exhalation to occur through the nose and mouth, which allows for voicing and speech. However it is important to note that an infant or child who has a tracheostomy due to upper airway obstruction may not be able to tolerate a speaking valve due to compromised airway patency. The otolaryngologist, SLP, and/or respiratory therapist (RT) could measure transtracheal pressure via manometry in order to determine airway patency or the ability for the child to exhale adequately through the nose and mouth [10].

Anatomy and Physiology of Normal Swallowing

Swallowing is a complex, dynamic activity requiring neuromuscular timing and coordination involving the oral, pharyngeal, and esophageal phases and is highly impacted by bolus volume and consistency [11, 12] (Table 3.1). Six cranial nerves

Table 3.1 Normal swallowing anatomy and physiology

Location	Structures	Muscles	Physiology
Oral phase	Lips Teeth Hard palate/ maxilla Soft palate Uvula Mandible Tongue Sulci (anterior and lateral) Faucial arches Salivary glands	Lips and cheeks:	Lips and cheeks:
		Orbicularis oral⇒	Rounds and closes lips
		Buccinators ⇒	Compresses cheeks
		Levator labii superioris alaeque nasi⇒	Elevates upper lip
		Levator labii superioris ⇒	Elevates upper lip
		Levator anguli oris⇒	Lifts the corners of the mouth
		Depressor anguli oris ⇒	Depresses the corners of the mouth
		Depressor labii inferioris⇒	Lowers the bottom lip
		Zygomaticus major	Elevates the mouth and draws outward
		Zygomaticus minor	Pulls upper lip backward, upward, and outward
		Risorius	Pulls the angle of the mouth back laterally
		Mentalis	Protrusion of the lower lip and wrinkling of the chin
		Mastication: Masseter	*Mastication:* Elevates the mandible Protrudes the mandible Most powerful muscle of mastication
		Temporalis	Elevates the mandible Retracts the mandible

(continued)

Table 3.1 (continued)

Location	Structures	Muscles	Physiology
		Lateral pterygoid	Depresses the mandible Protrudes the mandible Lateral movement of the mandible
		Medial pterygoids	Lateral movement of the jaw Elevates the mandible
		Tongue: *Intrinsic* Superior longitudinal Inferior longitudinal Transverse Vertical	Tongue: *Intrinsic* Alter tongue shape
		Extrinsic Genioglossus Hyoglossus Styloglossus Palatoglossus	*Extrinsic* Protruding, depressing the tongue Depresses and retracts the tongue Tongue elevation and retraction Elevates the posterior portion of the tongue
		Floor of mouth: Mylohyoid	*Floor of mouth:* Elevated the hyoid bone, tenses the floor of mouth
		Geniohyoid	Pulls hyoid bone anteriorly and superiorly Widens the pharynx
		Stylohyoid	Elevates and retracts the hyoid bone
		Anterior belly of the digastric	Elevates hyoid bone and depresses the mandible
		Posterior belly of digastric	Elevates hyoid bone

Table 3.1 (continued)

Location	Structures	Muscles	Physiology
Pharyngeal phase	*Pharynx* Soft palate Tongue base Valleculae Posterior pharyngeal walls Lateral pharyngeal walls Epiglottis Pyriform sinuses Mandible Hyoid bone Thyroid cartilage Cricoid cartilage *Larynx* Aryepiglottic folds Arytenoid cartilage False vocal cords True vocal cords	Palatoglossus	Elevates the posterior portion of the tongue Draws the soft palate inferiorly Assists in pressure generation of swallow
		Palatopharyngeus	Elevates the larynx Narrows the pharynx
		Levator veli palatini	Pulls the velum up and back toward the posterior pharyngeal wall
		Tensor veli palatini	Opens Eustachian tube during swallowing
		Superior constrictor Medial constrictor Inferior constrictor	Contract to propel bolus through the pharynx
		Cricopharyngeal muscle (most inferior structure of the pharynx)	Maintains UES closure at rest, opens during swallowing
		True vocal cords	
		Vocalis	Shortens/lengthens vocal cords
		Thyroarytenoid muscle	Shortens/relaxes the vocal cords
		Posterior cricoarytenoid muscle	Vocal cord abduction for respiration
		Lateral cricoarytenoid	Vocal cord adduction for voicing and swallowing
		Transverse and oblique arytenoid	Vocal cord adduction for voicing and swallowing
		Suprahyoid muscles (anterior and posterior belly of digastric, mylohyoid, geniohyoid, stylohyoid)	Elevate the larynx (with the stylopharyngeus)
		Infrahyoid muscles (thyrohyoid, omohyoid, sternohyoid, sternothyroid)	Depress the larynx
Esophageal phase	Upper esophageal sphincter esophagus Lower esophageal sphincter	Upper one third of the esophagus: made up of striated muscle Middle one third of the esophagus: made up of both striated and smooth muscles Lower one third: made up of smooth muscle	Peristaltic wave via relaxation and contraction

Table 3.2 Cranial nerves

Cranial nerve	Sensory	Motor
Trigeminal V	Anterior two third sensation of tongue Pain, temperature, and tactile to the face, forehead, mucous membranes of the nose and mouth, teeth Deep pressure and kinesthetic to the teeth. Gums, hard palate, TMJ	Muscles of mastication (masseter, temporalis, lateral pterygoid, medial pterygoids) Tenses the palate via tensor veli palatine Elevates the larynx via anterior digastric, mylohyoid
Facial VII	Anterior two third of the tongue for taste Nasopharynx	Labial closure and rounding (orbicularis oris) Pulling cheeks inward (buccinators) Elevates the larynx (digastric and stylohyoid)
Glossopharyngeal IX	Posterior one third of the tongue taste and sensation Velar sensation Pharynx Faucial pillars Gag reflex	Laryngeal elevation and anterior movement via stylopharyngeus Superior pharyngeal constrictor Velopharyngeal closure
Vagus X	Velar sensation Tongue base Pharynx Larynx Subglottal	Constricts the pharynx Tenses the palate (tensor veli palatini) Abducts/adducts vocal cords via recurrent laryngeal nerve Elevates the back of the tongue (palatoglossus) Esophageal contraction of smooth muscles
Accessory XI	N/A	Assists in elevation of the soft palate assists in innervation of intrinsic laryngeal muscles
Hypoglossal XII	N/A	Tongue movement (protrusion, retraction, depressing, cupping). All intrinsic muscles of the tongue and all but one extrinsic muscle of the tongue (palatoglossus)

play a role in swallowing and include V (trigeminal), VII (facial), IX (glossopharyngeal), X (vagus), XI (accessory), and XII (hypoglossal) (Table 3.2). Typical duration for the oral phase of swallowing is 1–2 seconds, and duration of the pharyngeal phase is <1 second [13].

Historically, it was believed that only the brainstem centers were responsible for controlling swallowing; however, later studies emphasized the importance of the cerebral cortex during this action [14, 15]. The oral, pharyngeal, and esophageal phases of swallowing are controlled by central pattern-generating circuitry of the brainstem and peripheral reflexes. The central pattern generators of the brainstem control the timing of swallowing, and the peripheral involvement depends on sensory feedback through reflexes of the pharynx and esophagus. The brainstem nuclei that mediate the oral, pharyngeal, and esophageal phases of swallowing include the trigeminal nucleus, reticular formation, nucleus tractus solitarius, nucleus ambiguous, dorsal motor nucleus, and ventromedial nucleus [16].

Oral Phase

During the oral preparatory phase of the swallow, labial compression reduces anterior spillage and promotes oral containment. Labial compression is important for spoon clearance, labial rounding for straw drinking, and retraction/compression movement during mastication.

Next, tension in the buccal musculature closes off the lateral sulcus and prevents food particles from falling laterally into the sulcus between the mandible and the cheek [11].

The tongue is divided into the oral portion and the pharyngeal portion, and the oral tongue is under cortical and voluntary neural control [11]. The sensory receptors in the tongue control sensation of the bolus and taste. Tongue movements include tongue cupping (important for bottle feeding), as the sides of the tongue seal against the lateral alveolus for bolus holding. The oral cavity is sealed anteriorly by elevation of the tongue tip and posteriorly by the soft palate and tongue contact. The tongue elevates anteriorly and posteriorly to propel the bolus to the pharynx. As food viscosity increases, the pressure of the tongue against the palate increases. Adequate oral strength and range of motion help ensure that there is limitation to no oral residue remaining in the oral cavity after swallowing [11, 17].

Pharyngeal Phase

Two critical roles of the pharyngeal phase of swallowing are to (1) generate enough pressure to propel the bolus through the pharynx and upper esophageal sphincter (into the esophagus) and (2) airway protection, closure of the larynx to prevent penetration or aspiration. Laryngeal penetration is when liquid or food enters the airway but does not move below the vocal cords. Aspiration occurs when food or liquid passes below the vocal cords into the trachea. During the pharyngeal stage, the soft palate elevates and contacts the lateral and posterior walls of the pharynx, closing the nasopharynx at about the same time that the bolus head comes into the pharynx. Soft palate elevation prevents bolus regurgitation into the nasal cavity. The base of the tongue retracts (involuntary control from the brainstem but also can be placed under some volitional control) to contact the bulging posterior pharyngeal walls. The pharyngeal constrictor muscles contract sequentially from the top to the bottom, squeezing the bolus downward, and the larynx elevates and the epiglottis protects the airway [11, 17].

There are several airway protective mechanisms preventing aspiration of the foreign materials to the trachea before or during swallowing. The vocal folds close to seal the glottis, the arytenoids tilt forward to contact the epiglottic base, the hyoid bone and larynx are elevated and pulled anteriorly upward and forward, and the epiglottis tilts backward to seal the laryngeal vestibule [11, 17].

Opening of the upper esophageal sphincter (UES) is essential for the bolus entry into the esophagus. The UES is closed at rest during respiration and opens during swallowing due to relaxation of the cricopharyngeus muscle, hyolaryngeal excursion, and pressure of the descending bolus [11].

Esophageal Phase

The esophagus is a muscular tube from the lower part of the UES to the lower esophageal sphincter (LES). The UES is tensed at rest and opens during the swallow to allow for passage of the bolus from the pharynx into the esophagus. The lower esophageal sphincter is also tensed at rest to prevent regurgitation from the stomach, relaxes during a swallow, and allows the bolus passage to the stomach. The cervical esophagus (upper one third) is mainly composed of striated muscle, but thoracic esophagus (lower two thirds) is smooth muscle. Through peristalsis the bolus moves through the esophagus. Material moves from the UES to the LES within 8–20 seconds by a peristatic wave, regulated by the autonomic nervous system. Gravity assists peristalsis in upright position [11, 17].

Feeding/Swallowing for Patients with Craniofacial Microsomia (CFM)

Dysphagia is a feeding/swallowing impairment that includes any phases of the swallow (oral, pharyngeal, or esophageal). Children present with dysphagia from one or more of the following etiologies:

1. Neurologic (i.e., prematurity, central nervous system conditions)
2. Respiratory and other conditions (i.e., respiratory syncytial virus, bronchopulmonary dysplasia, cardiac disease)
3. Anatomic abnormalities of the aerodigestive tract (i.e., craniofacial abnormalities, vocal fold hypomobility, laryngeal cleft)
4. Gastrointestinal (i.e., reflux)
5. Other or unknown [18–23]

Children with dysphagia are at increased risk for developing respiratory compromise, failure to thrive, feeding refusal, and stressful interactions with their caregivers [18]. The goals for feeding/swallowing treatment are to implement evidence-based

Table 3.3 Feeding/swallowing for patients with CFM and potential areas of difficulty

Craniofacial diagnosis	Characteristics	Potential impact on feeding
Craniofacial microsomia	Mandibular hypoplasia	Inefficient sucking due to restricted mandibular excursion
	Upper airway anomalies/OSA	Disorganized suck, swallow, and breathe sequence – -may result in instability or aspiration
	Unilateral pharyngeal weakness	Pharyngeal residue on VFSS on the affected side
	Cleft lip	Incomplete lip seal
	Cleft palate	Nasopharyngeal regurgitation Impaired intraoral pressure for suction when bottle feeding Breast feeding can be extremely challenging
	Extracranial anomalies	Prolonged feeding times, fatigue Risk of vocal cord injury s/p cardiac repair GI discomfort or reflux

strategies to *reduce* the risk of complications from dysphagia, preserve pulmonary integrity, and identify the method of intervention which is least likely to cause an adverse event (i.e., aspiration or pneumonia) [24].

The prevalence of feeding/swallowing difficulties in patients with CFM ranges from 42% to 83% [25]. Anatomic anomalies of the jaw, palate, and cranial nerves in patients with CFM can contribute to oropharyngeal phase dysfunction [26]. Children with CFM with and without a cleft can present with impaired bolus control, delayed swallowing initiation, nasopharyngeal regurgitation, post-swallow stasis/residue, and aspiration in VFSS [26]. In addition, some children with CFM can have extra cranial anomalies including CNS, cardiac, gastrointestinal, kidney, or skeletal. Given these risk factors, it is important that an infant or child with CFM be closely monitored for dysphagia (Table 3.3).

Given the wide phenotypic presentation associated with CFM, the assessment and treatment of feeding/swallowing are highly individualized. If concerns arise a speech/language pathologist should be consulted for an assessment and intervention for impaired latch or extraction of fluid from bottle nipple, coughing with oral feeds, instability with oral feeds, prolonged feeding times, and stridor/gulping with oral feeds. Below are characteristics that may be present in a child with CFM and descriptions of how that could impact feeding/swallowing (Table 3.4).

Mandible

Mandibular hypoplasia is present in 89–100% of patients with CFM [26]. More severe hypoplasia showed more difficulty to form an appropriate bolus than less severe hypoplasia, which can result in premature spillage of the bolus and possible aspiration [26]. Structural anomalies such as mandibular hypoplasia can impact

Table 3.4 Feeding impairment and intervention for patients with CFM

Feeding impairment	Intervention strategy
Nasal regurgitation	Modify positioning to near upright May benefit from elevated side-lying
Incomplete lip seal during bottle or breast feeding	Wide-based nipple can help occlude space
Inability to compress the nipple	Squeeze bottles to gently assist with extraction of fluid and closely monitor the patient for anterior spillage, signs of stress, or signs/symptoms of dysphagia
Poor suction strength/inability to create negative pressure for fluid extraction	Use specialized nipple (extracts with up/down movement)
Poor coordination of suck-swallow-breathe	Side-lying positioning External pacing or regulation Slow-flow nipple
Fatigue during feeding and/or underlying cardiac issues	Use of small, frequent feedings Change flow rate Increase caloric density of feeds
Aspiration of thin liquids on instrumental examination	Thickened liquids if proven successful

extraction of fluid when bottle feeding in infancy due to restriction of the mandible [25]. Infants with significant micrognathia may benefit from specialty bottles which extract fluid with up/down compression rather than suction.

At 12 months of age, the child transitions to intake of regular solids. Mastication can be impaired in patients with CFM secondary to mandibular hypoplasia, which can be a risk for aspiration or choking. Craniofacial bony abnormalities are associated with underdeveloped masticatory muscles [27].

Poor Coordination of Respiration/Swallowing

Upper airway obstruction seen in patients with CFM can compromise oral feeding [2]. Babies with CFM may present with tachypnea, stridor, and increased work of breathing due to difficulty adequately breathing during the challenging task of oral feeding. The ideal rhythm for bottle feeding is suck-swallow-breathe (SSB), occurring approximately once every second or 60 times a minute during bottle feeding. Impaired coordination of breathing and swallowing can result in oxygen desaturations or bradycardia during feeding, and the baby may benefit from strategies such as pacing/regulation [28, 29].

Some patients require high-flow nasal cannula support for respiratory compromise or noninvasive positive pressure ventilation which can increase pressure from above and could compromise the child's ability to close the airway adequately during a swallow resulting in misdirection of part of the bolus into the airway [30]. A patient may require enteral feeding at that time which can include nasogastric tube, orogastric tube, or gastrostomy tube. If there is a concern for emesis, the feeding tube could bypass the stomach to the jejunum. Once a patient is oral feeding, quality of the feeding is critical. Volume is a by-product of a "quality feeding" where there is physiologic stability, good state regulation, and endurance [28, 29].

Infants and children who have been intubated (prolonged or emergent) may present with airway swelling, vocal cord injury, or tracheal injury which can compromise oral feeding [24]. Palate remodeling could also result, leading to velopharyngeal incompetence [31, 32]. The clinician must consider the following: Was the intubation emergent? Were there multiple attempts to achieve successful intubation? Did the patient self-extubate? Was intubation prolonged?

Misdirection of the Bolus into the Airway: Laryngeal Penetration and Aspiration

Laryngeal penetration is defined as material entering the airway *but does not pass below the vocal cords*. Aspiration is defined as *passage of material below the vocal cords* [11]. Misdirection of the bolus into the airway (penetration or aspiration) is a symptom of a physiologic swallowing impairment [33], and aspiration can occur before the swallow secondary to oral control impairment or impaired timing/coordination, during the swallow secondary to incomplete closure of the laryngeal vestibule, or after the swallow secondary to weakness/impaired range of motion (associated with residue). Thin liquids flow quickly through the oropharynx and can be challenging to swallow safely for patients with dysphagia. Thus, liquids are the most frequently aspirated material in children, and greater than 90% of the time aspiration is silent [34]. If there is a concern that a patient has dysphagia and strategies during bedside treatment are not successful, an instrumental swallow examination could be performed to allow for visualization of the structures and swallowing physiology. The two instrumental swallowing assessments are Videofluoroscopic Swallow Study (VFSS)/Modified Barium Swallow Studies and Fiberoptic/Flexible Endoscopic Evaluation of Swallowing. VFSS allows for views of the oral, pharyngeal, and esophageal phases of the swallow, whereas the VFSS assesses anatomy and physiology of the nasopharynx, hypopharynx, and larynx (Figs. 3.1, 3.2, and 3.3).

Strategies are used during VFSS and FEES to help guide the thin liquid bolus away from the airway and into the esophagus, and the strategies will vary depending on the type/etiology of the dysphagia. These strategies can include changing the flow rate, bolus size, and positioning (i.e., side-lying, chin down, head turn, head tilt) (Fig. 3.4).

When strategies are not successful in eliminating aspiration, thickened liquids (if proven to be swallowed safely) may be recommended. Thickening liquids slows oropharyngeal transit time while creating a more cohesive bolus, which makes the liquid easier to control and minimizes the risk of aspiration before the swallow [35]. In addition, thickening can increase timing/duration of UES opening and amount of

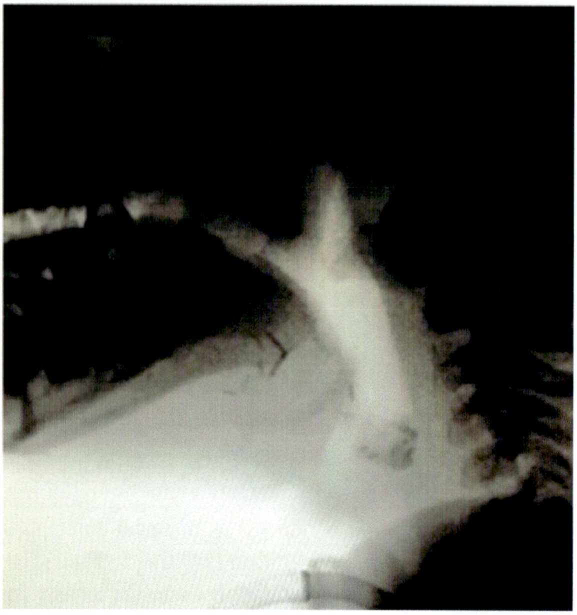

Fig. 3.1 VFSS lateral view

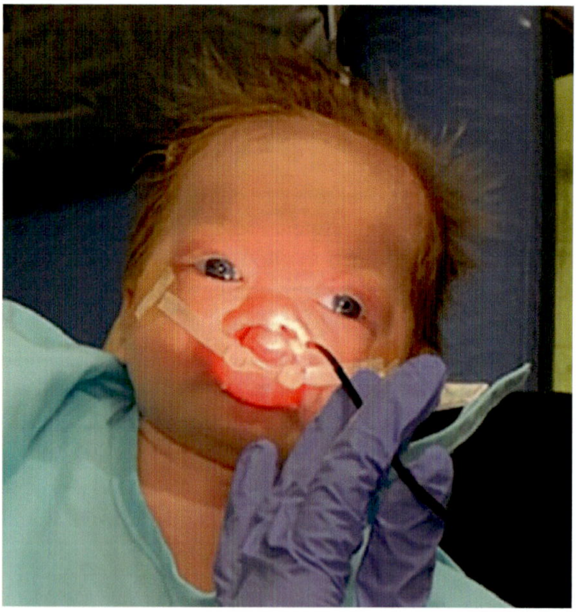

Fig. 3.2 FEES

hyolaryngeal movement [12, 36]. However, there can be negative consequences associated with thickened liquids, including refusal leading to dehydration, cost of the thickening agent, accessibility of commercial thickeners, inconsistent achievement of target viscosity, and a negative impact on the child's immature digestive tract [37].

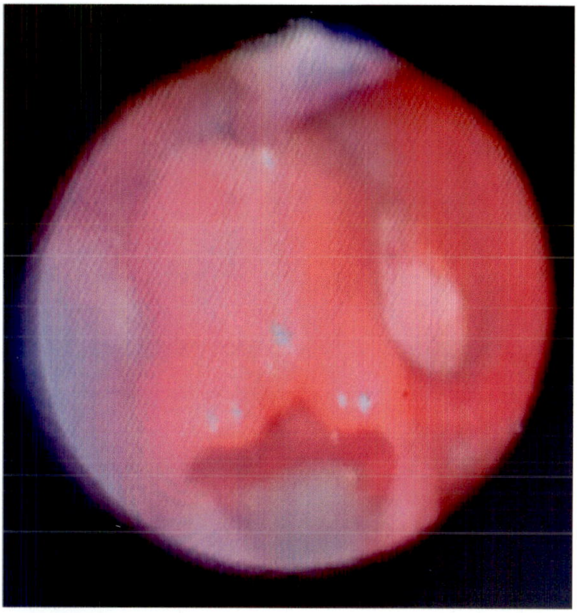

Fig. 3.3 FEES

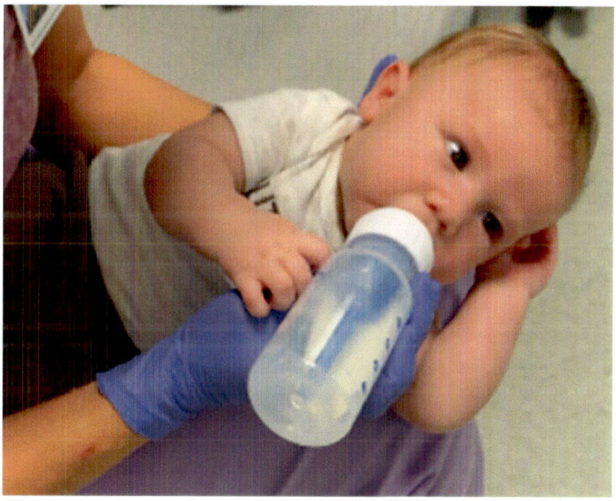

Fig. 3.4 Side-lying

Pharyngeal Weakness

Movement of the lateral pharyngeal wall of the affected side can be reduced in patients with CFM [25]. Decreased pharyngeal constriction can result in ineffective bolus propulsion and/or pharyngeal residue, which can place the patient at risk for aspiration after the swallow. The speech/language pathologist can confirm if the residue is unilateral or bilateral by switching from lateral to anterior-posterior view during a VFSS and then implement strategies to improve swallow function (Fig. 3.5).

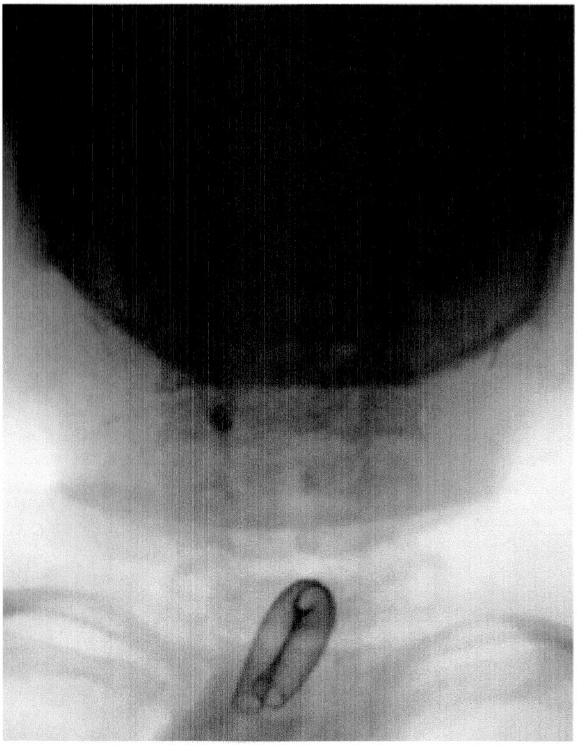

Fig. 3.5 VFSS A–P view

Cleft Palate and Nasopharyngeal Regurgitation

Patients with CFM with a cleft lip/palate have been shown to have a higher likelihood of nasogastric feeding tube dependence at some point, which can impact development of swallowing [26]. Suction strength/intraoral pressure can be severely impaired if the patient also has a cleft palate. For bottle feeders, there are a variety of nipple and bottle shapes, sizes, and characteristics that can help facilitate efficient oral feeding. Specialty bottle nipples allow for extraction of fluid from up/down movement of the jaw, rather than suction, and squeeze bottles to allow for the feeder to compensate for the infant's inability to extract fluid independently. Nasopharyngeal regurgitation is present in a patient with a cleft palate, and approximately 20% of children will require a secondary intervention for velopharyngeal insufficiency post-cleft palate repair [38]. Infants with nasopharyngeal regurgitation may benefit from a more upright feeding position [39].

Extracranial Anomalies That Impact Swallowing

Patients with CFM can present with extracranial anomalies including CNS, cardiac, gastrointestinal, kidney, or skeletal involvement. Patients with cardiac involvement might present with tachypnea that can compromise the ability to coordinate suck-swallow-breathe [40]. Infants with cardiac abnormalities can also present with fatigue and poor endurance during oral feeding. After cardiac repair the patient could present with vocal cord impairment if the recurrent laryngeal nerve was compromised during surgery. Patients with gastrointestinal issues may have reduced interest in oral feeding. Patients with reflux can place a patient in discomfort after feed or, worse, risk for secondary aspiration of emesis.

Normal Speech and Language Development

The first 3 years of a child's life are critical in the developmental of speech and language skills. In infancy, babies are exposed to various stimuli, including sounds, sights, and speech/language from others. Communication occurs early on in infancy, such as crying to communicate a need, engaging or making eye contact, and reacting to certain sounds heard in the environment. While children may vary in their development of speech and language, there is a typical progression or timetable of speech and language skills that children follow (Table 3.5).

Table 3.5 Normal speech and language development

Receptive speech and language	Expressive speech and language
Birth–1 year Startles to loud sounds *Smiles when a caregiver speaks/ recognizes his/her voice Tracks or turns head in the direction of sounds (toys, music) Begins to understand words for objects or people (*mommy, car.*) Responds to commands/questions such as "no" and "come here" Engages in games like peek-a-boos	*Birth–1 year* Coos Cries change for different needs Smiles Babbles (i.e., *ta, ma, papapa*) Laughs Makes sounds to communicate when happy or upset Points to objects Uses gestures like waving bye, reaching for "up," and shaking his head "no" Imitates different speech sounds Says one or two words, like *hi, dog, dada, mama*, or *uh oh*
1–2 years Identifies body parts Follows one-step commands, like "roll the ball" Responds to simple questions, like "where's mommy?" Points to pictures in a book when you name them	*1–2 years* Increases word repertoire Uses new sounds such as *p, b, m, h*, and *w* Starts to name objects or pictures Asks questions, like "what's that?" Produces one- to two-word utterances

(continued)

Table 3.1 (continued)

Receptive speech and language	Expressive speech and language
2–3 years Understands opposites, like up-down Follows two-step directions, like "get the spoon and put it on the table" Understands new vocabulary easily	*2–3 years* Can name most familiar objects Uses new sounds such as *k, g, f, t, d*, and *n* Uses location words such as *in, on*, and *under* Combines two to three words or produces short sentences By age 3, speech is generally understandable Asks "why?
3–4 years Responds when a sound is heard from another room Understands colors, like *red, blue*, and *green* Understands shapes, like *circle* and *square*	*3–4 years* Answers simple "wh-" questions Says rhyming words, like *hat-cat* Uses pronouns, like *I, you*, and *me* Uses plural words, like *toys* Speech is understood by most people Asks "when" and "how" questions Combines four words together (with some errors) "I went to school"
4–5 years Understands words for order, like *first, next*, and *last* Understands words for time, like *yesterday, today*, and *tomorrow* Follows three-step directions Hears and understands most of what she hears at home and in school	*4–5 years* Uses all speech sounds in words. May make mistakes on sounds that are harder to say, like *l, s, r, v, z, ch, sh*, and *th* Responds to "What did you say?" Names letters and numbers Tells a short story Engages in a conversation

American Speech- Language- Hearing Association
https://www.asha.org/public/speech/development/chart/

Speech and Language Development for a Child with CFM

Children with CFM have anomalies and comorbidities that can increase their risk for speech, language, communication deficits, and neuropsychological deficits [41, 42]. Approximately 75–80% of children with CFM have some degree of hearing impairment, most commonly conductive hearing loss, although sensorineural hearing loss can also be noted in approximately 10% of children with CFM [43, 44]. Children with features of CFM can demonstrate variable anomalies associated with hearing loss including external ear abnormalities, aural atresia, and Eustachian tube dysfunction [43]. Although most children with microtia have unilateral external ear malformations, they are at risk for bilateral hearing loss [1, 43]. Children with CFM should have a comprehensive hearing assessment within the first 6 months of age to identify hearing loss and assess the type and severity of hearing impairment [1]. Amplification options should be tailored to the degree of hearing loss, nature, and laterality of hearing loss. Amplification can be beneficial for children with even a mild hearing loss, and academic accommodations can be implemented [45].

Severe to profound hearing loss can be associated with higher prevalence of delays in speech articulation, receptive and expressive language delay, learning disabilities, and poorer communication and social skills [43]. Whether or not mild or unilateral hearing loss can impact speech and language development is debatable [43].

In addition to the risk of delay with hearing loss, children can present with delays or impairment due to facial nerve palsy, asymmetric soft palate movement, orofacial clefting, malocclusion, tongue anomalies, and/or muscular deficiencies [42, 44, 46, 47]. These structural factors may impact articulation, speech intelligibility, vocal quality, and/or resonance [42].

Children with CFM may present hypernasality and nasal emissions due to velopharyngeal dysfunction (VPD) associated with one or more of the following categories: structural deficits (cleft palate), physiologic (neuromotor), or mislearning of articulation [38]. A submucous cleft palate can result in VPD if the velum is too short to adequately contact the posterior pharyngeal wall [38]. A speech/language pathologist can address accurate articulatory placement for speech sounds and correct errors associated with mislearning.

Children with CFM can be at higher risk of delayed language and neurodevelopmental milestones, particularly for patients with combined microtia and mandibular hypoplasia [41, 48, 49]. Deficits can be particularly noted in receptive vocabulary [47]. Children with CFM have complex healthcare needs and ongoing speech, language, and hearing monitoring throughout development [42].

Case Studies

Case Study #1

ZG was born at 34.4 weeks gestation with Goldenhar syndrome characterized by microtia (no external auditory canal), mandibular hypoplasia on R side, cleft lip, high arched and short palate, right sided macrostomia, R ear moderate to severe conductive hearing loss on newborn hearing screening and ABR. Her ECHO, RBUS, spinal films were normal. She presented with oxygen desaturations after delivery so she was intubated for 1 day and then placed on supplemental O2 via NC. PSG revealed 19 obstructive, 45 central, and 3 mixed apneas. There were 44 obstructive and 0 central hypopneas, giving an overall Apnea/Hypopnea Index (AHI) of 19.1 events/hour. The Obstructive AHI was 11.4 events/hour. The Central AHI was 7.7 events/hour. She also had tracheobronchomalacia and laryngomalacia and underwent a supraglottoplasty which resolved the stridor but did not help with her O2 desaturations. Five months later she had jaw surgery (rib graft, expanded jaw), and her oxygenation improved and desaturations resolved. She also underwent placement of gastrostomy tube (G-tube) at that time. Swallowing improved after surgery as well, and her subsequent VFSS revealed no aspiration with thin liquids. She fed best with the Dr. Brown's specialty feeder (compression extraction) with a preemie nipple. After so much time without oral feeding, she had difficulty with interest and endurance, and given her G-tube feeding schedule, her mother felt that she did not have an appetite. G-tube feeds were adjusted/compressed, and she has more interest now in orally feeding. Foods and drinks were offered prior to her bolus feeds when her appetite was the greatest.

Case Study #2

ES is a 7- month-old fraternal twin born at 36.3 weeks of gestation with craniofacial microsomia which was not diagnosed prenatally (perinatologist noted a "recessed chin" only). After birth she presented with features of CFM including with L microtia (L hearing loss) and mandibular hypoplasia. The lip and palate were intact without clefting. She had increased work of breathing with suprasternal retractions requiring supplemental oxygen via nasal cannula. She had stridor concerning for laryngomalacia, but endoscopy was compromised by her narrow airway (the epiglottis and tongue compromising the view of her larynx). Supraglottoplasty was planned several times under sedation but discontinued, and given that her breathing and stridor improved over time, she did not require surgical intervention. After admission to the NICU, she presented with oxygen desaturation during oral feeding, so she relied on an orogastric feeding tube for nutrition and hydration. She transitioned from continuous enteral feeding to bolus feeds, but given emesis the feeds ran over 2 hours Q3. She was discharged home with OG tube taking small-volume expressed breast milk, 5 ml, for practice. She had a gastrostomy tube placed at 10 weeks of age. She had an apnea monitor at home but did not have any events. PSG showed OSA AHI of 16.6, and pulmonology put her on oxygen during the day and night. A tracheostomy was discussed, but she was able to avoid that surgery with improvement from supplemental O2. Follow-up PSG was normal, and she was able to wean from O2, with only a home pulse ox to monitor oxygen saturations. She received outpatient SLP through the craniofacial clinic and advanced oral intake to 70 ml in 20 minutes via Dr. Brown's specialty feeder (compression extraction) using preemie nipple. At 4 months of age, she regressed and became significantly aversive to oral. Weight gain was a challenge, and her enteral feeds were closely monitored. Nutrition increased her calories from 20 kcal to 22 kcal. She started to have worsening emesis at ~5 months of age, and G-tube schedule was changed to continuous feeds overnight and bolus during the day. She is currently practicing oral feeds of expressed breast milk via Dr. Brown's specialty feeder with level 1 nipple and has not initiated intake of purees. She has not yet had an instrumental swallow study. She is less verbal than her twin sister and is starting early intervention soon.

References

1. Heike CL, Hing AV, Aspinall CA, Bartlett SP, Birgfeld CB, Drake AF, et al. Clinical care in craniofacial microsomia: a review of current management recommendations and opportunities to advance research. Am J Med Genet C: Semin Med Genet. 2013, November;163(4):271–82.
2. Caron CJJM, Pluijmers BI, Joosten KFM, Mathijssen IMJ, Van Der Schroeff MP, Dunaway DJ, et al. Obstructive sleep apnoea in craniofacial microsomia: a systematic review. Int J Oral Maxillofac Surg. 2015;44(5):592–8.
3. Cloonan YK, Kifle Y, Davis S, Speltz ML, Werler MM, Starr JR. Sleep outcomes in children with hemifacial microsomia and controls: a follow-up study. Pediatrics. 2009;124(2):e313–21.
4. Kholdani C, Fares WH, Mohsenin V. Pulmonary hypertension in obstructive sleep apnea: is it clinically significant? A critical analysis of the association and pathophysiology. Pulm Circ. 2015;5(2):220–7.
5. Cohen SR, Levitt CA, Simms C, Burstein FD. Airway disorders in hemifacial microsomia. Plast Reconstr Surg. 1999;103(1):27–33.
6. Katz ES, D'Ambrosio CM. Pathophysiology of pediatric obstructive sleep apnea. Proc Am Thorac Soc. 2008;5(2):253–62.
7. Dehlink E, Tan HL. Update on paediatric obstructive sleep apnoea. J Thorac Dis. 2016;8(2):224.
8. Luna-Paredes C, Antón-Pacheco JL, Hernández GG, Gimeno AM, García AIR, Recuero IIG. Screening for symptoms of obstructive sleep apnea in children with severe craniofacial anomalies: assessment in a multidisciplinary unit. Int J Pediatr Otorhinolaryngol. 2012;76(12):1767–70.
9. Khansa I, Hall C, Madhoun LL, Splaingard M, Baylis A, Kirschner RE, Pearson GD. Airway and feeding outcomes of mandibular distraction, tongue-lip adhesion, and conservative management in Pierre Robin sequence: a prospective study. Plast Reconstr Surg. 2017;139(4):975e–83e.
10. Brooks L, Figueroa J, Edwards T, Reeder W, McBrayer S, Landry A. Passy muir valve tolerance in medically complex infants and children: are there predictors for success? Laryngoscope. 2020;130(11):E632–9.
11. Logemann JA. Evaluation and treatment of swallowing disorders. Pro ed, Austin Texas; 1998.
12. Dantas RO, Kern MK, Massey BT, Dodds WJ, Kahrilas PJ, Brasseur JG, Cook IJ, Lang IM. Effect of swallowed bolus variables on oral and pharyngeal phases of swallowing. Am J Phys. 1990;258(5):G675–81.
13. Perlman AL, Luschei ES, Du Mond CE. Electrical activity from the superior pharyngeal constrictor during reflexive and nonreflexive tasks. J Speech Lang Hear Res. 1989;32(4):749–54.
14. Jestrović I, Coyle JL, Sejdić E. Decoding human swallowing via electroencephalography: a state-of-the-art review. J Neural Eng. 2015;12(5):051001.
15. Martin RE, Sessle BJ. The role of the cerebral cortex in swallowing. Dysphagia. 1993;8(3):195–202.
16. Lang IM. Brain stem control of the phases of swallowing. Dysphagia. 2009;24(3):333–48.
17. Matsuo K, Palmer JB. Anatomy and physiology of feeding and swallowing: normal and abnormal. Phys Med Rehabil Clin N Am. 2008;19(4):691–707.
18. Lefton Greif MA. Pediatric dysphagia. Phys Med Rehabil Clin N Am. 2008;19(4):837–51.
19. Gewolb IH, Vice FL. Abnormalities in the coordination of respiration and swallow in preterm infants with bronchopulmonary dysplasia. Dev Med Child Neurol. 2006;48(07):595–9.
20. Khoshoo V, Edell D. Previously healthy infants may have increased risk of aspiration during respiratory syncytial viral bronchiolitis. Pediatrics. 1999;104(6):1389–90.
21. Sheikh S, Allen E, Shell R, Hruschak J, Iram D, Castile R, McCoy K. Chronic aspiration without gastroesophageal reflux as a cause of chronic respiratory symptoms in neurologically normal infants. Chest J. 2001;120(4):1190–5.
22. Arvedson JC. Assessment of pediatric dysphagia and feeding disorders: clinical and instrumental approaches. Dev Disabil Res Rev. 2008;14(2):118–27.

23. Brooks L. Treatment for dysphagia: a speech language pathologist's perspective. In: Ongkasuwan J, Chiou E, editors. Pediatric dysphagia. Cham: Springer; 2018.
24. Coyle JL. Dysphagia following prolonged endotracheal intubation: is there a rule of thumb?. SIG 13 Perspectives on Swallowing and Swallowing Disorders (Dysphagia). 2014;23(2):80–6.
25. Caron CJJM, Pluijmers BI, Joosten KFM, Mathijssen IMJ, Van Der Schroeff MP, Dunaway DJ, et al. Feeding difficulties in craniofacial microsomia: a systematic review. Int J Oral Maxillofac Surg. 2015;44(6):732–7.
26. van de Lande LS, Caron CJ, Pluijmers BI, Joosten KF, Streppel M, Dunaway DJ, et al. Evaluation of swallow function in patients with craniofacial microsomia: a retrospective study. Dysphagia. 2018;33(2):234–42.
27. Huisinga-Fischer CE, Zonneveld FW, Vaandrager JM, Prahl-Andersen B. Relationship in hypoplasia between the masticatory muscles and the craniofacial skeleton in hemifacial microsomia, as determined by 3-D CT imaging. J Craniofac Surg. 2001;12(1):31–40.
28. Shaker C. Cue-based feeding in the NICU: using the infant's communication as a guide. Neonatal Netw. 2013;32(6):404–8.
29. Ross ES, Philbin MK. Soffi: an evidence-based method for quality bottle-feedings of preterm, ill, and fragile infants. J Perinat Neonatal Nurs. 2011;25(4):349–59.
30. Ferrara L, Bidiwala A, Sher I, Pirzada M, Barlev D, Islam S, Rosenfeld W, Crowley CC, Hanna N. Effect of nasal continuous positive airway pressure on the pharyngeal swallow in neonates. J Perinatol. 2017;37:398–403.
31. Rotschild A, Dison PJ, Chitayat D, Solimano A. Midfacial hypoplasia associated with long-term intubation for bronchopulmonary dysplasia. Am J Dis Child. 1990;144(12):1302–6.
32. Tutor JD. Dysphagia and aspiration in the pediatric patient. SIG 13 Perspectives on Swallowing and Swallowing Disorders (Dysphagia). 2001;10(2):6–9.
33. Martin-Harris B, Brodsky MB, Michel Y, Castell DO, Schleicher M, Sandidge J, et al. MBS measurement tool for swallow impairment—MBSImp: establishing a standard. Dysphagia. 2008;23(4):392–405.
34. Arvedson J, Rogers B, Buck G, Smart P, Msall M. Silent aspiration prominent in children with dysphagia. Int J Pediatr Otorhinolaryngol. 1994;28(2–3):173–81.
35. Logemann JA, Gensler G, Robbins J, Lindblad AS, Brandt D, Hind JA, et al. A randomized study of three interventions for aspiration of thin liquids in patients with dementia or Parkinson's disease. J Speech Lang Hear Res. 2008;51(1):173–83.
36. Lazarus CL, Logemann JA, Rademaker AW, Kahrilas PJ, Pajak T, Lazar R, Halper A. Effects of bolus volume, viscosity, and repeated swallows in nonstroke subjects and stroke patients. Arch Phys Med Rehabil. 1993;74(10):1066–70.
37. Woods CW, Oliver T, Lewis K, Yang Q. Development of necrotizing enterocolitis in premature infants receiving thickened feeds using SimplyThick®. J Perinatol. 2012;32(2):150–2.
38. Pryor LS, Lehman J, Parker MG, Schmidt A, Fox L, Murthy AS. Outcomes in pharyngoplasty: a 10-year experience. Cleft Palate Craniofac J. 2006;43(2):222–5.
39. Miller CK, Madhoun LL. Feeding and swallowing issues in infants with craniofacial anomalies. Perspectives of the ASHA Special Interest Groups. 2016;1(5):13–26.
40. Barlow SM. Oral and respiratory control for preterm feeding. Curr Opin Otolaryngol Head Neck Surg. 2009;17(3):179.
41. Cohen MS, Samango-Sprouse CA, Stern HJ, Custer DA, Vaught DR, Saal HM, et al. Neurodevelopmental profile of infants and toddlers with oculo-auriculo-vertebral spectrum and the correlation of prognosis with physical findings. Am J Med Genet. 1995;60(6):535–40.
42. Collett BR, Chapman K, Wallace ER, Kinter SL, Heike CL, Speltz ML, Werler M. Speech, language, and communication skills of adolescents with craniofacial microsomia. Am J Speech Lang Pathol. 2019;28(4):1571–81.
43. Mitchell RM, Saltzman BS, Norton SJ, Harrison RG, Heike CL, Luquetti DV, Sie KCY. Hearing loss in children with craniofacial microsomia. Cleft Palate Craniofac J. 2017;54:656–63.
44. Carvalho GJ, Song CS, Vargervik K, Lalwani AK. Auditory and facial nerve dysfunction in patients with hemifacial microsomia. Arch Otolaryngol Head Neck Surg. 1999;125:209–12.

45. Walker EA, Holte L, McCreery RW, Spratford M, Page T, Moeller MP. The influence of hearing aid use on outcomes of children with mild hearing loss. J Speech Lang Hear Res. 2015;58(5):1611–25.
46. Strömland K, Miller M, Sjögreen L, Johansson M, Joelsson BM, Billstedt E, et al. Oculo-auriculo-vertebral spectrum: associated anomalies, functional deficits and possible developmental risk factors. Am J Med Genet A. 2007;143A:1317–25.
47. Chen EH, Reid RR, Chike-Obi C, Minugh-Purvis N, Whitaker LA, Puchala J, Bartlett SP. Tongue dysmorphology in craniofacial microsomia. Plast Reconstr Surg. 2009;124(2):583–9.
48. Speltz ML, Wallace ER, Collett BR, Heike CL, Luquetti DV, Werler M. Intelligence and academic achievement of adolescents with craniofacial microsomia. Plast Reconstr Surg. 2017;140:571–80.
49. Collett BR, Speltz ML, Cloonan YK, Leroux BG, Kelly JP, Werler MM. Neurodevelopmental outcomes in children with hemifacial microsomia. Arch Pediatr Adolesc Med. 2011;165:134–40.

Chapter 4
Extracraniofacial Manifestations of Craniofacial Microsomia

Jessica S. Lee and Paul W. Kloostra

Introduction

Craniofacial microsomia (CFM) represents a spectrum of congenital malformations of the craniofacial structures in the first and second branchial arches, with 5–30% of patients manifesting with asymmetric bilateral involvement [1, 2]. Although the term craniofacial microsomia suggests that the affected structures solely pertain to the structures of the head and neck, many extracraniofacial manifestations are associated with CFM and are important to recognize for accurate diagnosis and management. As with many other craniofacial anomalies, patients with CFM require longitudinal care by a multidisciplinary craniofacial team consisting of craniofacial surgeons (oral and maxillofacial surgery, otolaryngology, and/or plastic surgery), neurosurgeons, nursing, nutritionists, oral and maxillofacial surgery and otolaryngology (when either is not the primary craniofacial surgeon), orthodontists, pediatric dentists, pediatricians, psychologists, social workers, and speech pathologists. This chapter provides an overview of the extracraniofacial systems that may be involved, the associated diagnoses within each system, physical exam findings, and imaging available to initiate a workup, or rules out a suspected diagnosis. However, it is beyond the scope of this chapter to discuss the various nuances of each diagnosis and its management but should be used to direct the reader toward the many other resources available for a more in-depth discussion.

J. S. Lee
Northeast Facial and Oral Surgery Specialists, Florham Park, NJ, USA

Former Pediatric Cleft and Craniofacial Surgery Fellow, Cleft and Craniofacial Center, Charleston Area Medical Center, Women & Children's Hospital, Charleston, WV, USA
e-mail: drlee@nefoss.com

P. W. Kloostra (✉)
Cleft and Craniofacial Surgery, CAMC Cleft and Craniofacial Center, Charleston Area Medical Center Women & Children's Hospital, Charleston, WV, USA
e-mail: paul.kloostra@camc.org

D. M. Yates, M. R. Markiewicz (eds.), *Craniofacial Microsomia and Treacher Collins Syndrome*, https://doi.org/10.1007/978-3-030-84733-3_4

Etiology

Several theories have been proposed to explain the etiology of CFM, including the disturbance of vascular development within the first and second branchial arches during the first 6 weeks of gestation, teratogen exposure, and/or an error in migration of neural crest cells responsible for the formation of craniofacial structures. With the use of a mouse model, Poswillo demonstrated some of the phenotypic anomalies seen in CFM by causing vascular disruption of the stapedial artery in utero resulting in the destruction of local and regional differentiating craniofacial tissues [3–5]. Exposure to teratogens, such as thalidomide and retinoic acid, has been documented to produce craniofacial anomalies similar to that of CFM, including extracraniofacial manifestations [6, 7]. Accutane (13-*cis*-retinoic acid) is known to destroy neural crest cells and disrupt their migration resulting in craniofacial anomalies resembling CFM and Treacher Collins syndrome, based on timing of gestational exposure [6, 8, 9]. A study by Lammer et al. (1985) demonstrated a characteristic pattern of anomalies in 21 infants exposed to isotretinoin during the first trimester involving craniofacial, cardiac, thymic, and central nervous system structures [10], suggesting a deleterious effect on cephalic neural crest cell activity observed in patients with CFM.

A genetic basis for CFM has also been well documented in the literature where autosomal dominant and recessive patterns of transmission have been described in families with features of CFM with a large case series reporting a positive history of 50% of patients. Variability in penetrance and expression along with heterogeneity is likely the reason for the wide phenotypic spectrum observed in CFM [11].

The exact etiology of CFM remains a subject of debate and is likely secondary to a multifactorial process including both genetic and environmental factors resulting in a wide spectrum of phenotypic variability.

Classification of Craniofacial Microsomia

Several classification systems of CFM have been proposed. In 1969, Pruzansky classified mandibular anomalies of CFM into three types, I through III, based on the severity of hypoplasia of the ramus and condyle [12]. This classification system was later modified by Kaban et al. (1988) where type II was subdivided to IIA and IIB, to clarify the degree of mandibular function and location of the temporomandibular joint apparatus, which would then determine the necessary surgical correction, if any [13]. This modified classification of mandibular anomalies was included in the OMENS classification system, first conceived by Vento et al. (1991), to include other craniofacial manifestations of CFM in which each letter represents one of the five major manifestations: *O* for orbital distortion, *M* for mandibular hypoplasia, *E* for ear anomaly, *N* for nerve involvement, and *S* for soft tissue deficiency [14]. Owing to the frequent association with cardiac, skeletal, and central nervous systems, the OMENS classification was modified by Horgan et al. (1995) to include extracraniofacial manifestations of CFM and expanded to the OMENS+ (plus) designation [15].

Extracraniofacial Anomalies Associated with Craniofacial Microsomia

A review of the literature suggests that up to 55% of patients with craniofacial microsomia demonstrate extracraniofacial differences [15–18]. Several studies have demonstrated a higher rate of association between specific organ systems (e.g., skeletal, central nervous system, cardiac) and CFM, while other systems did not demonstrate as strong of an association (e.g., pulmonary, gastrointestinal) [15–17, 19]. Syndromologists typically consider an anomaly to be associated with a diagnosis if it occurs in at least 10–15% of patients [15, 20]. Based on this definition, associated extracraniofacial manifestations of CFM include vertebral (24.3–35.5%), cardiac (18.5–33.1%), central nervous system (10.4–18.2%), developmental (8–73%), and genitourinary (10.5–15.8%). Other organ systems, such as gastrointestinal and pulmonary, were less frequently associated, with a prevalence of only in 7–11.6% and 3–9%, respectively [15–17, 19] (Table 4.1). Given the common association of extracraniofacial anomalies with CFM, it is essential that CFM patients are screened with a comprehensive history, prenatal imaging, and postnatal physical examination with imaging.

Table 4.1 Incidence of extracraniofacial findings associated with craniofacial microsomia [15–17, 19, 24, 26, 29, 44]

System	Prevalence	Diagnoses
Vertebral	24.3–35.5%	Scoliosis Hemivertebrae Block vertebrae Vertebral agenesis Failure of vertebral fusion Cervical spine instability Rib anomalies
Cardiac	18.5–33.1%	Atrial septal defect Ventricular septal defect Valvular defects Patent ductus arteriosus Tetralogy of Fallot Pulmonary valve stenosis Transposition of great arteries Dextrocardia

(continued)

Table 4.1 (continued)

System	Prevalence	Diagnoses
Central nervous system	10.4–18.2%	Neural tube defects (e.g., encephalocele) Corpus callosum agenesis/hypoplasia Intracranial lipomas Hydrocephaly Ventriculomegaly Cerebral hypoplasia Arnold-Chiari malformations Intellectual disability Speech and language delay Neuropsychomotor delay
Genitourinary	10.5–15.8%	Renal agenesis/aplasia Renal ectopia Hydronephrosis Ureteral anomalies Vesicoureteral reflux Hypospadias Cryptorchidism
Gastrointestinal	7–11.6%	Esophageal atresia with or without tracheoesophageal fistula Anorectal stenosis/atresia Imperforate anus Diaphragmatic hernia Umbilical hernia
Respiratory	3–9%	Choanal atresia Laryngomalacia Tracheomalacia Tracheal stenosis Lobar anomaly of lung Lung hypoplasia

Vertebral and Central Nervous System

Vertebral anomalies are the most frequent extracraniofacial manifestations associated with CFM with a prevalence of 24.3–35.5% [15–17, 19]. The most common anomalies include scoliosis, hemivertebrae, block vertebrae (Fig. 4.1), and rib anomalies. Less commonly associated manifestations include vertebral agenesis, failure of vertebral fusion, and cervical spine instability, such as atlanto-axial subluxation.

The prevalence of central nervous system (CNS) anomalies is reported to be between 10.4% and 18.2% [15–17, 19]. The most common structural anomalies of the CNS include neural tube defects (e.g., encephalocele), agenesis or hypoplasia of the corpus callosum, intracranial lipomas, Arnold-Chiari malformations, hydrocephaly, ventriculomegaly, cerebral hypoplasia, and microcephaly [15, 16, 18,

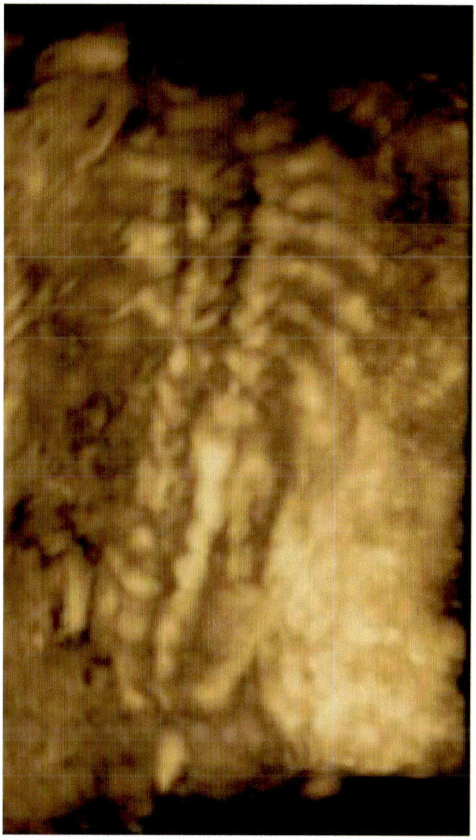

Fig. 4.1 3D ultrasound demonstrating fused/block vertebrae

21–31]. A higher prevalence of developmental disorders, such as intellectual disability, language, speech, or neuropsychomotor delay, has also been associated with CFM when compared to the general population [32–34]. Some CNS anomalies may be detected prenatally via α-fetoprotein (AFP) concentrations in maternal serum and sonography which may detect such conditions as neural tube defects, hydrocephalus, and agenesis of the corpus callosum [35, 36].

Physical exam findings related to vertebral anomalies include torticollis, shortening, and/or decreased flexibility of the neck and asymmetric shoulder height. The lower back should be examined for hypertrichosis, skin tags, dimples, sinus tracts, and lipomas which are suggestive of underlying intraspinal anomalies. The thorax should be examined for symmetry and rib size anomalies. In older children, the spine and thorax should also be examined while the patient is bending forward to evaluate for size and symmetry. The vertebrae should also be examined for deformities and disruptions in the curvature of the spine [37].

Physical exam findings significant for CNS anomalies include sacral dimples, port wine stain, genitourinary, vertebral anomalies, and micro- or macrocephaly. Sacral cutaneous dimple over the midline of the back (Fig. 4.2), dermal sinus, port

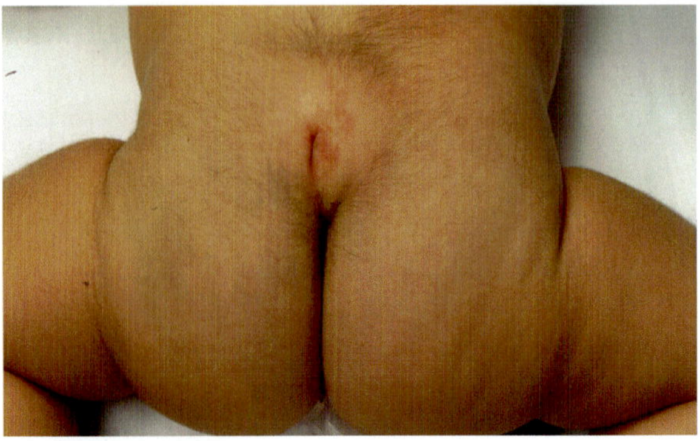

Fig. 4.2 Deep sacral dimple

wine stain, focal hirsutism, lower extremity anomalies, and anal and genitourinary anomalies may suggest the presence of an underlying neural tube defect [38, 39]. Patients with micro- or macrocephaly will demonstrate a head circumference greater than two standard deviations from the mean. Head circumference should be measured and tracked with a centile growth chart [35]. Microcephaly should be monitored for developmental delay, while macrocephaly should be evaluated and monitored for signs and symptoms of hydrocephalus including irritability, seizures, somnolence, vomiting, loss of muscle strength, or tone.

A neurological exam should include evaluation of lower extremity reflexes, sensation, strength, and symmetry. Suspected limb atrophy should be further assessed with limb length and calf circumference. Lower extremity findings may indicate the presence of a long-standing neurologic anomaly, such as tethered cord syndrome or diastematomyelia, which may respond to operative intervention [37]. The presence of vertebral anomalies on clinical exam should raise suspicion for possible intraspinal pathology.

Imaging may be indicated in any patient with positive physical exam findings, as well as for tracking growth over time and helping anticipate future progression [37]. Posteroanterior and lateral radiographs of the thoracolumbosacral spine, including the pelvis, should be obtained with inspection of the entire spine for signs of pathology, as dysplastic vertebrae are often non-contiguous [37].

Suspicious findings on plain films should be further characterized with CT and/or MRI. CT and MR imaging unfortunately possess inherent risks including ionizing radiation and possible need for sedation in young children, respectively. However, vertebral anomalies are commonly associated with CFM; Buckley and Guille (2010) reported a high risk of occult intraspinal anomalies, including tethered cords and diastematomyelia [37, 40, 41]. Trenga et al. (2016) also found a higher incidence of spinal cord anomalies in patients with complex bony malformations (>2 vertebra involved) when compared to less complex bony malformations [42]. Similarly, some CNS anomalies, such as agenesis of the corpus callosum or intracranial lipomas, may not be apparent on clinical exam [26]. Renkema et al. (2018) reported a notable disparity of the prevalence of CNS anomalies among studies that routinely obtained CT or MR imaging (42–69%) and those that did not (2–29%) [15, 16, 18, 21–31, 43].

Due to the high incidence of occult vertebral and CNS pathology, routine screening of CFM patients with CT and/or MRI seems warranted, especially for those not previously evaluated, and investigation of concerning findings on history and physical exam. In addition, it is reasonable to include a complete view of the head, vertebrae, and spine when obtaining advanced imaging. As always, the prudent surgeon should use his or her best clinical judgment to weigh the risk, benefits, and alternatives of additional imaging with each patient's unique presentation.

Developmental Disorders

Screening for developmental disorders with timely diagnosis is crucial, as children with CFM have a higher prevalence of intellectual disability (18–58%), language or speech delay (8–68%), and neuropsychomotor delay (17–73%) [24, 26, 29, 44]. Screening for developmental delay in infants and toddlers from birth to age 5 should be assessed with a standardized screening tool (e.g., Center for Disease Control Milestone Checklist) which can assist with early detection, referral, and possible intervention [45]. However, assessment of development and psychosocial health cannot be limited to a single assessment and must be monitored regularly over time. Table 4.2 provides a summary of the recommended measures for psychosocial screening for children with craniofacial differences.

The diagnosis of intellectual disability (ID) requires impairments in both intellectual and adaptive functioning, which should take into account the child's age,

Table 4.2 Recommended measures for psychosocial screening for children with craniofacial differences [49]

Scale	Low cost/free	Proxy report	Self-report ages	Multiple languages	Items/scale	Paper (P) or computer (C)
PROMIS[a]	Free	X	8+	X	4–8 items/scale	P, C
CBCL/YSR	[b]	X	11+	X	120 items	P, C
PedsQL[c]	X	X	5+	X	5–8 items/scale	P, C
CLEFT-Q	Free	–	8+	X	7–12 items/13 scales	P
PedsQL family impact	X	–	Caregiver	X	3–6 items/scale	P, C
PAT-CV	[d]	–	Caregiver	–	3–20 items/scale; 8 scales	P, C

[a]PROMIS: Peer relationships, anxiety, depression, friendships, cognitive scales
[b]Replacement forms are inexpensive (~$1.50 per form); however, scoring program requires an initial investment
[c]PedsQL: Emotions, physical, social, school domains
[d]Requires an annual "use" fee of $350

culture language, and communication. ID may be assessed with various standardized assessment tools, such as the American Psychiatric Association's *Diagnostic and Statistical Manual of Mental Disorders*, 5th edition (DSM-5) and the American Association on Intellectual and Developmental Disabilities (AAIDD), which possess similar definitions of ID but differ in their definitions of severity [46].

Evaluation and management of speech and language delays in children include determining whether an impairment in communication skills exists, specifying the nature of any impairments, and initiate appropriate intervention strategies. Development of speech and language can be assessed with standardized screening tools, such as the CDC Milestone Checklist; however, caretakers should be aware that each child's developmental timeline may differ. If the child is not meeting expected milestones for speech and language, a comprehensive developmental evaluation, in addition to a speech and language evaluation, may be warranted.

The American Cleft Palate – Craniofacial Association (ACPA) Standards of Care require that all cleft and craniofacial teams have in place "a mechanism to initially and periodically assess and treat, as appropriate, the psychological and social needs of patients and families/caregivers and to refer for further treatment as necessary" and that "the team uses a process to evaluate its own performance with regard to patient assessment, treatment or satisfaction and to make improvements as a result of those evaluations." [47] The Americleft Psychosocial Group (APG) has identified measures that can be used efficiently within the context of a routine cleft or craniofacial team visit and encourages the use of valid and reliable measures that would allow for consistent assessment of psychosocial adjustment of children within teams and allow for comparisons of outcomes across teams [48].

The APG has identified measures within three major categories to properly address psychosocial needs of patients and families/caregivers which can be used routinely in the context of a cleft or craniofacial team visit: (1) family risk, (2) psychosocial adjustment, and (3) quality of life. The recommended measures address categories that are both generic (used with children with and without cleft and/or craniofacial anomalies) and specific to children with cleft and/or craniofacial anomalies. Further, they have identified measures that allow for both children (patients) to self-report and for their caregiver to report on these measures to include both perspectives "Heppner CE, April 27, 2020, Clinical audit and psychosocial screening in cleft and craniofacial teams, Personal communication".

Family risk measures can be assessed with the Pediatric Quality of Life Inventory Family Impact Module (PedsQL FIM) and the Psychosocial Assessment Tool-Craniofacial Version (PAT-CV) which are completed by caregivers and can be used as screening for families.

Psychosocial adjustment measures include both child (patient) and caregiver report instruments. The most widely used and internationally validated instrument is the Child Behavior Checklist (CBCL) which provides caregiver report forms for children 18 months of age into adulthood and self-report instruments beginning at 11 years of age. The Patient-Reported Outcomes Measurement Information System (PROMIS®) also utilizes child and caregiver report instruments which evaluates and monitors physical, mental, and social health in children and adults. This

National Institutes of Health (NIH) supported measurement tool is free of charge for all users "Heppner CE, April 27, 2020, Clinical audit and psychosocial screening in cleft and craniofacial teams, Personal communication".

The third major category of assessment recommended by the APG is quality of life. The Pediatric Quality of Life Inventory (PedsQL) is a generic measure of quality of life, assessing physical, emotional, social, and school functioning, with caregiver proxy report available beginning in infancy and child self-report available beginning at age 5. The CLEFT-Questionnaire (CLEFT-Q) is a cleft-specific measure completed only by the child beginning at age 8 and assesses the child's perception of appearance, speech, psychological adjustment, social functioning, and physical functioning in the area most likely to be affected by the cleft, drinking, and eating "Heppner CE, April 27, 2020, Clinical audit and psychosocial screening in cleft and craniofacial teams, Personal communication".

Patients with facial differences, including CFM, are at risk for intellectual disability, speech and language delay, neuropsychomotor delay, poor self-esteem, maladaptive or poor coping skills, and poor home and community interactions. Ensuring our patients are treated within a multidisciplinary setting, screened early and regularly for developmental, speech and language, and psychosocial development, is imperative. The ideal comprehensive cleft and craniofacial team will include a social worker, speech language pathologist, and psychologist present at team meetings, but all teams must, at the very least, have access to these services when at-risk patients and/or families are identified with the aforementioned screening tools.

Cardiac

Cardiac anomalies are commonly observed in the CFM population with a prevalence rate of 18.5–33.1% [19]. The predominant cardiac anomalies include ventricular septal defects, atrial septal defects, valvular defects, patent ductus arteriosus, and Tetralogy of Fallot. Less common anomalies include pulmonary valve stenosis, transposition of the great arteries, and dextrocardia.

Diagnosis of cardiac anomalies may be possible with prenatal obstetric sonography, with the optimal age for screening being 18–22 weeks of gestation [49]. Advanced fetal echocardiography may be indicated if maternal risk factors such as fetal cardiac or non-cardiac abnormalities are suspected on obstetric ultrasound, such as increased nuchal translucency or congenital heart disease in a first-degree relative of the fetus [50]. While the cardiac screening exam, consisting of the four-chamber and outflow tract views, is designed to maximize the detection of heart anomalies during a second-trimester scan, some cardiac anomalies such as fetal arrhythmias, valvular insufficiency, obstruction, or cardiomyopathy may not be detected or present, until after 18–22 weeks of gestation [51–53]. A fetus diagnosed with CFM should prompt a high index of suspicion for cardiac defects and consideration for fetal echocardiography. When a fetal cardiac anomaly is diagnosed with fetal echocardiography, a referral should be made to a pediatric cardiologist before delivery, to discuss pre- and perinatal management.

Newborn examination should include visual inspection, auscultation, pulse oximetry, blood pressure, abdominal, and extremity exams. A newborn demonstrating central cyanosis should alert the physician to possible underlying congenital heart disease (CHD). Cardiac auscultation may demonstrate abnormal heart sounds (e.g., S3 gallop) or pathologic murmurs. Pulse oximetry should be used to screen for CHD as some newborns may be asymptomatic. Pre- and post-ductal pulse oximetry should be obtained to identify ductal-dependent lesions, as these infants are at increased risk for significant morbidity and mortality [54]. Blood pressure discrepancies measuring ≥10 mmHg higher in the upper extremity compared to the lower and diminished or absent pulses in the lower extremity are also suggestive of CHD [55]. Hepatomegaly in newborns where the liver edge is palpated more than 3 cm below the right costal margin may be seen in infants with heart failure secondary to CHD.

In the presence of a positive physical exam finding, screening should be continued with an electrocardiogram (EKG) and chest radiograph. While some lesions such as tricuspid atresia and pulmonary stenosis may present with specific EKG patterns, many cyanotic lesions will not be apparent on a neonatal EKG, and a high index of suspicion should be maintained even with a negative EKG. A chest radiograph should be obtained for a newborn with cyanosis or respiratory distress, assessing for non-cardiac causes, such as pneumothorax, pulmonary hypoplasia, or diaphragmatic hernia [56].

In the setting of positive physical exam findings, but negative EKG and/or chest radiograph, newborn echocardiography should be obtained. This can provide a definitive diagnosis of congenital heart defects with information on cardiac anatomy and function and should be performed in consultation with a pediatric cardiologist. An echocardiogram should be considered for first-line workup if signs and symptoms of a critical cardiac anomalies are present, such as shock, cardiomegaly, severe cyanosis, or respiratory distress concerning for pulmonary edema. The necessity, timing, and frequency of follow-up echocardiogram assessment should be made in conjunction with your pediatric cardiologist, guided by the nature and severity of the cardiac anomaly, presence of heart failure, anticipated timing and mechanism of progression, and the options available for intervention.

Extremity

Extremity anomalies are fairly common in CFM patients, with a prevalence rate of 11.6–20.7% [15, 16]. The most common include polydactyly, absent or anomalous thumb with or without radial dysplasia, and congenital hip dislocation. Other regions of the skeletal system may accompany extremity anomalies, such as the ribs and vertebrae, including the cervical spine (see section on "Vertebral and Central Nervous System").

Prenatal detection of extremity anomalies may not be demonstrated on ultrasound until the end of the second trimester or beginning of the third trimester as endochondral ossification occurs during the third trimester.

Physical exam of a newborn should include evaluation of height/length and upper and lower extremity morphology and lengths, along with the number and morphology of digits. Radial dysplasia encompasses a range of presentations from a minor, such as an isolated thumb anomaly, to more severe, such as the complete absence of the thumb and radius with severe ulnar bowing, elbow stiffness, and humeral hypoplasia (Fig. 4.3) [57, 58]. A shortened, unilateral lower extremity may be a sign of unilateral hip dislocation. The Ortolani and/or Barlow maneuvers may be used to evaluate the stability of the hips, where a palpable "clunk" may be elicited in the affected hip [59].

The underlying skeletal morphology associated with polydactyly, first-digit (thumb) hypoplasia, or first-digit agenesis with radial dysplasia can be assessed with pain radiography. Depending on the severity, treatment may include occupational and/or physical therapy, splinting and/or casting, or surgery.

Ultrasonography is the first-line imaging for suspected congenital hip dislocation in the first 4 or 6 months of life; however, it is technique sensitive. Radiographs are helpful in infants older than 4–6 months, when the femoral head and acetabulum are

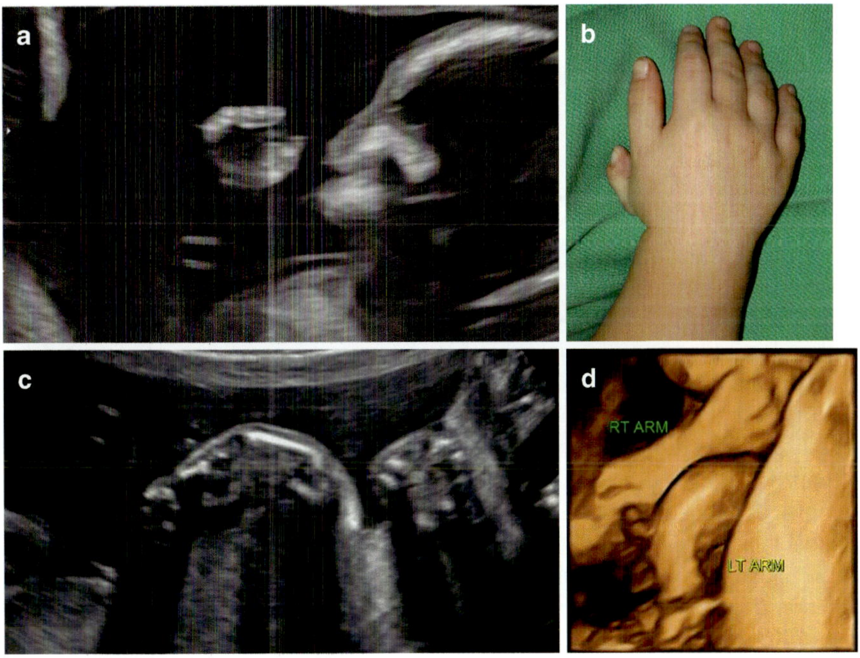

Fig. 4.3 (**a**) 2D ultrasound demonstrating polydactyly. (**b**) A clinical photo demonstrating radial polydactyly. (**c**) 2D ultrasound demonstrating radial hypoplasia. (**d**) 3D ultrasounds demonstrating radial hypoplasia

ossified. More advanced imaging such as CT or MRI are not typically useful in making the diagnosis but may aid in the evaluation of postsurgical reduction [60].

Infants born with or suspected of extremity anomalies should be referred to an orthopedic and/or plastic surgeon for further evaluation and management.

Genitourinary

Genitourinary anomalies occur in 10.5–15.8% of patients with CFM. The most common include renal agenesis or aplasia, renal ectopia, hydronephrosis, ureteral anomalies, vesicoureteral reflux (VUR), hypospadias, and cryptorchidism [15–17, 19].

Initial diagnosis of congenital genitourinary anomalies is possible with routine antenatal ultrasonography as fetal kidneys can be detected by the 12th to 15th week of gestation [61]. However, the renal cortex and medulla may not be distinct from each other until the 20th to 25th week of gestation [62]. Amniotic fluid volume can be assessed at or beyond 20 weeks of gestation with decreased amniotic fluid (oligohydramnios) being a positive predictor of abnormal fetal renal function and indicates bilateral fetal renal dysfunction or a poorly functioning solitary kidney [63].

Postnatal evaluation should include an abdominal exam, where a palpable mass may represent hydronephrosis secondary to obstructive uropathy. An enlarged bladder in a male infant, especially after voiding, is suggestive of bladder outlet obstruction (i.e., posterior urethral valves) [64]. A single umbilical artery is also associated with an increased risk of congenital genitourinary anomalies, particularly VUR [65]. Pulmonary evaluation in neonates with severe oligohydramnios is critical to rule out pulmonary hypoplasia with severe cases often requiring intensive supportive care after birth [66].

Postnatal evaluation of the genitourinary tract with renal ultrasonography is recommended in infants with renal malformation detected on antenatal ultrasound [67]. Routine ultrasonography should not be performed until after the infant returns to their birth weight to ensure volume repletion and increased renal plasma flow, glomerular filtration rate, and urine output, as this will avoid underestimating the severity of hydronephrosis compared to renal ultrasonography completed within the first 48 hours of life. In contrast, neonates with known bilateral renal involvement, solitary kidney, or a history of oligohydramnios should have a renal ultrasound completed within the first 24 hours of life due to their increased risk of severe renal anomaly and need for intervention [67]. Additional diagnostic tests such as serum creatinine and voiding cystourethrography (VCUG) may be obtained to assess renal function in patients with bilateral renal anomalies as well as serial ultrasounds to monitor renal growth and development. These findings should be discussed with a pediatric urologist and/or pediatric surgeon for the appropriate timing and management of congenital urologic anomalies.

Gastrointestinal

Extracraniofacial anomalies involving the gastrointestinal (GI) system are relatively uncommon with a prevalence of 7–11.6% in CFM patients [15, 16, 19]. The most common GI anomalies reported include esophageal atresia (EA) with possible tracheoesophageal fistula (TEF), anorectal stenosis or atresia, imperforate anus, diaphragmatic hernia, and umbilical hernia.

Congenital GI anomalies may be first detected on a standard obstetric ultrasound during the second or third trimester which may demonstrate polyhydramnios with a small or collapsed stomach, suspicious for esophageal atresia [68–70]. However, it may be difficult to diagnose esophageal atresia if it is associated with a tracheoesophageal fistula, which allows amniotic fluid to flow into the stomach, resulting in relatively normal stomach and amniotic volumes [71]. Congenital diaphragmatic hernias (CDH) may also be diagnosed via prenatal ultrasound with the majority of cases detectable by 24 weeks of gestation, or later, detection prior to 24 weeks is associated with greater severity and may require further workup and/or referral to a fetal surgeon to prevent or reverse pulmonary hypoplasia and restore adequate lung development for neonatal survival [72, 73].

Anorectal atresia may be identified as early as 12 weeks of gestation with dilated loops of fetal bowel seen on prenatal ultrasound [74], but more recent studies demonstrate that the absence of a "target sign" on prenatal ultrasound may be the most important sign of anorectal malformation [74–78].

The newborn abdominal exam should first evaluate overall size and appearance, noting defects in the abdominal wall and assessing for distension. A scaphoid abdomen with the absence of breath sounds on the ipsilateral side is suggestive of a congenital diaphragmatic hernia. Palpation of the abdomen should be completed to assess for defects of the abdominal wall and abdominal masses, which require further workup.

Esophageal atresia (EA) is an interruption of esophageal continuity, often associated with tracheoesophageal fistula (TEF) [79]. The classification of the various relationships between esophageal atresia and tracheoesophageal fistula was first described by Vogt (1929) and modified by Gross (1953) (Fig. 4.4) [80, 81]. A neonate with isolated esophageal atresia (Gross Type A) generally present with excessive drooling, choking, and inability to feed. Gross Type B, C, and D represents a combination of EA with TEF: EA with proximal TEF (Type B), EA with distal TEF (Type C), or EA with proximal and distal TEF (Type D) [81]. These combinations place the newborn at risk for aspiration of food, saliva, and/or gastric acid. Gross Type E, also known as an H-type TEF, consists of an intact esophagus with TEF, often less symptomatic and diagnosed later in life. Infants with a Type E anomaly often present with a long-standing history of recurring aspiration and multiple episodes of pneumonia [82].

Finally, the anus should be inspected for presence and position. However, patency cannot be assumed until verified by passing of meconium, usually by 48 hours of

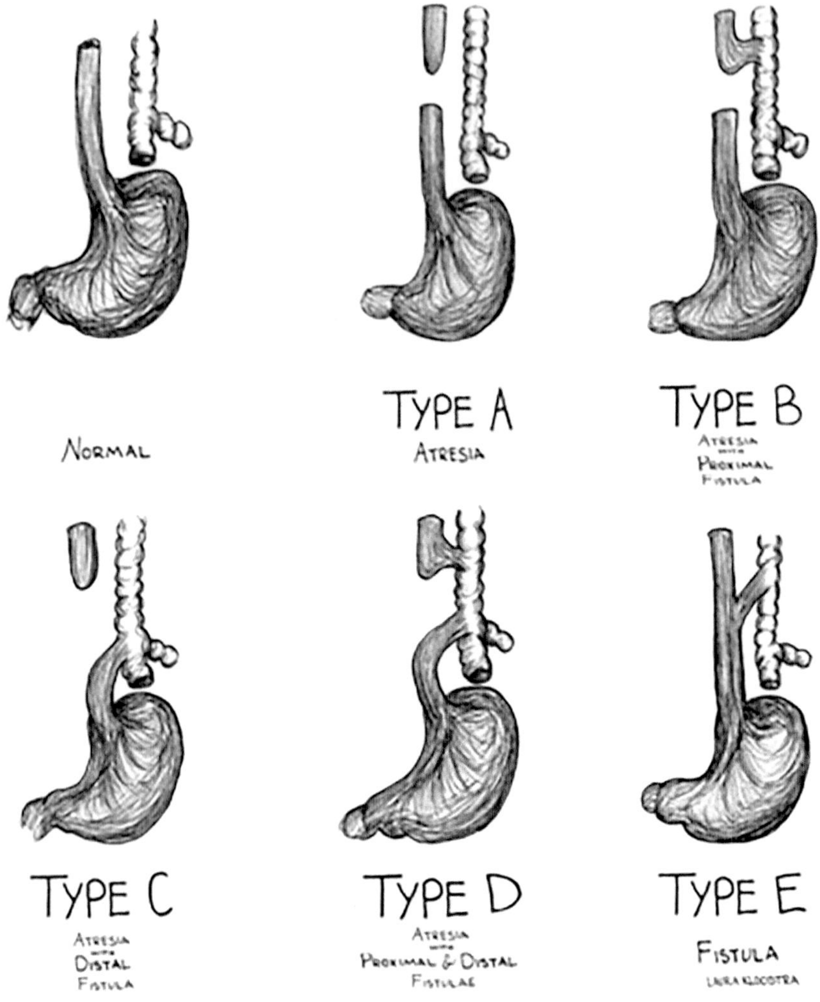

Fig. 4.4 Gross classification of tracheoesophageal malformation

life, and failure to pass meconium in the setting of progressive abdominal distension, refusal to feed, and vomiting should be investigated for possible anorectal atresia or stenosis [83]. Atresia or stenosis may not be apparent on initial exam in infants with a normal external anus; however, it may be confirmed with inability to pass a rectal temperature probe 2–3 cm from the anal verge. When anorectal atresia or stenosis is suspected clinically in the setting of poor feeding or no passage of meconium, plain radiographs of the abdomen should be obtained [84],

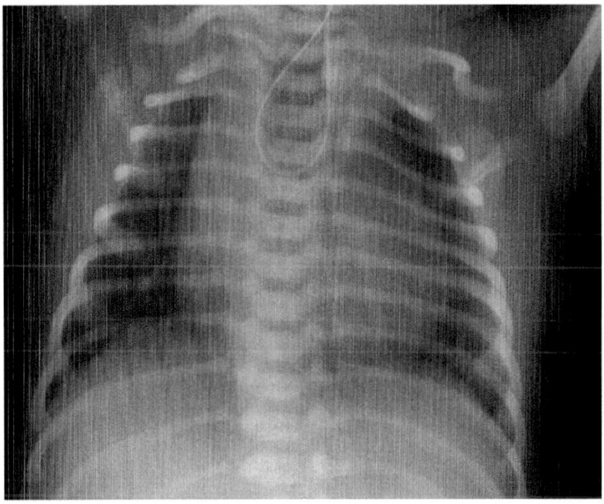

Fig. 4.5 Supine AP chest plain film demonstrating catheter coiling in the distal esophagus

demonstrating colonic obstruction. If the diagnosis of an atresia or stenosis is suspected but not demonstrated on plain film radiography, a barium enema should be obtained [85–87].

Suspected esophageal atresia can be confirmed by obtaining a chest radiograph after attempting to pass a catheter into the stomach more than 15 cm. Gross Types A–D (Fig. 4.5) will demonstrate the catheter curled in the proximal esophageal pouch, whereas Type E, consisting of a continuous esophagus with TEF, will not. The presence of air in the proximal stump of the esophagus is suggestive of Type A (no fistula) or B (proximal fistula), and gastric air suggests the presence of a distal fistula as in Type C or D. A barium swallow study with passage of contrast from the esophagus into the tracheobronchial tree confirms the presence of a proximal fistula (Type B, D, or E). Type E fistulas can be difficult to diagnose and may require esophageal endoscopy and bronchoscopy. CT is generally not necessary; however, three-dimensional virtual bronchoscopy may be beneficial for surgical planning [88].

Umbilical hernias are asymptomatic and spontaneously resolve within the first 5 years of life and may be observed if they demonstrate progressive decrease in umbilical ring size. However, some hernias may interfere with feeding and become incarcerated or strangulated if the hernia contains bowel, and, although rare, an incarcerated umbilical hernia is a surgical emergency. Umbilical rings that are greater than 1.5 cm in diameter and do not decrease in size, or elicit symptoms are a relative indication for surgical repair [89, 90].

Suspected congenital diaphragmatic hernias (CDH) that have not already been diagnosed in utero should be evaluated with chest radiography, which will demonstrate herniation of abdominal contents into the thoracic cavity (Fig. 4.6) [91]. If undiagnosed CDH is suspected, radiographic evaluation should not be delayed, as

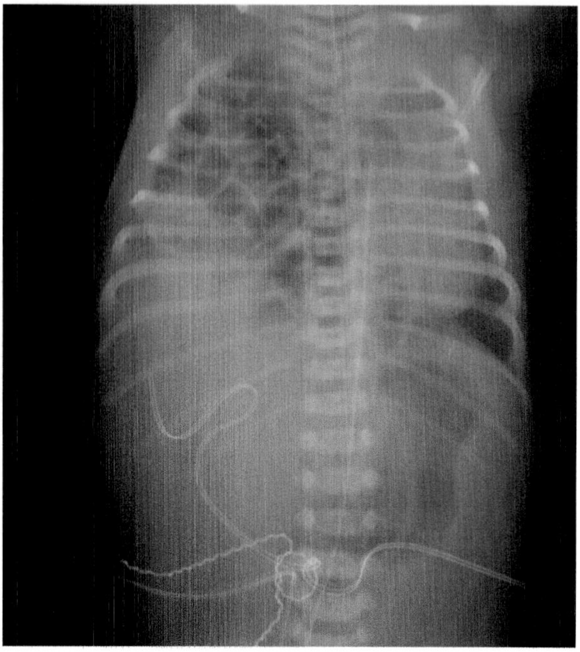

Fig. 4.6 Supine AP pain film demonstrating gastric contents within the right chest

most patients develop respiratory distress. Severe cases often require endotracheal intubation or even extracorporeal membrane oxygenation (ECMO) [92–94].

Suspected or confirmed gastrointestinal anomalies should be followed up with a pediatric otolaryngologist and pediatric gastroenterologist and/or surgeon for further workup with possible intervention.

Respiratory

Although fairly uncommon, respiratory system anomalies may accompany patients born with CFM with a prevalence rate of 3–9% [15, 16, 19]. The most common anomalies include pulmonary hypoplasia choanal atresia, laryngomalacia, tracheomalacia, and tracheal stenosis.

Prenatal ultrasound may confirm the presence of pulmonary hypoplasia, especially in the setting of congenital diaphragmatic hernia or oligohydramnios. Other respiratory anomalies, however, are not well characterized with prenatal ultrasound.

Respiratory system anomalies may be apparent soon after birth. Many, including pulmonary hypoplasia, present with non-specific signs and symptoms such as tachypnea, retractions, respiratory distress, hypoxemia, and/or cyanosis. A newborn in respiratory distress should be managed according to standard guidelines relative to gestational age.

Children with choanal atresia may vary in presentation depending on the extent of involvement, as they can present unilaterally or bilaterally. Those born with unilateral choanal atresia, which represent two-thirds of cases, typically present later in life with unilateral nasal discharge and/or obstruction [95, 96]. Infants born with bilateral choanal atresia typically present with noisy breathing, upper airway obstruction, or cyanosis that worsens with feeding and improves with crying. Choanal atresia should be suspected if a number 5 or 6 French catheter cannot be passed through the nasal fossa into the oropharynx with a distance of at least 32 mm [97].

Laryngomalacia in a newborn will often manifest with intermittent, low-pitched, "wet" inspiratory stridor and may be louder when feeding or sleeping [98, 99]. Tracheomalacia will present with different symptoms based on location and severity. Intrathoracic lesions typically present with a barking and croup-like cough, whereas extrathoracic lesions will present with an inspiratory stridor. Tracheal stenosis may demonstrate an inspiratory stridor or expiratory wheeze refractory to bronchodilator therapy [100].

Chest radiography is typically the first-line imaging modality obtained for infants with a suspected respiratory anomaly, differentiating between cardiac and pulmonary causes such as pneumothorax, pulmonary hypoplasia, and/or diaphragmatic hernia [56]. Infants with pulmonary hypoplasia may demonstrate a diffuse haziness and coarse interstitial pattern on their chest radiograph, reflecting atelectasis or inflammation, with low or normal lung volumes. Suspected choanal atresia can be confirmed with CT, typically demonstrating narrowing of the posterior nasal cavity at the level of the pterygoid plate [101]. Tracheal anomalies, however, are not well visualized with plain film radiography or CT. While CT and MRI "virtual tracheobronchoscopy" have been reported as viable options for the assessment of tracheal stenosis, a multidetector CT is needed to provide both end-inspiratory and end-expiratory images to demonstrate the dynamic change in tracheomalacia [101–105].

A child with suspected respiratory anomalies including choanal atresia, tracheal stenosis, tracheomalacia, or laryngomalacia should be referred to a pediatric otolaryngologist for full endoscopic evaluation.

Conclusion

Extracraniofacial manifestations should be suspected in children born with craniofacial microsomia as up to 55% of patients are likely to demonstrate these findings. A systematic approach to each extracraniofacial organ system is recommended to work up or rule out various suspected diagnoses. As with the care for craniofacial manifestations of CFM, multidisciplinary and longitudinal care is often required for these extracraniofacial diagnoses as well.

References

1. Posnick JC. Craniofacial and maxillofacial surgery in children and young adults. 1st ed. Philadelphia: Saunders; 2000. p. 419–45.
2. Posnick JC. Orthognathic surgery: principles and practice. St. Louis: Saunders; 2014. p. 1095–158.
3. Poswillo D. The pathogenesis of the first and second branchial arch syndrome. Oral Surg Oral Med Oral Pathol. 1973;35:302–28.
4. Poswillo D. Hemorrhage in development of the face. Birth Defects Orig Artic Ser. 1975;11:61–81.
5. Poswillo. The embryological basis of craniofacial dysplasia. Postgrad Med J. 1977;53:517.
6. Johnston MC, Bronsky PT, Millicovsky G. Embryology of the head and neck. In: McCarthy JG, editor. Plastic surgery, vol. 4. Philadelphia: WB Saunders; 1990. p. 2410–95.
7. Johnston MC, Bronsky PT. Animal models for human craniofacial malformations. J Craniofac Genet Dev Biol. 1991;11:227–91.
8. Sulik KK, Johnston MC, Smiley SJ, Speight HS, Jarvis BE. Mandibulofacial dysostosis: a new proposal for its pathogenesis. Am J Med Genet. 1987;27:359–72.
9. Sulik KK, Smiley SJ, Turey TA, Speight HS, Johnston MC. Pathogenesis of cleft palate in Treacher Collins, Nager, and Miller syndromes. Cleft Palate J. 1989;26:209–15.
10. Lammer EJ, Chen DT, Hoar RM, et al. Retinoic acid embryopathy. N Engl J Med. 1985;313:837–41.
11. McCarthy JG, Grayson BH, Hopper RA, Tepper OM. Craniofacial microsomia. In: Neligan P, Rodriguez E, Losee E, editors. Craniofacial, head and neck surgery and pediatric plastic surgery, 3rd ed of Plastic surgery, vol. 3. Edinburgh: Elsevier Health Sciences; 2012. p. 761–91.
12. Pruzansky S. Not all dwarfed mandibles are alike. Birth Defects. 1969;1:120–9.
13. Kaban LB, Moses MH, Mulliken JB. Surgical correction of hemifacial microsomia in the growing child. Plast Reconstr Surg. 1988;82(1):9–19.
14. Vento AR, LaBrie RA, Mulliken JB. The O.M.E.N.S. classification of hemifacial microsomia. Cleft Palate Craniofac J. 1991;28:68–76.
15. Horgan JE, Padwa BL, LaBrie RA, Mulliken JB. OMENS-Plus: analysis of craniofacial and extracraniofacial anomalies in hemifacial microsomia. Cleft Palate Craniofac J. 1995;32:405–12.
16. Barisic I, Odak L, Loane M, et al. Prevalence, prenatal diagnosis and clinical features of oculo-auriculo-vertebral spectrum: a registry-based study in Europe. Eur J Hum Genet. 2014;22(8):1026–33.
17. Caron CJJM, Pluijmers BI, Wolvius EB, et al. Craniofacial and extracraniofacial anomalies in craniofacial microsomia: a multicenter study of 755 patients' [published correction appears in J Craniomaxillofac Surg. 2017 Nov;45(11):1906]. J Craniomaxillofac Surg. 2017;45(8):1302–10.
18. Rollnick BR, Kaye CI, Nagatoshi K, Hauck W, Martin AO. Oculoauriculovertebral dysplasia and variants: phenotypic characteristics of 294 patients. Am J Med Genet. 1987;26(2):361–75.
19. Renkema RW, Caron CJJM, Pauws E, et al. Extracraniofacial anomalies in craniofacial microsomia: retrospective analysis of 991 patients. Int J Oral Maxillofac Surg. 2019;48(9):1169–76.
20. Gorlin RJ, Jue KL, Jacobson NP, Goldschmidt E. Oculoauriculovertebral dysplasia. J Pediatr. 1963;63:991–9.
21. Beleza-Meireles A, Hart R, Clayton-Smith J, Oliveira R, Reis CF, Venaˆncio M, Sá J, Cunha E, Pires LM, Carreira IM, Scholey R, Wright R, Urquhart JE, Briggs TA, Kerr B, Kingston H, Metcalfe K, Donnai D, Newman WG, Saraiva JM, Tassabehji M. Oculo-auriculo-vertebral spectrum: clinical and molecular analysis of 51 patients. Eur J Med Genet. 2015;58:455–65.
22. Shokeir MH. The Goldenhar syndrome: a natural history. Birth Defects Orig Artic Ser. 1977;13(3C):67–83.

23. Strömland K, Miller M, Sjögreen L, Johansson M, Joelsson BM, Billstedt E, Gillberg C, Danielsson S, Jacobsson C, Andersson-Norinder J, Granström G. Oculo-auriculo- vertebral spectrum: associated anomalies, functional deficits and possible developmental risk factors. Am J Med Genet A. 2007;143A:1317–25.
24. Tasse C, Böhringer S, Fischer S, Lüdecke HJ, Albrecht B, Horn D, Janecke A, Kling R, König R, Lorenz B, Majewski F, Maeyens E, Meinecke P, Mitulla B, Mohr C, Preischl M, Umstadt H, Kohlhase J, Gillessen-Kaesbach G, Wieczorek D. Oculo-auriculo-vertebral spectrum (OAVS): clinical evaluation and severity scoring of 53 patients and proposal for a new classification. Eur J Med Genet. 2005;48:397–411.
25. Johansson M, Billstedt E, Danielsson S, Strömland K, Miller M, Granström G, Flodmark O, Råstam M, Gillberg C. Autism spectrum disorder and underlying brain mechanism in the oculoauriculovertebral spectrum. Dev Med Child Neurol. 2007;49:280–8.
26. Rosa RF, Graziadio C, Lenhardt R, Alves RP, Paskulin GA, Zen PR. Central nervous system abnormalities in patients with oculo-auriculo vertebral spectrum (Golden- har syndrome). Arq Neuropsiquiatr. 2010;68:98–102.
27. Pegler JR, Soares DC, Quaio CR, Fernandes N, Oliveira LA, Honjo RS, Bertola DR, Kim CA. Clinical description of 41 Brazilian patients with oculo-auriculo-vertebral dysplasia. Rev Assoc Med Bras. 2016;62:202–6.
28. Touliatou V, Fryssira H, Mavrou A, Kanavakis E, Kitsiou-Tzeli S. Clinical manifestations in 17 Greek patients with Goldenhar syndrome. Genet Couns. 2006;17:359–70.
29. Cohen MS, Samango-Sprouse CA, Stern HJ, Custer DA, Vaught DR, Saal HM, Tifft CJ, Rosenbaum KN. Neurodevelopmental profile of infants and toddlers with oculo-auriculo-vertebral spectrum and the correlation of prognosis with physical findings. Am J Med Genet. 1995;60:535–40.
30. Aleksic S, Budzilovich G, Greco MA, McCarthy J, Reuben R, Margolis S, Epstein F, Feigin I, Pearson J. Intracranial lipomas, hydrocephalus and other CNS anomalies in oculoauriculo-vertebral dysplasia (Goldenhar–Gorlin syndrome). Childs Brain. 1984;11:285–97.
31. Engiz O, Balci S, Unsal M, Ozer S, Oguz KK, Aktas D. 31 cases with oculoauriculo- vertebral dysplasia (Goldenhar syndrome): clinical, neuroradiologic, audiologic and cytogenetic findings. Genet Couns. 2007;18:277–88.
32. Beange H, Taplin JE. Prevalence of intellectual disability in northern Sydney adults. J Intellect Disabil Res. 1996;40(Pt 3):191–7.
33. Leonard H, Petterson B, Bower C, Sanders R. Prevalence of intellectual disability in Western Australia. Paediatr Perinat Epidemiol. 2003;17:58 67.
34. McConkey R, Mulvany F, Barron S. Adult persons with intellectual disabilities on the island of Ireland. J Intellect Disabil Res. 2006;50(Pt 3):227–36.
35. Verity C, Firth H, ffrench-Constant C. Congenital abnormalities of the central nervous system. J Neurol Neurosurg Psychiatry. 2003;74:i3–8.
36. Grimme JD, Castillo M. Congenital anomalies of the spine. Neuroimaging Clin N Am. 2007;17(1):1–16.
37. Buckley PS, Guille JT. Evaluation of the patient with a congenital spinal deformity. Semin Spine Surg. 2010;22:113–7.
38. Guggisberg D, Hadj-Rabia S, Viney C, et al. Skin markers of occult spinal dysraphism. Arch Dermatol. 2004;140:1109–15.
39. Robinson AJ, Russell S, Rimmer S. The value of ultrasonic examination of the lumbar spine in infants with specific reference to cutaneous markers of occult spinal dysraphism. Clin Radiol. 2005;60:72–7.
40. Prahinski JR, Polly DW, McHale KA, et al. Occult intraspinal anomalies in congenital scoliosis. J Pediatr Orthop. 2000;20:59–63.
41. Suh SW, Sarwark JF, Vora A, et al. Evaluating congenital spine deformities for intraspinal anomalies with magnetic resonance imaging. J Pediatr Orthop. 2001;21:525–31.

42. Trenga AP, Singla A, Feger MA, Abel MF. Patterns of congenital bony spinal deformity and associated neural anomalies on X-ray and magnetic resonance imaging. J Child Orthop. 2016;10(4):343–52.
43. Rooryck C, Souakri N, Cailley D, Bouron J, Goizet C, Delrue MA, Marlin S, Lacombe FD, Arveiler B. Array-CGH analysis of a cohort of 86 patients with oculoauriculovertebral spectrum. Am J Med Genet A. 2010;152A:1984–9.
44. Renkema RW, Caron CJJM, Wolvius EB, et al. Central nervous system anomalies in craniofacial microsomia: a systematic review. Int J Oral Maxillofac Surg. 2018;47(1):27–34.
45. Center for Disease Control and Prevention Developmental Milestones. https://www.cdc.gov/ncbddd/actearly/milestones/index.html. Accessed 31 Mar 2020.
46. American Psychiatric Association. Diagnostic and Statistical Manual of Mental Disorders, Fifth Edition, American Psychiatric Association, Arlington 2013; American Association of Intellectual and Developmental Disabilities (AAIDD), Definition of Intellectual Disability, available at: http://aaidd.org/intellectual-disability/definition. Accessed on 13 Apr 2020.
47. The American Cleft Palate - Craniofacial Association. Standards for approval of cleft palate and craniofacial teams. https://acpa-cpf.org/wp-content/uploads/2019/04/Standards-2019-Update.pdf. Accessed 29 Apr 2020.
48. Crerand CE, Conrad AL, Albert M, et al. The Americleft psychosocial outcomes project: a multicenter approach to advancing psychosocial outcomes for youth with cleft lip and palate. Clin Pract Pediatr Psychol. 2017;5(1):65–76.
49. Friedman KG, Sleeper LA, Freud LR, et al. Improved technical success, postnatal outcome and refined predictors of outcome for fetal aortic valvuloplasty. Ultrasound Obstet Gynecol. 2018;52:212.
50. Donofrio MT, Moon-Grady AJ, Hornberger LK, et al. Diagnosis and treatment of fetal cardiac disease: a scientific statement from the American Heart Association. Circulation. 2014;129:2183.
51. International Society of Ultrasound in Obstetrics and Gynecology, Carvalho JS, Allan LD, et al. ISUOG Practice Guidelines (updated): sonographic screening examination of the fetal heart. Ultrasound Obstet Gynecol. 2013;41:348.
52. Committee on Practice Bulletins-Obstetrics and the American Institute of Ultrasound in Medicine. Practice Bulletin No. 175: ultrasound in pregnancy. Obstet Gynecol. 2016;128:e241.
53. Rasiah SV, Publicover M, Ewer AK, et al. A systematic review of the accuracy of first-trimester ultrasound examination for detecting major congenital heart disease. Ultrasound Obstet Gynecol. 2006;28:110.
54. Schultz AH, Localio AR, Clark BJ, et al. Epidemiologic features of the presentation of critical congenital heart disease: implications for screening. Pediatrics. 2008;121:751.
55. Duff FD, McNamara DG. History and physical examination of the cardiovascular system. In: Garson A, Bricker JT, Fisher DJ, Neish SR, editors. The science and practice of pediatric cardiology. Baltimore: Williams and Wilkins; 1998. p. 693.
56. Report of the New England regional infant cardiac program. Pediatrics. 1980;65:375.
57. Bednar MS, James MA, Light TR. Congenital longitudinal deficiency. J Hand Surg. 2009;34(9):1739–47.
58. Murphy GRF, Logan M, Smith G, Sivakumar B. RADIATE - radial dysplasia assessment, treatment and aetiology: protocol for the development of a core outcome set using a Delphi survey. Trials. 2019;20(1):339. Published 2019 Jun 10.
59. Shaw BA, Segal LS, SECTION ON ORTHOPAEDICS. Evaluation and referral for developmental dysplasia of the hip in infants. Pediatrics. 2016;138
60. Desai AA, Martus JE, Schoenecker J, Kan JH. Spica MRI after closed reduction for developmental dysplasia of the hip. Pediatr Radiol. 2011;41:525.
61. Dugoff L. Ultrasound diagnosis of structural abnormalities in the first trimester. Prenat Diagn. 2002;22:316.
62. Cohen HL, Cooper J, Eisenberg P, et al. Normal length of fetal kidneys: sonographic study in 397 obstetric patients. AJR Am J Roentgenol. 1991;157:545.

63. Leibovitch L, Kuint J, Rosenfeld E, et al. Short-term outcome among term singleton infants with intrapartum oligohydramnios. Acta Paediatr. 2012;101:727.
64. Macpherson RI, Leithiser RE, Gordon L, Turner WR. Posterior urethral valves: an update and review. Radiographics. 1986;6:753.
65. Murphy-Kaulbeck L, Dodds L, Joseph KS, Van den Hof M. Single umbilical artery risk factors and pregnancy outcomes. Obstet Gynecol. 2010;116:843.
66. Shrem G, Nagawkar SS, Hallak M, Walfisch A. Isolated oligohydramnios at term as an indication for labor induction: a systematic review and meta-analysis. Fetal Diagn Ther. 2016;40:161.
67. Baskin LS. Postnatal management of fetal hydronephrosis. In: Post TW, editor. UpToDate. Waltham: UpToDate. Accessed on 30 Mar 2020.
68. Estroff JA, Parad RB, Share JC, Benacerraf BR. Second trimester prenatal findings in duodenal and esophageal atresia without tracheoesophageal fistula. J Ultrasound Med. 1994;13:375.
69. Kalache KD, Wauer R, Mau H, et al. Prognostic significance of the pouch sign in fetuses with prenatally diagnosed esophageal atresia. Am J Obstet Gynecol. 2000;182:978.
70. Sase M, Asada H, Okuda M, Kato H. Fetal gastric size in normal and abnormal pregnancies. Ultrasound Obstet Gynecol. 2002;19:467.
71. Shulman A, Mazkereth R, Zalel Y, et al. Prenatal identification of esophageal atresia: the role of ultrasonography for evaluation of functional anatomy. Prenat Diagn. 2002;22:669.
72. Flake AW. Fetal surgery for congenital diaphragmatic hernia. Semin Pediatr Surg. 1996;5:266.
73. Doyle NM, Lally KP. The CDH Study Group and advances in the clinical care of the patient with congenital diaphragmatic hernia. Semin Perinatol. 2004;28:174.
74. Bean WJ, Calonje MA, April CN, Geshner J. Anal atresia: a prenatal ultrasound diagnosis. J Clin Ultrasound. 1978;6:111–2.
75. Lee MY, Won HS, Shim JY, et al. Sonographic determination of type in a fetal imperforate anus. J Ultrasound Med. 2016;35:1285–91. Perlman S, Bilik R, Leibovitch L, et al. More than a gut feeling — sonographic prenatal diagnosis of imperforate anus in a high-risk population. Prenat Diagn. 2014;34:1307–11.
76. Vijayaraghavan SB, Prema AS, Suganyadevi P. Sonographic depiction of the fetal anus and its utility in the diagnosis of anorectal malformations. J Ultrasound Med. 2011;30:37–45.
77. Ochoa JH, Chiesa M, Vildoza RP, et al. Evaluation of the perineal muscular complex in the prenatal diagnosis of anorectal atresia in a high-risk population. Ultrasound Obstet Gynecol. 2012;39:521–7.
78. Rohrer L, Vial Y, Gengler C, Tenisch E, Alamo L. Prenatal imaging of anorectal malformations - 10-year experience at a tertiary center in Switzerland. Pediatr Radiol. 2020;50(1):57–67.
79. Spitz L. Oesophageal atresia. Orphanet J Rare Dis. 2007;2:24. Published 2007 May 11.
80. Vogt EC. Congenital esophageal atresia. AJR Am J Roentgenol. 1929;22:463–5.
81. Gross RE. The surgery of infancy and childhood. Philadelphia: WB Saunders; 1953.
82. Pinheiro PF, Simões e Silva AC, Pereira RM. Current knowledge on esophageal atresia. World J Gastroenterol. 2012;18(28):3662–72.
83. Loening-Baucke V, Ken Kimura MD. Failure to pass meconium: diagnosing N eonatal intestinal obstruction. Am Fam Physician. 1999 Nov 1;60(7):2043–50.
84. American College of Radiology Appropriateness Criteria for Vomiting in Infants Protocol.
85. Lee C-H, Chou M-C, Yeh H-M. Rectal atresia with rectourethral fistula: a rare anomaly. World J Pediatr. 2007;3(2):150–1.
86. Berrocal T, Lamas M, Gutiérrez J, Torres I, Prieto C, del Hoyo ML. Congenital anomalies of the small intestine, colon, and rectum. Radiographics. 1999;19(5):1219–36.
87. Sato Y, Pringle KC, Bergman RA, Yuh WT, Smith WL, Soper RT, et al. Congenital anorectal anomalies: MR imaging. Radiology. 1988;168(1):157–62.
88. Fitoz S, Atasoy C, Yagmurlu A, et al. Three-dimensional CT of congenital esophageal atresia and distal tracheoesophageal fistula in neonates: preliminary results. AJR Am J Roentgenol. 2000;175(5):1403–7.

89. Zens T, Nichol PF, Cartmill R, Kohler JE. Management of asymptomatic pediatric umbilical hernias: a systematic review. J Pediatr Surg. 2017;52:1723.
90. Brandt ML. Pediatric hernias. Surg Clin North Am. 2008;88:27.
91. Sakurai M, Donnelly LF, Klosterman LA, Strife JL. Congenital diaphragmatic hernia in neonates: variations in umbilical catheter and enteric tube position. Radiology. 2000;216:112.
92. Frenckner B, Ehrén H, Granholm T, et al. Improved results in patients who have congenital diaphragmatic hernia using preoperative stabilization, extracorporeal membrane oxygenation, and delayed surgery. J Pediatr Surg. 1997;32:1185.
93. Wilson JM, Lund DP, Lillehei CW, Vacanti JP. Congenital diaphragmatic hernia--a tale of two cities: the Boston experience. J Pediatr Surg. 1997;32:401.
94. Downard CD, Wilson JM. Current therapy of infants with congenital diaphragmatic hernia. Semin Neonatol. 2003;8:215.
95. Szeremeta W, Parikh TD, Widelitz JS. Congenital nasal malformations. Otolaryngol Clin N Am. 2007;40:97.
96. Hengerer AS, Brickman TM, Jeyakumar A. Choanal atresia: embryologic analysis and evolution of treatment, a 30-year experience. Laryngoscope. 2008;118:862.
97. Myer CM 3rd, Cotton RT. Nasal obstruction in the pediatric patient. Pediatrics. 1983;72:766.
98. Smith JL 2nd, Sweeney DM, Smallman B, Mortelliti A. State-dependent laryngomalacia in sleeping children. Ann Otol Rhinol Laryngol. 2005;114:111.
99. Amin MR, Isaacson G. State-dependent laryngomalacia. Ann Otol Rhinol Laryngol. 1997;106:887.
100. Sánchez I, Navarro H, Méndez M, et al. Clinical characteristics of children with tracheobronchial anomalies. Pediatr Pulmonol. 2003;35:288.
101. Kwong KM. Current updates on choanal atresia. Front Pediatr. 2015;3:52. Published 2015 Jun 9.
102. Wallis C, Alexopoulou E, Antón-Pacheco JL, et al. ERS statement on tracheomalacia and bronchomalacia in children. Eur Respir J. 2019;54:1900382.
103. Lee EY, Boiselle PM. Tracheobronchomalacia in infants and children: multidetector CT evaluation. Radiology. 2009;252:7.
104. Heyer CM, Nuesslein TG, Jung D, et al. Tracheobronchial anomalies and stenoses: detection with low-dose multidetector CT with virtual tracheobronchoscopy – comparison with flexible tracheobronchoscopy. Radiology. 2007;242:542.
105. Desir A, Ghaye B. Congenital abnormalities of intrathoracic airways. Radiol Clin N Am. 2009;47:203.

Chapter 5
Management of the Mandibular Deformity in the Growing Patient with Craniofacial Microsomia

Cory M. Resnick and Bonnie L. Padwa

Treatment of the Growing Child

Craniofacial surgeons initially concentrated on the correction of end-stage deformities in older children and adults. Advances in anesthetic and surgical techniques and in understanding the pathogenesis of craniofacial anomalies encouraged earlier intervention for certain malformations during growth. The hypothesis was that operative correction of a craniofacial malformation in the growing child would normalize the functional matrix, thereby optimizing future growth potential by placing structures in a more anatomical position and improving function. In theory, this would minimize secondary deformity and distortion by releasing restricted growth of adjacent skeletal structures. Moreover, early intervention can improve appearance, body image, and socialization of the child.

The goal of treatment of CFM in childhood is to achieve improved function and optimal facial symmetry and aesthetics when craniofacial growth is complete. The treatment approach is dictated by mandibular skeletal type (Kaban types I, IIA, IIB, and III), presence of a midface deformity (cant of the maxillary occlusal plane and piriform rims), age (chronological, dental, skeletal), and psychosocial development

C. M. Resnick (✉) · B. L. Padwa
Harvard School of Dental Medicine and Harvard Medical School, Boston, MA, USA

Department of Plastic and Oral Surgery, Boston Children's Hospital, Boston, MA, USA
e-mail: Cory.resnick@childrens.harvard.edu; Bonnie.padwa@childrens.harvard.edu

D. M. Yates, M. R. Markiewicz (eds.), *Craniofacial Microsomia and Treacher Collins Syndrome*, https://doi.org/10.1007/978-3-030-84733-3_5

Table 5.1 General assessment principles by age and skeletal type

Skeletal type	Deciduous	Mixed	Permanent
Type I	Skin tag removal	Functional appliance	Presurgical orthodontics
		Mandibular elongation osteotomy/distraction	Bimaxillary surgery
		Creation of posterior open bite	
Type IIA	As above	As above	As above
		Functional appliance	
		Mandibular distraction	
Type IIB	As above	Construction of ramus, condyle, glenoid fossa	Presurgical orthodontics
		Creation of posterior open bite	Bimaxillary surgery
		Level occlusal plane	Construction of temporomandibular joint
Type III	As above	Construction of ramus, condyle, glenoid fossa	As above
		Creation of posterior open bite	
		Level occlusal plane	

From: Kaban LB, Padwa BL, Mulliken JB: *J Oral Maxillofac Surg* 56:628–638, 1998

of the child. (Table 5.1 provides a summary of general assessment principles by age and skeletal type [1].)

In the growing child, the first goal is to surgically create an open bite on the affected side by elongation and rotation of the mandible to the midline. The open bite must be maintained and controlled to permit leveling of the occlusal plane by vertical maxillary growth on the affected side. Success depends on the potential for vertical growth of the midface and maxillary alveolus as the deciduous teeth are shed and the permanent teeth erupt. Therefore, a child with CFM must be in the mixed dentition to benefit from early management. The protocol is not applicable after the permanent teeth have erupted because vertical midfacial and dentoalveolar growth is essentially complete by this time.

Treatment should proceed in a stepwise fashion, conforming to a predictable sequence with several sequential phases consisting of some or all of the following: functional appliance treatment, early orthodontic treatment, early mandibular operation (including ramus and fossa construction if necessary), immediate postsurgical dental appliance to support graft remodeling or regenerate consolidation, comprehensive orthodontic treatment, treatment of the end-stage skeletal deformity in non-growing patients, and soft tissue augmentation.

Functional Appliance Treatment

Impaired mandibular growth may be the result of absent or reduced condylar cartilage proliferation and reduced protrusive action of the condyle due to the absolute or relative absence of lateral pterygoid muscle function on the condylar head. A functional orthodontic appliance that enhances the neuromuscular environment, promotes mandibular and maxillary growth, and expands the soft tissue envelope on the affected side may be used in young patients with CFM. The appliance is a removable acrylic orthodontic activator with guide planes and shields that is constructed to hold the affected side of the mandible in a lowered and protrusive position. The appliance stimulates bone apposition in the ramus-condyle unit and coronoid process by substituting for the normal translatory and protrusive motion produced by the lateral pterygoid muscle. The degree of deformity and patient compliance greatly affect the outcome of functional appliance therapy. Response to functional appliance therapy has been shown to be beneficial in patients with type I CFM.

A study of 15 type I CFM patients showed that, during treatment with a functional appliance, the affected side increased in size more than the unaffected side in four children, by an amount equal to the unaffected side in four children, and slightly less than the unaffected side in seven children. However, no significant mean difference between the groups in growth of the two sides in the sample occurred [2]. A similar response was reported by Melsen et al. [3]

If the response to functional appliance therapy is good, then it may be possible to avoid surgical lengthening of the mandibular ramus on the affected side in patients with type I mandibles, provided the angulation of the maxillary occlusal plane is acceptable. In type IIA CFM, a similar presurgical treatment phase may be beneficial [3, 4]. Advocates of presurgical orthopedic therapy are of the opinion that even when a functional appliance does not avoid the need for mandibular lengthening procedures, the appliance produces a soft tissue environment that has a reduced tendency for postoperative skeletal relapse.

Early Orthodontic Treatment

In patients with CFM, there may be delayed tooth eruption and dental anomalies, and crowding of the dentition is common [5]. Orthodontic treatment in childhood focuses on control of tooth eruption and prevention or correction of dentoalveolar adaptations to the asymmetrical position of the maxilla and mandible. The orthodontist should be actively involved in the treatment of children with CFM throughout their growth period.

Early Mandibular Operation and Immediate Postsurgical Dental Appliance

Operative correction of the mandibular skeletal deformity is indicated in some children. Mandibular lengthening and creation of an open bite on the affected side during the mixed dentition allow vertical growth of the midface on that side, permitting the maxilla to meet the new position of the mandible. In turn, the secondary deformity of maxillary occlusal plane canting that occurs when interceptive treatment is not employed may be decreased or avoided. This can theoretically prevent the need for a Le Fort I osteotomy after completion of skeletal growth.

In type I, IIA, and some IIB patients, the mandible is elongated and rotated to the correct midline. The mandible can be elongated using either conventional orthognathic surgical methods or by distraction osteogenesis (DO).

Conventional orthognathic techniques include a vertical ramus osteotomy, often combined with a coronoidectomy on the affected side, or an inverted L osteotomy, leaving the condyle on the affected side in position. The proximal and distal fragments are secured using rigid fixation. A compensatory releasing osteotomy may be required on the unaffected side to allow the mandible to rotate passively to the new position without excessive torquing of the condyle on the unaffected side; this is usually not required in young children.

The standard procedure for distraction osteogenesis (DO) includes creation of a mandibular ramus osteotomy. A distraction device is fixed to the lateral aspect of the ramus and is secured to the bone on either side of the osteotomy. Numerous distraction devices are commercially available, all permitting a gradual separation of bone fragments. The ideal device is technically easy to apply, completely buried (avoiding the cutaneous pin tracks associated with transcutaneously placed pins and externally located devices), and easily removed following the period of distraction and retention. To obtain the most predictable outcomes, three-dimensional treatment planning should be used to allow precise positioning of the osteotomy and proper orientation and fixation of the device to the bony segments (Fig. 5.1).

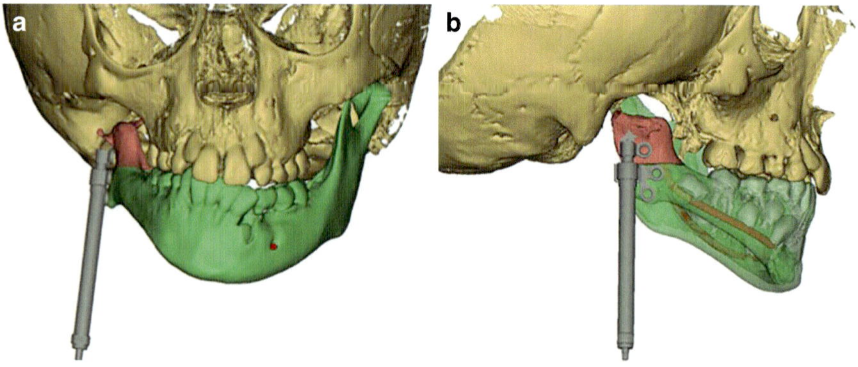

Fig. 5.1 Three-dimensional plan for distraction osteogenesis of the right ramus using a semi-buried unidirectional device. Note the proximal segment in red. (Reproduced with permission from: Resnick et al. [42])

Ilizarov [6] recommended a 5-day latency period to permit soft tissue healing prior to the beginning of distraction, a principle extrapolated from the orthopedic experience of distracting long bones. Animal models [7] as well as human studies of mandibular distraction [8] have shown no difference in outcomes when the latency period is eliminated. As such, many craniofacial surgeons have eliminated the latency period from the DO protocol and instead begin the distraction phase immediately following osteotomy and device placement [9]. Distraction commences at a rate of 1–2 mm per day, spreads over two to four activations, and continues until the desired mandibular expansion is achieved. This end point is based on clinical examination and follow-up radiographs correlated with three-dimensional treatment planning. Clinical examination ensures correction of the asymmetry and presence of an open bite on the affected side. During the first 3–4 days of distraction, the proximal fragment may move posteriorly and superiorly until it becomes fully seated in the glenoid fossa or against a stop at the skull base; mandibular lengthening may not be appreciated on clinical examination at this stage. The distraction period is then followed by a retention period of 6–8 weeks or at least two times the number of millimeters of distraction in days, to allow the regenerate to consolidate [10]. Ultrasonography can be used to assess bone consolidation during the retention period, if desired [11, 12]. Following the consolidation period, the distraction device is removed.

DO has a number of advantages compared to conventional techniques: mandibular lengthening occurs with minimal morbidity, need for bone grafting and donor site morbidity are eliminated, operative time is decreased, and hospital length of stay is shortened. Additionally, initial observational studies and animal models suggested that soft tissue expansion occurs simultaneously with bone lengthening [13, 14]. This provides a soft tissue environment that may permit greater long-term skeletal stability. However, several recent longitudinal follow-up studies have shown that the mandibular asymmetry usually recurs over time and that additional operations to correct skeletal asymmetry are often necessary [15–18].

With both conventional osteotomies and DO, no operation is performed on the maxilla in a growing child; an open bite created on the affected side is maintained and regulated by the use of an orthodontic appliance to allow for eruption of the teeth and vertical growth of the maxilla, thus leveling the maxillary occlusal plane (Fig. 5.2) [19–22].

If the ramus has been lengthened by distraction, the appliance should be fitted on the final day of distraction and worn throughout the period of consolidation. If the ramus has been lengthened by conventional osteotomy or ramus construction, the appliance should be fitted as soon as possible following the operation. The orthodontic appliance is first used as a bite block to maintain the open bite for 3–6 months after the operation. Then eruption of the maxillary teeth and vertical growth of the maxilla on the affected side are directed by gradually reducing the maxillary side of the appliance over the next 1–2 years. Finally, the open-bite closure is completed by active orthodontic movement of the maxillary teeth, thus leveling the maxillary occlusal plane.

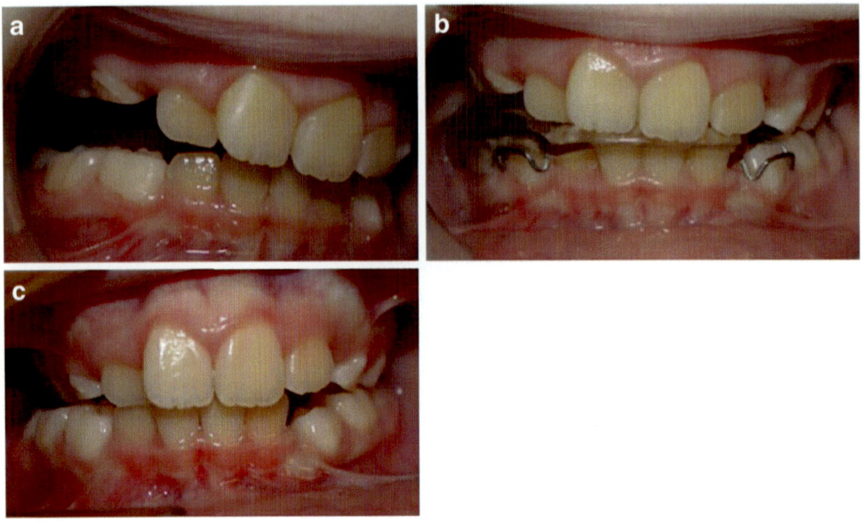

Fig. 5.2 (**a**) Occlusal photo at the end of distraction, demonstrating intended right posterior open bite. (**b**) Orthodontic appliance guides the eruption of the teeth and vertical growth of the maxilla. (**c**) Occlusion after removal of dental appliance, demonstrating eruption of maxillary dentition on the affected side to close the open bite. (Reproduced with permission from: Resnick et al. [42])

In many patients with type IIB and in all patients with type III deformities, there is insufficient ramus available for the use of conventional osteotomies. Similarly, DO cannot be used because this technique requires enough available bone to fix the device and a glenoid fossa or flat surface at the skull base to act as a stop for movement of the proximal bone fragment. Therefore, the mandibular ramus and TMJ must be constructed with an autologous graft or flap. Costochondral grafts or vascularized free fibula flaps are used most commonly for this purpose (Fig. 5.3). The new TMJ is constructed to be symmetrical with the opposite joint, as lateral and posterior as possible. The creation of an open bite and the use of an orthodontic appliance to control maxillary growth and eruption of the maxillary teeth are otherwise the same.

Costochondral grafts have long been the gold standard for mandibular reconstruction in young patients [23, 24] because they have an excellent track record of viability and stability [25]. A small cartilaginous cap is harvested with the costal bone and used as the articulating surface. The long-term prognosis depends on symmetrical growth between the normal side and the constructed ramus-condyle unit. Ramus-condyle units that have been constructed with costochondral grafts often elongate during facial growth allowing symmetry to be maintained [26], though overgrowth and undergrowth are possible [27, 28]. CCGs are primarily composed of cortical bone and rely on recipient tissues for revascularization [29]. Postoperative resorption, therefore, is common, and, in some cases, complete graft loss occurs over time. Furthermore, the grafted bone is thin and does not respond well to

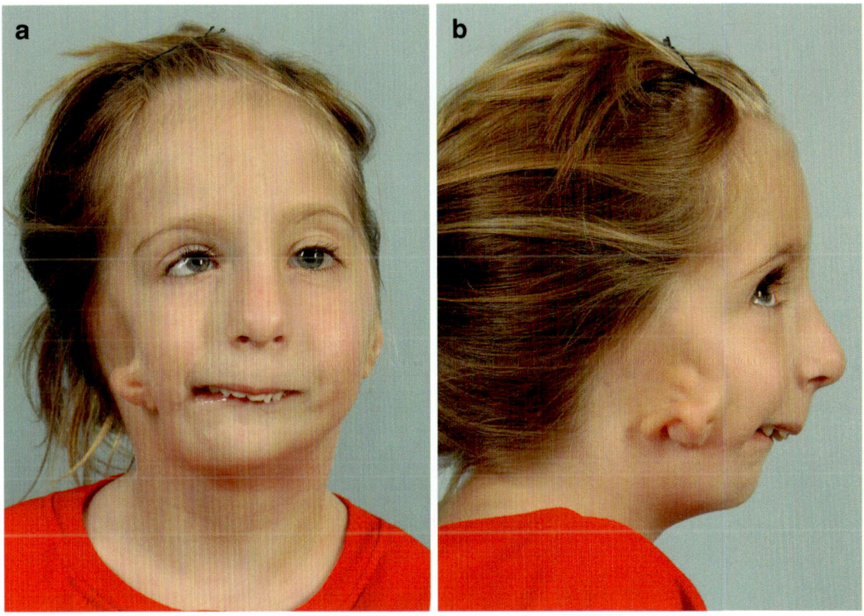

Fig. 5.3 A 6-year-old girl with right predominant hemifacial microsomia and a Kaban-Pruzansky type III mandible. (**a**, **b**) Preoperative photographs showing mandibular deviation to the right, retrognathia, microtia, and soft tissue insufficiency. (**c–e**) Type III mandible with minimal ramus on the right side. (**f**) Virtual repositioning of the mandible to provide occlusion on the left side and create a right posterior open bite. A surgical splint is fabricated to dictate this planned position during the operation. (**g**) A free fibula flap is virtually positioned with one osteotomy to facilitate the planned mandibular position and mimic the contralateral mandibular contour which has been transposed on to the affected side (green). (**h**, **i**) Planned fibula flap position. (**j**) A surgical guide is fabricated to dictate the length and internal osteotomy of the fibula flap. (**k**) Intraoperatively, the fibula flap is harvested, the internal osteotomy performed, and a miniplate applied to provide the planned contours, while the flap remains attached to the vascular pedicle. (**l**) The fibula flap is harvested and an AlloDerm™ (Allergan, Inc., Parsippany NJ), and cap is applied to serve as the articulating surface. (**m**) The flap is inserted, contoured, and secured to the native mandible with lag screws. (**n**) Microvascular anastomoses are performed to the facial artery and the external jugular vein. (**o**) After flap insertion and removal of the occlusal splint, the planned occlusion has been achieved. (**p**, **q**) Postoperative CT demonstrating the position of the flap. (**r**, **s**) One-month postoperative photographs showing improved projection and symmetry of the mandible. (**t**) One-year postoperative photograph, just prior to beginning ear construction. (Reproduced with permission from: Resnick [43])

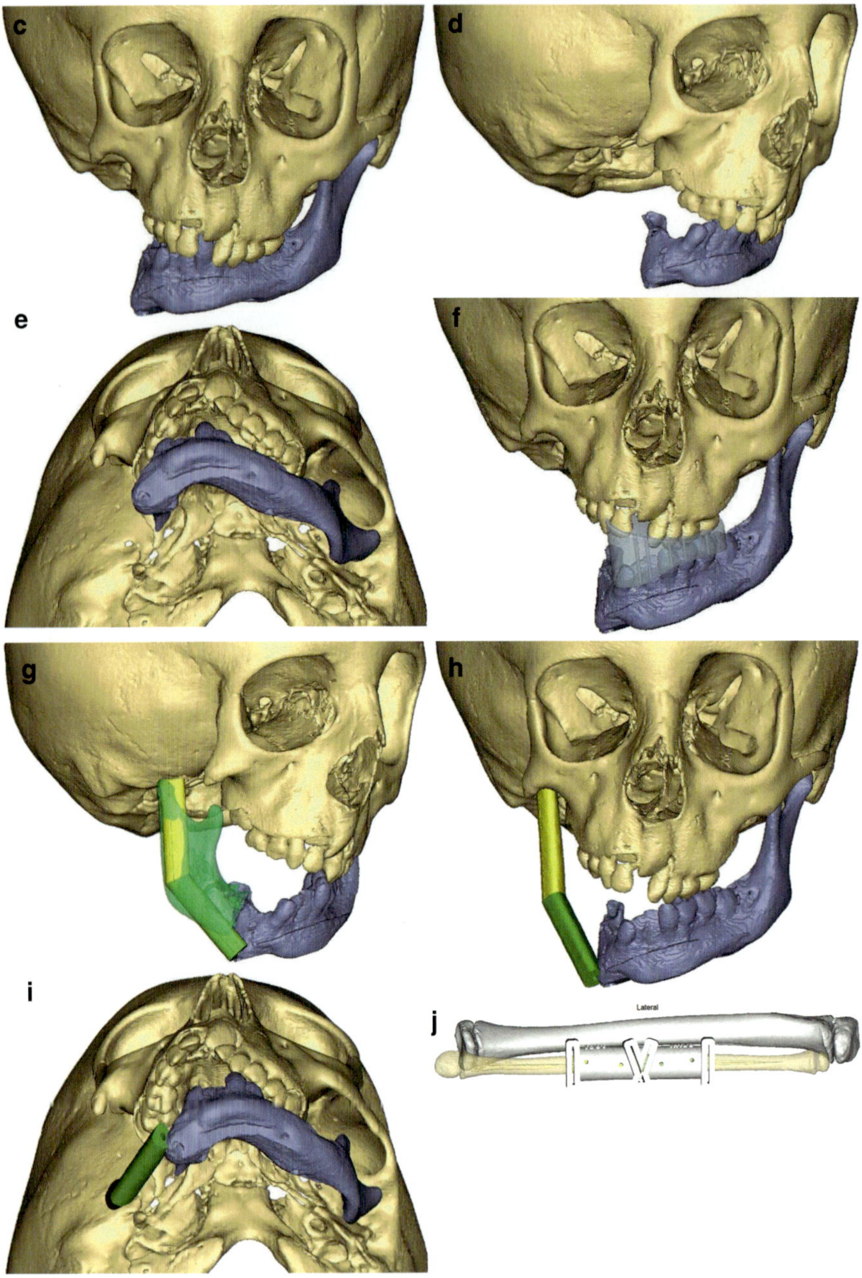

Fig. 5.3 (continued)

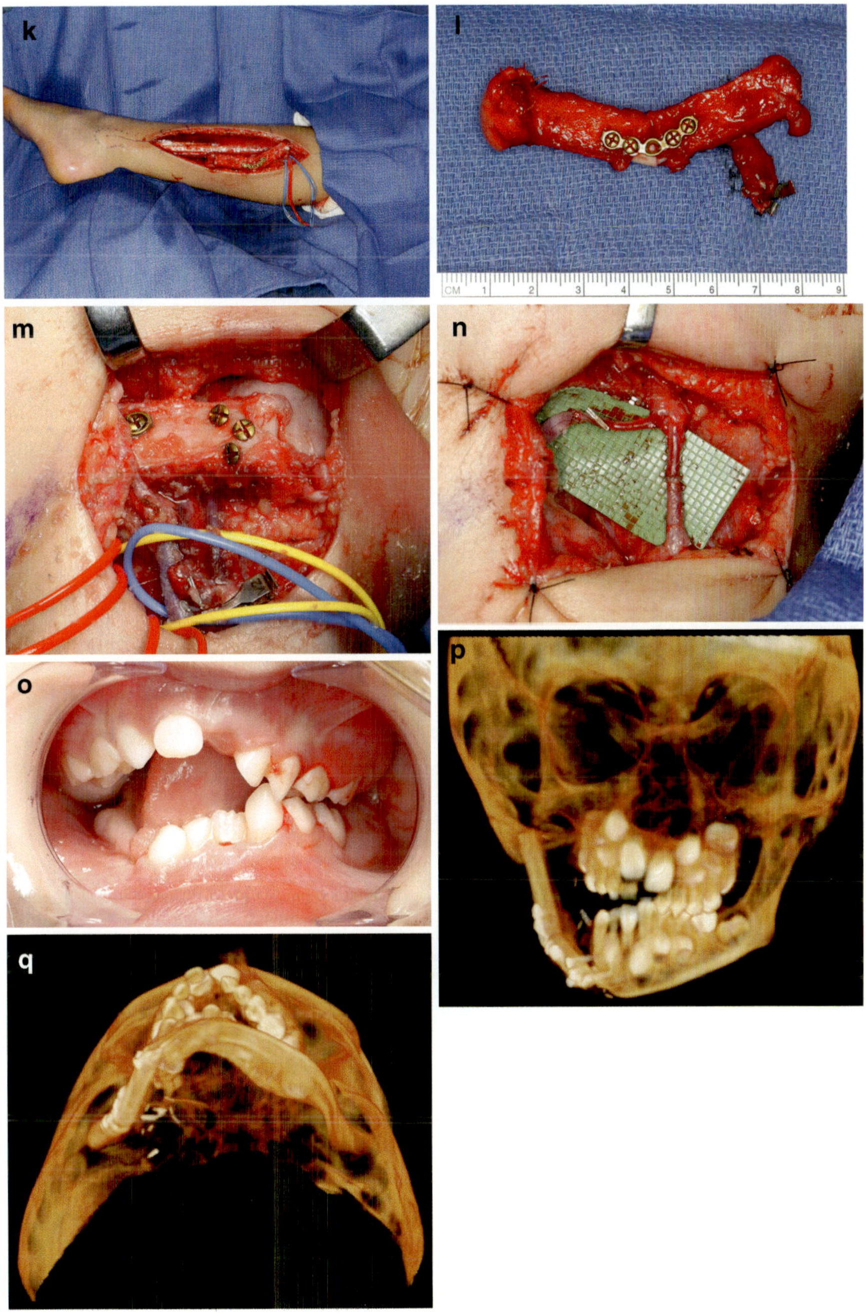

Fig. 5.3 (continued)

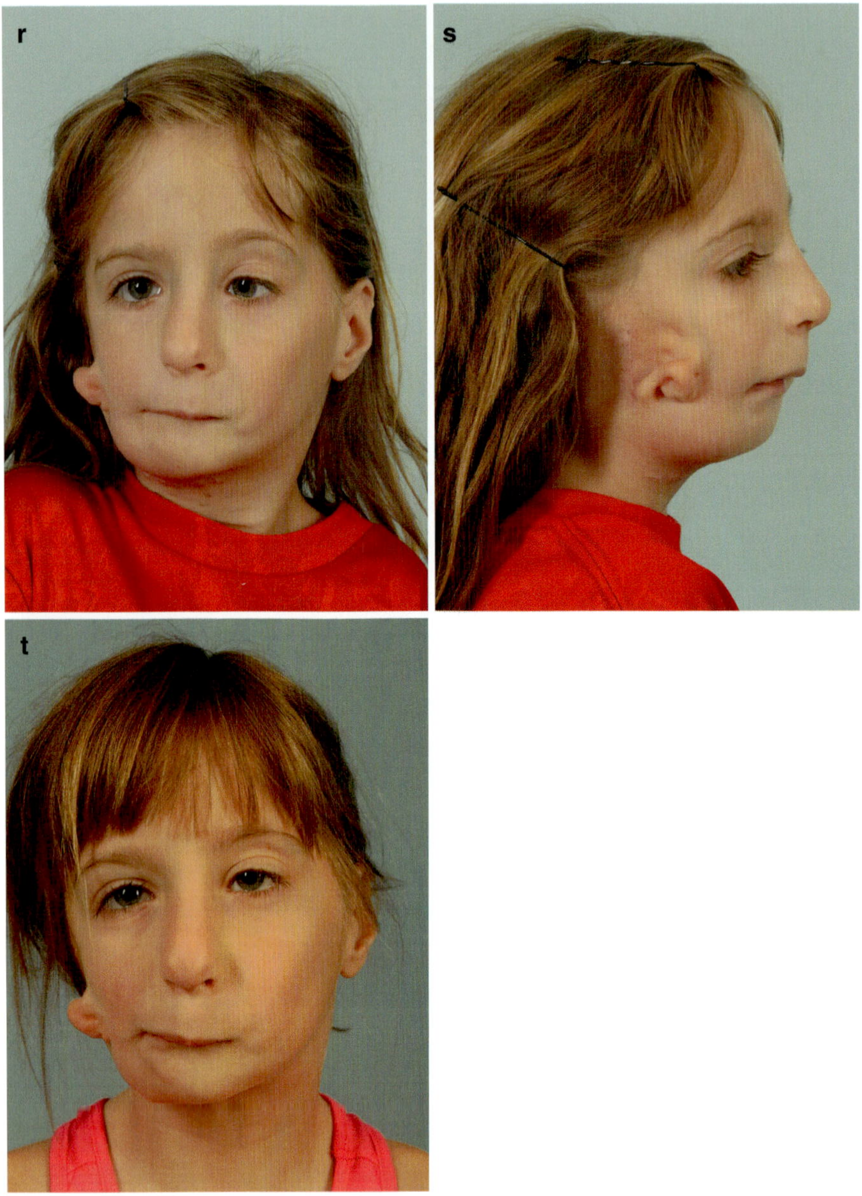

Fig. 5.3 (continued)

contouring osteotomies or distraction osteogenesis if necessary after completion of craniofacial growth to correct asymmetry [30].

The free fibula flap is an alternative to CCG for mandibular construction [31]. The attributes of this flap include a large amount of available donor bone, a consistent bone shape allowing for osteotomies within the flap to create a more natural shape, a robust blood supply, less resorption compared with grafts, and a favorable response to future distraction osteogenesis if needed [31, 32]. The free fibula flap may have growth potential in skeletally immature patients [5, 33]. The outcome of free fibula flaps for ramus-condyle unit construction has variable results with observational studies suggesting a lack of growth potential [34, 35] and others showing that the flaps do elongate during growth [36].

A disappointing complication that has been associated with construction using free fibula flaps in patients with CFM is ankylosis. Resnick and colleagues reported that 63% (5 of 8) of their patients with CFM (mean age 8.8 years) who had construction of the ramus condyle unit with a fibula developed ankylosis over a 7.3-year follow-up [37]. The patients that developed ankylosis were skeletally immature at the time of construction. This is in contrast to Santamaria et al.'s series of ten patients with HFM who had a free fibula flap for ramus construction at a mean age of 7.2 years [31]. None of their patients developed ankylosis over the 45.4 months of mean follow-up period. The operative technique described is similar in both studies, except that Santamaria et al. did not use intermaxillary fixation intraoperatively. One possible explanation for the significant difference in ankylosis rates between the studies is that Resnick et al. attempted to improve symmetry and posterior facial height by rotating the mandible to the midline and in a counterclockwise direction. They established the best-fit dental occlusion and fixed this position intraoperatively with intermaxillary fixation and an occlusal splint while the fibula was inserted. The ramus lengthening and midline correction on the affected side might have caused the fibula to be pushed superiorly into the fossa particularly in younger patients who did not undergo a compensatory releasing osteotomy on the contralateral (unaffected) side. The lack of intraoperative intermaxillary fixation in the report by Santamaria and colleagues indicates that they may not have repositioned the mandible and that the fibula may therefore have been placed in a passive position, exerting less pressure on the fibula against the fossa. The tight abutment of the articulating surface of the fibula and the skull base in those patients in the Resnick series who did not undergo contralateral releasing osteotomies may have contributed to their high rate of ankylosis. When this construction is used, it is best to avoid close approximation of the articulating flap surface and the skull base. This can be accomplished either by inserting the fibula in a passive position and planning to use distraction osteogenesis in the future to achieve symmetry and occlusal correction or by creating a contralateral releasing osteotomy to allow the mandible to rotate while minimizing upward pressure on the fibula at the time of the construction. Given the variability in the growth of the fibula and the chance of ankylosis, these patients should be followed closely for recurrent asymmetry and treated if necessary with a secondary lengthening procedure.

The results of treatment of growing children with CFM using conventional methods are mixed. Kaban et al. at Boston Children's Hospital reported 20 patients with CFM who underwent treatment during growth [21]. They were separated into two groups: group 1 (type I or IIA, $n = 10$) and group 2 (type IIB or III, $n = 10$). Group 1 patients were treated with a mandibular osteotomy with or without a bone graft to lengthen the mandibular ramus and rotate the mandible to the midline, followed by the use of an orthodontic appliance as discussed earlier. Group 2 patients had construction of the ramus-condyle unit and, as necessary the temporomandibular joint, with costochondral grafts or iliac crest grafts with costochondral junctions. The average follow-up was 50.9 months (group 1) and 45 months (group 2). In all children the midface grew vertically to close the surgically created open bite, and the maxillary occlusal plane was leveled without an osteotomy. Of the patients with type I or IIA (group 1), followed to completion of growth ($n = 9/10$), none required a maxillary osteotomy or a second procedure to lengthen the mandible. Of the patients with type IIB or III (group 2) who were followed to growth completion, none required a maxillary osteotomy, but four required a second mandibular elongation procedure in the late mixed dentition or early teen years.

Padwa et al. at Boston Children's Hospital retrospectively studied midfacial growth in patients ($n = 33$) with type IIB and III CFM after early construction with costochondral grafts [38]. Patients who had symmetrical growth of the constructed ramus and condyle (42%) had leveling of the intergonial angles and occlusal planes. Patients whose constructed rami grew but, at a diminished rate relative to the normal side (42%), remained asymmetrical with some improvement in but not complete leveling of the maxillary occlusal plane. Those who had minimal growth of the graft (16%) had an increase in the maxillary and mandibular deformities (increase in occlusal cant and intergonial angle).

Vargervik and Ousterhout at the University of California, San Francisco, reported continued growth of the lengthened mandible in the majority of ten patients with CFM followed until growth was completed [2]. In three of their patients, however, growth of the affected side did not keep pace with the normal side and facial asymmetry recurred, requiring a second mandibular lengthening procedure that also involved a maxillary osteotomy.

Longitudinal studies of CFM patients treated with DO in the mixed dentition have demonstrated that the majority of patients experience recurrence of their facial asymmetry and require additional procedures after the completion of skeletal growth. Meazzini et al. studied eight patients with type I and II mandibular deformities who had DO at a mean age of 5.6 years [15]. By postoperative year 5, all patients demonstrated recurrent asymmetry, with a mean return of 77% of the original asymmetry between the affected and unaffected sides.

In 2009 Nagy et al. published a meta-analysis which included 13 studies of early mandibular DO for CFM and concluded that there was a lack of statistical evidence to support DO as a single-stage treatment for the facial asymmetry associated with CFM [39]. Recently, Pluijmers et al. published another meta-analysis of early CFM treatment including bone graft construction and DO. In the patients who had a bone graft, more than 50% experienced recurrent asymmetry [18]. While the study design did not permit calculation of a relapse rate for patients who had DO, the analysis found that most patients had recurrence of the asymmetry after DO. Not surprisingly, recurrent asymmetry occurred least frequently in patients with type I mandibles. The best long-term results were achieved in those patients who had early grafting followed by distraction of the graft in adolescence. Some studies also suggested that early intervention can reduce negative psychosocial effects associated with having facial asymmetry. Based on these observations, the authors of this analysis concluded that single-stage correction should be delayed until the completion of skeletal growth and that a staged approach with both an early intervention and a final correction at skeletal maturity should be considered in patients with type IIB and III mandibles.

There has been a recent trend in the temporomandibular joint surgery community to favor total alloplastic joint replacement over autologous reconstruction of destroyed joints. As a result of the success of these alloplasts, this technique is beginning to expand to pediatric and congenital mandibular construction. Initial concerns about longevity of these joints and utility in young patients have been quelled by emerging long-term evidence of their success [40]. Alloplastic constructs have the advantages of complete customizability via virtual planning, ability to achieve large vertical and horizontal changes, and predictable and stable mandibular construction that allows precision in maxillary repositioning without the expected settling and remodeling that occurs postoperatively in autologous constructs. In growing patients, one must continue to consider the very long timeline of expected use of this joint with still unknown longevity after 20 years and possible need to upsize the condylar components during and after growth. Some surgeons have suggested performing an osteotomy in the native mandibular body to advance the mandible as necessary to compensate for growth asymmetry after an alloplastic joint has been placed during growth, to avoid the need to exchange joint components for larger versions [41].

In summary, it appears that early treatment should not be considered definitive treatment for the facial asymmetry seen in CFM. Early intervention may be useful as a component of a staged approach to asymmetry correction and may be indicated to reduce the psychosocial burden of facial asymmetry during the childhood years. Future advances in techniques and materials may improve outcomes.

References

1. Vargervik K. Comprehensive surgical and orthodontic management of hemifacial microsomia. In: Facial clefts and craniosynostosis: principles and management. Philadelphia: Saunders; 1995.
2. Vargervik K, Ousterhout DK, Farias M. Factors affecting long-term results in hemifacial microsomia. Cleft Palate J. 1986;23 Suppl 1:53–68.
3. Melsen B, Bjerregaard J, Bundgaard M. The effect of treatment with functional appliance on a pathologic growth pattern of the condyle. Am J Orthod Dentofacial Orthops. 1986;90(6):503–12.
4. Harvold EP, Vargerik K, Cherici G. Treatment of hemifacial microsomia. New York: AR Liss; 1983.
5. Cohen MM. Variability versus “incidental findings” in the first and second branchial arch syndrome: unilateral variants with anophthalmia. Birth Defects Orig Artic Ser. 1971;7(7):103–8.
6. Ilizarov GA. Clinical application of the tension-stress effect for limb lengthening. Clin Orthop Relat Res. 1990;250:8–26.

7. Troulis MJ, Glowacki J, Perrott DH, Kaban LB. Effects of latency and rate on bone formation in a porcine mandibular distraction model. J Oral Maxillofac Surg. 2000;58(5):507–13; discussion 514.
8. Hollier LH, Higuera S, Stal S, Taylor TD. Distraction rate and latency: factors in the outcome of pediatric mandibular distraction. Plast Reconstr Surg. 2006;117(7):2333–6.
9. Resnick CM. Precise osteotomies for mandibular distraction in infants with Robin sequence using virtual surgical planning. Int J Oral Maxillofac Surg. 2018;47(1):35–43.
10. Swennen G, Schliephake H, Dempf R, Schierle H, Malevez C. Craniofacial distraction osteogenesis: a review of the literature: part 1: clinical studies. Int J Oral Maxillofac Surg. 2001;30(2):89–103.
11. Thurmüller P, Troulis M, O'Neill MJ, Kaban LB. Use of ultrasound to assess healing of a mandibular distraction wound. J Oral Maxillofac Surg. 2002;60(9):1038–44.
12. Troulis MJ, Coppe C, O'Neill MJ, Kaban LB. Ultrasound: assessment of the distraction osteogenesis wound in patients undergoing mandibular lengthening. J Oral Maxillofac Surg. 2003;61(10):1144–9.
13. Lawler ME, Hansen GM, Williams WB, et al. Serial histologic and immunohistochemical changes in anterior digastric myocytes in response to distraction osteogenesis. J Oral Maxillofac Surg. 2012;70(1):168–78.
14. Molina F, Ortiz MF. Mandibular elongation and remodeling by distraction: a farewell to major osteotomies. Plast Reconstr Surg. 1995;96(4):825–40; discussion 841-842.
15. Meazzini MC, Mazzoleni F, Gabriele C, Bozzetti A. Mandibular distraction osteogenesis in hemifacial microsomia: long-term follow-up. J Craniomaxillofac Surg. 2005;33(6):370–6.
16. Meazzini MC, Mazzoleni F, Bozzetti A, Brusati R. Comparison of mandibular vertical growth in hemifacial microsomia patients treated with early distraction or not treated: follow up till the completion of growth. J Craniomaxillofac Surg. 2012;40(2):105–11.
17. Ascenço ASK, Balbinot P, Junior IM, D'Oro U, Busato L, da Silva Freitas R. Mandibular distraction in hemifacial microsomia is not a permanent treatment: a long-term evaluation. J Craniofac Surg. 2014;25(2):352–4.
18. Pluijmers BI, Caron CJJM, Dunaway DJ, Wolvius EB, Koudstaal MJ. Mandibular reconstruction in the growing patient with unilateral craniofacial microsomia: a systematic review. Int J Oral Maxillofac Surg. 2014;43(3):286–95.
19. Kaban LB, Mulliken JB, Murray JE. Three-dimensional approach to analysis and treatment of hemifacial microsomia. Cleft Palate J. 1981;18(2):90–9.
20. Murray JE, Kaban LB, Mulliken JB. Analysis and treatment of hemifacial microsomia. Plast Reconstr Surg. 1984;74(2):186–99.
21. Kaban LB, Moses MH, Mulliken JB. Correction of hemifacial microsomia in the growing child: a follow-up study. Cleft Palate J. 1986;23 Suppl 1:50–2.
22. Kaban LB, Moses MH, Mulliken JB. Surgical correction of hemifacial microsomia in the growing child. Plast Reconstr Surg. 1988;82(1):9–19.
23. Kumar P, Rattan V, Rai S. Do costochondral grafts have any growth potential in temporomandibular joint surgery? A systematic review. J Oral Biol Craniofac Res. 2015;5(3):198–202.
24. Poswillo D. Experimental reconstruction of the mandibular joint. Int J Oral Surg. 1974;3(6):400–11.
25. Mulliken JB, Ferraro NF, Vento AR. A retrospective analysis of growth of the constructed condyle-ramus in children with hemifacial microsomia. Cleft Palate J. 1989;26(4):312–7.
26. Perrott DH, Umeda H, Kaban LB. Costochondral graft construction/reconstruction of the ramus/condyle unit: long-term follow-up. Int J Oral Maxillofac Surg. 1994;23(6 Pt 1):321–8.
27. Guyuron B, Lasa CI. Unpredictable growth pattern of costochondral graft. Plast Reconstr Surg. 1992;90(5):880–6; discussion 887–889.
28. Munro IR, Phillips JH, Griffin G. Growth after construction of the temporomandibular joint in children with hemifacial microsomia. Cleft Palate J. 1989;26(4):303–11.
29. Resnick CM. Temporomandibular joint reconstruction in the growing child. Oral Maxillofac Surg Clin North Am. 2018;30(1):109–21.

30. Corcoran J, Hubli EH, Salyer KE. Distraction osteogenesis of costochondral neomandibles: a clinical experience. Plast Reconstr Surg. 1997;100(2):311–5; discussion 316-317.
31. Santamaría E, Morales C, Taylor JA, Hay A, Ortiz-Monasterio F. Mandibular microsurgical reconstruction in patients with hemifacial microsomia. Plast Reconstr Surg. 2008;122(6):1839–49.
32. Hidalgo DA. Fibula free flap: a new method of mandible reconstruction. Plast Reconstr Surg. 1989;84(1):71–9.
33. Zhang WB, Liang T, Peng X. Mandibular growth after paediatric mandibular reconstruction with the vascularized free fibula flap: a systematic review. Int J Oral Maxillofac Surg. 2016;45(4):440–7.
34. Phillips JH, Rechner B, Tompson BD. Mandibular growth following reconstruction using a free fibula graft in the pediatric facial skeleton. Plast Reconstr Surg. 2005;116(2):419–24; discussion 425-426.
35. Guo L, Ferraro NF, Padwa BL, Kaban LB, Upton J. Vascularized fibular graft for pediatric mandibular reconstruction. Plast Reconstr Surg. 2008;121(6):2095–105.
36. Temiz G, Bilkay U, Tiftikçioğlu YÖ, Mezili CT, Songür E. The evaluation of flap growth and long-term results of pediatric mandible reconstructions using free fibular flaps. Microsurgery. 2015;35(4):253–61.
37. Resnick CM, Genuth J, Calabrese CE, Taghinia A, Labow BI, Padwa BL. Temporomandibular joint ankylosis after ramus construction with free fibula flaps in children with hemifacial microsomia. J Oral Maxillofac Surg. 2018;76(9):2001.e2001–15.
38. Padwa BL, Mulliken JB, Maghen A, Kaban LB. Midfacial growth after costochondral graft construction of the mandibular ramus in hemifacial microsomia. J Oral Maxillofac Surg. 1998;56(2):122–7; discussion 127–128.
39. Nagy K, Kuijpers-Jagtman AM, Mommaerts MY. No evidence for long-term effectiveness of early osteodistraction in hemifacial microsomia. Plast Reconstr Surg. 2009;124(6):2061–71.
40. Wolford LM, Mercuri LG, Schneiderman ED, Movahed R, Allen W. Twenty-year follow-up study on a patient-fitted temporomandibular joint prosthesis: the Techmedica/TMJ Concepts device. J Oral Maxillofac Surg. 2015;73(5):952–60.
41. Mercuri LG, Swift JQ. Considerations for the use of alloplastic temporomandibular joint replacement in the growing patient. J Oral Maxillofac Surg. 2009;67(9):1979–90.
42. Resnick CM, Kaban LB, Padwa BL. Hemifacial microsomia: the disorder and its surgical management. In: Brennan PA, Schliephake H, Ghali GE, Cascarini L, editors. Maxillofacial surgery. 3rd ed. St. Louis: Elsevier; 2017. p. 870–93.
43. Resnick CM. TMJ reconstruction in the growing child. Oral Max Surg Clin North Am. 2018;30:109–21.

Chapter 6
Surgical Management of Hemifacial Microsomia with Temporomandibular Joint Malformation

Larry M. Wolford

Learning Aims

1. Understand hemifacial microsomia (HFM) relative to the nature of this congenital deformity as well as the clinical, radiographic, and diagnostic characteristics.
2. Realize the surgical treatment options that have been used to manage HFM, particularly in reference to TMJ reconstruction.
3. Review the literature on application of techniques to reconstruct the TMJ and correct the associated HFM dento-skeletal-facial deformity.
4. Be aware that patient-fitted total joint prosthesis provides superior outcomes relative to stability, function, and quality of treatment compared to autogenous bone grafts for TMJ reconstruction in the HFM patient.
5. Know the surgical protocol and sequencing for surgical correction of the severe HFM patient with patient-fitted total joint prosthesis in conjunction with orthognathic surgery and facial augmentation.

Introduction

Hemifacial microsomia (HFM) is a specific condition of unilateral incomplete or hypoplastic development of the facial soft tissues and skeleton. HFM is the second most common facial birth defect after cleft lip and palate with an estimated occurrence rate of 1 in 5600 live births. It is also known as Goldenhar's syndrome,

L. M. Wolford (✉)
Clinical Professor of Oral and Maxillofacial Srugery and Orthodontics, Texas A&M University College of Dentistry, Private Practice; Baylor University Medical Center, Dallas, TX, USA
e-mail: lwolford@drlarrywolford.com

D. M. Yates, M. R. Markiewicz (eds.), *Craniofacial Microsomia and Treacher Collins Syndrome*, https://doi.org/10.1007/978-3-030-84733-3_6

oculo-auriculo-vertebral spectrum, otomandibular dysostosis, lateral facial dysplasia, and branchial arch syndrome. HFM occurs sporadically in most cases and can be considered as a nonspecific symptom complex that is etiologically and pathogenetically heterogeneous. Extreme variability of expression is characteristic of this disorder [1, 2].

Classification

There are several proposed classifications that identify the severity of this syndrome, but for the purpose of this chapter, the classification system proposed by Pruzansky in 1969 and later modified by Mulliken and Kaban in 1987 will be used [3]. This assigns HFM patients to one of four categories based on size and function of the temporomandibular joint (TMJ). Type I is a small mandible with normal TMJ morphology. Type IIa is a ramus with abnormal size and shape, but the glenoid fossa maintains its position, whereas Type IIb is a ramus and TMJ with abnormal size, shape, and function and is displaced outside of the plane of the contralateral side. Type III describes an absent condyle, ramus, and TMJ. This classification system may be the most useful to the surgeon in the preoperative evaluation, diagnosis, and treatment planning because of its simplicity and inclusion of TMJ anatomy and function.

Clinical and Imaging Features

The features of HFM patients, depending on the degree of expression, may include some or all of the following characteristics: (1) unilateral hypoplasia or absence of the mandibular condyle, ramus, and body; (2) retruded mandible and chin deviated toward the ipsilateral side; (3) high occlusal plane angle facial morphology; (4) hypoplasia of the ipsilateral maxilla, zygomatico-orbital complex, and temporal bone including the absence of the zygomatic arch and glenoid fossa; (5) ipsilateral soft tissue deficiency affecting the muscles, subcutaneous and glandular tissues, nerves, and skin; (6) decreased ipsilateral facial height; (7) Class II skeletal and occlusal relationship; (8) premature occlusal contact on the ipsilateral side; (9) transverse cant in the occlusal plane and skeletal structures; (10) ipsilateral hypoeruption of the teeth and partial anodontia; (11) eye, ear, and vertebral anomalies; and (12) decreased oropharyngeal airway and sleep apnea in cases with significant expression and mandibular retrusion (Figs. 6.1a–c and 6.2a, b). Facial deformity and asymmetry usually worsen with growth. The contralateral TMJ articular disc may become anteriorly displaced induced by the abnormal condylar rotation caused by the mandibular asymmetry and the functional overload on the contralateral joint. Typical TMJ symptoms may accompany the contralateral TMJ disc displacement such as TMJ pain, headaches, myofascial pain, ear symptoms, clicking/popping, etc.

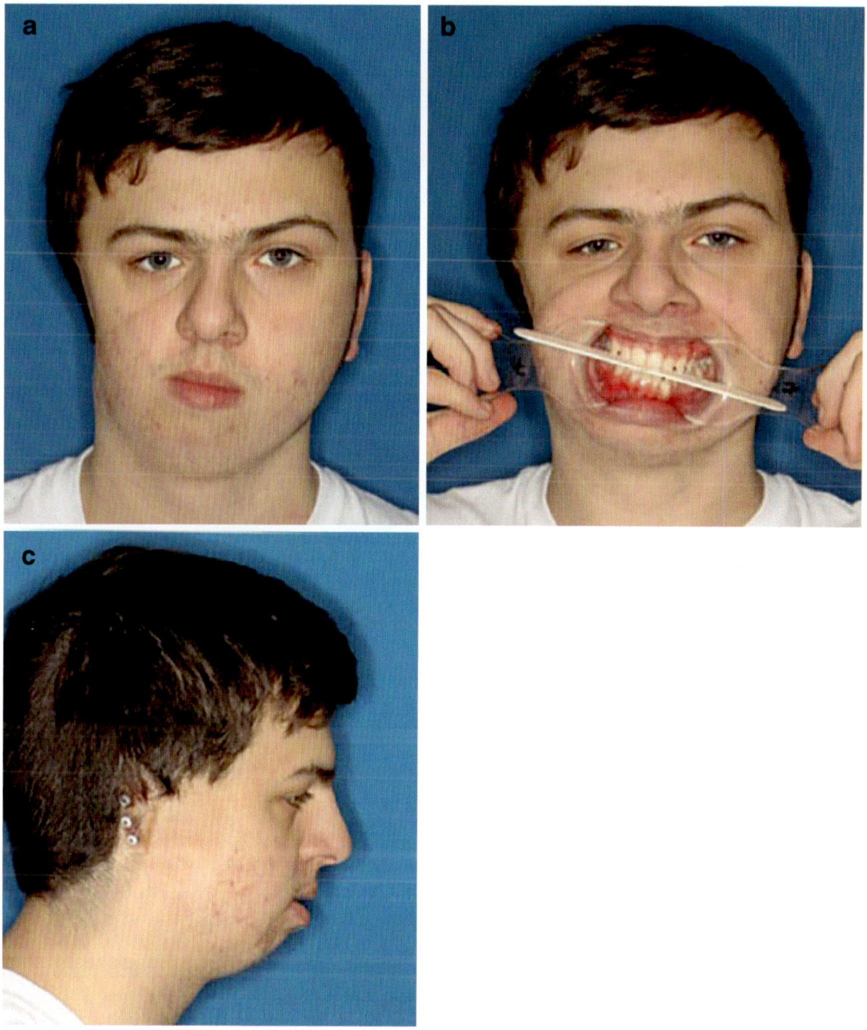

Fig. 6.1 (**a**) A 17-year-old male with right-sided hemifacial microsomia. Facial structures including the nose, maxilla, and mandible are shifted significantly off toward the right side. (**b**) The severe transverse cant in the occlusal plane is noted as well as the shift of the dental midlines and chin off to the right side. (**c**) Profile demonstrates a high occlusal plane angle facial morphology and a severely retruded mandible

CBCT scan will provide a lateral cephalometric radiograph, panogram, TMJ tomograms, and 3-D imaging to be used to analyze and quantify the antero-posterior, transverse, and vertical hard and soft tissue dimensional differences relative to the left to right sides. The use of 3-D CT scans and virtual surgical planning (VSP) is advocated to obtain more consistent and predictable surgical outcomes. MRI evaluation will demonstrate the deformed or absent TMJ of the ipsilateral side, while the contralateral TMJ may show a displaced disc.

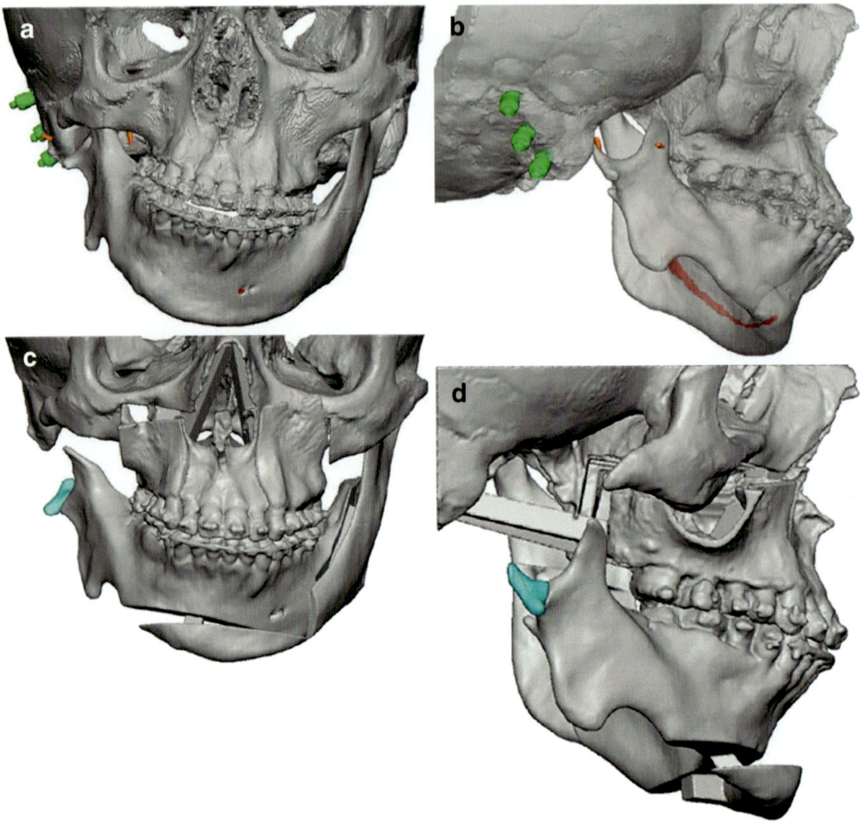

Fig. 6.2 (**a**) CT scan with the TMJ Concepts protocol was acquired and a 3-D computer model generated. The significant facial asymmetry is noted. (**b**) Right profile view shows the absence of the right zygomatic arch, fossa, and the severely deformed right condyle. There is a significant difference in the vertical heights of the mandible at the inferior border. (**c**) VSP has been completed with advancement of the maxillo-mandibular complex, leveling of the occlusal plane, shifting of the skeletal structures toward the left with an augmentation genioplasty. (**d**) Significant downward and forward rotation of the maxillo-mandibular complex is seen. The vertical gap between the temporal bone and the ramus is noted. The blue residual condyle will be removed to allow better adaptation of the patient-fitted prosthesis to the ramus. A coronoidectomy will be required to facilitate the vertical lengthening and advancement of the mandible

Less-involved HFM deformities with a healthy functional ipsilateral TMJ can usually be treated with orthognathic surgery and facial augmentation if indicated. However, HMF deformities commonly have a unilateral distorted, hypoplastic, or absent TMJ structure requiring TMJ reconstruction in conjunction with orthognathic surgery to provide optimal stable and predictable functional and esthetic outcomes. There are two primary methods to reconstruct the TMJ: autogenous bone grafts (i.e., costochondral graft, sternoclavicular graft) and alloplastic TMJ total joint prosthetic devices. Understanding the nature of the HFM deformity, the timing of reconstruction, the surgical treatment options including TMJ reconstruction and orthognathic surgery, and the outcome predictability and stability will enable the surgeon to apply this knowledge to optimally treat HFM and similar deformities. This chapter will focus on the more complex HMF cases with absent TMJs that are not amendable to conventional orthognathic surgery.

Autogenous Bone Grafts (ABGs)

The most common sources for autogenous bone grafts (ABGs) to reconstruct the ipsilateral condyle in HFM are costochondral grafts (CCG, Fig. 6.3) followed by sternoclavicular grafts (SCGs, Fig. 6.4). Vascularized fibula grafts could be

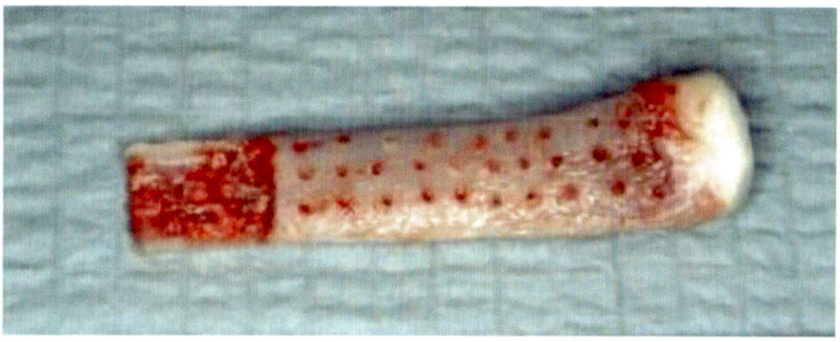

Fig. 6.3 Costochondral graft harvested and prepared for implantation. The multiple holes were placed to enhance revascularization of the graft

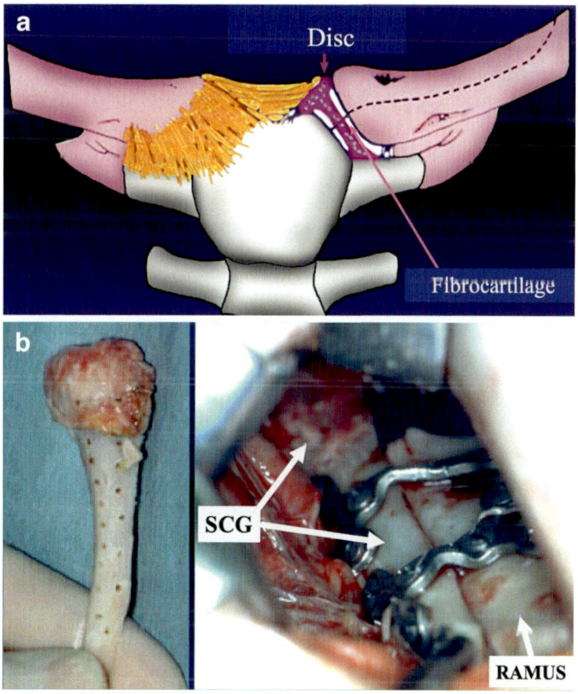

Fig. 6.4 (**a**) The sternoclavicular graft (SCG) is harvested from the upper half of the clavicle and includes harvesting the articular disc overlying the graft to provide better function of the reconstructed TMJ. (**b**) The graft is prepared and in this case inserted along the posterior border of the mandible. In HFM patients without a fossa, it may be better to place the graft on the medial side of the ramus with the head of the graft against the base of the skull, avoiding the necessity to reconstruct a fossa. The multiple holes in the cortex were placed to enhance revascularization of the graft

considered when bone and soft tissue deficiencies are severe requiring bone and soft tissue replacement, but this is rarely indicated. For growth center transplants if required in younger patients, CCG or SCG may provide growth potential, although unpredictable. An additional method advocated by some to reconstruct the ipsilateral mandible is distraction osteogenesis.

Indications for condylar reconstruction using ABG include the following: (1) non-functional TMJ related to deformed or absent TMJ condyle, (2) zero to one of the previous TMJ surgeries (for free grafts), (3) good vascular bed (for free grafts), (4) both hard and soft tissues are required (vascularized fibula graft), (5) growth center transplant indicated (CCG or SCG), (6) custom-fitted total joint prosthesis unavailable, (7) allergy to all metals in total joint prosthesis, (8) requires relatively minimal repositioning of the dento-skeletal structures, and (9) patient preference.

Contraindications for free ABG include (1) multiply operated TMJ (two or more previous failed TMJ surgical procedures), (2) connective tissue autoimmune disease or systemic inflammatory disease, (3) previously failed TMJ allografts, (4) conditions causing decreased vascularization and prolonged healing, (5) polyarthropathies, and (6) concomitant TMJ and orthognathic surgery indicated, requiring significant movement of the dento-skeletal structures.

Advantages of using ABG are (1) native bone readily available, (2) growth potential (CCG or SCG), (3) articular disc attached to graft (SCG), and (4) vascularized fibula graft available for requirement of major hard and soft tissue replacement.

Disadvantages of ABG are as follows: (1) requires graft harvest significantly increasing the operating time, (2) donor site morbidity, (3) grafts subject to physiological loading with possible subsequent bone remodeling or resorption, (4) grafts can bend, warp, and fracture, (5) cannot predictably correct significant dento-craniofacial deformities, (6) unpredictable growth, and (7) difficult to control occlusion.

Costochondral Grafts (CCGs)

CCG grafts (Fig. 6.3) for many years were the most popular and published ABG technique to reconstruct the TMJ for HFM, ankylosis, or other TMJ pathologies [3–8]. It is relatively easy to harvest and stabilize to the ramus. The costochondral junction fits nicely into the glenoid fossa, if there is a fossa present. Often HFM patients will not have an ipsilateral zygomatic arch or glenoid fossa. Some surgeons suggest reconstructing the fossa with bone grafting in order to place the CCG into a stable relationship [7]. This is usually not necessary if the CCG is placed on the medial side of the ramus where it can articulate on the base of the skull, eliminating the need for reconstructing a fossa. The CCG does have growth potential, but it is very unpredictable. The CCG can exhibit no growth or commonly will demonstrate significant over growth, as the CCG grows more like the rib than the TMJ. The elasticity and flexibility of the CCG, often because of the thin cortex, present a structure that when stressed or loaded excessively can bend, warp, or fracture resulting in the positional shifting of the mandible and occlusion, with larger skeletal movements increasing that risk. CCGs also have a significant risk of TMJ ankylosis.

Kaban et al. [4] advocated early treatment of HMF patients with Type I, IIa, and some Type IIb patients with mandibular osteotomies. The costochondral graft has been popular for reconstruction of the ipsilateral TMJ in the young Type IIb and III HFM patients due to the growth center at the costochondral junction and for reconstruction of the glenoid fossa [3–8]. However other articles demonstrated that rib graft growth is unpredictable with either no growth or significant overgrowth, creating a deformity that required additional surgery [5, 6].

CCG grafts are falling out of favor as a recent international survey by Hawkins et al. [9], in 2019 reported that 95.5% of responding surgeons prefer alloplastic TMJ replacement for end-stage TMJ pathology over CCG.

Sternoclavicular Grafts (SCGs)

SCG may function better than CCG for autogenous reconstruction of the TMJ as it has a very thick cortex, lots of medullary bone, and an articular disc attached to the condylar head (Fig. 6.4a). The upper half of the clavicle is harvested along with the articular disc attached to the upper head of the clavicle providing a more normal functioning condyle. For Types IIb and III HFM patients with an absent fossa, the SCG usually fits best by placement on the medial side of the ramus, articulating beneath the skull base or positioned along the posterior border of the mandible if there is a fossa present (Fig. 6.4b). The SCG grows more like a mandibular condyle, when used as a growth center transplant, but growth is unpredictable. The SCG is much stronger with minimal elasticity and flexibility as compared to the CCG, with less susceptibility to excessive loading that could bend, warp, or fracture the graft, thus providing better predictability and stability than CCG. However, it is susceptible to bony remolding when loaded as in large mandibular advancements that could affect occlusal stability. The primary complication is post-surgical clavicle fracture, as the donor site is significantly weakened by the harvest and may take a minimum of 6 months to regain significant strength [10, 11].

Wolford et al. [10] in 1994 demonstrated the use of the sternoclavicular graft (SCG) to reconstruct the HMF patient with the absent TMJ and to lengthen the mandible on the affected side. The upper half of the clavicle and associated portion of the articular disc were harvested (Fig. 6.4). The mandible was advanced as predetermined, and the graft was secured against the medial side of the residual ramus/body secured with bone screws and the condylar head seated against the base of the skull (see Case Presentation #1; Figs. 6.5, 6.6, 6.7, 6.8, and 6.9), or the graft was positioned against the posterior border of the ramus (Fig. 6.4b) if a fossa is present. This grafting system provided a better normal growth potential and stability as compared to a CCG. The graft will either grow relatively normally or exhibit deficient growth, but has not been observed to overgrow. Wolford [10] recommended the use

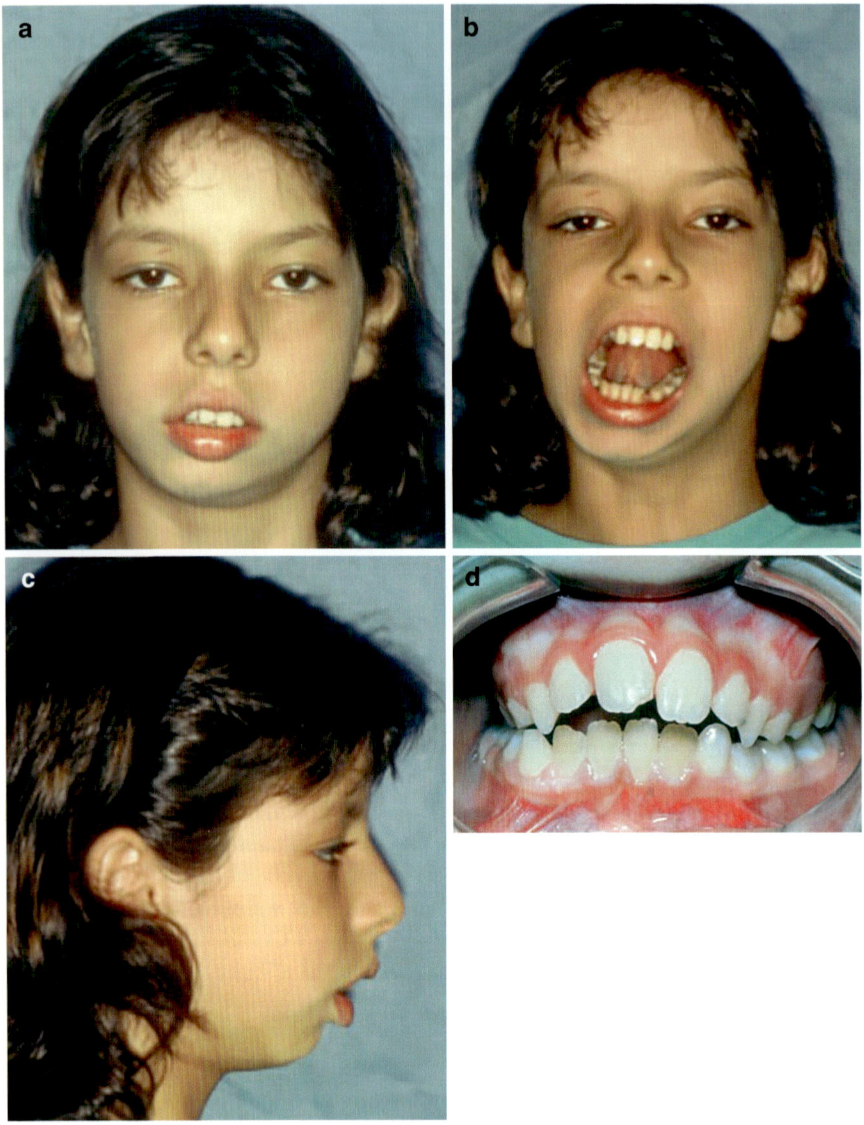

Fig. 6.5 *Case #1:* A 10-year-old female with right-sided HFM and associated significant dentofacial deformity: (**a**, **b**) frontal view, (**c**) profile view, and (**d**) occlusal view with the significant transverse occlusal cant

of the SCG after the age of 6 years, as the clavicle is too small at an earlier age to provide adequate bone for grafting the mandible as well as enough integrity to support the remaining clavicle during the healing phase.

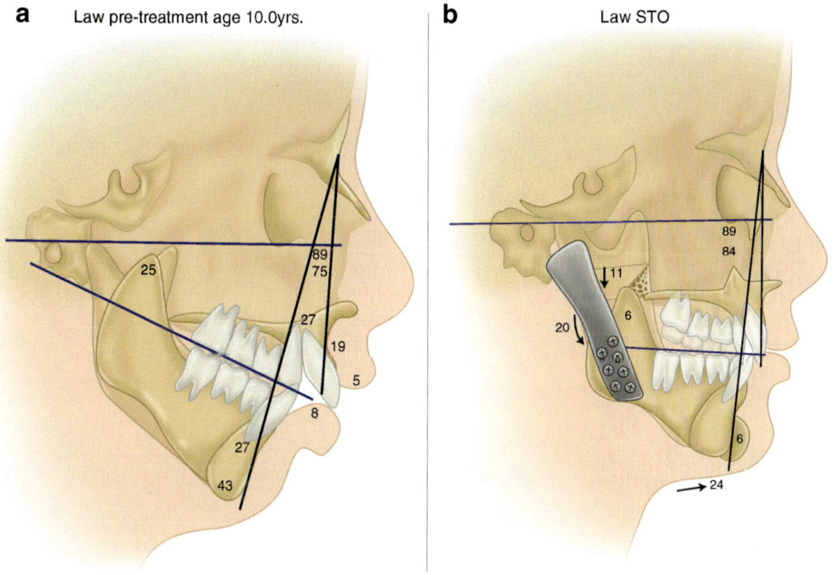

Fig. 6.6 *Case #1:* (**a**) Cephalometric analysis shows the anterior mandibular hypoplasia and high occlusal plane angle facial deformity. (**b**) Prediction tracing illustrates the planned surgery including reconstruction of the right TMJ, mandibular advancement, and vertical elongation with the SCG and a left-side inverted "L" osteotomy to permit a counterclockwise rotation for advancement and transverse leveling of the mandible. Since this patient had no fossa on the right side, the SCG was placed on the medial side of the ramus and articulated with the cranial base. Posterior open bites were created and closed with orthodontics

Vascularized Fibula Grafts

Vascularized fibula grafts have been documented for use in HFM patients [12]. The fibula graft can be a viable autogenous alternative where there is gross deficiency in bone and soft tissue, vascularly compromised recipient site, and/or major volumes of bone and soft tissue replacement are required. The fibula graft does leave an unsightly scar and bony deformity at the donor site. Although this graft system has been successful in some cases of HFM and for other conditions requiring mandibular reconstruction, there are significant risks with early and late morbidities including chronic donor site sensory disturbance (67%), chronic pain (26%), gait disturbance (20%), chronic lower limb weakness (20%) such as limited walking or stair climbing ability, limited toe mobility, donor site cosmetic deformity, and malocclusion (22%) [13]. Ankylosis is a major complication occurring in 63% of HFM patients receiving these grafts [12]. These risks must be carefully weighed before considering this method of HFM reconstruction.

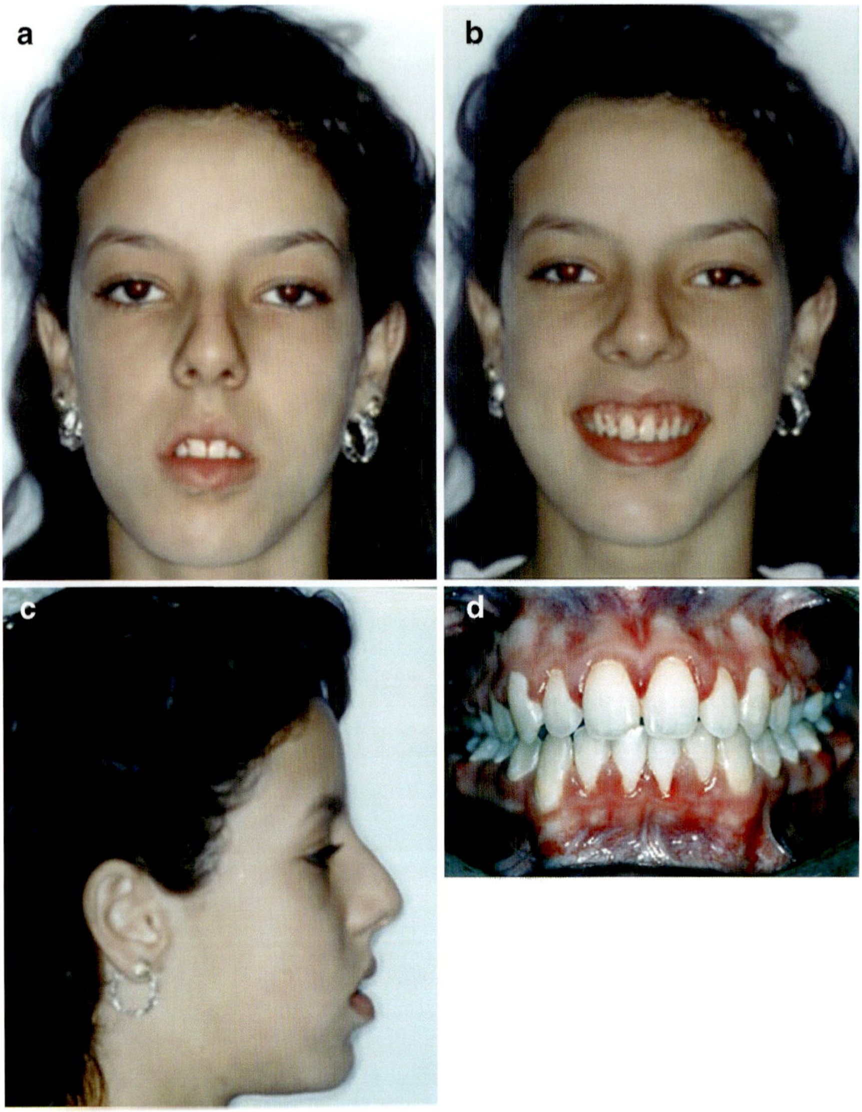

Fig. 6.7 *Case #1:* (**a**–**d**) Normal growth of the graft occurred, and the patient was followed until age 18 demonstrating the maintenance of the facial symmetry, although there were presurgical issues with maxillary vertical hyperplasia to be addressed

Distraction Osteogenesis

Distraction osteogenesis (DO) has become popular more recently, particularly in treating HFM and similar types of deformities [13–19]. This requires placing a distraction device, performing an osteotomy, and then distraction of the segments to

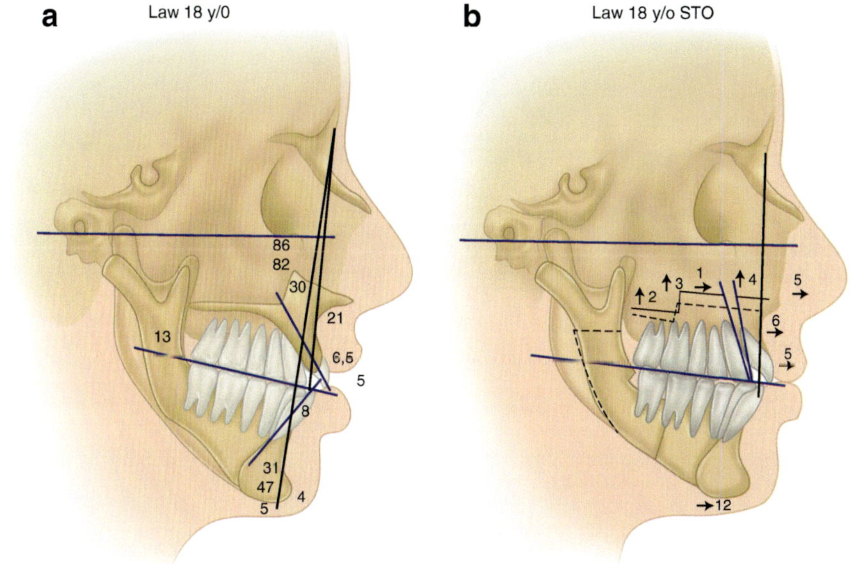

Fig. 6.8 *Case #1:* (**a**) Cephalometric analysis of the patient at age 18 years illustrating maxillary vertical hyperplasia but transverse symmetry. (**b**) Prediction tracing illustrates the surgical changes to be accomplished to maximize the functional and esthetic outcome. Double-jaw orthognathic surgery was performed including bilateral mandibular ramus osteotomies and maxillary osteotomies

produce new bone, increasing ramus/body length while protracting the mandible forward. This technique may eliminate the requirement for bone harvest. It is most applicable when the TMJ is still present and functional although it may be hypoplastic. It does not improve the growth potential of the mandible but can lengthen the mandible decreasing the degree of deformity. It requires at least two operations; the first procedure to place the distraction device and perform the osteotomy and the second operation to remove the device. It may be difficult to control the vector of distraction. Extra-oral distraction devices can create significant facial scaring. Intraoral devices may cause significant fibrosis of the masseter muscle and around the mandible because of the two surgeries required for placement and removal of the device, making subsequent reconstruction surgery more difficult, and jaw function could be adversely affected. Significant dento-craniofacial deformity cannot be corrected concomitantly. The neo-condyle may be quite small and narrow mediolaterally, creating a significant increased load to the neo-condyle. These patients commonly require additional orthognathic and possibly TMJ reconstruction procedures to achieve satisfactory outcomes. Ascenco et al. [19] evaluated 33 HFM patients treated with distraction at an average age of 7.3 years with 5–15 years of follow-up. Recurrence of facial asymmetry occurred in 30 (91%) of the patients with all requiring orthognathic surgery. The authors concluded that bone distraction

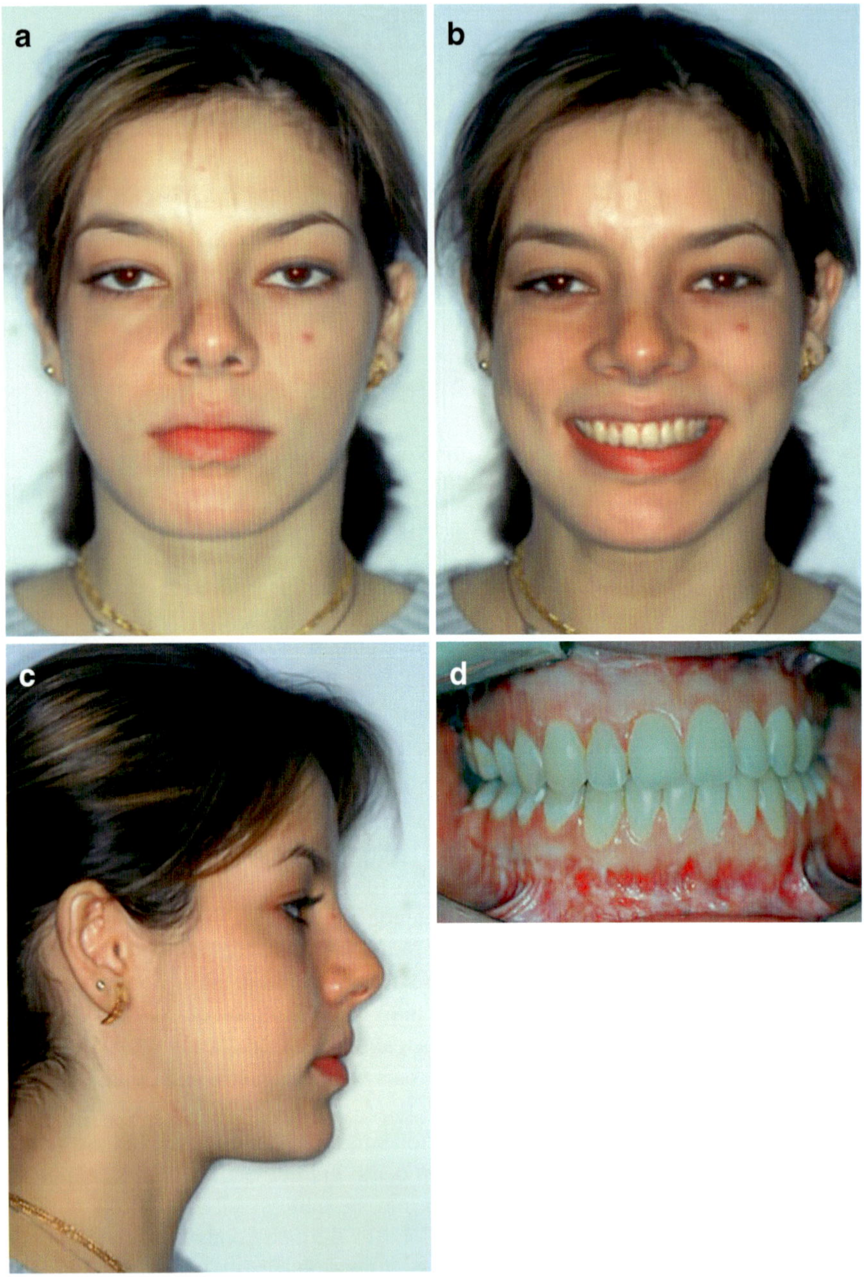

Fig. 6.9 *Case #1:* The patient is seen 2 years post-double-jaw orthognathic surgery demonstrating a good functional and esthetic outcome: (**a**, **b**) frontal views, (**c**) profile, and (**d**) occlusion

for HFM patients will require subsequent orthognathic surgery. TMJ ankylosis is also a significant risk with DO techniques.

Patient-Fitted TMJ Total Joint Prosthesis

There are two TMJ total joint prosthesis (TJP) systems in the USA approved by the Food and Drug Administration (FDA) for TMJ reconstruction: TMJ Concepts (Ventura, CA, USA) and Biomet Microfixation (Jacksonville, FL, USA). For application to HFM, a patient-fitted prosthesis is superior to a stock device.

Biomet Microfixation System

The Biomet Microfixation TMJ replacement system is a stock device (off-the-shelf) with several sizes to choose from for fossa and mandibular components. Biomet patient-fitted devices are not FDA approved for use in the USA but are available in other countries. Clinical trials for the stock device were initiated in 1995 and granted FDA approval in 2005. The ramus component is composed of a chromium cobalt alloy, but the side toward the ramus has a titanium coating to help with osseointegration. The ramus component is available in three lengths, 45, 50, and 55 mm, which limit adaptation for HFM patients. There are three basic styles including standard, offset, and narrow. The fossa component is composed of dense ultra-high-molecular-weight polyethylene (UHMWPE), with three fossa sizes to choose from including small, medium, and large. This is metal-on-polyethylene articulation, which is the gold standard in orthopedics. The mandibular component is stabilized to the ramus with 2.7-mm-diameter screws, and the polyethylene fossa component is secured to the lateral rim of the fossa with 2.0-mm-diameter screws. There is no osseointegration of the fossa component and no posterior stop in the fossa, rendering the standard stock prosthesis unsuitable for reconstruction of the HFM patient. The literature has demonstrated good outcomes using the stock device for indicated TMJ pathology [20–25]. Aagaard [26] has shown success using the patient-fitted Biomet device for TMJ reconstruction of end-stage TMJ pathology, but there are no reports on use for the HFM patients. The patient-fitted prosthesis does have a posterior stop on the fossa component, but no osseointegration. For HFM patients with the absence of the zygomatic arch and glenoid fossa, where the fossa component must be adapted to the temporal bone, this device is not recommended because of potential for screw loosening related to the thin temporal bone, unfavorable anatomical morphology, and lack of osseointegration of the device.

TMJ Concepts System

Developed originally in 1989 by Techmedica, Inc. (Camarillo, CA, USA) and since 1997 manufactured by TMJ Concepts, Inc. (Ventura, CA, USA), this patient-fitted TMJ total joint prosthesis is manufactured to meet the patient's specific anatomical requirements for TMJ reconstruction and mandibular repositioning. The fossa component is made of a commercially pure titanium (CPT) shell and four layers of CPT mesh bonded to the shell. UHMWPE is bonded to the titanium mesh to function as the articulating surface. The CPT mesh allows the fossa component to be fixated to the zygomatic arch, or the temporal bone if the arch and fossa are missing, with screws and provides a framework for osseointegration maximizing the long-term stability of the fossa component. The fossa component has a posterior stop to provide a centric relation position for the condylar head of the prosthesis, which is essential when the TMJ TJP is combined with orthognathic surgical procedures and particularly for reconstruction of the HFM patient. The mandibular ramus component is made of titanium alloy with a condylar head of cobalt-chromium-molybdenum alloy. This device provides a metal-on-polyethylene articulation which is the gold standard for orthopedic joint reconstruction. The titanium alloy composition of the mandibular component provides osseointegration with the underlying bone of the ramus. The TMJ Concepts TJP provides the ability to reconstruct the TMJ and advance the mandible and concomitantly perform orthognathic surgery at the same operation.

Virtual Surgical Planning (VSP)

Presurgery, a CT scan is acquired following the specific TMJ Concepts CT acquisition protocol. The CT data is sent to 3-D Systems (Littleton, CO) to develop a 3-D computer model of the patient's anatomical structures (Fig. 6.2a, b). The application of computer-assisted surgical simulation with virtual surgical planning (VSP) for cases requiring TMJ reconstruction with patient-fitted TJP and orthognathic surgery has significantly improved treatment quality by decreasing the preoperative workup time and increasing the accuracy of surgical preparation, and subsequent surgery. VSP is performed on the computer model, placing the maxilla and mandible into the planned final post-surgical position and occlusion (Fig. 6.2c, d). The indicated condylectomy (if any condylar remnant remains) and any necessary bony recontouring of the fossa or ramus can be done virtually (Fig. 6.2d). A 3-D stereolithic model is constructed with the maxilla and mandible in their final post-surgery position and sent to TMJ Concepts to manufacture the patient-fitted TJP (Fig. 6.10a, b) [27, 28]. HFM patients may be missing the zygomatic arch and glenoid fossa. The fossa component, therefore, can be designed to fit against the temporal bone where it can be fixated with bone screws with subsequent osseointegration (Fig. 6.3a,b). Extreme care must be exercised as the temporal bone in this area may be extremely thin,

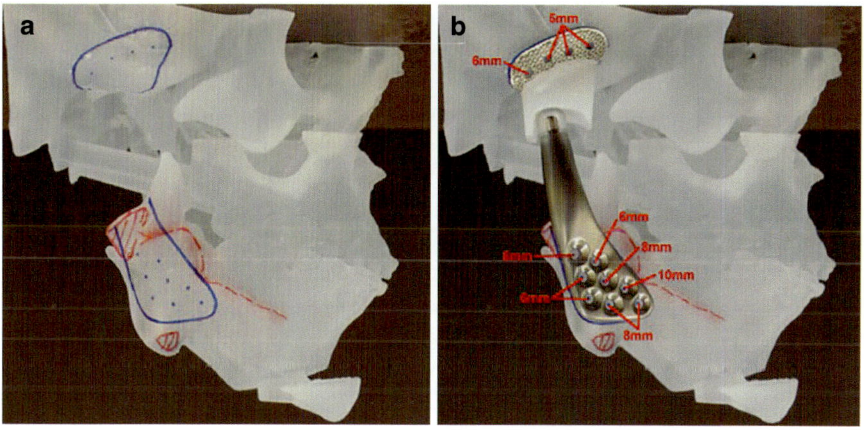

Fig. 6.10 (**a**) The 3-D stereolithic model demonstrates the outline of the fossa component on the temporal bone and also the outline of the mandibular component. The maxilla will be down grafted on the right side to level the transverse occlusal plane. Augmentation genioplasty is included. (**b**) The patient-fitted total joint prosthesis is shown on the model. The fossa component will be stabilized to the temporal bone with four bone screws. The titanium mesh will allow osteointegration of bone to stabilize the fossa component. Note the posterior stop on the fossa, necessary to support the prosthesis and mandible in its new position

1–2 mm. Drilling the holes for screw placement must be done very delicately to avoid damage to the dura and other middle cranial structures.

Two weeks prior to surgery, the final dental models are prepared. This usually requires one mandibular dental model and two maxillary models if the maxilla is to be segmentalized (one sectioned and used to establish the surgical occlusion and an uncut model). These models are sent to 3-D Systems for incorporation into the computer model for construction of the surgical splints. Two splints are produced: an intermediate splint used to reposition the mandible into its final position for stabilization of the contralateral mandibular ramus sagittal split osteotomy and for placement of the ipsilateral TMJ TJP, and a final palatal splint to stabilize the segmented maxilla (if indicated). Upon completion of manufacture by TMJ Concepts, the TMJ prosthesis is forwarded to the hospital, and the dental models and splints are forwarded to the surgeon.

Surgical Management of HFM Patients

Presurgical orthodontic preparation is usually required to obtain the best occlusal outcome.

The most consistently predictable treatment outcomes functionally and esthetically for the HFM (Type IIB and III) patients are achieved by reconstructing the TMJs and advancing the maxillo-mandibular complex in a counterclockwise direction with a patient-fitted TJP and orthognathic surgery. The TMJ Concepts system is the prosthesis of choice because of the material selection, patient-fitted design to meet the patient's specific anatomical requirements, presence of a defined posterior stop in the fossa component, and osseointegration of the fossa and mandibular components (Fig. 6.10a, b). For the HFM patient, a contralateral mandibular ramus sagittal split osteotomy is performed to aid in repositioning the mandible, and the indicated maxillary osteotomies are completed as well as any other adjunctive procedures (turbinectomies, nasoseptoplasty, genioplasty, rhinoplasty, etc.). All procedures can be done at one operation or separated into two or more operations if the surgeon prefers. Additional secondary reconstruction procedures to correct residual bony and soft tissue deficiencies may be necessary in more complex HFM cases using bone grafts, synthetic bone, alloplastic implants, etc. to build up the residual deformed skeletal structures as well as soft tissue reconstruction to fill out the soft tissue defects using fat grafts, tissue flaps, free vascularized grafts, and so on.

Surgical Sequencing

The surgical sequencing used by the author for treating HFM patients is outlined in Table 6.1. Since HFM cases can usually benefit from counterclockwise rotation of the maxillo-mandibular complex to get the best functional and esthetic outcome [29–32], repositioning the mandible first with the TJP and contralateral sagittal split osteotomy (before the maxillary osteotomies are performed) simplifies the model surgery, and splint construction improves the accuracy of the patient's surgery and outcome as compared to the traditional orthognathic surgical sequencing of performing the maxillary osteotomies first [33]. Performing the counterclockwise rotation of the mandible first will create posterior open bites, being greater on the ipsilateral side as the transverse cant of the mandibular occlusal plane is also corrected. If segmentalization of the maxilla is required to optimize the occlusion, a palatal splint is indicated to stabilize the upper arch and allow maximum interdigitation of the occlusion as the maxilla is stabilized [32]. Any ancillary procedures are then performed.

Patients with HMF commonly have sleep apnea issues as a result of the retruded mandible, decreased oropharyngeal airway, and/or nasal airway obstruction. Counterclockwise rotation of the maxillo-mandibular complex with advancement of the mandible is highly effective and predictable in opening the oropharyngeal airway. In conjunction with correcting any nasal airway obstruction (e.g., turbinectomies, nasoseptoplasty) post-surgery, these patients will have significant improvement in the airway and elimination of sleep apnea [34–36].

Table 6.1 Surgical sequencing for hemifacial microsomia requiring patient-fitted total joint prosthesis

1. Contralateral disc repositioning if displaced (Mitek anchor technique) through an endaural or preauricular incision
2. Ipsilateral side endaural or preauricular incision if the ear is present or adjacent to where the TMJ would be if the ear is severely deformed, mal-positioned, or absent. Dissect down to the temporal bone and beneath the cranial base
3. Ipsilateral condylectomy if condylar remnant present
4. Ipsilateral coronoidectomy if coronoid process present and detach the temporalis muscle
5. Submandibular approach to expose the hypoplastic mandibular angle/body and to detach the masseter and medial pterygoid muscles
6. Recontour ramus if indicated from the stereolithic model preparation
7. Mobilize the mandible with downward and forward traction
8. Contralateral mandibular ramus sagittal split osteotomy
9. Insert intermediate splint and apply MMF
10. Application of rigid fixation to contralateral mandibular ramus osteotomy. Closure of the intraoral incision
11. Placement of ipsilateral total joint prosthesis
12. Reattach masseter muscle(s) to the angle of the mandible and close submandibular incision
13. TMJ fat graft (harvested from the abdomen, buttock, or elsewhere) and pack around the articulation area of the prosthesis. Closure of incision
14. Remove MMF and intermediate splint
15. Maxillary osteotomies through vestibular incision, mobilization, segmentation, and placement of palatal stabilizing splint
16. Intranasal procedures if indicated (turbinectomies, nasal septoplasty, etc.)
17. MMF, maxillary stabilization with bone plates and bone or synthetic bone grafting, alar base cinch suture, and V-Y closure of vestibular incision
18. Remove IMF, check occlusion, and place light elastics
19. Other indicated procedures, i.e., genioplasty, rhinoplasty, facial augmentation, etc.
20. Secondary surgery when required for facial augmentation or other procedures to maximize functional and esthetic outcome

Surgical Protocol

The surgical procedures are done under general anesthesia with nasoendotracheal intubation. The HFM surgical sequencing is outlined in Table 6.1. The patient is prepared for surgery, and a Tegaderm dressing applied over the mouth and nose to seal off while performing the TMJ procedures. For the HFM patients with a contralateral TMJ disc displacement, an endaural incision is made, and disc repositioned and stabilized with the Mitek Mini Anchor (Mitek Products Inc. Westwood, MA) technique [37, 38]. The ipsilateral side is approached via an endaural or preauricular incision if the ear is present or adjacent to where the TMJ would be if the ear is severely deformed, mal-positioned, or absent. The zygomatic arch may be absent as well as the glenoid fossa; therefore the dissection is carried down to the temporal bone anterior to the internal meatus and extended medially beneath the cranial base to develop a pocket and foundation to place the patient-fitted fossa component. The superior aspect of the ramus is identified if present. A condylectomy is performed if there is a remnant that would interfere with the placement of the prosthesis. A coronoidectomy is performed if present. If the coronoid is severely hypoplastic or absent, the hypoplastic temporalis muscle, if present, is reflected from the remnant of the coronoid process.

An ipsilateral submandibular incision is made to expose the hypoplastic ramus/body, and the hypoplastic pterygo-masseteric sling is reflected off the mandible. A subperiosteal tunnel is created over the ramus to connect to the base of the temporal bone. The ipsilateral mandible is then mobilized so it can be repositioned downward and forward to advance the mandible to its new position; this is a critical aspect for the success of the surgery. If the mandible is not completely stripped of all its attachments and fully mobilized, an adequate position of the mandible may not be achieved. The soft tissues surrounding the mandible (skin and muscles) will usually stretch to accommodate large advancements. Any bony modifications to the fossa, temporal bone, or ramus/body of the mandible are completed as determined from the 3-D stereolithic model surgery workup.

The face is draped with sterile towels, Tegaderm incised, and oral cavity entered to perform a contralateral mandibular ramus sagittal split osteotomy using Wolford's modified technique [39, 40]. The mandible is mobilized, and a prefabricated intermediate occlusal splint is placed to position the mandible into its final predetermined position. Maxillo-mandibular fixation (MMF) is applied; the contralateral mandibular sagittal split osteotomy is stabilized with a bone plate and screws, and the incision closed. The face is re-prepped and resealed with a Tegaderm dressing, and the surgeon changes gloves and gown. The fossa component of the patient-fitted TMJ Concepts prosthesis is placed through the endaural/preauricular or temporal incision and secured to the lateral rim of the fossa if present or temporal bone with 4–5, 2-mm-diameter, 4-mm-length screws. The mandibular component is inserted through the submandibular incision, and the condyle seated into the fossa component against the posterior flange and secured to the ramus/body with 8–9, 2-mm-diameter bicortical screws. Fat is harvested from the abdomen through an umbilicus or suprapubic incision or from the buttock and packed around the fossa/condyle articulating area to prevent heterotrophic bone and scar tissue formation [41–44]. The incisions are closed.

MMF and the occlusal splint are removed. Through a maxillary vestibular incision, the maxillary osteotomies are completed. The maxilla is down-fractured, mobilized, and segmented when indicated, and palatal splint is secured in place. Intranasal procedures such as turbinectomies and/or nasal septoplasty are performed if indicated to eliminate pre-existing nasal airway obstruction. The new occlusion is established and secured with MMF. Four bone plates and screws are used to stabilize the maxilla with at least two screws above and two screws below the osteotomy site for each plate. Autogenous or synthetic bone grafts are placed into the osseous gaps in the lateral maxillary walls. An alar base cinch suture is placed to redefine nasal width, and the incision closed in a V-Y fashion [45]. MMF is removed, and light elastics applied to guide the occlusion and decrease stress on the muscles of mastication. Adjunctive procedures such as genioplasty, rhinoplasty, and so on are then completed. It is recommended that additional ipsilateral hard and soft tissue augmentation be performed at a secondary operation.

Periarticular Fat Grafts

With any of the TMJ reconstruction procedures using ABG or the alloplastic TMJ joint prosthesis, the placement of fat grafts around the articulating areas of the new joint significantly improves the treatment outcomes. The rationale for placing autologous fat grafts around the ABG or TJP is to obliterate the dead space surrounding the graft or prosthesis, thus preventing the formation and subsequent organization of a blood clot. Creating this physical barrier, the fat grafts serve to reduce the differentiation of pluripotential cells and prevent the formation of extensive fibrosis and heterotopic calcification at the TMJ articulation.

Wolford et al. [41–44] have previously reported a technique in which fat grafts harvested from the abdomen or buttock were packed around the articulating components of the total joint prosthesis. This technique significantly decreased the postoperative incidence of peri-implant fibrosis and heterotopic/reactive bone formation. Patients with fat grafts were shown to do better clinically with less pain and increased jaw function compared to similar patients reconstructed without fat grafts. Prior to the use of fat grafts, approximately 35% of patients with total joint prostheses required additional surgery to remove heterotopic/reactive bone and dense fibrosis that developed around the prostheses causing pain as well as limited TMJ and jaw function. Using the fat grafts has reduced reoperation to less than 2% for heterotrophic bone and fibrosis. Wolford also described the use of fat grafts to replace the deficient soft tissues in HFM patients on the ipsilateral side of the face [46].

Age of Surgical Intervention

The patient's age and symptoms can affect the treatment protocol. For instance, a HFM patient under the age of 12 years with severe hypoplasia and malformation or absence of the TMJ may benefit from a growth center transplant, using a CCG [3–5] or sternoclavicular graft [10, 11]. CCGs are unpredictable relative to growth and stability and often significantly overgrow creating a dentofacial deformity [5, 6]. Sternoclavicular grafts tend to have a better growth potential similar to normal TM growth and better stability than a rib graft [10]. With either graft system, there is a possibility that the grafts will not grow, overgrow, resorb, or fracture during the initial healing phase.

Another option for early intervention is the use of distraction osteogenesis [13–19]. This technique has shown mixed results in the literature with the problem that it requires multiple operations to place and remove the distractors, and it can lead to difficulty in controlling the vector of distraction. Lengthening of the ramus under the pressure of the pterygo-masseteric sling may be difficult to accomplish and may significantly overload the already hypoplastic TMJ causing further degenerative changes and risk of ankylosis. Orthognathic surgery is usually necessary following completion of growth to maximize the functional and esthetic results.

Predictability of results and limiting correction of the jaw and TMJ-related deformities to one major operation can best be achieved by waiting until growth is relatively complete, provided that the patient is functionally and psychologically stable. Females usually have the majority of their facial growth (98%) complete by the age of 15 years, and males by the age of 17–18 years [47]. Since asymmetric growth is a component of HFM and some required orthognathic surgical procedures may have further adverse effects on subsequent facial growth, performing orthognathic surgery during the growing years may result in the need for additional surgery at a later time to correct asymmetry, antero-posterior discrepancy, and malocclusion that may develop during the completion of growth.

There are definite indications for early surgery such as requirement for growth center transplant (i.e., rib or sternoclavicular grafts) or distraction, to correct masticatory dysfunction, airway obstruction, sleep apnea, and psychological factors. Wolford et al. have previously published on maxillary and mandibular orthognathic surgery and the effects on growth, with age consideration guidelines for surgical intervention [48–50], as well as age consideration and surgical treatment protocols for the common TMJ pathological conditions [51]. HFM patients have one side of the mandible with a normal-growing condyle that rarely requires TMJ reconstruction; thus the recommendation to wait until growth of that condyle is complete to achieve predictable treatment outcomes with one surgical intervention for correction of the TMJ, skeletal, occlusal, and airway issues.

Early treatment with a patient-fitted TMJ TJP can also be considered during growth as it is more stable and predictable than CCG or SCG, but without growth potential. Over-correction with the TJP may be indicated by over-advancing and creating an ipsilateral posterior open bite. This may require additional surgery after cessation of normal growth. This could require changing out the mandibular component for a longer component verses additional orthognathic surgery.

Outcome Studies

Relative to the HFM patient, there are important studies relative to the various surgical technique outcomes, and of particular interest are comparison studies evaluating the outcomes between ABG and TJP for TMJ reconstruction.

Comparative Studies: Autogenous Bone Grafts Versus Alloplastic TMJ Reconstruction

There have been a few comparison studies of autogenous tissues versus total joint prostheses.

Henry and Wolford [52] in 1993 reported a study of 107 patients in whom autogenous tissue grafts or Techmedica TJP were placed to reconstruct the TMJs severely damaged by failed Vitek Inc. Proplast/Teflon TMJ devices. A 4-year follow-up subjective and objective evaluation of pain, occlusal stability, and jaw function reported the percentages of successful outcomes for each autogenous tissue graft (costochondral, 12%; sternoclavicular, 21%; dermal, 8%; temporal fascia, 13%; temporal fascia with mandibular sagittal split osteotomies, 31%; auricular cartilage, 25%). The Techmedica TMJ TJP had an 86% success. Although this was a different TMJ pathology than HFM, it showed superiority of TMJ TJP over autogenous tissues.

Freitas et al. [53] in 2002 compared outcomes for costochondral grafts, sternoclavicular grafts, and total joint prostheses. They evaluated 12 patients with 24 operated joints. Six patients received costochondral grafts or sternoclavicular grafts, and six patients received TMJ Concepts total joint prostheses. The follow-up ranged from 48 to 58 months. The total joint prostheses provided statistically significant better objective and subjective outcomes, decreased the operating room time, and produced significantly better skeletal and occlusal stability particularly when the maxilla and mandible were advanced.

Wolford et al. [54] in 2010 evaluated 13 patients with TMJ ankylosis with the age range of 5–15 years. Four patients received CCGs, six SCGs, and three TJPs with a follow-up of 2–13 years. Seven of the 13 patients had fat grafts packed around the reconstructed TMJs. Of the four CCGs, three grafts demonstrated excessive overgrowth. None of these CCGs had fat placed around them, and all four re-ankylosed. Four patients received SCGs and had fat grafts packed around the articulating area of the grafts. There was no re-ankylosis in this group, and they had good jaw function, although decreased translation ability. Two of the SCGs did not receive fat grafts and both re-ankylosed. With the SCGs, bony remolding occurred under increased loading to the joints with mandibular advancement resulting in occlusal changes. Three patients received TJPs with fat packed around the prostheses. There was no re-ankylosis nor mandibular relapse. The TJP incisal opening presurgery ranged from 2 to 29 mm, and post-surgery ranged from 35 to 52 mm, demonstrating good outcomes. The use of fat grafts packed around the articulation area of the SCGs and around the TJP prevented re-ankylosis of the TMJs.

Saeed et al. [55] in 2002 evaluated 49 patients with 66 CCGs and 50 patients with 68 TJPs using the Christensen system (TMJ, Inc. Golden, CO, USA) with metal on-metal articulation. The mean follow-up ranged from 43 to 49 months, and the mean age was 38 years. The authors reported complications in 27 patients with CCG and 34 patients that received the TJP. However, the authors reported 26 of 49 CCG patients (53%) required reoperation, whereas only 6 of 50 TJP patients (12%)

required reoperation. The TJP provided better subjective and objective outcomes. The authors recommended TJP in cases of ankylosis, multiply operated joints, and previously failed alloplastic implants.

Key Points
These comparative studies demonstrate the following:

1. TJPs provide better outcomes relative to pain, function, stability, and esthetics compared to autogenous bone grafts.
2. With the use of TJP, concomitant TMJ and orthognathic surgery can be performed at the same operation with highly predictable outcomes relative to skeletal and occlusal stability, function, esthetics, and decrease in pain.
3. TJPs work better in poorly vascularized tissues compared to free autogenous grafts.
4. Packing fat grafts around the articular area of the autogenous grafts or TJP decreases the risk of heterotopic bone formation and ankylosis, increases function, and decreases pain.

TMJ Concepts Outcome Studies

There have been more than 150 papers published in reference to the use of the TMJ Concepts TJP. The efficacy of TMJ Concepts TJP has been well documented in the literature by numerous studies including those by Wolford et al. [52–54, 56, 57] and Mercuri et al. [58–60]

Coleta et al. [61] in 2008 evaluated 47 female patients for surgical stability after bilateral TMJ reconstruction using TMJ Concepts TJP, TMJ fat grafts, and counterclockwise rotation of the maxillo-mandibular complex with the mandible advancing an average of 18.4 mm. At an average follow-up of 40.6 months, the surgical results remained very stable (no relapse).

Pinto et al. [62] in 2008 evaluated the same 47 female patients for pain and dysfunctional outcomes. Significant improvements (37–52%) were observed for TMJ pain, headaches, jaw function, diet, and disability. Jaw opening increased 14%. These two studies showed that patients with end-stage TMJ pathology could be treated in one operation with TMJ Concepts TJP, fat grafts, and correction of an associated dentofacial deformity with good stability and improvement in pain and TMJ function.

Although the life expectancy of the TMJ Concepts TJP is unknown, Wolford et al. [63] published a 21-year follow-up study of 56 patients who had received the Techmedica TJP between 1989 and 1993. There were statistically significant improvements for incisal opening, jaw function, TMJ pain, and diet, with 85.7% of the patients reporting significant improvement in their quality of life. There were no reports of device removal due to material wear or failure.

TMJ Total Joint Prosthesis in Treating Hemifacial Microsomia Patients

Wolford et al. [64] in 2012 introduced the use of TMJ Concepts total joint prosthesis for the treatment of HFM. They evaluated six HFM patients treated with this surgical protocol. The average age at surgery was 23.5 years (range from 14 years to 39 years), and the average follow-up was 6 years and 2 months (range from 1 year to 11.4 years). For all subjective parameters including facial pain, headaches, TMJ pain, jaw function, diet, and disability, all patients improved or remained the same. Incisal opening improved from 36.3 to 39.2 mm. The mean surgical changes showed the forward horizontal movement of anterior nasal spine (ANS) was 1.3 mm, upper incisor tip (U1T) advanced 7.4 mm, lower incisor tip (L1T) 8.9 mm, point B 14.8 mm, pogonion (Pog) 18.6 mm, and menton (Me) 17.5 mm. The occlusal plane angle (OPA) decreased by a mean −12.3°. Post-surgical stability analysis demonstrated point A, PNS, and U1T moved approximately 1 mm posteriorly at long-term follow-up. All mandibular anatomical points remained very stable as did the OPA with virtually no change at 6 years post-surgery. Two patients (33%) had concomitant contralateral disc displacement repaired with the Mitek anchor technique with good outcomes.

Polley et al. [65] in 2019 reported on a multicenter study of ten HFM patients treated with reconstruction of the ipsilateral side with TMJ Concepts total joint prosthesis, contralateral mandibular ramus osteotomy, and Le Fort I osteotomy. The cases were reported to have good outcomes with improved incisal opening, stable occlusion, and improved facial balance. However, no cephalometric evaluation for surgical change and stability or subjective evaluation relative to pain, diet, disability, or quality of life was reported.

Case Presentations

Case #1 This 10-year-old female had right sided-HFM, Kaban Type III, with absent right TMJ (Figs. 6.5a–d and 6.6a). She was treated at 10 years old with a right TMJ and mandibular reconstruction with a SCG and a left ramus inverted "L" osteotomy and genioplasty to advance the mandible in a counterclockwise rotation creating posterior open bites, significantly greater on the right side to level the mandible horizontally (Fig. 6.6b). Post-surgery, the occlusion was leveled orthodontically. She grew symmetrically post-surgery with active growth of the SCG equal to the contralateral side through the age of 18 years (Figs. 6.7 and 6.8a). At 18 years old, routine double-jaw orthognathic surgery was performed to correct the residual dentofacial deformity to maximize the functional and esthetic result (Fig. 6.8b). The patient is seen 2 years post-orthognathic surgery (Fig. 6.9a–d). Maximal incisal opening was 38 mm, excursive movement to the right 5 mm, to the left 3 mm, no pain issues, and a stable Class I occlusion. Although this case had a great result relative to growth of the SCG and nice functional and esthetic result, some cases with SCG grafts have compromised outcomes relative to deficient growth of the graft.

Case #2 This 28-year-old male had right-sided HFM, Kaban Type III (Figs. 6.11a–f and 6.12a). He had 15 prior jaw and facial surgeries including 3 failed CCGs to reconstruct the right TMJ, previous double-jaw orthognathic surgery with an aug-

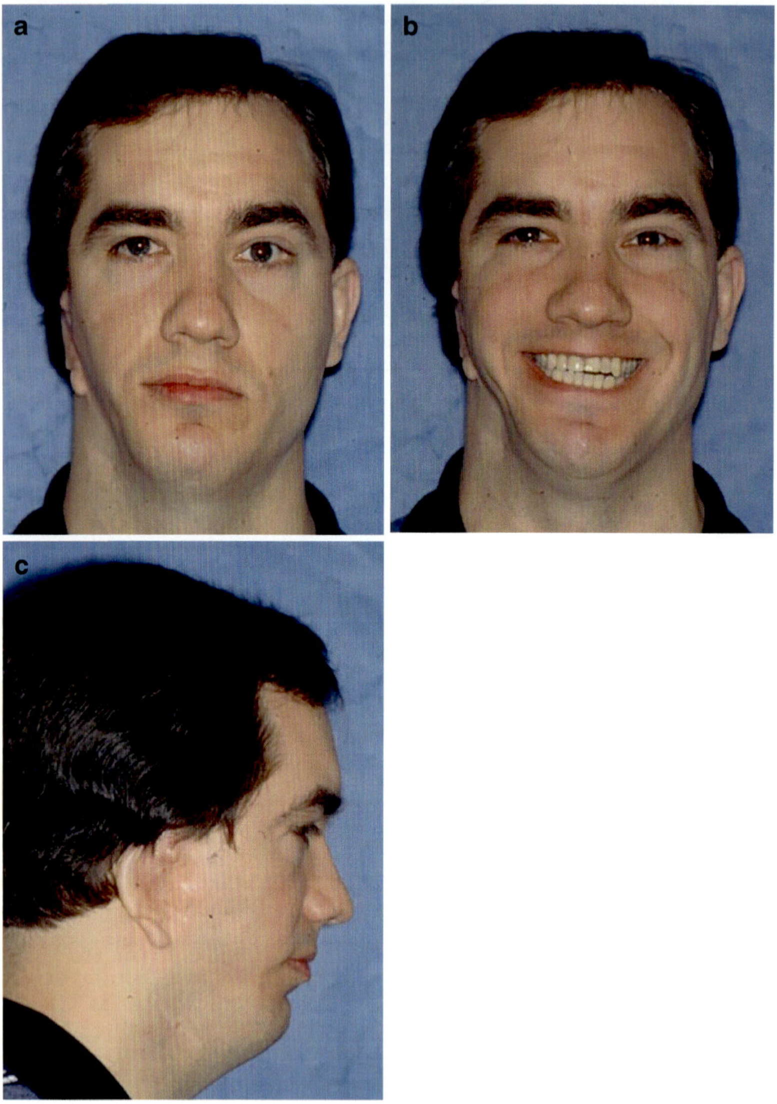

Fig. 6.11 *Case #2:* (**a**–**c**) A 28-year-old male with right-sided HFM (Kaban Type III), maxillomandibular hypoplasia and asymmetry and nasal airway obstruction. (**d**–**f**) Class II cuspid relationship on the right with anterior and left posterior open bite and a transverse cant of the occlusal plane. Surgical procedures included right TMJ reconstruction and counterclockwise rotation mandibular advancement with patient-fitted total joint prosthesis; left mandibular sagittal split osteotomy; multiple maxillary osteotomies; fat graft around right TMJ prosthesis; and partial turbinectomies, nasoseptoplasty, A–P reduction genioplasty, and removal of deformed right ear

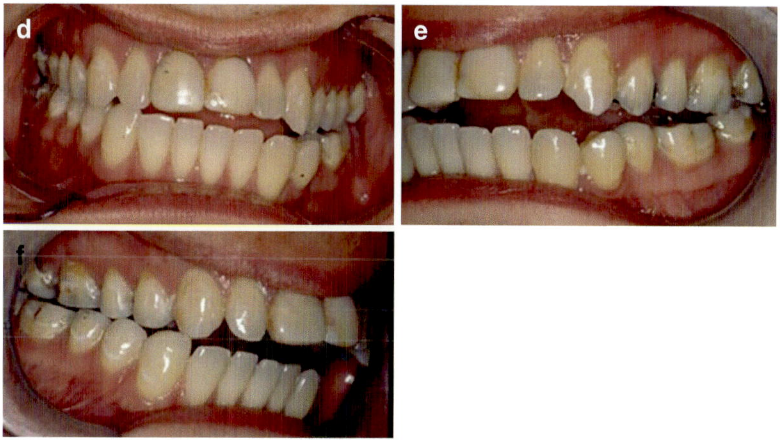

Fig. 6.11 (continued)

mentation genioplasty, and multiple right ear surgeries. His MIO was 50 mm, right lateral excursion 6 mm, and left 2 mm; maxillary dental midline was 2 mm to the right, mandibular dental midline 4 mm to the right, and the chin was shifted 10 mm to the right and retruded 15 mm. He occluded only on the right posterior teeth and had an anterior and left posterior open bite with a Class II occlusion on the right side. He had a transverse skeletal and soft tissue deficiency on the right side of 15–20 mm compared to the left side. There was a transverse cant of the occlusal plane with the right cuspid 5 mm higher compared to the left cuspid. Presurgery facial pain/headache was 5 (0 = no pain and best function; 10 = worst pain imaginable and no function), left TMJ pain 7, jaw function 6, diet 4, and disability 0. Presurgical orthodontics included aligning and leveling the arches. Surgery included the following: (1) reconstruct right TMJ and counterclockwise rotation and mandibular advancement with TMJ Concepts patient-fitted total joint prosthesis, (2) right TMJ fat graft harvested from the abdomen, (3) left TMJ articular disc reposition with a Mitek Anchor, (4) left mandibular ramus sagittal split osteotomy, (5) multiple maxillary osteotomies with counterclockwise rotation, (6) A–P reduction genioplasty, (7) bilateral partial turbinectomy, (8) nasoseptoplasty, and (9) removal of deformed right ear (Fig. 6.12b, c). At a secondary procedure, he had osseointegrated implants placed in the right temple area with a right prosthetic ear constructed. The patient is seen at 4 years post-surgery (Fig. 6.13a–f) with improved facial balance. His MIO was 45 mm, right lateral excursion 2 mm, left lateral excursion 2 mm, pain 0, headaches 0, jaw function 3, and diet 3. Surgical stability and occlusion remained stable.

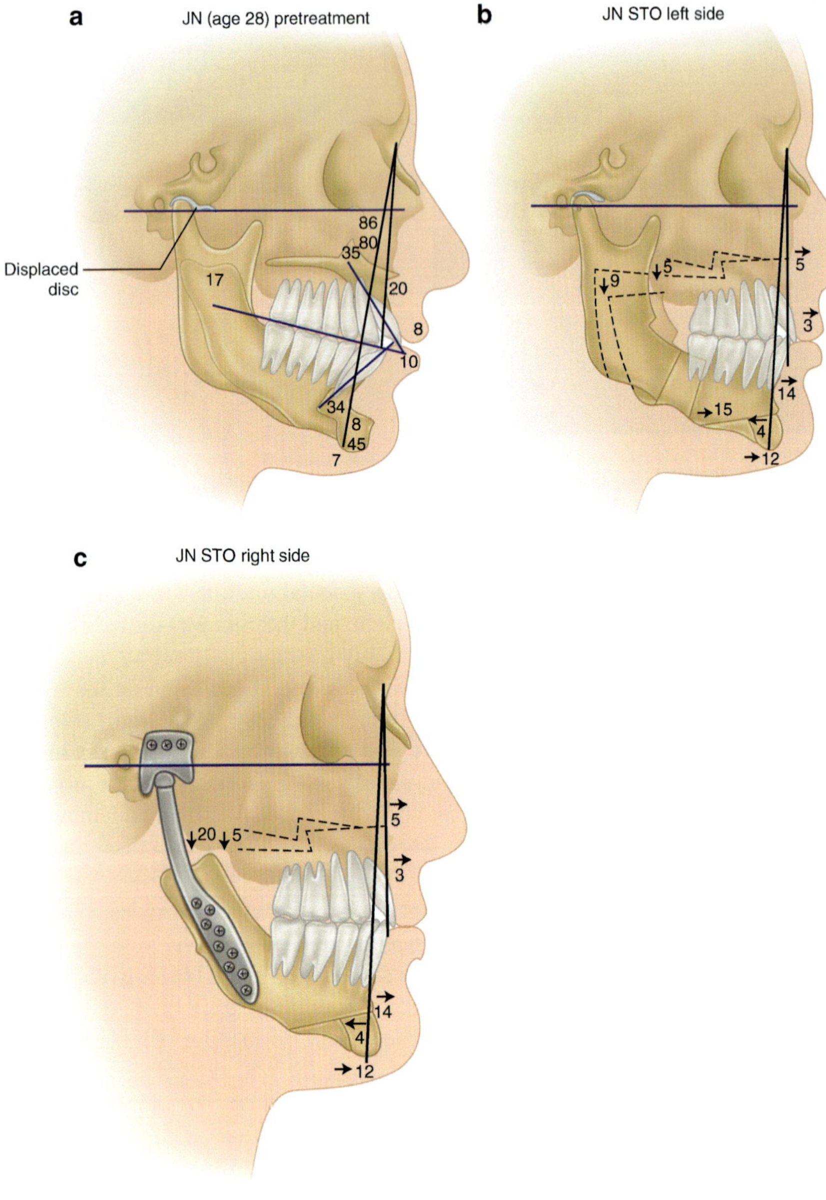

Fig. 6.12 *Case #2:* (**a**) Cephalometric analysis shows the retruded mandible and maxilla with a high occlusal plane angle. (**b**, **c**) Prediction tracings demonstrate the significant counterclockwise rotation of the maxillo-mandibular complex of the mandible on the left side advanced with a sagittal split osteotomy and on the right side the mandible advanced and lengthened vertically with the TMJ Concepts TJP

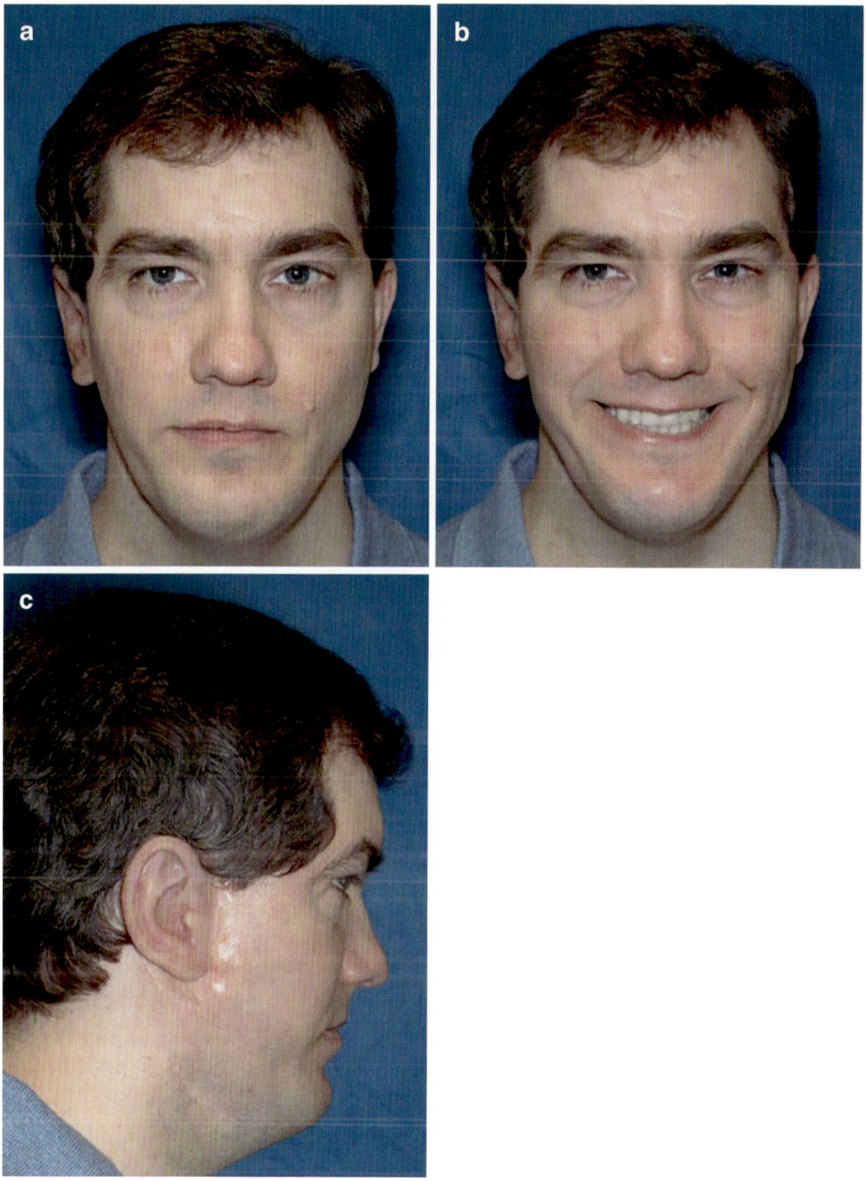

Fig. 6.13 *Case #2:* (**a–c**) The patient is seen 4-years post-surgery with improved facial balance and excellent surgical stability. (**d–f**) He has a stable Class I occlusion. He was pain-free with improved jaw function and esthetics

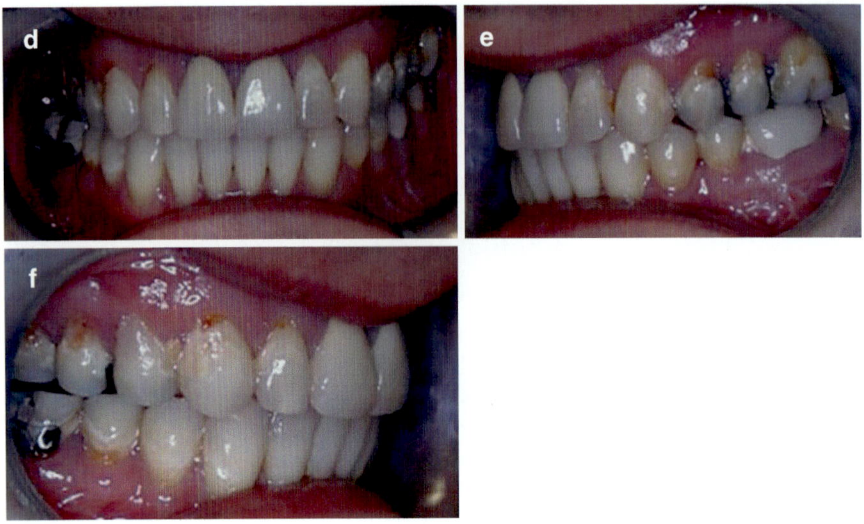

Fig. 6.13 (continued)

Case #3 This 15-year-old female was born with left-sided Goldenhar HFM, Kaban Type III, left transverse facial cleft, and cleft palate (Figs. 6.14a–f and 6.15a). She had several previous surgeries including repair of a left transverse facial cleft at 5 months and cleft palate repair at 1 year. A SCG and cranial bone grafts for reconstruction of the left ramus and TMJ joint were performed at age 6 years. Although the graft took, it did not grow (Fig. 6.16a). Presurgery MIO was 33 mm, right excursion 1 mm, left excursion 5 mm, facial pain/headache 0, TMJ pain 0, jaw function 1, diet 1, and disability 0. AP chin deficiency was 20 mm, mandibular dental midline was 7 mm, and chin midline 14 mm to the left. Presurgical orthodontics aligned and leveled the arches. At age 15 years, she was surgically treated with left TMJ reconstruction and mandibular counterclockwise rotation advancement with TMJ Concepts patient-fitted total joint prosthesis including simultaneous reconstruction of the left ramus with cranial bone grafts (Fig. 6.16b–d), left TMJ fat graft harvested from the abdomen, right mandibular ramus sagittal split osteotomy, multiple maxillary osteotomies, and nasal turbinectomies (Fig. 6.15b). A secondary surgical stage was performed at age 16 that included a sliding genioplasty to augment her chin and a fat graft to the left side of the face to augment the soft tissue defect (Fig. 6.17a–d). The patient is seen at 4 years post-surgery (Figs. 6.15c and 6.18a–f) with improved facial balance and function; MIO was 35 mm, right lateral excursion 1 mm, left excursion 3 mm, facial pain/headaches and TMJ pain 0, jaw function 1, diet 0, disability 0, and facial nerve function was unchanged compared to presurgery.

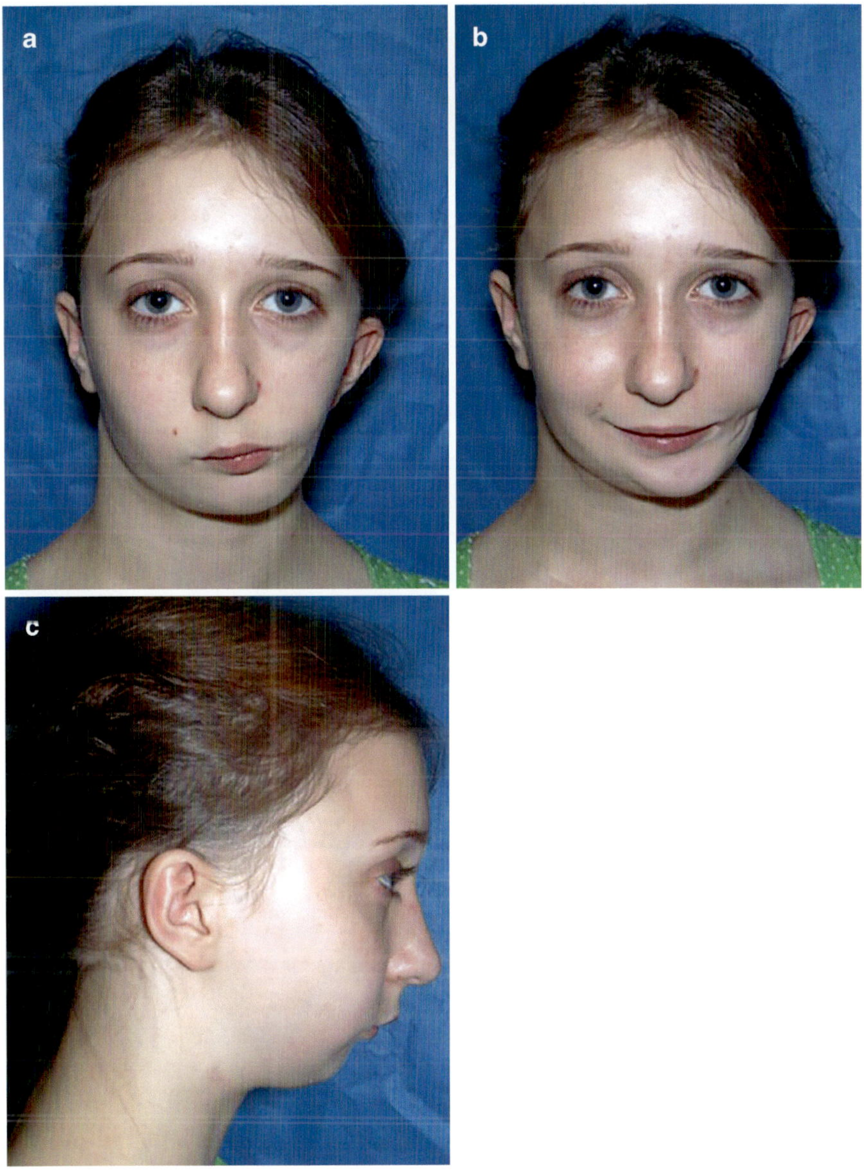

Fig. 6.14 *Case #3:* (**a–c**) A 15-year-old female with left-sided HFM (Kaban Type III), repaired transverse facial cleft, maxillo-mandibular hypoplasia and asymmetry, nasal airway obstruction, and (**d–f**) Class II end-on occlusion and transverse cant of the occlusal plane. Surgical procedures included the following: (Stage 1) Left TMJ reconstruction mandibular advancement with total joint prostheses, right mandibular sagittal split osteotomy, multiple maxillary osteotomies, fat graft around left TMJ prosthesis, and partial turbinectomies. (Surgery Stage 2) AP augmentation osseous genioplasty, fat graft to left mandibular facial area, and reposition left ear

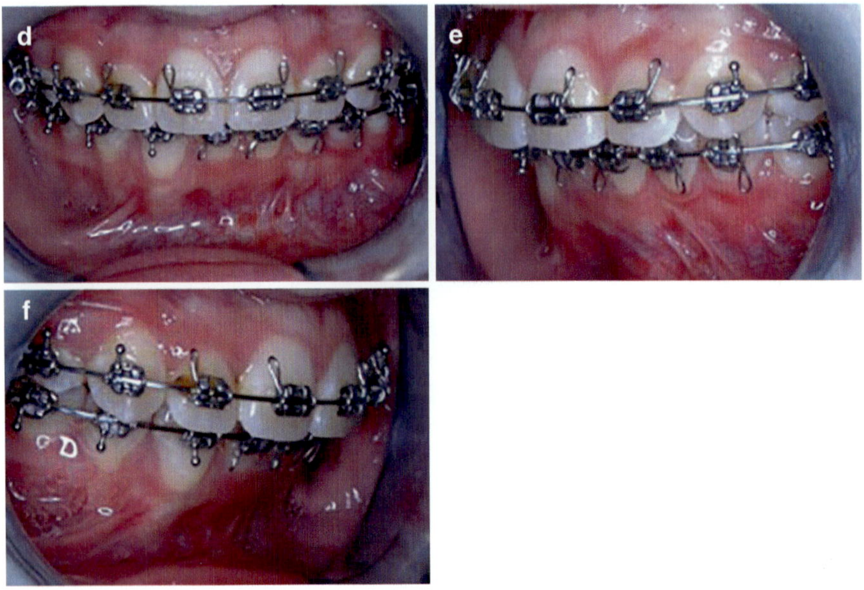

Fig. 6.14 (continued)

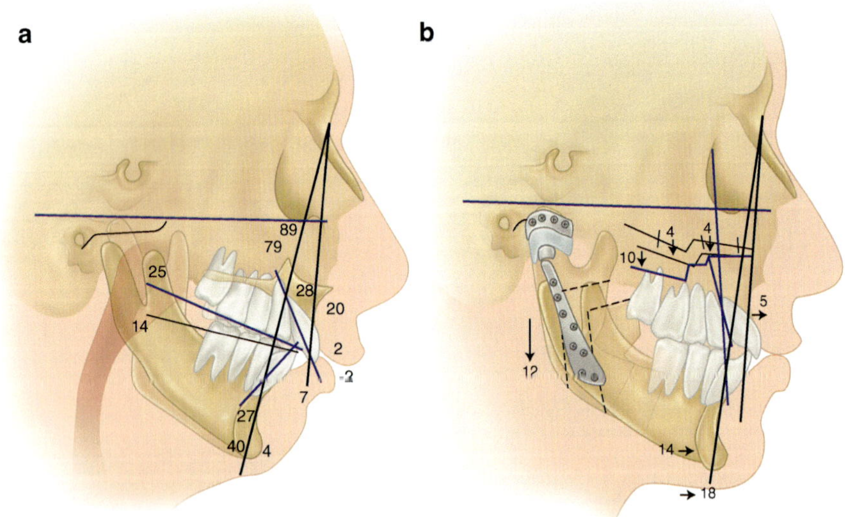

Fig. 6.15 *Case #3:* (**a**) Presurgery lateral cephalogram shows the vertical asymmetry and significant retrusion of the mandible and maxilla. Green lines represent the right side and red lines the left side. (**b**) Prediction tracing demonstrates the proposed surgical treatment outcome. (**c**) A 4-year follow-up radiograph shows the patient maintained good stability of the jaw structures

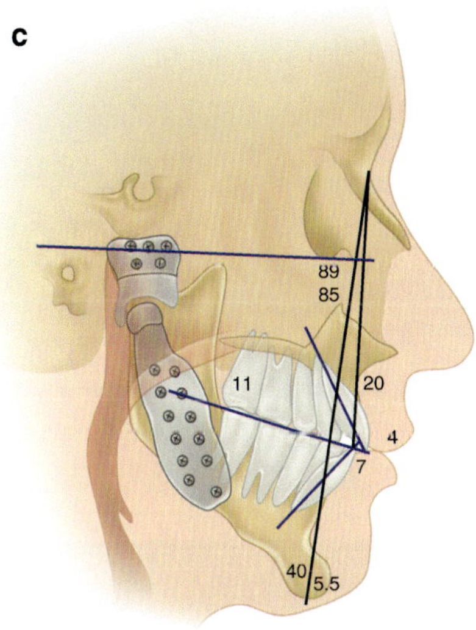

Fig. 6.15 (continued)

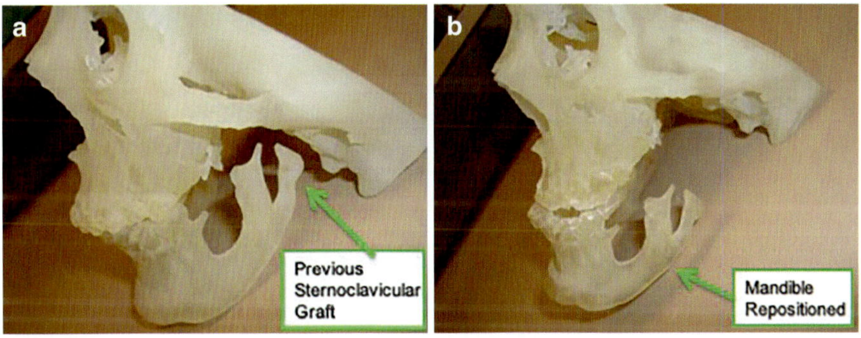

Fig. 6.16 *Case #3:* (**a**) 3-D stereolithic model depicting the patient's anatomy. The SCG was placed at age 6 years but did not grow. (**b**) The mandible was mobilized and repositioned in a counterclockwise direction to lengthen the ramus as well as advanced and transversely level the mandibular occlusal plane. (**c**) The left ramus was to be reconstructed with cranial bone grafts, and the pink wax-up demonstrates the expected size, shape, and positioning of the grafts. The TJP would be constructed on the wax-up. (**d**) TMJ Concepts manufactured a patient-fitted prosthesis to accommodate the patient's specific anatomical requirements which included the concomitant cranial bone grafts to reconstruct the left ramus in conjunction with the other orthognathic surgical procedures

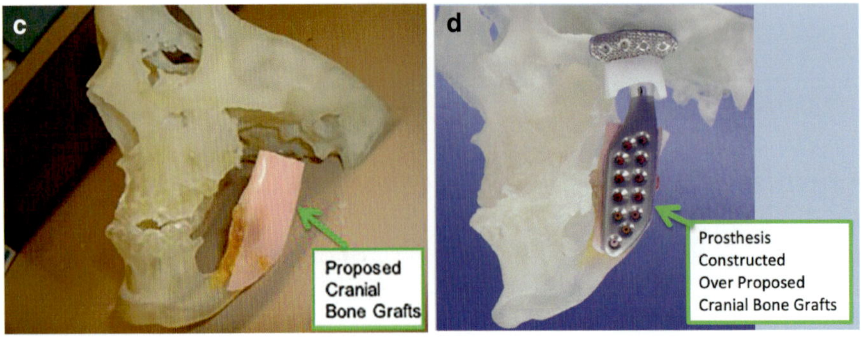

Fig. 6.16 (continued)

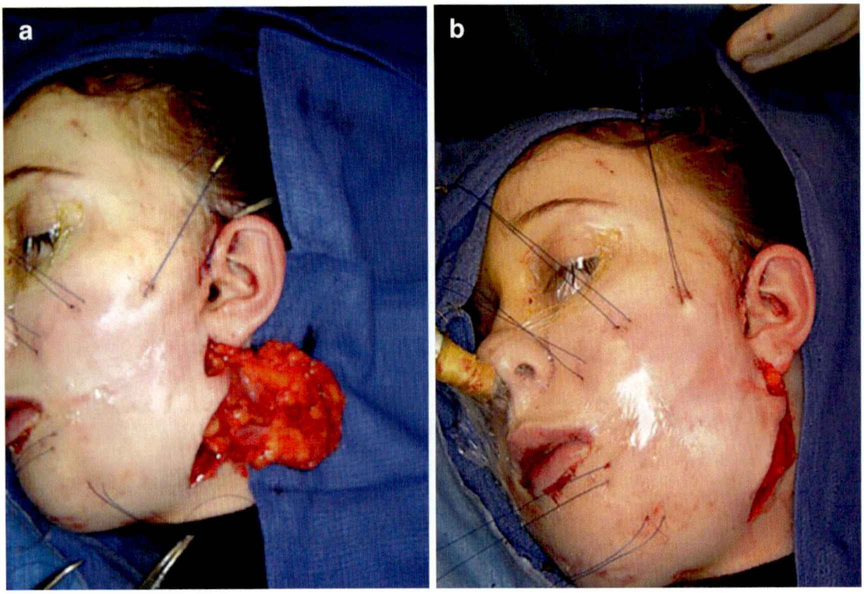

Fig. 6.17 *Case#3:* Following Stage 1 surgery, there was still a significant deficiency in soft tissue in the left side of the face. (**a**) A retromandibular incision was made, and soft tissues undermined creating a pocket of predetermined size to accommodate the fat graft. An abdominal fat graft was harvested and transplanted into the left side of the face. Sutures are passed at the extension of the tissue pocket dissection and attached to the fat graft to aid in delivery. (**b**) The fat graft has been delivered into position with the aid of the traction sutures which are maintained for 7–10 days. (**c**, **d**) The patient is seen 1-week post-surgery. The cotton balls on the cheek indicate areas of traction sutures to extend the graft and minimize the tendency for it to "ball-up" in the cheek

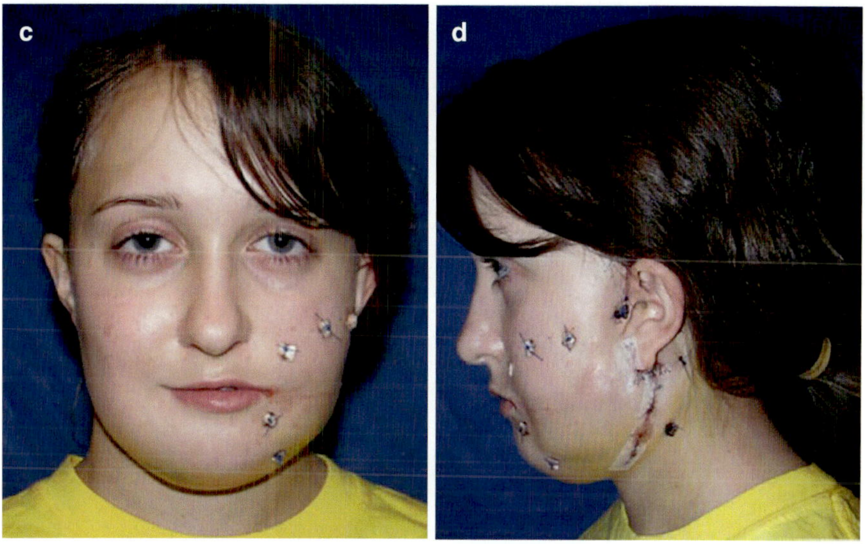

Fig. 6.17 (continued)

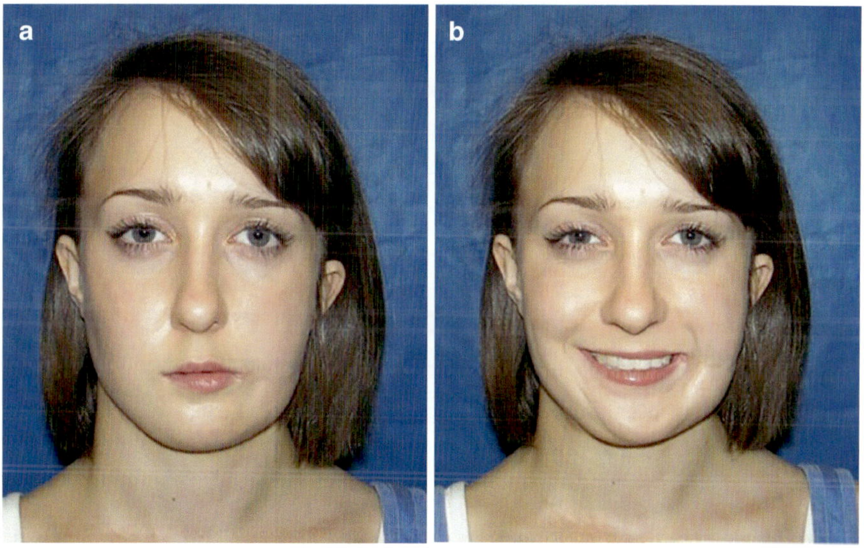

Fig. 6.18 *Case #3:* (**a–c**) The patient was seen 4 years and 2 months post-surgery demonstrating significantly improved facial balance with good jaw and TMJ function. (**d–f**) She has maintained a stable Class I occlusion

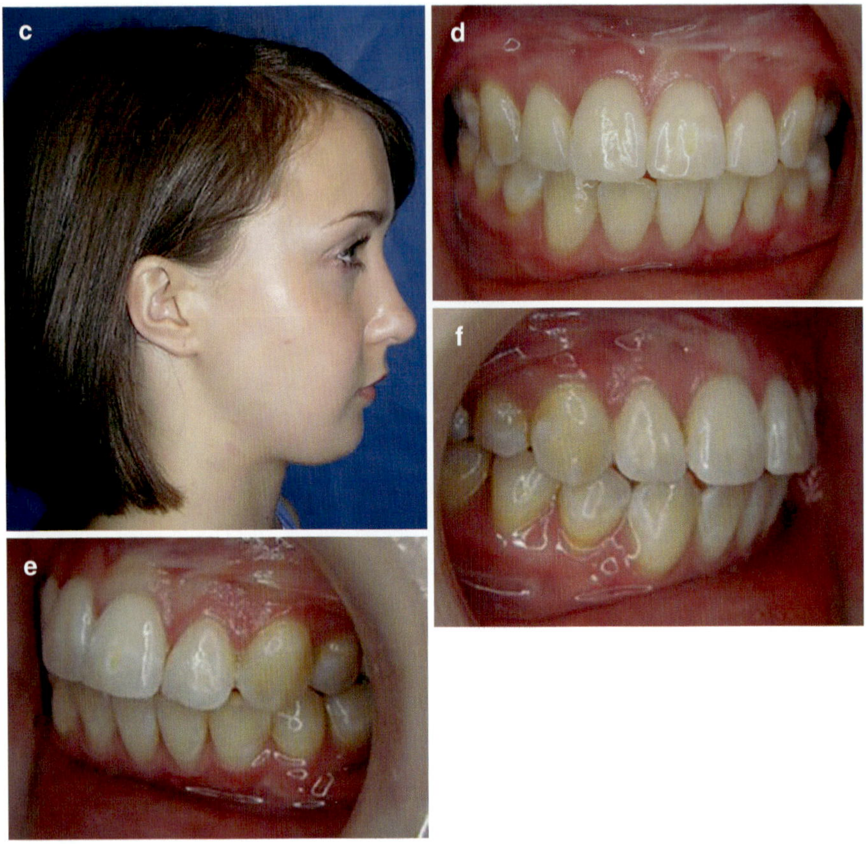

Fig. 6.18 (continued)

Summary

Many options have been proposed for surgical correction of Kaban Type IIB and III HFM patients. For many years the most popular technique to reconstruct the deformed or absent TMJ was ABG including CCG and SCG, but results are not predictable and stable when the maxilla and mandible require surgical repositioning, particularly advancement and vertical lengthening of the ipsilateral ramus. Distraction osteogenesis has also become popular to lengthen the hypoplastic mandible and works best with an existing ipsilateral TMJ. The distraction vectors may be difficult to control, and most cases will require secondary orthognathic surgery to optimize the functional and esthetic outcomes. The literature shows that ABGs are not reliable in providing predictable treatment outcomes relative to stability of skeletal and occlusal relationships, particularly if performed concomitant with orthognathic surgery, as significant relapse can be expected related to graft remodeling, flexibility, warping, fracture, extended healing time, loading, and biological responses. In addition, there can be significant donor and recipient site complications.

The TMJ Concepts patient-fitted TJP in conjunction with orthognathic surgery for TMJ and jaw reconstruction is a valid option for patients with HFM. Research has clearly demonstrated that TMJ and orthognathic surgery can be safely and predictably performed at the same operation to surgically correct the facial deformities associated with HFM [64, 65] but does necessitate the correct diagnosis and treatment plan as well as requires the surgeon to have expertise in both TMJ and orthognathic surgery. The application of computer-assisted surgical simulation with virtual surgical planning (VSP) for cases requiring TMJ reconstruction with patient-fitted TJP and orthognathic surgery has significantly improved treatment quality by decreasing the preoperative workup time and increasing the accuracy of surgical preparation and subsequent surgery [25, 26].

Corrective surgical procedures for HFM can be performed in childhood if indicated for functional, psychological, or airway issues such as growth center transplants (CCG, SCG) or distraction. Patient-fitted TJP can also be considered as there is less chance of complications compared to AGB. Any of these procedures done in childhood will require additional surgery at a later time for optimal functional and esthetic outcomes. In order to do one-stage surgery for the TMJ reconstruction and orthognathic surgery phase, it would be best to delay until 15 years old for females and 17–18 for males when at the end of pubertal growth. Using TMJ TJP in conjunction with orthognathic surgery provides the patient with a better, more predictable, and functional result compared to multiple-staged ABG reconstructions done early. No other surgical technique is able to provide the amount of mandibular advancement, ramus lengthening, and stability as the patient-fitted TMJ TJP to correct the severely deformed HFM patient.

Conclusion

TMJ Concepts TJPs are superior to ABGs for TMJ reconstruction in the HFM patient population for the following reasons: (1) no bone harvest required eliminating donor site morbidity; (2) osseointegration of the TMJ Concepts fossa and mandibular components provides long-term stability; (3) posterior stop on the fossa component stabilizes the joint, jaw position, and occlusion; (4) concomitant orthognathic surgery can be performed at the same time as the TMJ is reconstructed with predictable outcomes even with large skeletal changes and advancements; (5) fat grafts packed around the articulating area of the prostheses improve outcomes relative to decreased pain, improved jaw function, and decreased requirement for repeat surgery; (6) highly predictable outcomes relative to skeletal and occlusal stability, TMJ and occlusal function, esthetics, and improvement in the airway; and (7) a 20-year follow-up study on TMJ Concepts TJP demonstrated improvements in pain, jaw function, diet, incisal opening, and quality of life, with no removal of devices secondary to failure or wearing out.

References

1. Grabb WC. The first and second branchial arch syndrome. Plast Reconstr Surg. 1965;36:485.
2. Gorlin RJ, Cohen MM Jr, Hemekam RCM. Syndromes of the head and neck. 4th ed. Oxford Universe Press; New York, 2001. p. 790–7.
3. Miliken JB, Kaban LB. Analysis and treatment of hemifacial microsomia in childhood. Clin Plast Surg. 1987;14:91–100.
4. Kaban LB, Moses MH, Mulliken JB. Surgical correction of hemifacial microsomia in the growing child. Plast Reconstr Surg. 1988;82:9.
5. Ware WH, Brown SL. Growth centre transplantation to replace mandibular condyles. J Maxillofac Surg. 1981;9:50.
6. Peltomaki T, Quevedo LA, Jeldes G, Ronning O. Histology of surgically removed overgrown osteochondral rib grafts. J Craniomaxillofac Surg. 2002;30:355.
7. Munro IR, Phillips JH, Griffin G. Growth after construction of the temporomandibular joint in children with hemifacial microsomia. Cleft Palate J. 1989;26:303.
8. Mulliken JB, Ferraro NF, Vento RA. A retrospective analysis of growth of the constructed condyle-ramus in children with hemifacial microsomia. Cleft Palate J. 1989;26:312.
9. Hawkins A, Mercuri LG, Miloro M. Are rib grafts still used for temporomandibular joint reconstruction? J Oral Maxillofac Surg. 2020;78:195–202.
10. Wolford L, Cottrell D, Henry C. Sternoclavicular grafts for TMJ reconstruction. J Oral Maxillofac Surg. 1994;52:119–28.
11. Resnick CM, Genuth J, Calabrese CE, Taghinia A, Labow BI, Padwa BL. Temporomandibular joint ankylosis after ramus construction with free fibula flaps in children with hemifacial microsomia. J Oral Maxillofac Surg. 2018;76(9):2001.e1–2001.e15. PMID: 29852140.
12. Singh V, Bhagol A, Verma A, Kumar I. Reconstruction of ankylosed TMJ: sternoclavicular grafting as an approach to management. Int J Oral Maxillofac Surg. 2011;40:260–5.
13. Skamoto Y, Nakajima H, Ogata H, Kishi K. The use of mandibular body distraction in hemifacial microsomia. Ann Maxillofac Surg. 2013;3:178–81.
14. Nakajima H, Sakamoto Y, Tamada I, Ogata H, Kishi K, Sakamoto T. Maxillary-driven simultaneous maxillo-mandibular distraction for hemifacial microsomia. J Craniomaxillofac Surg. 2011;39:549–53.
15. Meazzini MC, Mazzoleni F, Gabriele C, Bozzetti A. Mandibular distraction osteogenesis in hemifacial microsomia: long-term follow-up. J Craniomaxillofac Surg. 2005;33:370–6.
16. Nada RM, Sugar AW, Wijdeveld MG, Borstlap WA, Clauser L, Hoffmeister B, et al. Eurocran distraction osteogenesis group. Current practice of distraction osteogenesis for craniofacial anomalies in Europe: a web based survey. J Craniomaxillofac Surg. 2010;38:83–9.
17. Paeng JY, Lee JH, Lee JH, Kim MJ. Condyle as the point of rotation for 3-D planning of distraction osteogenesis for hemifacial microsomia. J Craniomaxillofac Surg. 2007;35:91–102.
18. Scolozzi P, Herzog G, Jaques B. Simultaneous maxillo-mandibular distraction osteogenesis in hemifacial microsomia: a new technique using two distractors. Plast Reconstr Surg. 2006;117:1530–41
19. Ascenco ASD, Balbinot P, Junior IM, D'Oro U, Busato L, da Silva FR. Mandibular distraction in hemifacial microsomia is not a permanent treatment: a long-term evaluation. J Craniofac Surg. 2014;25:352–4.
20. Giannakopoulos HE, Sinn DP, Quinn PD. Biomet microfixation temporomandibular joint replacement system: a 3-year follow-up study of patients treated during 1995 to 2005. J Oral Maxillofac Surg. 2012;70(4):787–94; discussion 795–6.
21. Machon V, Hirjak D, Beno M, Foltan R. Total alloplastic temporomandibular joint replacement: the Czech-Slovak initial experience. Int J Oral Maxillofac Surg. 2012;41(4):514–7.

22. Leandro LF, Ono HY, Loureiro CC, Marinho K, Guevara HA. A ten-year experience and follow-up of three hundred patients fitted with the Biomet/Lorenz microfixation TMJ replacement system. Int J Oral Maxillofac Surg. 2013;42(8):1007–13.
23. Dimitroulis G. Comparison of the outcomes of three surgical treatments for end-stage temporomandibular joint disease. Int J Oral Maxillofac Surg. 2014;43(8):980–9.
24. Westermark A. Total reconstruction of the temporomandibular joint. Up to 8 years of follow-up of patients treated with Biomet((R)) total joint prostheses. Int J Oral Maxillofac Surg. 2010;39:951–5.
25. Sanovich R, Mehta U, Abramowicz S, Widmer C, Dolwick MF. Total alloplastic temporomandibular joint reconstruction using Biomet stock prostheses: the University of Florida experience. Int J Oral Maxillofac Surg. 2014;43(9):1091–5.
26. Aagaard E, Thygesen T. A prospective, single-centre study on patient outcomes following temporomandibular joint replacement using a custom-made Biomet TMJ prosthesis. Int J Oral Maxillofac Surg. 2014;43(10):1229–35.
27. Movahed R, Teschke M, Wolford LM. Protocol for concomitant temporomandibular joint custom-fitted total joint reconstruction and orthognathic surgery utilizing computer- assisted surgical simulation. J Oral Maxillofac Surg. 2013;71:2123–9.
28. Wolford LM. Computer-assisted surgical simulation for concomitant temporomandibular joint custom-fitted total joint reconstruction and orthognathic surgery. In: Sullivan S, editor. Techniques in orthognathic surgery, Atlas of the oral & maxillofacial surgery clinics, vol. 24; 2016. p. 55–66.
29. Wolford LM, Chemello PD, Hilliard FW. Occlusal plane alteration in orthognathic surgery. J Oral Maxillofac Surg. 1993;51:730.
30. Wolford LM, Chemello PD, Hilliard FW. Occlusal plane alteration in orthognathic surgery part I: effects on function and esthetics. Am J Orthod Dentofac Orthop. 1994;106:304.
31. Chemello PD, Wolford LM, Buschang MS. Occlusal plane alteration in orthognathic surgery-part II: long-term stability of results. Am J Orthod Dentofac Orthop. 1994;106:434.
32. Wolford LM, Goncalves JR. Surgical planning in orthognathic surgery and outcome stability. In: Brennan PA, Schliephake H, Ghali GE, Cascarini L, editors. Maxillofacial surgery. 3rd ed. St. Louis: Elsevier Inc.; 2017. p. 1048–126.
33. Cottrell DA, Wolford LM. Altered orthognathic surgical sequencing and a modified approach to model surgery. J Oral Maxillofac Surg. 1994;52:1010.
34. Mehra P, Wolford LM. Surgical management of obstructive sleep apnea. Proc (Bayl Univ Med Cent). 2000;13:338.
35. Mehra P, Downie M, Pitta MC, Wolford LM. Pharyngeal airway space changes after counterclockwise rotation of the maxillo mandibular complex. Am J Orthod Dentofac Orthop. 2001;120:154.
36. Goncalves JR, Buschang PH, Goncalves DG, Wolford LM. Postsurgical stability of oropharyngeal airway changes following counter-clockwise Maxillo-mandibular advancement surgery. J Oral Maxillofac Surg. 2006;64:755.
37. Wolford LM, Cottrell DA, Karras SC. Mitek Mini Anchor in maxillofacial surgery. Proceedings of SMST-94, the First International Conference on Shape Memory and Superelastic Technologies, 1995, Monterey, CA. MIAS: 477–482.
38. Mehra P, Wolford LM. The Mitek Mini Anchor for TMJ disc repositioning: surgical technique and results. Int J Oral Maxillofac Surg. 2001;30:497.
39. Wolford LM, Davis WM Jr. The mandibular inferior border split: a modification in the sagittal split osteotomy. J Oral Maxillofac Surg. 1990;48:92.
40. Wolford LM. The influence of osteotomy design on the bilateral mandibular ramus sagittal split osteotomy. J Oral Maxillofac Surg. 2015;73:1994–2004.
41. Wolford LM, Karras SC. Autologous fat transplantation around temporomandibular joint total joint prostheses: preliminary treatment outcomes. J Oral Maxillofac Surg. 1997;55:245–51.

42. Wolford LM, Morales-Ryan CA, Garcia-Morales P, Cassano DS. Autologous fat grafts placed around temporomandibular joint total joint prostheses to prevent heterotopic bone formation. Proc (Bayl Univ Med Cent). 2008;21:248.
43. Wolford LM, Cassano DS. Autologous fat grafts around temporomandibular joint (TMJ) total joint prostheses to prevent heterotopic bone. In: Shiffman MA, editor. Autologous fat transfer. Berlin Heidelberg: Springer; 2010. p. 361–82.
44. Mercuri LG, Ali FA, Woolson R. Outcomes of total alloplastic replacement with periarticular autogenous fat grafting for management of reankylosis of the temporomandibular joint. J Oral Maxillofac Surg. 2008;66(9):1794–803.
45. Guymon M, Crosby DR, Wolford LM. The alar base cinch suture to control nasal width in maxillary osteotomies. Int J Adult Orthodon Orthognath Surg. 1988;2:89.
46. Reiche-Fischel O, Wolford LM, Pitta M. Facial contour reconstruction using an autologous free fat graft: a case report with 18-year follow-up. J Oral Maxillofac Surg. 2000;58:103.
47. Riolo ML, Moyers RE, McNamara JA, Hunter WS. An atlas of craniofacial growth: cephalometric standards from the university school growth study, the University of Michigan. Ann Arbor: University of Michigan; 1974. p. 105–6.
48. Wolford LM, Karras SC, Mehra P. Considerations for orthognathic surgery during growth, part 1: mandibular deformities. Am J Orthod Dentofac Orthop. 2001;119:95.
49. Wolford LM, Karras SC, Mehra P. Considerations for orthognathic surgery during growth, part 2: maxillary deformities. Am J Orthod Dentofac Orthop. 2001;119:102.
50. Wolford LM, Rodrigues DB. Orthognathic considerations in the young patient and effects on facial growth. In: Preedy VR, editor. Handbook of growth and growth monitoring in health and disease. New York: Springer; 2012. p. 1789–808.
51. Wolford LM, Rodrigues DB. Temporomandibular joint (TMJ) pathologies in growing patients: effects on facial growth and development. In: Preedy VR, editor. Handbook of growth and growth monitoring in health and disease. New York: Springer; 2012. p. 1809–28.
52. Henry CH, Wolford LM. Treatment outcomes for TMJ reconstruction after Proplast- Teflon implant failure. J Oral Maxillofac Surg. 1993;51:352–8.
53. Frietas R, Mehra P, Wolford L. Autogenous versus alloplastic TMJ reconstructionin rheumatoid-induced TMJ disease. J Oral Maxillofac Surg. 2002;58:43.
54. Wolford L, McPhillips A, Rodrigues D. TMJ ankylosis in children: comparison of 3 methods of joint reconstruction. J Oral Maxillofac Surg. 2010;68:e57.
55. Saeed N, Henscher R, McLeod N, Kent J. Reconstruction of the TMJ: autogenous compared to alloplastic. Br J Oral Maxillofac Surg. 2002;40:296–9.
56. Wolford LM, Cottrell DA, Henry CH. Temporomandibular joint reconstruction of the complex patient with the Techmedica custom-made total joint prosthesis. J Oral Maxillofac Surg. 1994;52:2.
57. Wolford LM, Pitta MC, Reiche-Fischel, Franco PF. TMJ concepts/Techmedica custom-made TMJ total joint prosthesis: 5-year follow-up. Int J Oral Maxillofac Surg. 2003;32:268.
58. Mercuri LG, Wolford LM, Sanders B, White RD, Hurder A, Henderson W. Custom CAD/CAM total temporomandibular joint reconstruction system: preliminary multicenter report. J Oral Maxillofac Surg. 1995;53(2):106–15.
59. Mercuri LG, Wolford LM, Sanders B, White RD, Giobbie-Hurder A. Long-term follow-up of the CAD/CAM patient fitted total temporomandibular joint reconstruction system. J Oral Maxillofac Surg. 2002;60(12):1440–8.
60. Mercuri LG, Edibam NR, Giobbie-Hurder A. Fourteen-year follow-up of a patient-fitted total temporomandibular joint reconstruction system. J Oral Maxillofac Surg. 2007;65(6):1140–8.
61. Coleta KE, Wolford LM, Gonçalves JR, Pinto AS, Pinto LP, Cassano DS. Maxillo- mandibular counter-clockwise rotation and mandibular advancement with TMJ Concepts total joint prostheses: part I – skeletal and dental stability. Int J Oral Maxillofac Surg. 2009;38:126.
62. Pinto LP, Wolford LM, Buschang PH, Bernardi FH, Gonçalves JR, Cassano DS. Maxillo-mandibular counter-clockwise rotation and mandibular advancement with TMJ Concepts

total joint prostheses: part III – pain and dysfunction outcomes. Int J Oral Maxillofac Surg. 2009;38:326.

63. Wolford LM, Mercuri LG, Schneiderman ED, Movahed R, Allen W. Twenty-year follow-up study on a patient-fitted temporomandibular joint prosthesis: the Techmedica/TMJ concepts device. J Oral Maxillofac Surg. 2015;73(5):952–60.
64. Wolford LM, Bourland TC, Rodrigues D, Perez DE, Limoeiro E. Successful reconstruction of nongrowing hemifacial microsomia patients with unilateral temporomandibular joint total joint prosthesis and orthognathic surgery. J Oral Maxillofac Surg. 2012;70(12):2835–53.
65. Polley JW, Girotto JA, Fahrenkopf MP, Dietze-Fiedler ML, Kelly JP, Taylor JP, Lazarou SA, Demetriades NC. Salvage or solution: alloplastic reconstruction in hemifacial microsomia. Cleft Palate Craniofac J. 2019;56:896–901.

Chapter 7
Definitive Reconstruction of Associated Maxillomandibular Deformities in Craniofacial Microsomia

Fabio G. Ritto, Paul W. Orjuela, Kevin S. Smith, and Paul S. Tiwana

Introduction

Craniofacial microsomia (CFM) has a wide range of clinical presentations, and the treatment will be determined by a number of factors such as the patients' complaints, severity of the disease, and existing comorbidities. This chapter will discuss the definitive treatment for the CFM patient, and therefore it will address patients that have reached skeletal maturity or skeletal stability, where any residual growth that may occur will not compromise the surgical result.

Growing and Skeletal Maturity

Skeletal maturity is usually reached around 14–16 years old in girls and 15–17 years in boys [1]. Different studies have been performed to evaluate the potential growth of the affected mandibular side in a CFM patient. Most of the studies have shown that the asymmetry present at the early age is carried throughout the adolescence [2–5]. This means that the ramus is stable horizontally and vertically, even in the most dramatic type III cases. In 2020 Meazzini et al. [6] published a long-term study with 20 type III patients, 10 of which were submitted costochondral graft (CCG) reconstruction and 10 were not submitted to any surgical procedure. The authors concluded that restoring the height of the ramus with a CCG leads to an immediate restitution of facial symmetry, but in the long term, there is a return to the asymmetrical pattern. In the control group, the asymmetry was stable during years

F. G. Ritto · P. W. Orjuela · K. S. Smith· P. S. Tiwana (✉)
Department of Oral & Maxillofacial Surgery, The University of Oklahoma Health Sciences Center, Oklahoma City, OK, USA
e-mail: Fabio-Ritto@ouhsc.edu; Wilmer-Orjuela@ouhsc.edu; Kevin-Smith@oushc.edu; Paul-Tiwana@ouhsc.edu

D. M. Yates, M. R. Markiewicz (eds.), *Craniofacial Microsomia and Treacher Collins Syndrome*, https://doi.org/10.1007/978-3-030-84733-3_7

with no increase of the facial deformity. Therefore, it can be concluded that definitively treating the patient after skeletal maturity seems to be a reasonable treatment option, since it reduces the number of necessary procedures and eliminates growth as a stability factor.

Another philosophy states that the asymmetry is progressive, especially on the most severe type IIB and III cases, and that operating the mandible during mixed dentition would be more appropriate to correct the facial asymmetry [7, 8]. The surgery generates an open bite on the affected side that needs to be managed with an acrylic splint, so that the maxilla won't grow asymmetrically to compensate the open bite, which would generate a vertical asymmetry. The splint needs to be progressively trimmed to adjust to the maxillomandibular growth. The elongation of the mixed dentition mandible is achieved either by costochondral graft (CCG) reconstruction of the TMJ, which has several potential complications, or by distraction osteogenesis. Meazzini et al. [4] demonstrated that even though aesthetic and psychological advantages of early mandibular distraction osteogenesis are well accepted, early surgery should only be applied after careful patient selection and honest clarification of the long-term recurrence by a predetermined guided craniofacial growth pattern.

When patients are operated early on in life, the chances of them needing orthognathic surgery after reaching skeletal stability are relatively high. Therefore, it may be advantageous to follow these patients and defer the definitive treatment for the maxillomandibular deformities until after skeletal maturation.

For this reason, the authors' preferred approach in the treatment of CFM patient is to wait for skeletal maturity; personal experience and scientific data have demonstrated that this approach delivers the most favorable outcomes [9, 10].

Clinical Presentation

The malocclusion commonly seen in CFM is proportional to the degree of skeletal asymmetry. These patients are five times more likely to have missing teeth than the general populations. Usually the hypoplastic side will display crowding, crossbite, and inclination of incisors toward the affected side [11]. The craniofacial surgeon and orthodontist will have to establish clear communication in order to properly time dental extractions and dentoalveolar decompensation prior to surgery. Once the patient is orthodontically ready for surgery, the pre-operative workup will consist of a clinical examination, composite photos, imaging, and dental records. With the use of all acquired information, a surgical plan is designed as mentioned above; the surgical splints and guides are fabricated according to the specific plan.

The findings in the craniofacial microsomia patients are broad, depending on the severity, and may include angle class II anterior open bite; transverse cant in the occlusal plane and skeletal structures; hypoplasia or absence of mandibular condyle, ramus, and body on the affected side and decreased posterior facial height; diminished horizontal projection; retruded and deviated chin; hypoplastic maxilla, zygomatico-orbital complex, and temporal bone; hypoeruption and/or partial anodontia; and decreased airway volume and sleep apnea [12, 13]. The discrepancies created by the upward cant in the maxilla, gonial angles, and pyriform apertures are better appreciated in the coronal plane; planning the leveling of the discrepancies in this plane is a proper starting point [14].

The most important factor to be evaluated before determining the definitive treatment of the associated maxillofacial deformities is the health and stability of the temporomandibular joint. Notice that the shape of the TMJ components is not of paramount concern, since they will almost invariably have some degree of deformation.

As a general rule, healthy joints provide adequate function without eliciting pain. When this concept is applied to the temporomandibular joints, a stable and reproducible occlusion must be present, along with adequate range of motion and absence of joint pain. It is important however to differentiate articular disorders from muscular disorders, since the latter not necessarily interfere with the surgical stability. It is outside the scope of this chapter to discuss the diagnosis of temporomandibular disorders.

Adequate function for CFM patients can be considered when a mouth opening between 35 and 45 mm is present and protrusion and lateral movements between 5 and 10 mm can be achieved. Deviations during opening are normal in these patients, since there is usually a size discrepancy between the right and left joints. Active joint disease will usually present with pain, occlusal changes, cortical defects, subchondral cysts, and osteophytes. A thick cortical bone usually denotes a stable condyle.

Another important aspect on the clinical evaluation is the soft tissue. The skeletal asymmetry will be exacerbated due to soft tissue deficiency, which will range from thinner muscles to atrophy of all soft tissues that surround the facial bones (muscle, fascia, subcutaneous tissue, skin, and mucosa). In severe cases some muscles may be absent. Obtaining perfect skeletal symmetry after orthognathic surgery should be the goal, and Padwa et al. in 1997 [15] found that a four-degree asymmetry on the occlusal cant is the threshold for recognition by 90% of trained and untrained individuals and, therefore, a four-degree range seems to be a clear and reasonable goal to pursue. However, because of the soft tissue impairment, it is almost impossible to achieve perfect facial symmetry with skeletal surgery alone. Applying fillers to the soft tissue is a good alternative to improve facial balance after the skeletal surgery has been performed.

Treatment Plan

The concept of natural head position is extremely valuable on these patients, since it is difficult to find reliable anatomical landmarks to orient the head position. Gross head inclinations have to be adjusted during clinical evaluation and planning, but some degree of head tilting usually remains after surgery. Goldenhar patients often present with some degree of cervical spine involvement, which makes head positioning and planning even more difficult.

Virtual surgical planning (VSP) has a very important role in obtaining bone symmetry. Mounting models on a semi-adjustable articulator was a real challenge in this group of patients, because their external auditory canal is usually absent. The first thing to do in the virtual platform is to orient the CT volume according to the patient's natural head position, and different options have been described for that purpose [16–18]. There are different sequences that can be used when performing VSP, but the maxillary position is usually used as a reference to correct the occlusal plane cant, pitch, and yaw, and the mandible will follow the maxillary position.

After having the skeletal face reconstructed on the virtual platform, with the scanned dental arches superimposing the CT teeth, the first thing to do is set the final occlusion, driving the lower arch to match with the upper. To facilitate visualization, hide the mandible and focus on the maxillary position, but move both jaws while performing any movement. Start the planning by correcting the cant according to the facial evaluation, either by maxillary impaction or down grafting. After that align the upper arch midline with the facial midline, and adjust the yaw as necessary to obtain horizontal symmetry. Remember that moving the maxillomandibular complex to correct the yaw will influence both the buccal corridors and the outline of the face over the mandibular angles. Perform any vertical and anteroposterior corrections deemed necessary on the maxilla, and adjust the occlusal plane on the sagittal view. After the maxilla is in a good position, un-hide the mandible proximal segments and chin position. Further adjustments on the yaw, occlusal plane, and chin position might be accomplished to obtain the best possible facial balance.

Three-dimensional planning is extremely important, since the correction of one dimension will either positively or negatively affect the other two dimensions. For instance, when the mandible is rotated vertically to correct the occlusal cant, the distal segment on the non-affected side will push the proximal segment exacerbating the facial fullness. On the other hand, when a sagittal split osteotomy is used to rotate the mandible horizontally, correcting the lower midline, the ramus on the affected side will be pushed laterally by the distal segment, while the ramus on the contralateral side will move medially, improving the facial balance at the ramus level (Fig. 7.1).

Once the final plan is reached, the splints can be constructed virtually according to the surgeon's preference in terms of surgical sequence mandible or maxilla first. Since the TMJs are usually not stable, and it may be difficult to obtain records on centric relation, it seems more reasonable to start surgery on the mandible and then cut the maxilla. Customized guides such as cutting and positioning guides are extremely effective for transferring the VSP to the surgical scenario, but they require more complex softwares for the regular VSP ones and add extra costs that are usually not necessary for the conventional orthognathic cases, but are precious for the CFM patients.

Aligning the occlusal plane correctly in all three planes will not generate a symmetric face in the CFM patient. The mandible is small along the ramus, body, and symphysis, and further procedures are necessary to correct the facial balance. The

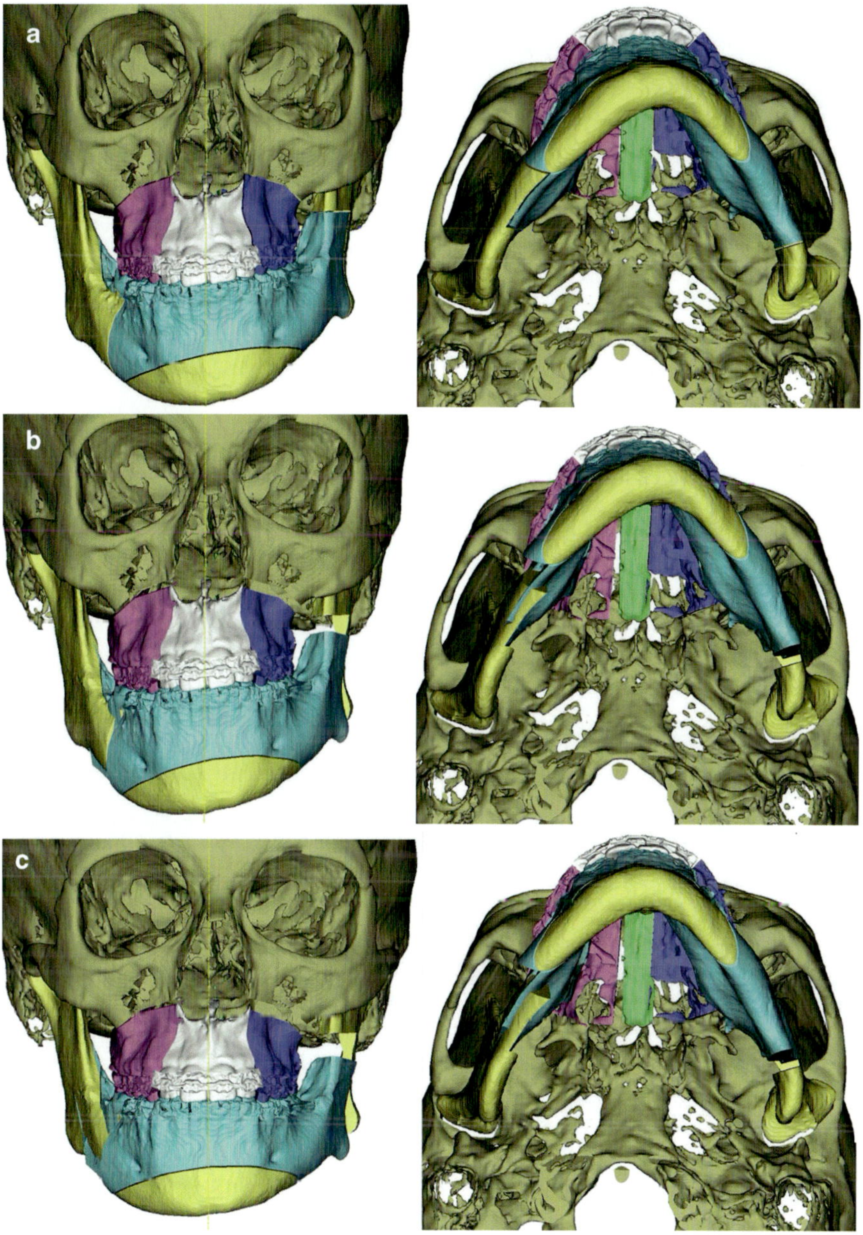

Fig. 7.1 Planning the maxillomandibular complex three-dimensional movements, frontal and submentovertex views: (**a**) initial view after the CT has been positioned according to the patient's natural head position; (**b**) the mandible is taken to the final occlusion against the maxilla; (**c**) the complex is rotated vertically to correct the cant and notice how the distal segment will push the proximal segment on the right side; (**d**) right proximal segment is rotated to accommodate the cant correction; (**e**) the complex is rotated horizontally to correct the yaw and notice how the mandibular body shifts to the left, filling the left body and angle region and allowing the right proximal segment to rotate back to its original position; and (**f**) right proximal segment is rotated to accommodate the yaw correction

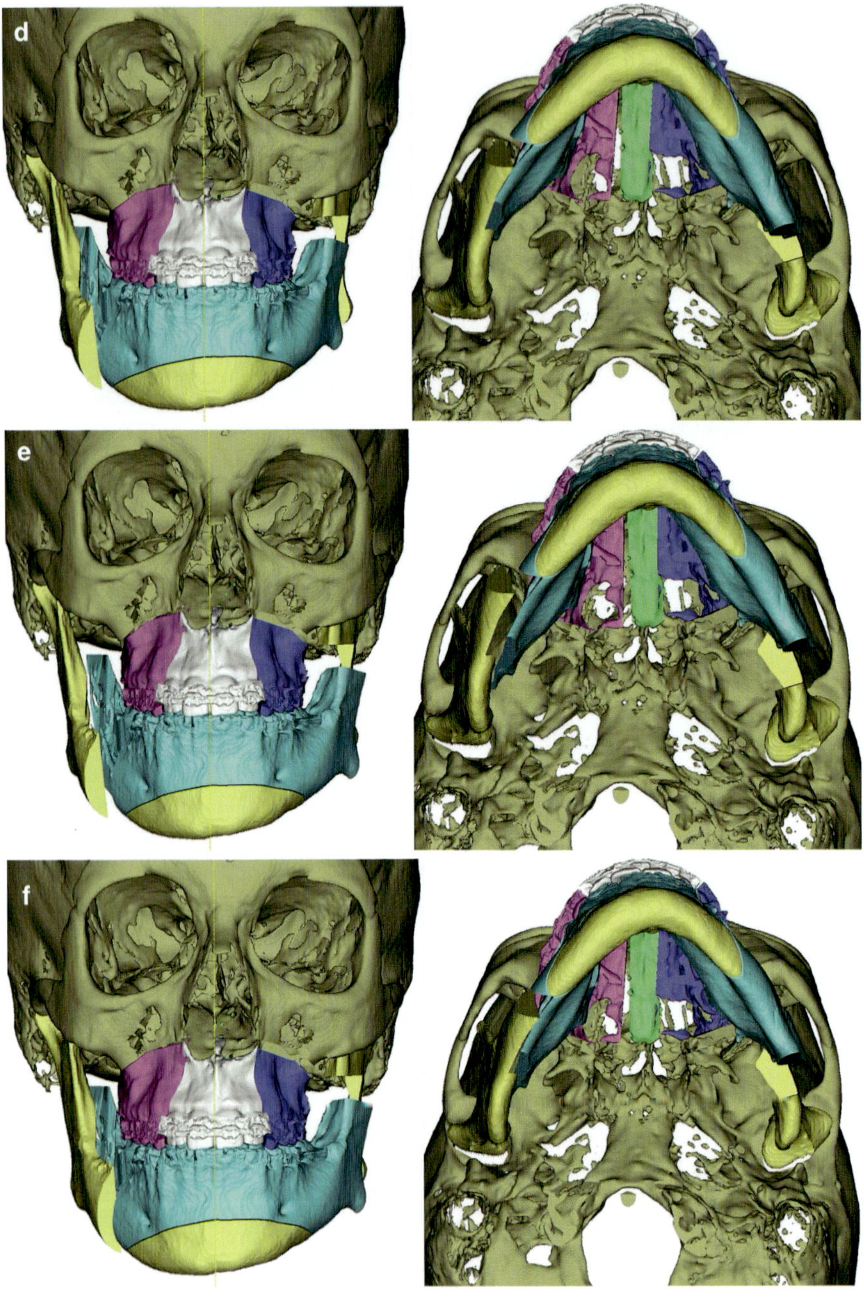

Fig. 7.1 (continued)

CT is the best image to obtain measurements, compare right and left sides, and plan for any necessary augmentation procedures. On top of that, the soft tissue atrophy may require the application of fillers to improve facial symmetry.

Treatment

After the patient reaches skeletal maturity, treatment is more predictable and resembles a regular orthognathic case. Orthodontic treatment should be established to remove dental compensations and allow for a complete skeletal correction of the deformity. These patients usually present with class II and anterior open bite malocclusion, maxillomandibular cant due to decreased facial height of the affected side, midline shifted to the affected side, and small symphysis, body, and ramus on the affected side. During the orthodontic treatment, compensations have to be eliminated and arches coordinated, which will further increase the malocclusion. It is important to avoid extrusive movements in an attempt to close the open bite because of two reasons: first, these movements are unstable and tend to relapse and reopen the bite, and second the extruded teeth hinder the surgeon from fully correcting the anterior open bite skeletally. If however the open bite is slightly increased during orthodontic treatment, any dental relapse that occurs after removing braces will be extrusive, increasing the long-term stability. Orthognathic surgery has been shown to be an effective and stable technique to treat the CM patients [19].

The first decision that needs to be made from a surgical standpoint is if the affected temporomandibular joint is reliable. If the TMJ needs to be reconstructed, we believe the best option for the skeletal mature patient is total joint replacement with a customized prosthetic device, which will be addressed elsewhere in this book. If TMJ is reliable, which is the case of most type I and IIa patients, the definitive treatment for the maxillomandibular deformities will consist of orthognathic surgery. Most types IIb and III will need temporomandibular joint reconstruction, and the current most reliable option for that is a total joint replacement (Fig. 7.2). There is still space for CCG or sternoclavicular grafts (SCG) in the growing patient, but due to the morbidity involved on the harvesting site and the lower predictability when compared to temporomandibular prosthesis, there seems to be very limited indications to perform a TJR with a costochondral graft in a non-growing patient. There may be a roll for CCG or SCG in countries with limited or no access to temporomandibular prosthesis or in patients with proven allergy to one of the prosthesis components, but those would be extreme exceptions.

The four techniques that need to be mastered to adequately treat the maxillomandibular deformities in craniofacial microsomia patient include Le Fort I maxillary osteotomy, sagittal split mandibular osteotomy, inverted L mandibular osteotomy, and genioplasty. Additional procedures such as iliac bone harvesting, bone augmentation with autogenous or alloplastic materials, and dermal fillers are also advantageous.

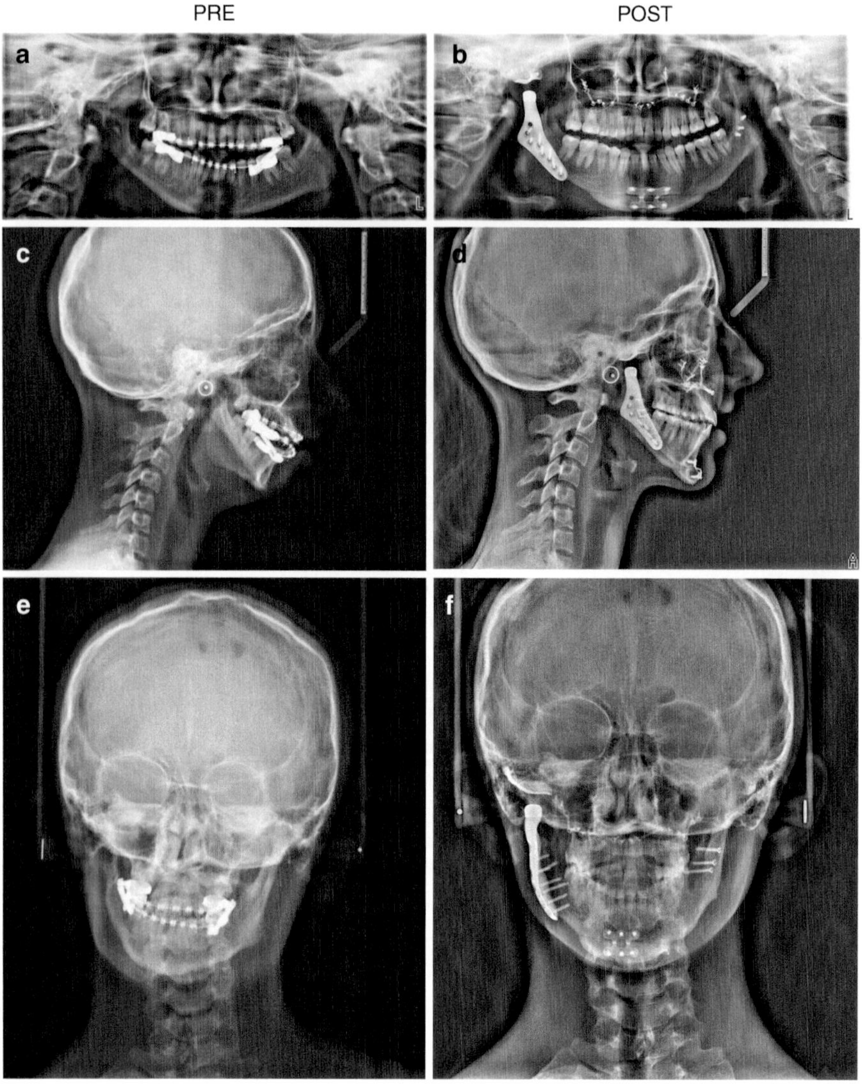

Fig. 7.2 (**a**–**f**) Patient with Kaban type IIB operated at skeletal maturity. Treatment: Le Fort I, (right) TMJ Concepts prosthesis, (left) sagittal osteotomy, and genioplasty

A Le Fort I osteotomy will be necessary to correct the maxillary position, usually by a combination of down grafting on the affected side, impaction on the contralateral side, and horizontal shifting to correct both midline yaw positions. The vertical movement is determined by the amount of teeth exposure – with the lip in repose and during smile – and by the desired occlusal plane rotation. Bone grafts are usually necessary to increase stability on the down-grafted side.

The mandible may be approached either by bilateral sagittal split osteotomies (BSSO) or by a combination of sagittal split osteotomy on the contralateral side and inverted L osteotomy on the affected side. Indications for the inverted L osteotomy have been described by Medeiros and Ritto [20], and the hemifacial patient may fill two of the three most common indications, including distorted anatomy and large advancement. The advantage of the inverted L is that it improves the mandibular angle outline and offers less risk to the inferior alveolar nerve. Disadvantages

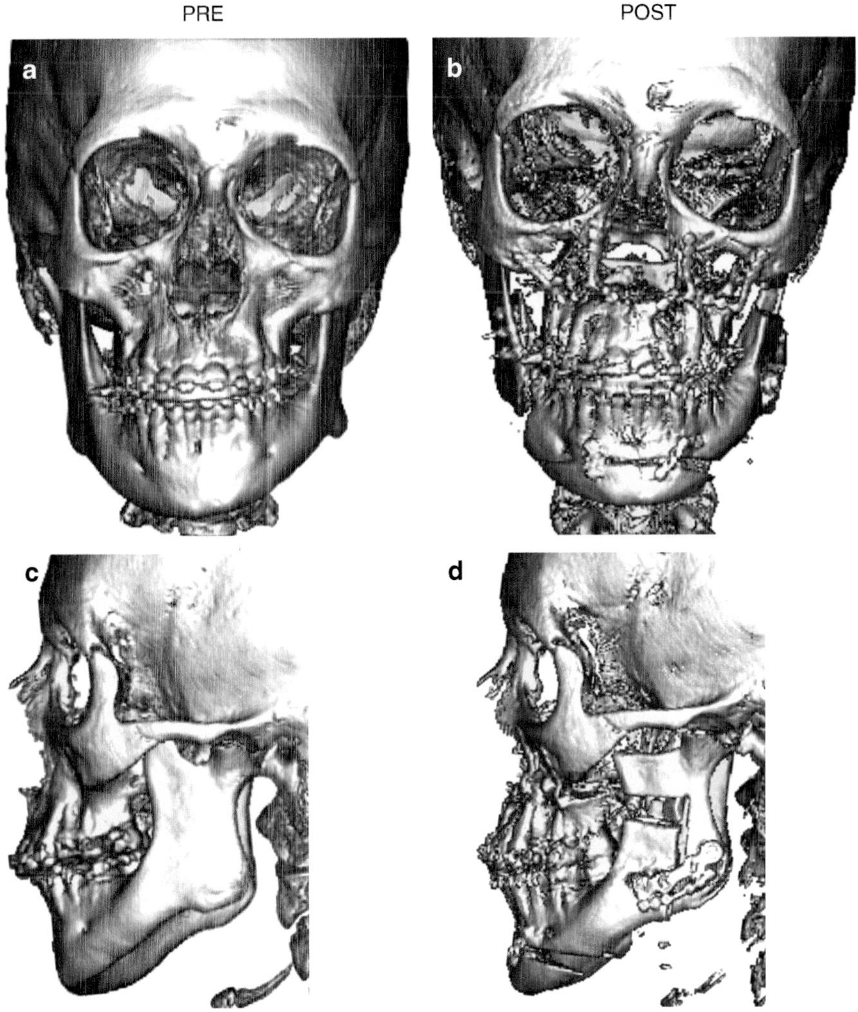

Fig. 7.3 (**a–g**) Patient with Kaban type I operated at skeletal maturity. Receives Le Fort I, (L) inverted L osteotomy, (R) sagittal osteotomy, and genioplasty. Grafted with bone harvested from the mandible. Notice on image (**b**) how the genioplasty is important to manage residual asymmetries after the maxillomandibular complex is adequately positioned. Image (**f**) shows the vertical measures of the pre-and post-operative mandibular angle position. Image (**g**) shows the pre-operative TMJ with abnormal shape but thick cortical bone

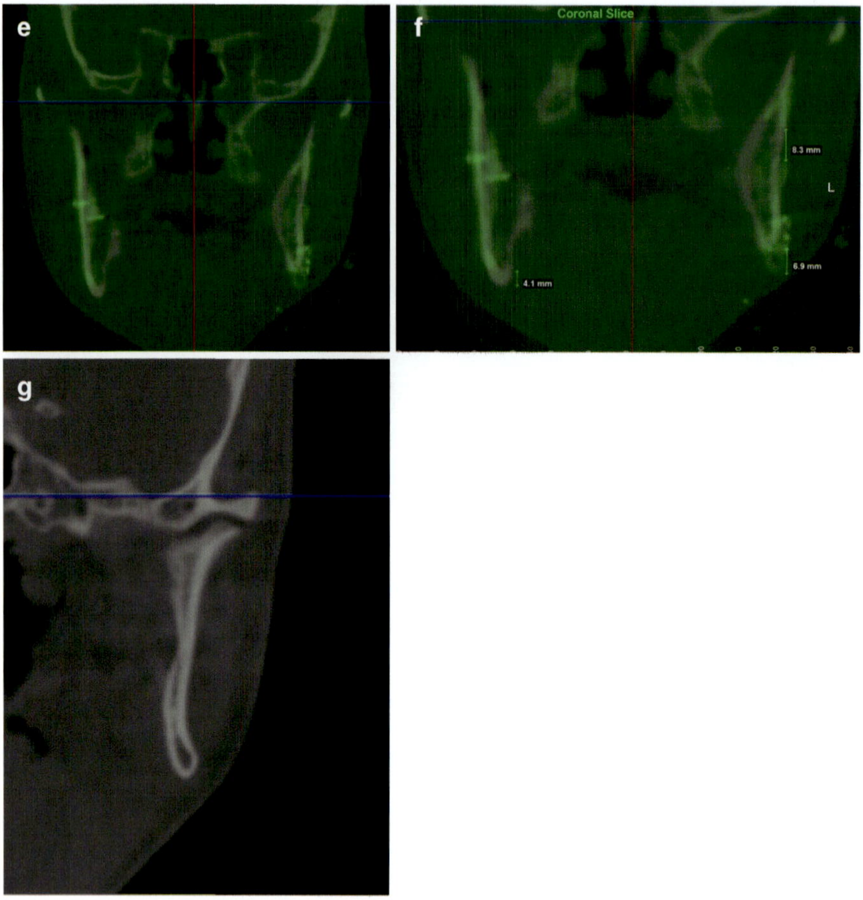

Fig. 7.3 (continued)

include external scar, risk of harming the marginal ramus of CN VII, and need for graft. See cases in Figs. 7.3 and 7.4.

Monasterio et al. (1997) [21] described a technique to perform maxillomandibular distraction osteogenesis (DO) for the hemifacial non-growing patient. The surgery involves performing a Le Fort I osteotomy preserving both the nasal septum connection to the maxilla and the pterygomaxillary junction on the non-affected side. An osteotomy is also performed on the affected mandibular ramus, and the distractor is installed. No procedure is accomplished on the contralateral ramus. After 5 days the patient is placed on maxillomandibular fixation, and the distractor is activated at a rate of 1 mm per day. The overall effect is rotation of the whole maxillomandibular complex. The authors concluded that simultaneous maxillary and mandibular distraction is the procedure of choice in patients with hemifacial microsomia over 14 years of age.

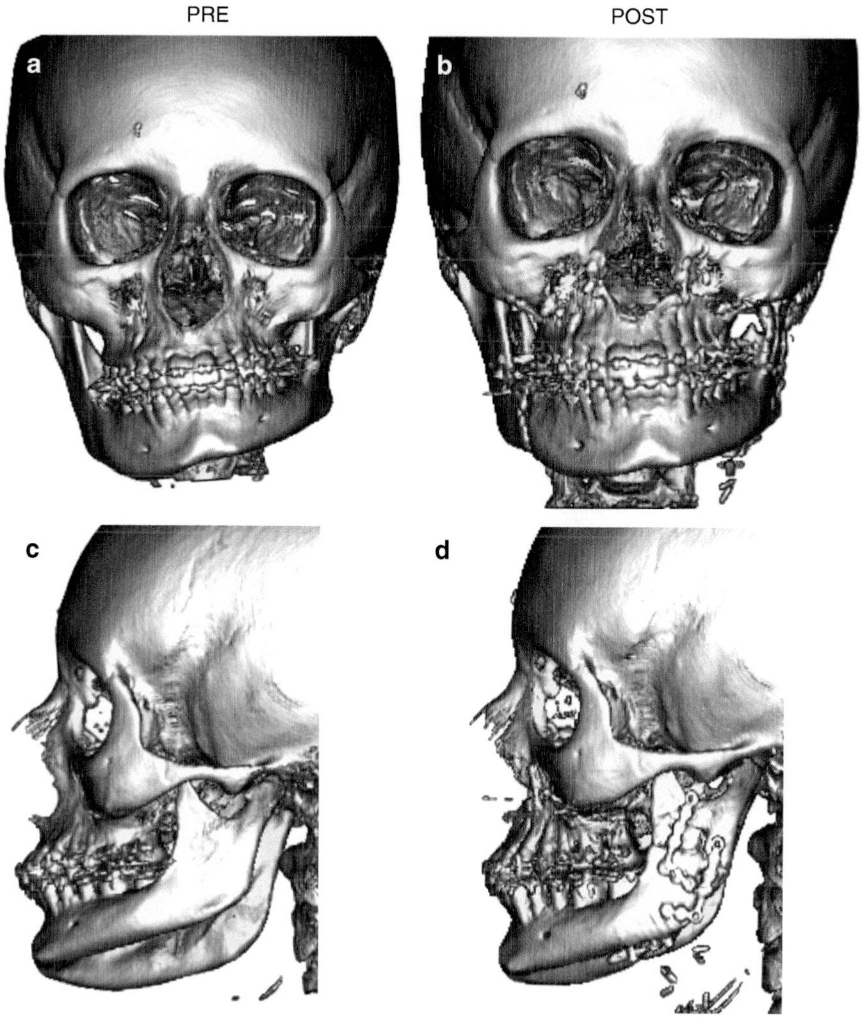

Fig. 7.4 (**a**–**g**) Patient with Kaban type I operated at skeletal maturity. Receives Le Fort I, (left) inverted L osteotomy, (right) sagittal osteotomy, and inferior border cortico-cancellous graft on the left body. Graft harvested from the hip. Image (**g**) shows the vertical measures of the pre- and post-operative mandibular angle position, the left side increased 10 mm and the right side reduced 2 mm

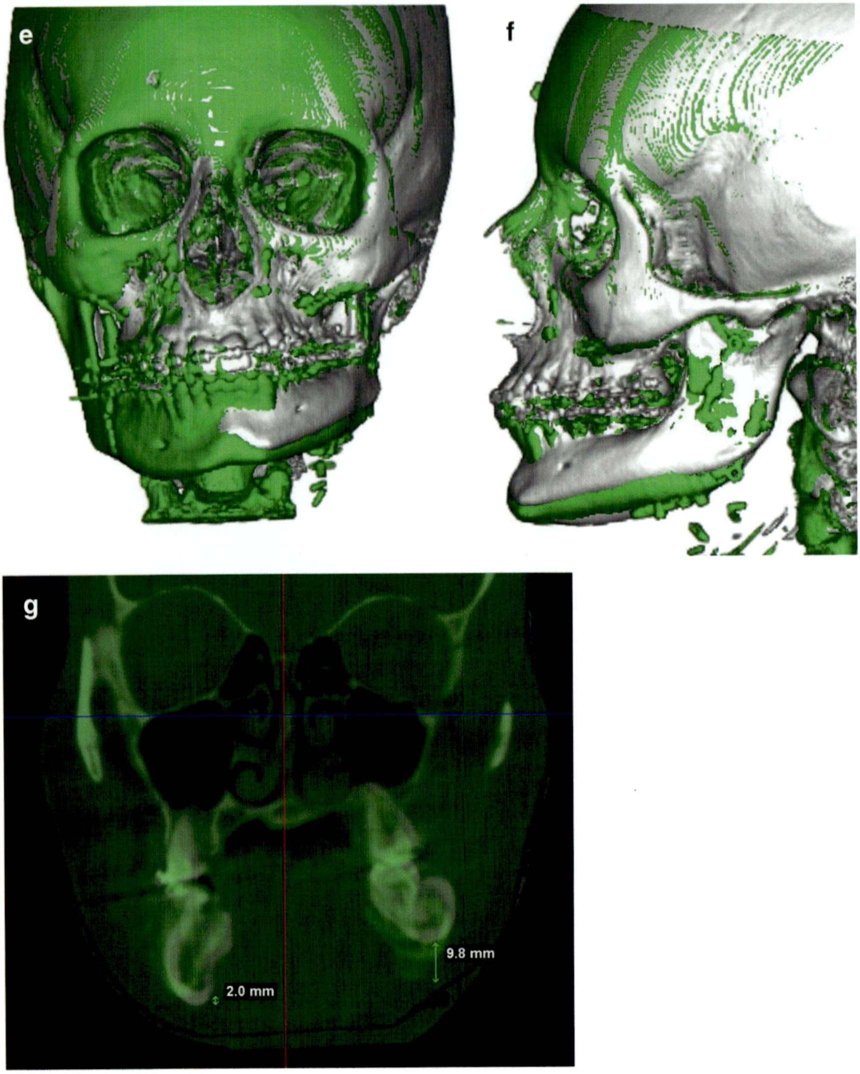

Fig. 7.4 (continued)

Modifications to this technique include performing a complete Le Fort I and fixating the non-affected side with titanium plate or wire. The exact position of the fixation device may vary according to the desired center of rotation. For instance, fixating close to the piriform rim will result in less down grafting of the maxilla and preservation of pre-operative teeth exposure, as opposed to fixating the zygomatico-maxillary buttress, which will result in greater facial elongation. Advantages of performing bimaxillary DO include good stability when correcting large vertical defects, no need for graft, and the fact that the correction can be continuously evaluated during the treatment [22].

The main problems with DO are that the surgical precision is lower than orthognathic surgery, and it does not allow to freely move the maxillomandibular complex three dimensionally. There is no control of the horizontal maxillary movement and no control of the occlusal plane rotation on the sagittal plane, the mandibular advancement is limited by the amount of ramus elongation, and the maxilla cannot be positioned superiorly; therefore teeth/gingiva exposure is always increased on the affected side and maintained or increased on the contralateral side. Also, the chin is not addressed by the DO, and future genioplasty is usually necessary. Liu et al. 2017 [23] performed a study and concluded that maxillomandibular DO with subsequent orthognathic surgery might be the best approach to achieve the most favorable results.

No matter how good the correction of the cant, pitch and yaw is, some asymmetry will still remain due to intrinsic mandibular deficiency on the affected side. Ramus, body, and mandibular symphysis are hypoplastic and will demand attention after the maxillomandibular complex has been corrected at the occlusal plane level. A genioplasty is required to correct the symphysis, and different augmentation procedures are usually necessary over the body and ramus region.

Ideally, during the pre-surgical orthodontic treatment, the midline of the lower teeth and chin will be aligned. Therefore, when the occlusal plane is adequately positioned, the midlines of the upper teeth, lower teeth, and symphysis will be aligned with the facial midline. The symphysis however is also hypoplastic on the affected side, and a genioplasty is required to rotate the chin vertically and/or horizontally. The amount of rotation can be easily calculated on the pre-operative CT scan, but transferring this three-dimensional movement to surgery can become very challenging depending on the complexity of the movement. Surgical guides are very helpful to adequately position the chin in these complex three-dimensional movements. This technique is also valuable to correct any anteroposterior deficiency that remains after the orthognathic surgery, improving the facial profile. Sometimes it may be advantageous to perform the genioplasty as a second procedure after the edema from the orthognathic surgery has resolved.

The hypoplastic mandibular body and ramus usually demand some augmentation procedure to obtain skeletal symmetry. This may be accomplished with autogenous or allogenic bone graft and alloplastic material. The advantage of the autogenous graft is that it is readily available and infection rate is very low. However it requires a second surgical site, and the resorption rate is unpredictable. Allogenic bone will spare the second surgical site but has a higher infection rate and can also resorb. Alloplastic materials such as porous polyethylene are excellent options since they dispense a second surgical site, can be easily adapted to reconstruct different mandibular regions, and do not resorb. Infection is the main concern with these implants, and they are preferably inserted from extra-oral wounds with gloves that haven't touched the mouth

Conclusion

Craniofacial microsomia patients require different levels of treatment according to the severity of the disease. The maxillomandibular reconstruction is essential to correct function and balance of the middle and lower facial thirds. Different techniques can be applied to obtain these goals, according to the clinical examination, including Le Fort I, BSSO, inverted L osteotomy, and genioplasty. Virtual surgical planning plays a major role in obtaining the best results and must be used in these patients. Finally, any remaining asymmetry after the maxillomandibular complex is adequately positioned can be addressed with bone and soft tissue augmentation procedures.

References

1. Costello BJ, Rivera RD, Shand J, Mooney M. Growth and development considerations for craniomaxillofacial surgery. Oral Maxillofac Surg Clin North Am. 2012;24(3):377–96.
2. Rune B, Sarnäs KV, Selvik G, Jacobsson S. Roentgen stereometry with the aid of metallic implants in hemifacial microsomia. Am J Orthod. 1983;84(3):231–47.
3. Polley JW, Figueroa AA, Liou EJ, Cohen M. Longitudinal analysis of mandibular asymmetry in hemifacial microsomia. Plast Reconstr Surg. 1997;99(2):328–39.
4. Meazzini MC, Mazzoleni F, Bozzetti A, Brusati R. Comparison of mandibular vertical growth in hemifacial microsomia patients treated with early distraction or not treated: follow up till the completion of growth. J Craniomaxillofac Surg. 2012;40(2):105–11.
5. Ongkosuwito EM, van Vooren J, van Neck JW, et al. Changes of mandibular ramal height, during growth in unilateral hemifacial microsomia patients and unaffected controls. J Craniomaxillofac Surg. 2013;41(2):92–7.
6. Meazzini MC, Battista VMA, Brusati R, Mazzoleni F, Biglioli F, Autelitano L. Costochondral graft in growing patients with hemifacial microsomia case series: long term results compared with non treated patients. Orthod Craniofac Res. 2020 Jun 8; https://doi.org/10.1111/ocr.12398. Online ahead of print.
7. Mulliken JB, Kaban LB. Analysis and treatment of hemifacial microsomia in childhood. Clin Plast Surg. 1987;14(1):91–100.
8. Padwa BL, Mulliken JB, Maghen A, Kaban LB. Midfacial growth after costochondral graft construction of the mandibular ramus in hemifacial microsomia. J Oral Maxillofac Surg. 1998;56(2):122–7.
9. Posnick JC. Hemifacial microsomia: evaluation and treatment. In: Posnick JC, editor. Craniofacial and maxillofacial surgery in children and young adults, vol. 20. Philadelphia: WB Saunders Co; 2000. p. 419–45.
10. Fattah AY, Caro C, Khechoyan DY, Tompson B, Forrest CR, Phillips JH. Cephalometric outcomes of orthognathic surgery in hemifacial microsomia. J Craniofac Surg. 2014;25(5):1734–9.
11. Monahan R, Seder K, Patel P, Alder M, Grud S, O'Gara M. Hemifacial microsomia. Etiology, diagnosis and treatment. J Am Dent Assoc. 2001;132(10):1402–8.
12. Wolford LM, Perez DE. Surgical management of congenital deformities with temporomandibular joint malformation. Oral Maxillofac Surg Clin North Am. 2015;27(1):137–54.
13. Posnick JC. Surgical correction of mandibular hypoplasia in hemifacial microsomia: a personal perspective. J Oral Maxillofac Surg. 1998;56(5):639–50.
14. Obwegeser HL. Correction of the skeletal anomalies of oto-mandibular dysostosis. J Maxillofac Surg. 1974;2(2–3):73–92.

15. Padwa BL, Kaiser MO, Kaban LB. Occlusal cant in the frontal plane as a reflection of facial asymmetry. J Oral Maxillofac Surg. 1997;55(8):811–6.
16. Schatz EC, Xia JJ, Gateno JJ, English JD, Teichgraeber JF, Garrett FA. Development of a technique for recording and transferring natural head position in 3 dimensions. J Craniofac Surg. 2010;(21):1452.
17. Xia JJ, McGrory JK, Gateno J, Teichgraeber JF, Dawson BC, Kennedy KA, et al. A new method to orient 3-dimensional computed tomography models to the natural head position: a clinical feasibility study. J Oral Maxillofac Surg. 2011;(69):584–91.
18. Bobek S, Farrell B, Choi C, Farrell B, Weimer K, Tucker M. Virtual surgical planning for orthognathic surgery using digital data transfer and an intraoral fiducial marker: the Charlotte method. J Oral Maxillofac Surg. 2015;(73):1143.
19. Luo E, Yang S, Wen D, Chen Q, Liao C, Fei W, Jing H. Bimaxillary orthognathic approach to correct skeletal facial asymmetry of hemifacial microsomia in adults. Aesthetic Plast Surg. 2016;40:400 9.
20. Medeiros PJ, Ritto F. Indications for the inverted-L osteotomy: report of 3 cases. J Oral Maxillofac Surg. 2009;67(2):435–44.
21. Ortiz MF, Molina F, Andrade L, Rodriguez C, Arregui JS. Simultaneous mandibular and maxillary distraction in hemifacial microsomia in adults: avoiding occlusal disasters. Plast Reconstr Surg. 1997;100:852–61.
22. Wang P, Yu W, Zhang Z, Li X, Ye B, Li J. Comprehensive consideration and design with the virtual surgical planning-assisted treatment for hemifacial microsomia in adult patients. J Craniomaxillofac Surg. 2018;46(8):1268–74.
23. Liu H, Zhang X, Liu L, Chen Q, Shao J, Luo E. Combined bimaxillary distraction osteogenesis associated with orthognathic surgery for hemifacial microsomia in adults. Aesthet Plast Surg. 2017;41(3):650–60.

Chapter 8
Orthodontic Considerations in the Craniofacial Microsomia Patients

Adriana Da Silveira and Pollyana Marques de Moura

Presentation and Diagnosis

Patients with craniofacial microsomia (CFM) typically display reduced growth and development of half of the face owing to abnormal development of the first and second branchial arches. CFM is also none as craniofacial microsomia (CFM). But for the purpose of this chapter, we will refer to the entity as CFM. This malformation sequence is usually unilateral but occasionally may involve both sides [1, 2]. A systematic review and meta-analysis carried out to determine the influence of gender and laterality on the incidence of CFM showed no significant difference between male and female rates. Also, the frequency of laterality was nearly equal; there was no clear evidence to prove any association between the laterality of CFM and gender [2, 3].

Patients with this condition have a striking appearance caused by progressive failure of the affected side to grow, which gives the involved side of the face a reduced dimension in all planes. In addition, aplasia or hypoplasia of the external ear (microtia) is common, and the ear canal is often missing. Delayed dental eruption and hypodontia on the affected side have also been reported [4]. From the orthodontist perspective, the best imaging tool is multidetector computed tomography (MDCT) or cone-beam computed tomography (CBCT). The primary radiographic finding is a reduction in the size of the bones on the affected side; additional findings are summarized on Table 8.1. The differential diagnosis involves ruling out

A. Da Silveira (✉)
Dell Children's Craniofacial Center, Dell Children's Medical Center, Private Practice, Austin, TX, USA
e-mail: acdasilveira@seton.org

P. M. de Moura
Private Practice, Dallas, TX, USA

D. M. Yates, M. R. Markiewicz (eds.), *Craniofacial Microsomia and Treacher Collins Syndrome*, https://doi.org/10.1007/978-3-030-84733-3_8

Table 8.1 Imaging features associated to CFM

Small to absent condyle
Fossa development proportional to condylar development and function
Decreased ipsilateral ramus and body development
Ramus and mandibular body development proportional to condylar development
Occlusal plane elevated on the involved side
Occasional cleft palate
Small zygomatic bone and arch
Hypoplasia of mastoid process
Orbit displaced laterally and inferiorly
Middle and external ear defects
The dentition on the affected side may show a reduction in the number or size of the teeth and delayed eruption pattern

of condylar hypoplasia associated with fracture of the condyle at birth or degenerative disease, radiation therapy during growth, and other syndromes such as Parry-Romberg syndrome.

The vast heterogeneity and phenotype require a classification system to assist the clinician to develop adequate therapeutic guidance [5]. One of the most widely used systems for preoperative assessment, due to its simplicity and inclusion of the anatomy and function of the TMJ in addition to its inherently therapeutic approach, was developed by Pruzansky [6] and expanded by Kaban et al. [7]. The classification categorizes CFM patients into four groups based on the size and function of the temporomandibular joint (TMJ): types I, IIA, IIB, and III. This classification system will be used in this chapter to discuss orthodontics' main concern, treatment strategies, and prognosis. The most common clinical issues related to the orthodontic intervention are summarized on Table 8.2.

A common problem in children with mandibular hypoplasia is upper airway obstruction. A retrospective review of 62 patients with CFM revealed a prevalence of 11.2%; this is double the incidence of OSA in the general pediatric population [8]. A systematic review of the literature on children with craniofacial microsomia showed a prevalence of OSA ranging from 7% to 67% [9]. These results are based on subjective measurements, such as questionnaires (i.e., the Pediatric Sleep Questionnaire, [10]), and on the retrospective evaluation of medical charts or are based on polysomnography performed in a small proportion of the group of patients studied.

Children with craniofacial conditions are at known risk for a variety of psychosocial problems, including low self-esteem, learning and speech problems, depression, anxiety, and negative social reactions from peers [11, 12]. In light of these risks, the American Cleft Palate-Craniofacial Association recommends periodic assessment of the psychosocial needs of children with craniofacial conditions and

Table 8.2 Clinical issues associated to CFM that require orthodontic management

Classification	Description	Clinical issues
Type I	All components are present but hypoplastic to varying degrees Temporomandibular joint is present but with reduced cartilage and joint space	The joint movement is normal, but there is reduced translation during jaw opening Possible discrepancies in the number and size of teeth Occlusal plan is elevated on the involved side Lower facial 1/3 is asymmetrical Dental midline may be compensated Possible sleep-breathing disorder
Type IIA	The condylar process is cone shaped and positioned anterior and medial of the normal position Coronoid process and gonial angle are well developed	An articulation that allows hinge but not translatory movement resulting in limited jaw opening Occlusal plan is elevated on the involved side Middle and lower facial 1/3 are asymmetrical Dental midline shifted to the affected side Possible discrepancies in the number and size of teeth Limited chewing Increased risk of dental caries Increased risk of sleep-breathing disorder
Type IIB	No condylar process that articulates with the temporal bone is present, but there is a coronoid process of varying size	An articulation that allows hinge but not translatory movement resulting in limited jaw opening Occlusal plan is elevated on the involved side Middle and lower facial 1/3 are asymmetrical Dental midline shifted to the affected side Possible discrepancies in the number and size of teeth Limited chewing Increased risk of dental caries Increased risk of sleep-breathing disorder
Type III	No condylar or coronoid process and no gonial angle area are present	Joint fails to develop, small or absent ramus, small mandibular body Limited jaw opening Occlusal plan is elevated on the involved side Middle and lower facial 1/3 are asymmetrical Dental midline shifted to the affected side Missing teeth Limited chewing Increased risk dental caries Higher risk of OSA

Mandibular retrognathic facial pattern, excessive overjet, open bite, and posterior and anterior crossbite may be present in all categories.

their families [13]. Improved facial appearance in childhood may have valuable psychosocial benefits; therefore early treatment of the hypoplastic mandible might be required to minimize facial asymmetry, to provide functional improvement, and to enhance body image development and peer acceptance.

Comprehensive Orthodontic Management

Preceding to the beginning of orthodontic treatment, a diagnosis of the patient's oral health condition must be made. The diagnosis gives rise to a treatment plan that addresses the patient's chief complaint: medical and dental history and dental, facial, skeletal, functional, and/or psychosocial problems. The treatment plan should be periodically reassessed throughout treatment with progress records taken as deemed appropriate by the clinician. This reassessment should take into consideration various limiting factors and establish short- and/or long-term objectives.

Overall, the orthodontic treatment plan includes the following strategies: (1) modifying the occlusion with a functional appliance and providing support for the mandibular muscles to function with a more symmetrically positioned mandible in anticipation of completing surgery on the abnormal side of the mandible; (2) early surgical intervention to correct the abnormal side, extending the mandible by distraction osteogenesis, or replacing the missing condyle with tissue that includes growth sites or growth center tissues such as a costochondral graft; (3) wait much later and not intervening in a young subject, hence decreasing the episodes of surgical intervention (see Chap. 7 on "Definitive Management"). A summary of treatment option based upon dentofacial development is presented on Table 8.3.

The usual protocol is a phase 1 orthodontic treatment to alleviate dental issues with a possible growth modification followed by a second phase of treatment when skeletal maturity is complete. This approach allows that this phase of treatment is final in which results of surgery can be better predicted. The severity of the bony hypoplasia will dictate the type of surgery used. In cases of Type I and II A, conventional orthognathic surgery can achieve great results. In cases of increased

Table 8.3 Summary of orthodontic treatment option based upon dentofacial development

Dentition and growth development	Treatment option
Primary	Fixed or removable space maintainer Extraction of primary teeth Orthopedic appliance
Mixed	Orthopedic appliance Fixed or removable orthodontic appliance
Permanent dentition with growth potential	Fixed orthodontic appliance adjunctive to distraction osteogenesis
Permanent dentition without growth potential	Fixed orthodontic appliance adjunctive to orthognathic surgery

deficiencies (Type IIB and III) different approaches may be used, including distraction osteogenesis, fibula free flap reconstruction, or costochondral graft reconstruction. If sleep apnea is present, when severe chewing or psychosocial is being affected, the team should consider treatment.

Attempt of Modification of Dentofacial Growth Using Orthopedic Treatment Approach

Reports from as early as the 1980s indicated that mild forms of CFM can be treated successfully by proper orthopedic and orthodontic intervention, fostering mandibular growth and reducing further need to orthognathic surgery [14–16]. However, those reports usually present mild and some moderately involved growing individuals (Type I, Type IIA) [18]. The treatment approach involves a nonsurgical orthopedic treatment with functional appliance (phase I) completed through fixed orthodontic treatment (phase II). A slight chin deviation, maximum mouth opening at a normal range, and both condyles showing proper transitory movements are required for a favorable scenario. For maintaining the results, long-term retention may be necessary. This involves fixed retainers and nighttime wearing of a functional appliance.

As described by [17], the functional appliances are made up in various combinations from three basic functional components. These components produce basal and dentoalveolar changes by acting on the following:

1. Eruption (bite planes)
2. Linguofacial muscle balance (shields or screens)
3. Mandibular repositioning (construction or working bite)

To benefit patients with CFM, the functional appliance must be designed to reposition the mandible downward, forward, and shifted to the unaffected side, producing a posterior open bite. The acrylic is progressively removed from the occlusal surface of the maxillary posterior teeth to allow overeruption for the purpose of leveling the occlusal plane. This approach must focus on:

1. Correcting the mandibular deviation and maxillary cant occlusion
2. Controlling the vertical growth pattern to prevent excessive mandibular clockwise rotation
3. Monitoring proper permanent dentition development
4. Achieving an aesthetical, functional, and stable occlusion

The use of the asymmetrical functional orthopedic appliance in growing patients with more severe CFM presentation (Type IIB and Type III) is limited due to the severity of the neuromuscular and soft tissue deficiency. Meazzini MC et al. [18] suggested that orthopedic treatment has little possibility of changing abnormality of early embryonic development such as CFM pattern. The authors pointed out that there is a peculiar type of mandibular asymmetry, often labeled in the literature as CFM, that might be an incorrect diagnosis; those case might be successfully treated with functional appliances.

Preoperative and postoperative treatment with a functional appliance has been recommended to improve muscle function and to stimulate growth of the soft and hard tissues (Vargervik K, Ousterhout DK, Farias M 1986; [16, 19]). Recently, in a pilot study, to solve mandibular canting and deviation, a hybrid treatment combining distraction osteogenesis of the mandibular ramus with a mandible-guided functional appliance was applied in early reconstructive therapy for CFM which was proposed by Wang Jie et al. [20]. The functional appliance was designed to augment autologous bone growth, navigate maxillary, and mandibular repositioning and stabilize the occlusal relationship during the entire distraction and consolidation period.

Long-Term Stability of Orthodontic Treatment Adjunctive to Surgical Interventions

Although various studies on long-term results were published in the last three decades, they usually report data on preadolescent children and are focused on surgical technique, and few information can be gathered in relation to the orthodontic intervention [21–26].

In order to analyze the dentofacial changes observed longitudinally, a 12-year-old girl, Type IIB CFM, undergone DO with an external device, was followed for 10 years by means of six Björk-type titanium implants placed bilaterally in the mandible. Marked lengthening was achieved during the active phase of mandibular distraction. The ratio between the ramus heights of the affected and normal sides improved significantly in the affected side's favor as the mandible was lengthened; however this ratio returned to its initial value after 10 years. The dental occlusion remained stable despite the changes in the occlusal plane canting and mandibular symmetry in the follow-up period. The authors concluded that although there was some growth at the affected side during the 10-year follow-up period, it was not enough to catch up with the growth of the condyle at the normal side. Therefore, the asymmetry relapsed because of the expected growth pattern in this growing craniofacial microsomia patient [25].

Case illustrations are provided below to establish the overall orthodontic treatment plan and management (Figs. 8.1, 8.2, 8.3, 8.4, 8.5, 8.6, 8.7, 8.8, 8.9, 8.10, 8.11, and 8.12).

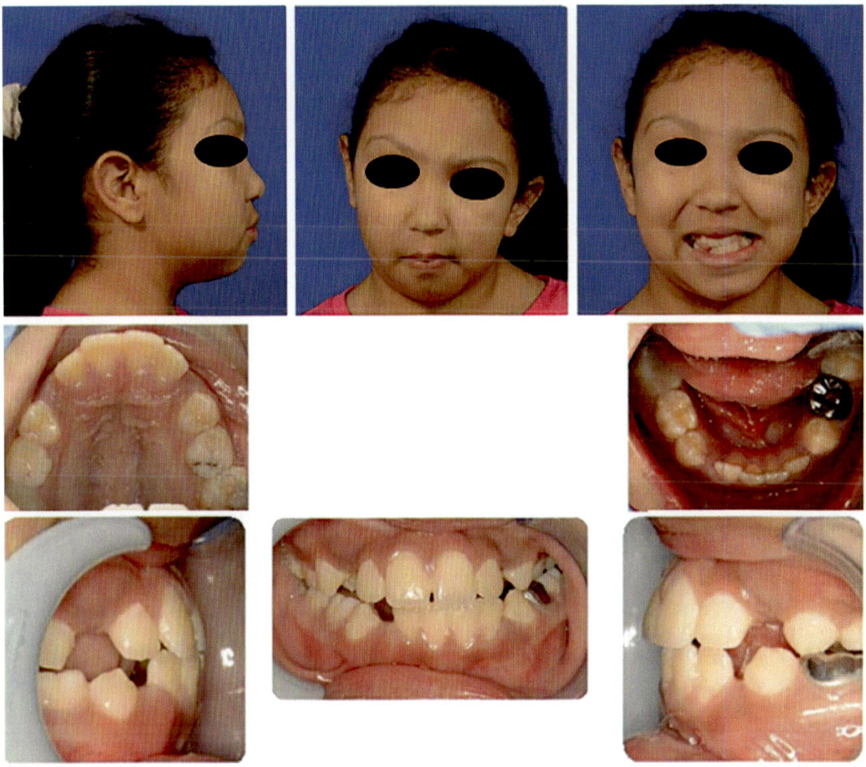

Fig. 8.1 Case 1, LG: Initial facial and intraoral photographs. Patient in late-mixed dentition presenting a mild Pruzansky-Kaban Type I hemifacial microsomia on the left side. The treatment objectives were established as follows: (1) coordinate the widths of the dental arches and (2) correct the canted occlusal plane and achieve dental Class I canine and molar relationships. Treatment plan: orthodontic treatment with fixed appliance

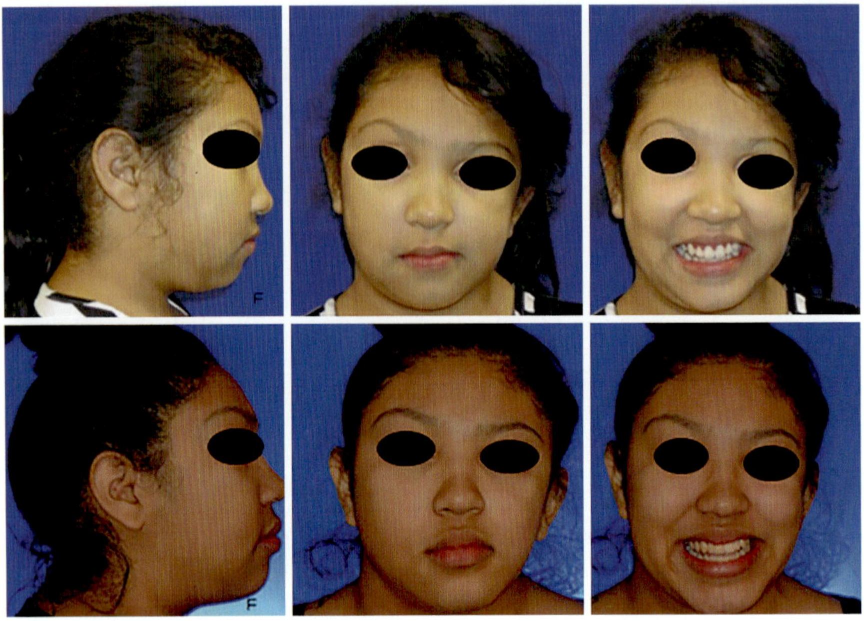

Fig. 8.2 Case 1, LG: Facial photographs. End of full braces therapy (first row): 5 years post retention. Note mild loss in the occlusal canting correction with subsequent growth. Severe jaw and facial asymmetries would be correct in the future with double-jaw surgery

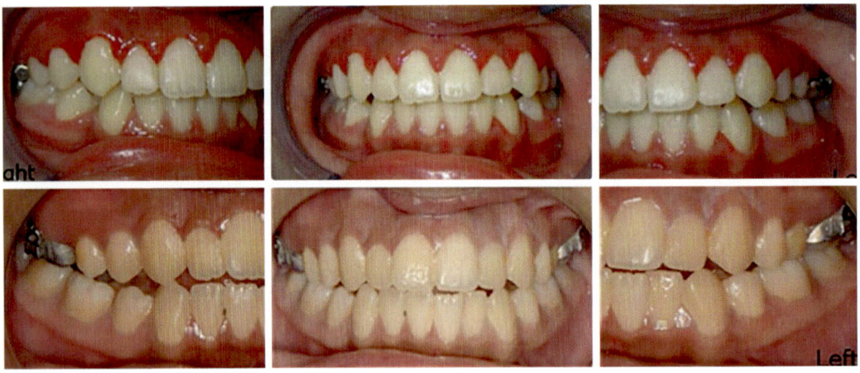

Fig. 8.3 Case 1, LG: End of full braces therapy (first row): 5 years post retention. Note loss of the vertical and transverse arch relationship with subsequent growth

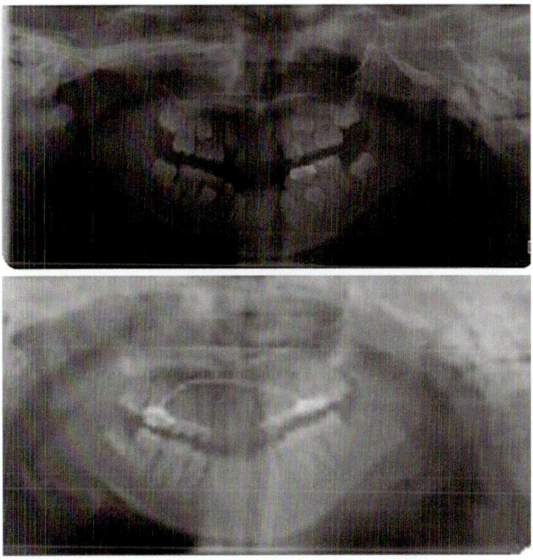

Fig. 8.4 Case 1, LG: Pre- and post-treatment panoramic images. All components of the TMJ are present but hypoplastic on the left side. Note transpalatal arch used as a fixed retainer attempting to prevent relapse of the posterior crossbite

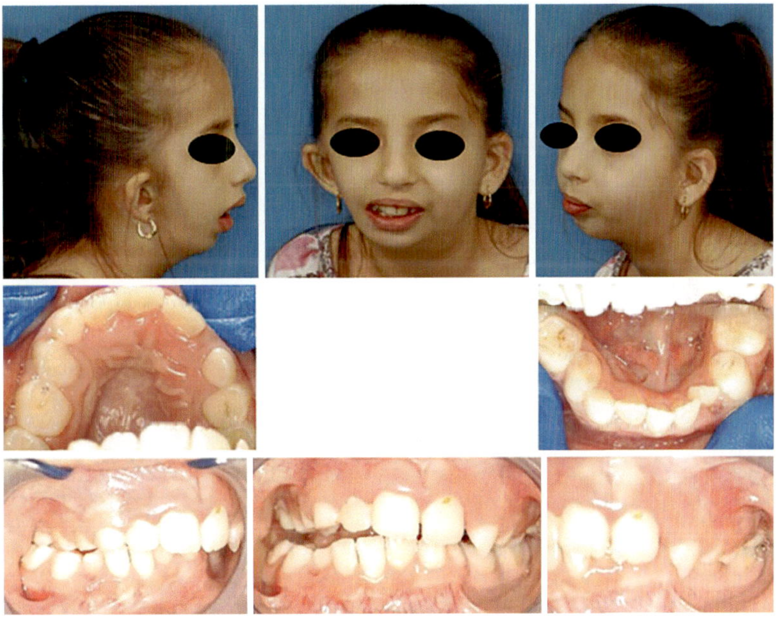

Fig. 8.5 Case 2, JE: Initial facial and intraoral photographs. A patient in mixed dentition presenting Pruzansky-Kaban Type IIB hemifacial microsomia on the right side. The patient expressed concern about his facial asymmetry. The treatment objectives were established as follows: (1) minimize the patient's facial asymmetry by coordinating the facial, maxillary, and mandibular dental midlines; (2) minimize the skeletal Class II anteroposterior jaw relationship; (3) coordinate the widths of the dental arches; and (4) correct the canted occlusal plane and achieve dental Class I canine and molar relationships. The patient was advised that multiple surgical interventions would be necessary to achieve treatment goals. Note posterior open bite on the right side. To free the vertical growth of the maxilla, an acrylic bite block was applied to maintain the upper and lower teeth apart

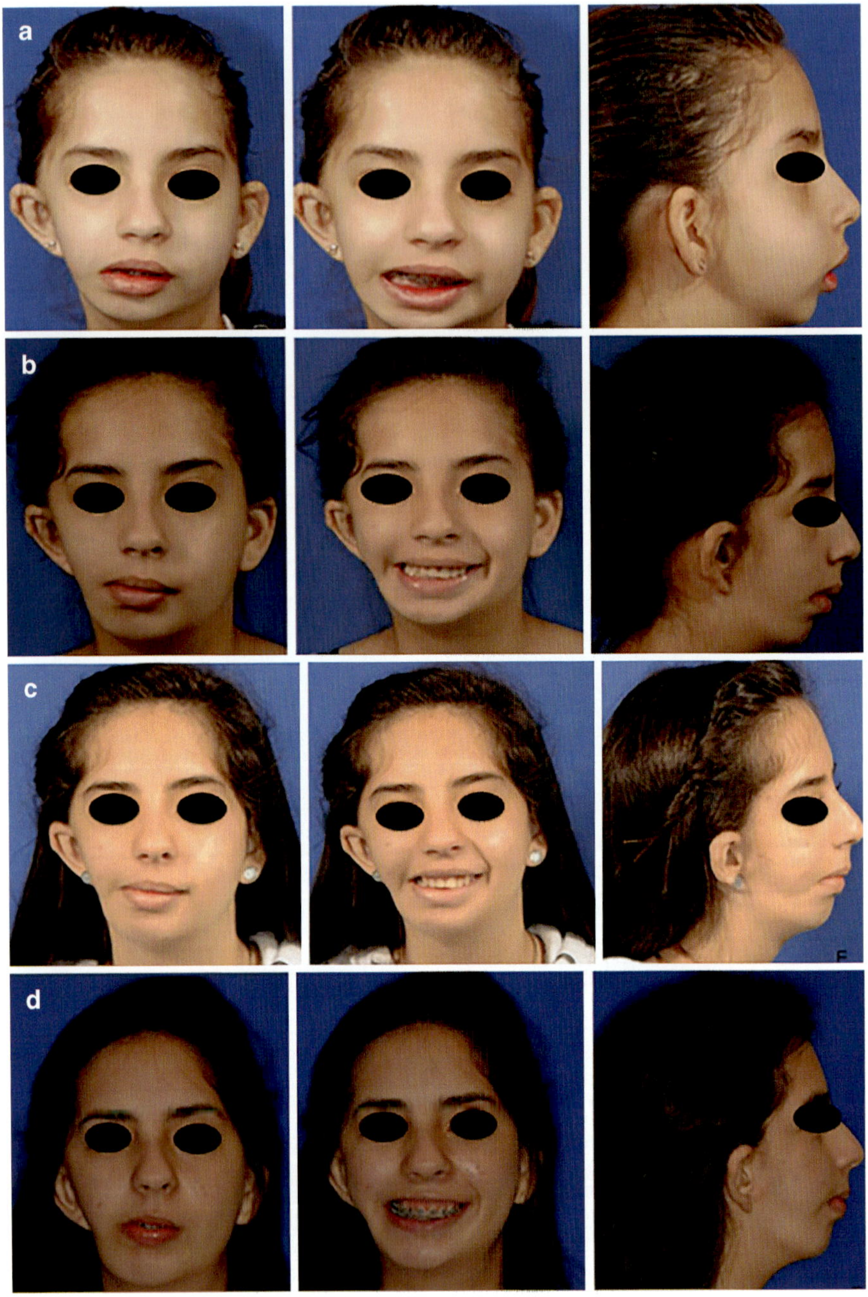

Fig. 8.6 Case 2, JE: Facial photographs. From top to bottom: (**a**) Pre-surgery orthodontic preparation (phase 1). (**b**) Post-surgery outcome (phase 1, 2010, Le Fort I with maxillary impaction to correct cant, mandibular sagittal split on the left side, right coronoidectomy). (**c**) Pre-ortho-treatment (phase 2). (**d**) Pre-surgery orthodontic preparation (phase 2). (**e**) Post-surgery (phase 2, 2015, mandibular reconstruction with free fibula flap, mandibular bilateral osteotomies, right inverted left mandibular osteotomy, left coronoidectomy, adjacent tissue transfer on the right-side face)

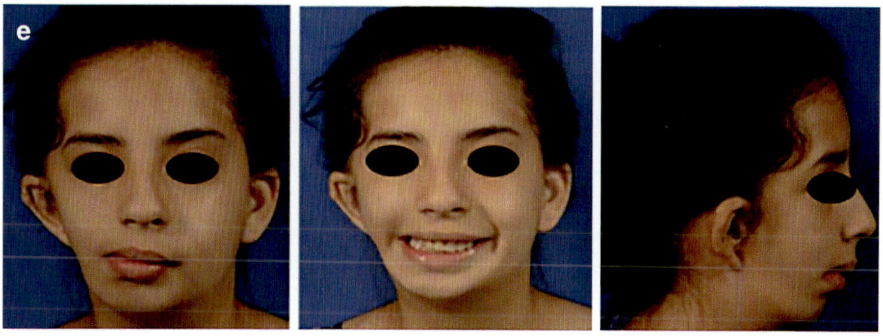

Fig. 8.6 (continued)

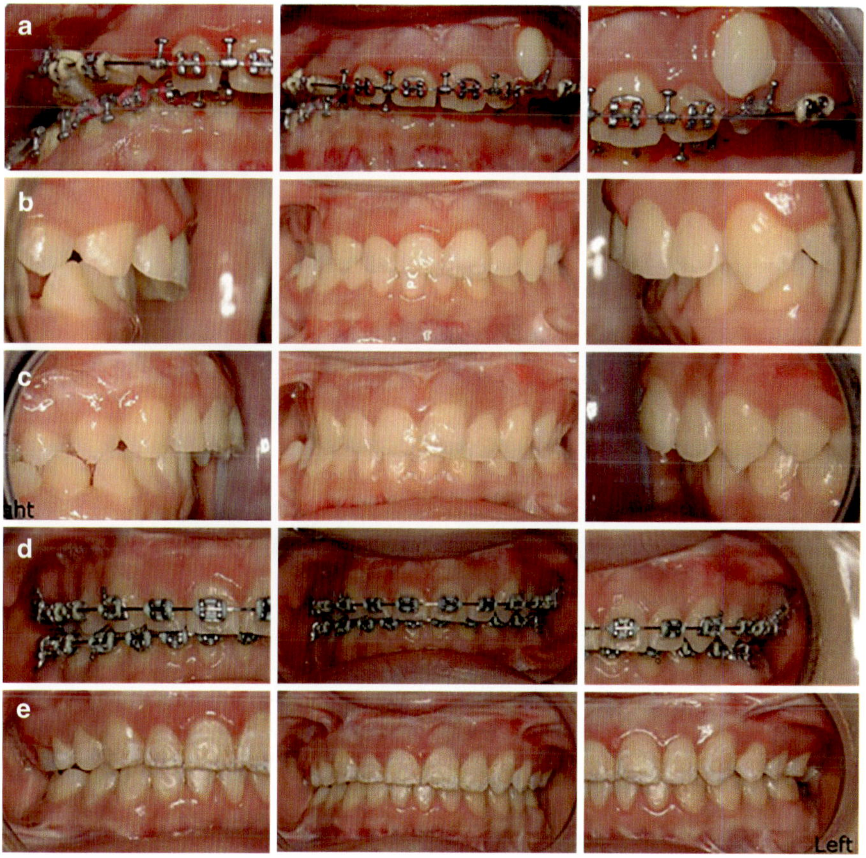

Fig. 8.7 Case 2, JE: Intraoral photographs. From top to bottom: (**a**) Pre-surgery orthodontic preparation (phase 1). (**b**) Phase 1 ortho-surgical intervention outcome. (**c**) Pre-orthodontic treatment (phase 2). (**d**) Orthodontic preparation for the final surgery (phase 2). (**e**) Final outcomes, after orthodontic treatment and post-surgery

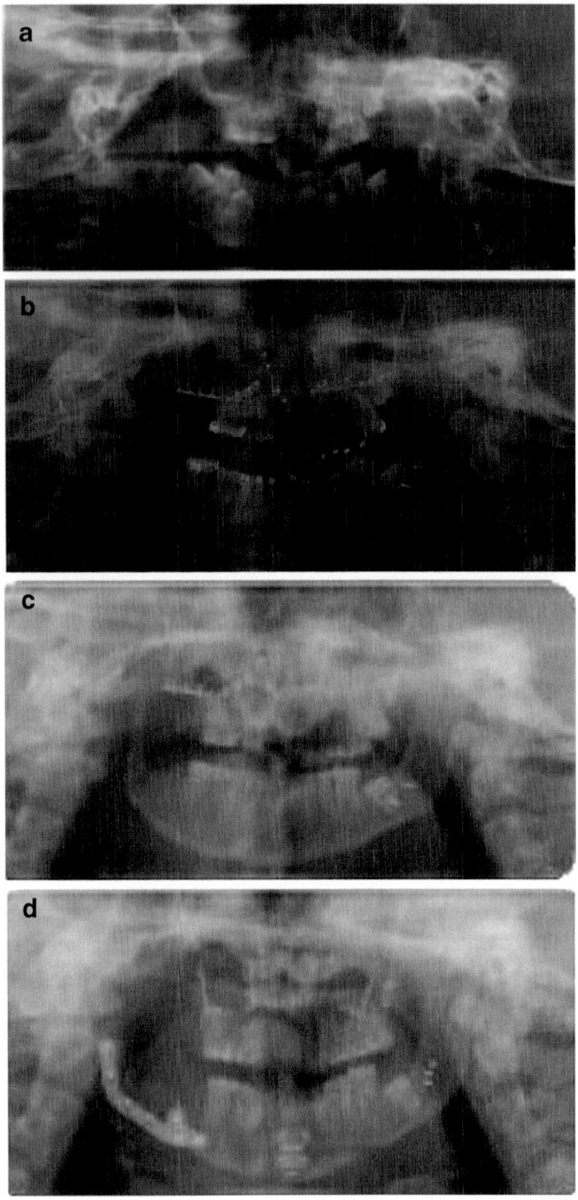

Fig. 8.8 Case 2, JE: Panoramic radiographs. Multiple two-jaw surgical interventions. Note impacted supernumerary tooth on the upper right side. Hypoplastic mandible on the right side. From top to bottom: (**a**) Initial phase 2 orthodontic treatment. (**b**) Post-surgery (phase 1). (**c**) Initial phase 2 orthodontic treatment. (**d**) Post-surgery (phase 2)

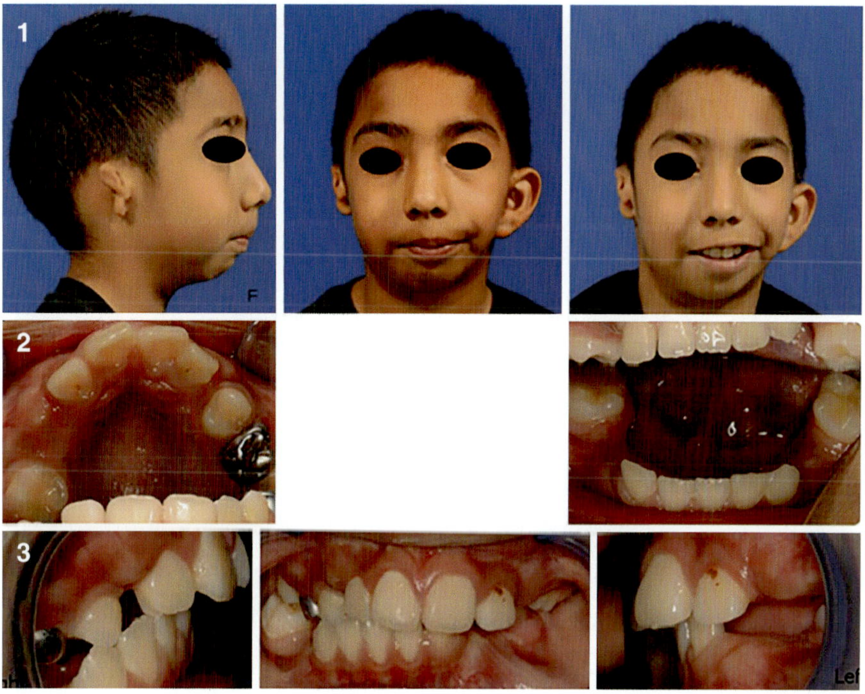

Fig. 8.9 Case 3, MV: Initial facial and intraoral photographs. The patient in late-mixed dentition presenting Pruzansky-Kaban Type IIA hemifacial microsomia on the right side. The patient expressed concern about his facial asymmetry and limited chewing. The treatment objectives were established as follows: (1) minimize the patient's facial asymmetry by lengthening the affected ramus, (2) coordinate the widths of the dental arches, and (3) minimize the canted occlusal plane and overjet. The patient was advised that a second orthodontic intervention would be necessary to prepare for the final orthognatic surgery

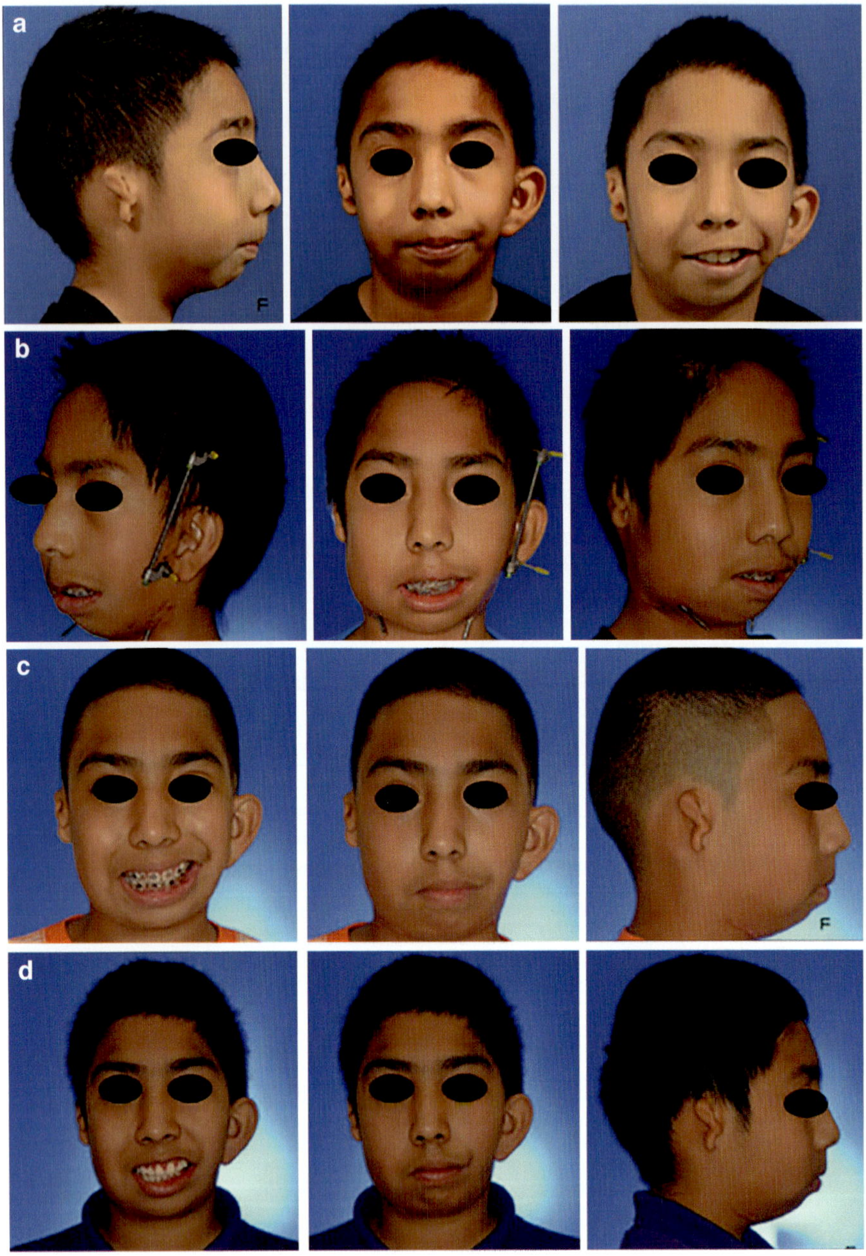

Fig. 8.10 Case 3, MV: Facial photographs. From top to bottom: (**a**, 2013) Pre-orthodontic treatment phase 1. (**b**, 2015) During orthodontic treatment, before distraction surgery. (**c**, 2015) During ortho-treatment after distraction surgery. (**d**, 2016) After phase 1 orthodontic treatment and distraction

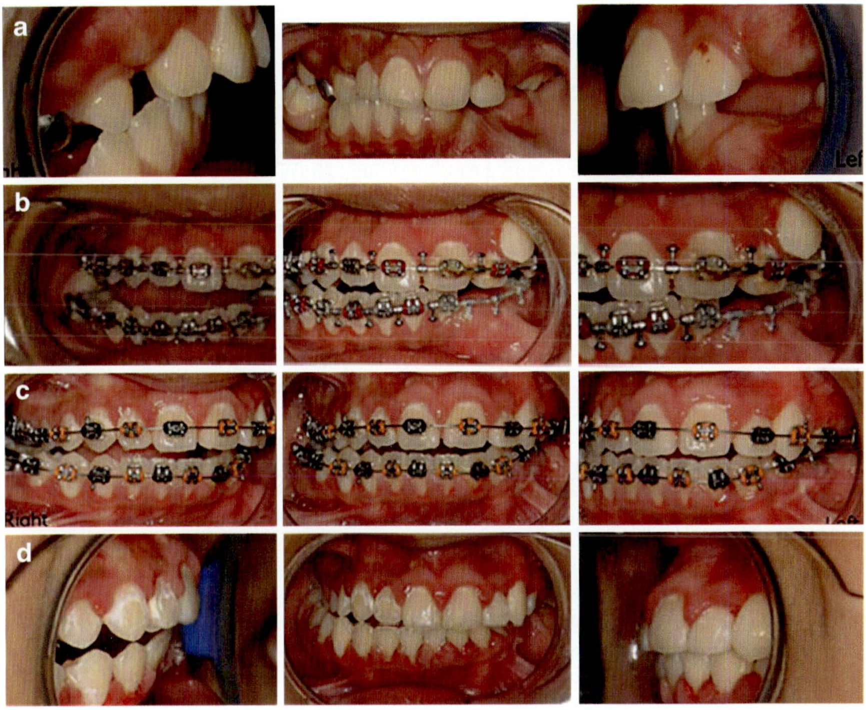

Fig. 8.11 Case 3, MV: Intraoral photographs. (**a**, 2013) Pre-orthodontic treatment phase 1. (**b**, 2015) During orthodontic treatment, before distraction surgery. (**c**, 2015) During ortho-treatment after distraction surgery. (**d**, 2016) After phase 1 orthodontic treatment and distraction

Fig. 8.12 Case 3, MV: Panoramic radiographs, pre- (**a**) and post-distraction (**b**) on the right side

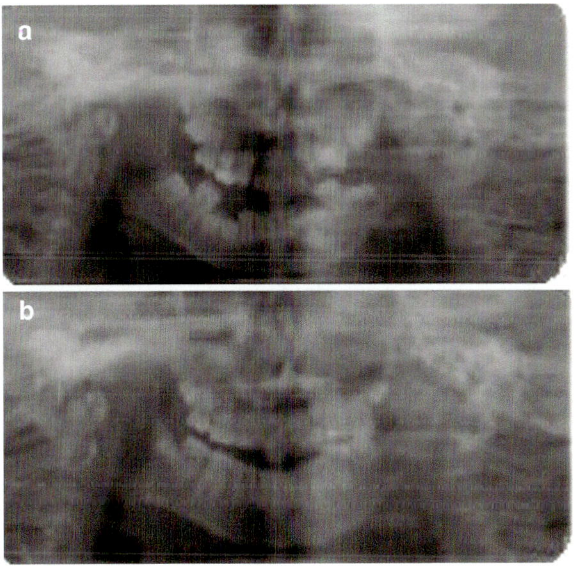

References

1. Johnson JM, Moonis G, Green GE, Carmody R, Burbank HN. Syndromes of the first and second branchial arches, part 2: syndromes. AJNR Am J Neuroradiol. 2001;32(2):230–7.
2. Xu S, Zhang Z, Tang X, Yin L, Liu W, Shi L. The influence of gender and laterality on the incidence of craniofacial microsomia. J Craniofac Surg. 2015;26(2):384–7.
3. Muñoz-Pedroza LA, Arenas-Sordo ML. Clinical features of 149 patients with facio-auriculo-vertebral Spectrum. Acta Otorrinolaringol Esp. 2013;64(5):359–62.
4. Maruko E, Hayes C, Evans CA, et al. Hypodontia in craniofacial microsomia. Cleft Palate Craniofac J. 2001;38:15–9.
5. White SC, Pharoah MJ. Oral radiology: principles and interpretation. Mosby; 2013, chapter 32. Elsevier, USA.
6. Pruzansky S. Not all dwarfed mandibles are alike. Birth Defects Orig Artic Ser. 1969;1:120–9.
7. Kaban LB, Moses MH, Mulliken JB. Surgical correction of craniofacial microsomia in the growing child. Plast Reconstr Surg. 1988;82:9–19.
8. Szpalski C, Vandergrift M, Patel PA, et al. Unilateral craniofacial microsomia: unrecognized cause of pediatric obstructive sleep apnea. J Craniofac Surg. 2015;26(4):1277–82.
9. Caron CJ, Pluijmers BI, Joosten KF, Mathijssen IM. Obstructive sleep apnoea in craniofacial microsomia: a systematic review. Int J Oral Maxillofac Surg. 2015;44(5):592–8.
10. Chervin RD, Hedger K, Dillon JE, Pituch KJ. Pediatric sleep questionnaire (PSQ): validity and reliability of scales for sleep-disordered breathing, snoring, sleepiness, and behavioral problems. Sleep Med. 2000;1(1):21–32.
11. Hunt O, Burden D, Hepper P, Johnston C. The psychosocial effects of cleft lip and palate: a systematic review. Eur J Orthod. 2005;27(3):274–85.
12. Stock NM, Feragen KB. Psycholocial adjustment to cleft lip and/or palate: a narrative review of the literature. Psychol Health. 2016;31(7):777–813.
13. American Cleft Palate Craniofacial Association. The parameters for evaluation and treatment of patients with cleft lip/palate or other craniofacial differences. December 2019. https://acpa-cpf.org/team-care/standardscat/parameters-of-care/.
14. Melsen B, Bjerrejaard J, Bundgaard M. The effect of treatment with functional appliance on a pathologic growth pattern of the condyle. Am J Orthod Dentofac Orthop. 1986;90(6):503–12.
15. Kaplan RG. Induced condylar growth in a patient with craniofacial microsomia. Angle Orthod. 1989;59:85–90.
16. Silvestri A, Natali G, Iannetti G. Functional therapy in craniofacial microsomia: therapeutic protocol for growing children. J Oral Maxillofac Surg. 1996;54:271–8.
17. Vig PS, Vig KW. Hybrid appliances: a component approach to dentofacial orthopedics. Am J Orthod Dentofac Orthop. 1986;90:273–85.
18. Meazzini MC, Caprioglio A, Garattini G, Lenatti L, Poggio CE. Hemandibular hypoplasia successfully treated with functional appliances: is it truly craniofacial Microsomia? Cleft Palate Craniofac J. 2008;45(1):50–6.
19. Ohtani J, Hoffman WY, Vargervik K, Oberoi S. Team management and treatment outcomes for patients with craniofacial microsomia. Am J Orthod Dentofac Orthop. 2012;141:S74–81.
20. Wang J, Yuan L, Liu J, Mao L, Xia L, Fang B. Craniofacial microsomia treated with a hybrid technique combining distraction osteogenesis and a mandible-guided functional appliance: pilot study. Am J Orthod Dentofac Orthop. 2019;155:801–11.
21. Molina F, Ortiz Monasterio F. Mandibular elongation and remodeling by distraction: a farewell to major osteotomies. Plast Reconstr Surg. 1995;96:825–40.
22. Trahar M, Sheffield R, Kawamoto H, Lee HF, Ting K. Cephalometric evaluation of the craniofacial complex in patients treated with an intraoral distraction osteogenesis device: a preliminary report. Am J Orthod Dentofac Orthop. 2003;124:639–50.

23. Baek SH, Kim S. The determinants of successful distraction osteogenesis of the mandible in craniofacial microsomia from longitudinal results. J Craniofac Surg. 2005;16:549–57.
24. Meazzini MC, Mazzoleni F, Canzi G, Bozetti A. Mandibular distraction osteogenesis in craniofacial microsomia. Long-term follow-up. J Craniomaxillofac Surg. 2005;33:370–6.
25. Işeri H, Kişnişci R, Altuğ-Ataç AT. Ten-year follow-up of a patient with craniofacial microsomia treated with distraction osteogenesis and orthodontics: an implant analysis. Am J Orthod Dentofac Orthop. 2008;134(2):296–304.
26. Pluijmers BI, Caron CJ, Dunaway DJ, Wolvius EB, Koudstaal MJ. Mandibular reconstruction in the growing patient with unilateral craniofacial microsomia: a systematic review. Int J Oral Maxillofac Surg. 2014;43(3):286–95.

Chapter 9
Management of Hearing Loss in Patients with Treacher-Collins Syndrome and Hemifacial Microsomia

Evan C. Cumpston, Andrea Sweetnam, and Brian Perry

Abbreviations

ABR	Auditory brainstem responses
CHL	Conductive hearing loss
HFMS	Hemifacial microsomia
MHL	Mixed hearing loss
OAE	Otoacoustic emissions
SNHL	Sensorineural hearing loss
TCS	Treacher-Collins syndrome

E. C. Cumpston
Department of Otolaryngology-Head & Neck Surgery, Resident at UT Health San Antonio, San Antonio, TX, USA
e-mail: cumpston@uthscsa.edu

A. Sweetnam
Pediatric and Cochlear Implant Audiologist at Southwest Ear, Nose, and Throat Consultants, El Paso, TX, USA

B. Perry (✉)
Department of Otolaryngology-Head & Neck Surgery, University of Texas-Rio Grande Valley, Edinburg, TX, USA
e-mail: brian.perry@utrgv.edu

D. M. Yates, M. R. Markiewicz (eds.), *Craniofacial Microsomia and Treacher Collins Syndrome*, https://doi.org/10.1007/978-3-030-84733-3_9

Background

Incidence of Outer Ear, Middle Ear, and Inner Ear Anomalies

Treacher-Collins Syndrome

The majority of malformations of the external and middle ear in patients with TCS are symmetric. Approximately 89% of patients have symmetric microtia of which 28% are classified as type I and 67% type II by the Marx classification (Table 9.1). All patients have abnormalities of the external auditory canals which is most commonly symmetric. Seventy-eight percent of patients have bilateral atresia, and 22% have bilateral stenosis. The middle ear cavity is hypoplastic and dysmorphic in nearly all patients. The ossicular chain is classified as dysplastic in 44% and absent in 56% of cases [2]. The cochlea is usually normal, but dysplasia of the lateral semicircular canal and vestibule may occur [3]. All patients were noted to have poorly pneumatized mastoids, and 22% of patients have an aberrant facial nerve course with facial nerve dysfunction, which has only been described as occurring unilaterally [2, 4].

Hemifacial Microsomia

Malformations of the external and middle ear with HFMS are predominantly asymmetric and with equal incidence in the right and left ears [5]. The incidence of anotia/microtia is reported between 66% and 100%, preauricular tags between 34% and 67%, and 60% of patients have ear canal atresia [6, 7]. The incidence of middle ear abnormalities is approximately 10%, and anatomic anomalies of the inner ear are not usually observed [5].

Incidence of Conductive Hearing Loss, Sensorineural Hearing Loss, and Mixed Hearing Loss

Treacher-Collins Syndrome

Conductive hearing loss (CHL) resulting from anatomic abnormalities of the external and middle ear structures accounts for the majority of hearing loss in patients with TCS, found in approximately 75% of patients. Some patients may also have

Table 9.1 Marx classification of microtia

Grade I	An abnormally small earlobe with all anatomical structures distinguishable
Grade II	An abnormally small earlobe with some anatomical structures distinguishable
Grade III	Only a rudiment of soft tissue is present, often a malformed lobule

Marx [1]

sensorineural hearing loss (SNHL) with approximately 10% of patients presenting with mixed hearing loss (MHL). Sensorineural hearing loss alone is uncommon occurring in approximately 1% of patients and is unilateral in 73% of patients [4]. Conductive hearing loss is generally symmetric with hearing differing by less than 10 dB [2].

Nearly all patients have bilateral hearing loss with an average hearing loss of 64.3 ± 8.5 dB. Of tested ears, approximately 17% have moderate CHL, 67% have moderately severe CHL, and approximately 17% have severe CHL. As anatomic abnormalities are generally symmetric, hearing between the two ears generally differs by less than 10 dB [2].

Hemifacial Microsomia

Overall, between 60% and 85% of patients with HFMS have hearing loss [6]. Conductive hearing loss is present in 40–60% of ears, sensorineural hearing loss in 20–30% of ears, and mixed hearing loss in 10% of ears. Normal hearing was present in 30% of ears, mild hearing loss was present in 30–40% of ears, moderate hearing loss was present in 20–50% of ears, and profound hearing loss in 10% of ears [5].

Evaluation and Workup

History and Examination

The majority of these children are either identified prenatally via ultrasound or on the immediate postpartum examination. Family history of craniofacial anomalies should be sought. Referral to genetics and the craniofacial team should be made immediately. Airway compromise should be assessed frequently. A complete head and neck examination should be performed to assess the status of the outer and middle ear anatomy, including patency of the ear canals and appearance of the tym panic membrane and ossicular chain. Cranial nerve examination should report the status of the facial nerve, as well as the oculomotor nerves, and gag reflex (sensory limb via cranial nerve IX, motor limb via cranial nerve X). Ophthalmologic exam should note any abnormalities.

Audiologic Assessment

Infants born in hospital facilities typically receive some type of universal newborn hearing screening (either OAE or AABR); however infants identified with anatomi cal malformations of the outer ear should be referred directly to a pediatric audiologist for a diagnostic evaluation according to the JCIH 2019 Position Statement [8]. The diagnostic audiological evaluation should include evoked auditory brainstem responses (ABR), evoked otoacoustic emissions (OAEs – either distortion product DPOAEs or transient evoked OAEs (TEOAEs), and high-frequency tympanometry when possible.

A patient with unilateral microtia or atresia needs to have the contralateral ear fully evaluated to verify hearing status because that is typically the better hearing ear. A screen only in the better ear can overlook a mild loss, high-frequency hearing loss, or reverse sloping loss. The ear with atresia cannot be able to be assessed with all measures because there is not an ear canal opening in which to place the testing probe, but it is possible to test via bone conduction to evaluate inner ear status. In the case of bilateral atresia, bone conduction ABR testing is recommended though it is difficult to obtain ear-specific data in this situation. Behavioral audiometry should be attempted once the baby is about 6–9 months old to start to obtain baseline behavioral hearing threshold data in patients with both unilateral and bilateral microtia/atresia. The patients with unilateral atresia need the opposite ear monitored every 4–6 months for any changes in hearing and to monitor middle ear function so prompt referral for medical intervention can be made if needed. Patients with either unilateral or bilateral atresia should also be referred as soon as possible to the local early intervention team for further evaluation and help with development of their communication and language skills [8]. The patient should also be referred to a craniofacial team if that has not already been done.

Additional Testing

Genetic evaluation and possible testing should be considered early on. Imaging of the temporal bones with CT can be done at a later date, as it does not change the initial management of these children. If planning otologic surgery (atresiaplasty, canalplasty), a high-resolution CT scan of the temporal bones should be performed to assess the location of the facial nerve, ventilation of the middle ear and mastoid, and the presence/absence of the ossicular chain.

Treatment

Conventional Hearing Aids

Due to the predominance of external ear malformations in these patients, conventional hearing aids have limited application. Even in patients who undergo reconstructive surgery, functional and audiologic outcomes are often disappointing with conventional hearing aids [9].

Bone Conduction Amplification Options

Bone conduction amplification should be considered as early as possible even in cases of unilateral atresia in order to provide good speech sound awareness to both ears which is needed for timely development of communication. Ideally amplification should be fit within the first month of life and no later than 6 months of age [8]. Most patients should be fit with bone conduction devices. In a study by Rosa et al., the pure tone average (PTA) in free field by bone conduction was 26.8 ± 4.1 dB with an estimated gain of 32.8 ± 8.3 dB [2].

Historically hearing aid companies modified behind-the-ear (BTE) hearings to connect with a cable to a bone conduction oscillator which was then fit on a headband or softband (Fig. 9.1). These hearing aids are no longer being manufactured by most US hearing aid companies because there are now alternative options from implant manufacturers to use their speech processor on softbands. Cochlear Americas has the Baha and Oticon Medical which makes the Ponto, both of which are easily fit on infants and young children using softbands.

Both companies offer surgical options once the patients are at least 5 years of age (see further explanation below). However, some families are undecided about what surgical interventions to choose and can opt for a SoundArc (Fig. 9.2) in lieu of the softband if they use a Baha.

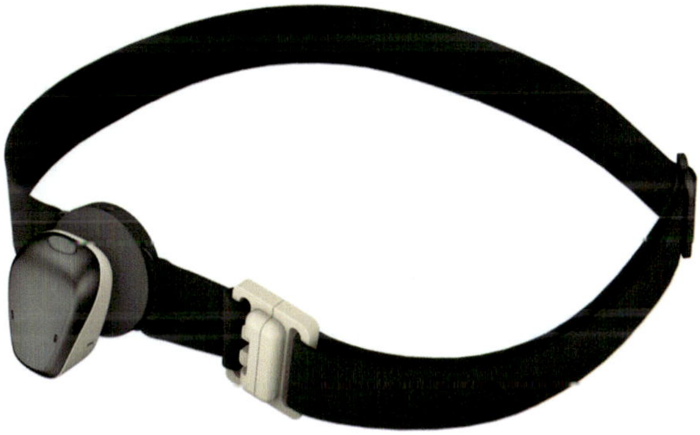

Fig. 9.1 Softband Baha courtesy of Cochlear Americas. (Image courtesy of Cochlear. © Cochlear Limited 2021. All rights reserved)

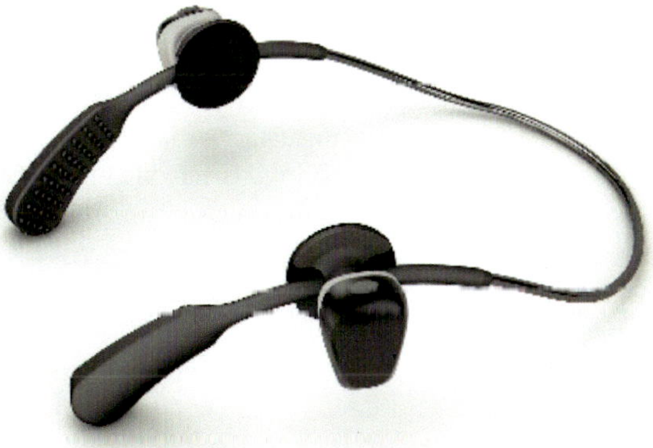

Fig. 9.2 Baha SoundArc. (Image courtesy of Cochlear. © Cochlear Limited 2021. All rights reserved)

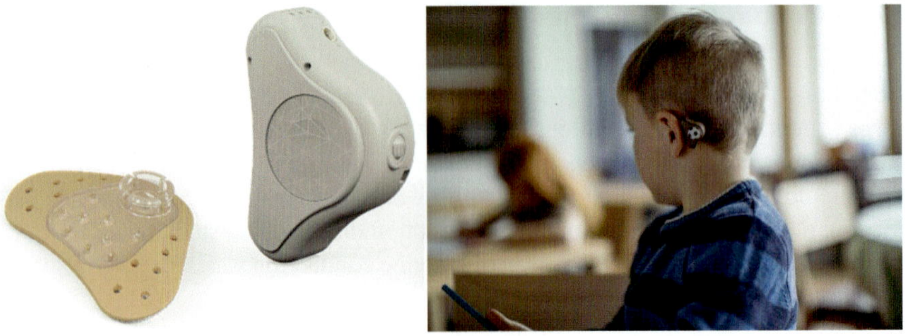

Fig. 9.3 ADHEAR. (Photos Courtesy of Med-El)

Another option is the MED-El ADHEAR (Fig. 9.3) which is a speech processor that can be used on a softband initially and later attached to the skin without the band using a medical grade adhesive.

Implanted Devices

In patients with TCS and HFMS, bone-anchored hearing devices are a very effective method of hearing implantation. The audiologic results of implanted conduction devices have been shown to have a PTA in free field 18.3 ± 1.3 dB with an estimated gain of 38 ± 5.5 dB. Advantages of bone-anchored hearing devices over conventional hearing aids are improved amplification and sound quality, improved bone conduction, as well as aesthetic appearance [2]. The FDA has approved several implantable bone conduction devices for children, and these include the Cochlear Baha and Osia, as well as the MED EL Bone Bridge. The Baha system has been approved in children since 1999. Two versions are in current use: an abutment system (Fig. 9.4) and an implantable magnetic system (Fig. 9.5). Both involve implanting a titanium pedestal into the mastoid or parietal bone, under a general anesthetic. Either a transcutaneous abutment (Baha Connect) or an implanted magnet (Baha Attract) is attached to the implanted pedestal. The child may begin to wear the hearing aid within a few weeks of the surgery.

The MED EL Bone Bridge (Fig. 9.6) and the Cochlear Osia (Fig. 9.7) are FDA approved over the age of 12 years. These both require implanting the hearing aid under the periosteum of the mastoid, and the microphone/receiver is attached via external magnet on the skin surface.

The use of middle ear implants has also been described in patients with TCS; however, further studies are needed to confirm audiologic outcomes as well as long-term follow-up to evaluate possible long-term adverse effects [10, 11]. These are not FDA approved for use in the United States.

Because severe to profound SNHL in patients with TCS and HFMS is rare and SNHL in these patients is most often unilateral, cochlear implantation in these

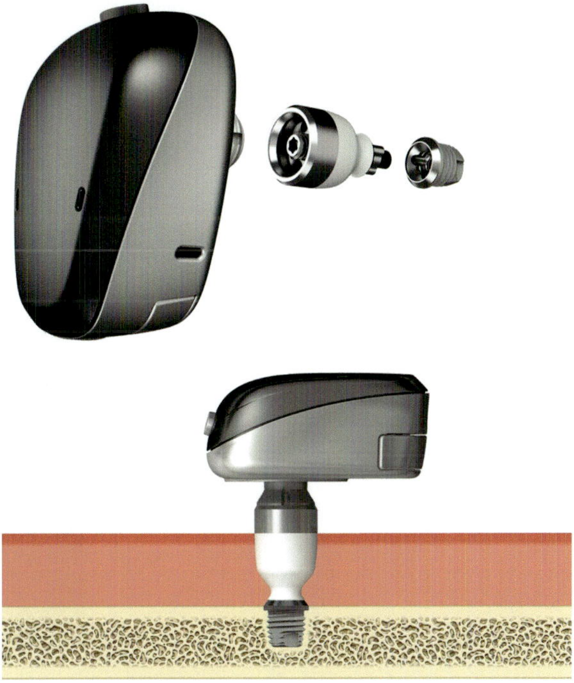

Fig. 9.4 Baha abutment system. (Image courtesy of Cochlear. © Cochlear Limited 2021. All rights reserved)

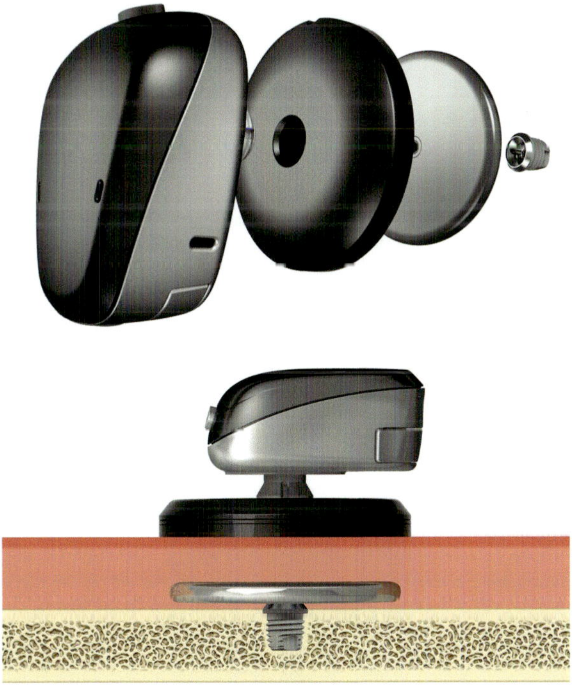

Fig. 9.5 Baha implantable magnetic system. (Image courtesy of Cochlear. © Cochlear Limited 2021. All rights reserved)

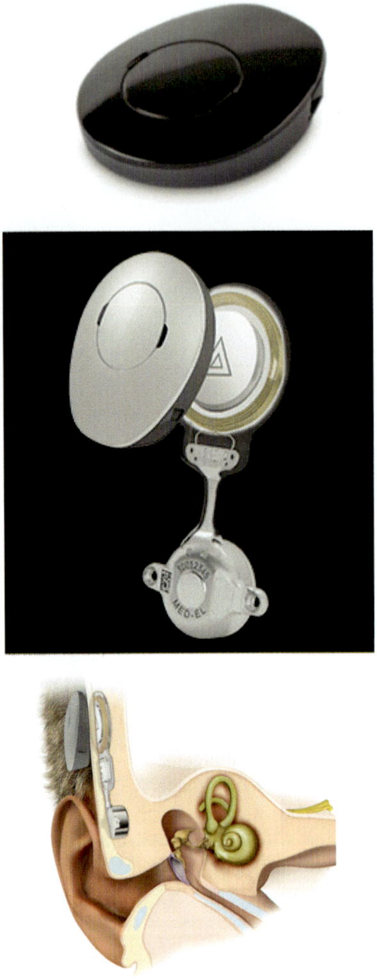

Fig. 9.6 MED EL bone bridge. (Image courtesy of Med-EL)

patients is rarely necessary. However, in patients' meeting criteria, cochlear implantation may be considered [10] and is quite effective.

Atresia Surgery

Ear canal reconstruction surgery is rarely indicated in TCS/HFMS due to the numerous associated abnormalities, including aberrant facial nerve location, dysmorphic ossicular chain, and hypo-pneumatization of the middle ear and mastoid. This surgery includes the creation of an ear canal and tympanic membrane through a post-auricular incision. A split-thickness skin graft is used to line the newly formed ear

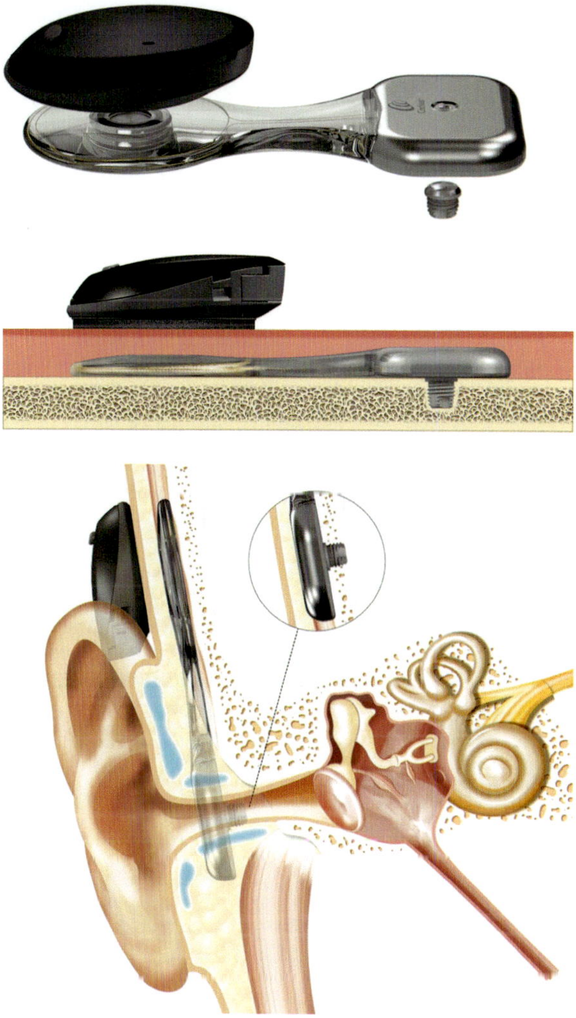

Fig. 9.7 Cochlear Osia. (Images courtesy of Cochlear. © Cochlear Limited 2021. All rights reserved)

canal and tympanic membrane [12]. Complications include sensorineural hearing loss, facial nerve injury, and restenosis requiring revision surgery.

References

1. Marx H. Die Missbildungen des Ohres. In: Henke F, Lubarsh O, editors. Handbuch der Spez Path Anatomie Histologie. Berlin: Springer; 1926. p. 620–5.
2. Rosa F, Coutinho MB, Ferreira JP, Sousa CA. Ear malformations, hearing loss and hearing rehabilitation in children with Treacher Collins syndrome. Acta Otorrinolaringol Esp (English Ed). 2016;67(3):142–7. https://doi.org/10.1016/j.otoeng.2016.05.001.

3. D'Arco F, Youssef A, Ioannidou E, et al. Temporal bone and intracranial abnormalities in syndromic causes of hearing loss: an updated guide. Eur J Radiol. 2020;123(June 2019):108803. https://doi.org/10.1016/j.ejrad.2019.108803.
4. Carvalho GJ, Song CS, Vargervik K, Lalwani AK. Auditory and facial nerve dysfunction in patients with hemifacial microsomia. Arch Otolaryngol Head Neck Surg. 1999;125(2):209–12. https://doi.org/10.1001/archotol.125.2.209.
5. Sleifer P, Gorsky NDS, Goetze TB, Rosa RFM, Zen PRG. Audiological findings in patients with oculo-auriculo-vertebral spectrum. Int Arch Otorhinolaryngol. 2013;19(1):5–9. https://doi.org/10.1055/s-0034-1390137.
6. Beleza-Meireles A, Hart R, Clayton-Smith J, et al. Oculo-auriculo-vertebral spectrum: clinical and molecular analysis of 51 patients. Eur J Med Genet. 2015;58(9):455–65. https://doi.org/10.1016/j.ejmg.2015.07.003.
7. Goetze TB, Sleifer P, Rosa RFM, da Silva AP, Graziadio C, Zen PRG. Hearing characterization in oculoauriculovertebral spectrum: a prospective study with 10 patients. Am J Med Genet A. 2017;173(2):309–14. https://doi.org/10.1002/ajmg.a.38017.
8. Year 2019 position statement: principles and guidelines for early hearing detection and intervention programs. J Early Hearing Detect Intervention. 4(2):1–44. https://doi.org/10.15142/fptk-b748.
9. Marres HAM. Hearing loss in the Treacher-Collins syndrome. Adv Otorhinolaryngol. 2002;61. ISSN: 0065-3071 Online ISSN: 1662-2847.
10. Tringali S, Pergola N, Ferber-Viart C, Truy E, Berger P, Dubreuil C. Fully implantable hearing device as a new treatment of conductive hearing loss in Franceschetti syndrome. Int J Pediatr Otorhinolaryngol. 2008;72(4):513–7. https://doi.org/10.1016/j.ijporl.2007.12.002.
11. Lesinskas E, Stankeviciute V, Petrulionis M. Application of the Vibrant Soundbridge middle-ear implant for aural atresia in patients with Treacher Collins syndrome. J Laryngol Otol. 2012;126(12):1216–23. https://doi.org/10.1017/S0022215112002344.
12. Jahrsdoerfer RA. Congenital atresia of the ear. Laryngoscope. 1978;9 Pt 3 Suppl 13:1–48.

Chapter 10
Microtia Reconstruction in Patients with Craniofacial Microsomia

Tania Kraai, Katherine Vandenberg, Sheryl Lewin, and Rosemary Seelaus

Introduction

The options for microtia reconstruction have vastly improved due to the innovation of dedicated surgeons and anaplastologists who have devoted their careers to this particularly challenging condition [1–6]. The goal of this chapter is to describe current protocols for reconstruction based on their work and the expertise of the authors with a focus on the three most common techniques: autologous cartilage, porous implant, and prosthetic ear reconstruction. All three of these techniques can achieve optimal results; however, expertise for a particular technique will influence the results. These techniques should only be undertaken by those who are dedicated to learning and caring for patients with complex auricular anomalies. The focus will be on timing, pearls to achieving an excellent result, and the pros and cons of different approaches to auricular reconstruction.

During the preoperative auricular reconstruction consultation, the surgeon should characterize the auricle and analyze the facial profile, noting the presence of asymmetry, hypoplastic tissue, consistency of the postauricular skin, presence of a canal, and the location of the hairline. Numerous classifications have been proposed to

T. Kraai (✉) · K. Vandenberg
University of New Mexico Health Science Centers, Department of Surgery, Albuquerque, NM, USA
e-mail: tkraai@salud.unm.edu; kvandenberg@salud.unm.edu

S. Lewin
Lewin Ear Reconstruction, Torrance, CA, USA
e-mail: slewin@lewinmd.com

R. Seelaus
The Craniofacial Center, Department of Surgery, University of Illinois at Chicago, Chicago, IL, USA
e-mail: rseelaus@uic.edu

D. M. Yates, M. R. Markiewicz (eds.), *Craniofacial Microsomia and Treacher Collins Syndrome*, https://doi.org/10.1007/978-3-030-84733-3_10

characterize the auricle [4, 7–13]. We find it most helpful to grade based on the increasing severity of the anomaly (see Fig. 10.1).

The protocol described in this chapter will focus more on severe congenital auricular deformities, i.e., grades II–IV. Grade I microtia is highly variable, and reconstruction in these cases needs to be tailored to each anomaly; there are various methods described to address these less severe anomalies [12, 14]. Each grade may be associated with a low-lying hairline, which is one of the more challenging characteristics associated with microtia. Table 10.1 lists several surgical techniques described in the literature that address a low hairline, which should be considered prior to making reconstructive recommendations.

The age, availability of sufficient costal cartilage, potential need for an implanted hearing device, and associated syndromes and comorbidities are also relevant during the presurgical consultation. Since the dominant vascular supply to the auricle and surrounding tissues may vary in patients with craniofacial microsomia, the vessels should be considered preoperatively by palpation or Doppler [44, 45]. The surgical approach should be modified based on relevant patient factors and their goals. Careful consideration of all options to address microtia is necessary, including the option to not reconstruct the ear as not all patients desire or benefit from reconstruction. The advantages and disadvantages of some of the most common microtia reconstruction techniques are summarized in Table 10.2.

Autologous Costal Cartilage Auricular Reconstruction

Numerous published approaches and entire books are dedicated to autologous cartilage microtia reconstruction [4, 11, 38, 46]. This chapter will provide a protocol with a focus on two-stage reconstruction as popularized by Drs. Nagata and Firmin while incorporating considerations from other techniques.

First-Stage Auricular Reconstruction Using Autologous Costal Cartilage

The first stage includes excision of the vestigial cartilage, transposition of the remnant lobule, harvesting and constructing a three-dimensional (3D) framework from autologous costal cartilage, and correct placement of the cartilaginous framework within the temporal pocket. Placement should be dictated by the contralateral auricle in unilateral cases. In severe forms of microtia, the external auditory canal may be displaced inferiorly and anteriorly making positioning of the reconstructed ear more challenging. Transposing or even closing the canal may be necessary for optimal positioning, but this carries the risk of recurrent external auditory canal infection or cholesteatoma. Careful consideration should be given in these cases with

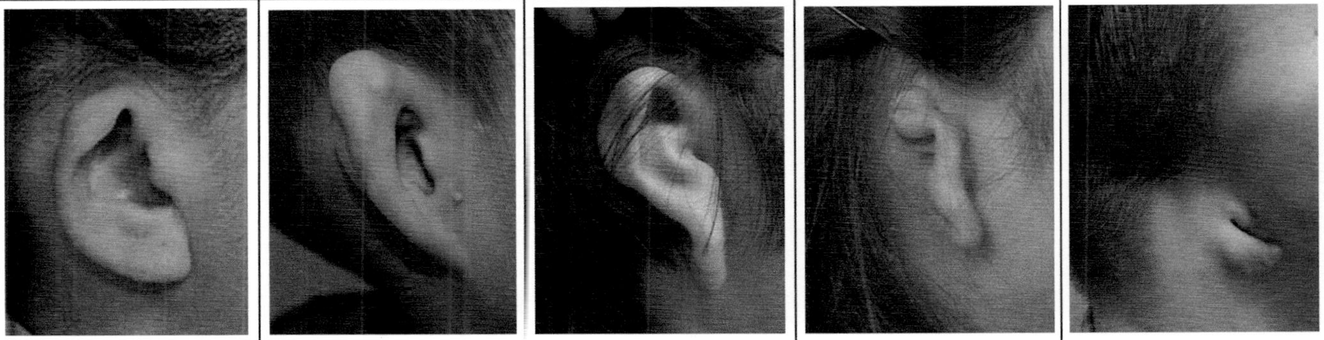

Grade I	Grade IIa	Grade IIb	Grade III	Grade IV
Upper 1/3rd ear anomalies. Near normal size. This anomaly varies widely.	Upper 1/2 ear anomalies; helix, antihelix and triangular fossa are absent or anomalous. The tragus, antitragus and concha cavum are near normal size but often over projected (Nagata's conchal type).	Upper 2/3rd ear anomalies; helix, antihelix, triangular fossa absent or anomalous, conchal bowl is constricted. The antitragus and tragus are variably formed (Nagata's small conchal type).	The lobule is vertically oriented, and the cartilage is very small with no other recognizable features (Nagata's lobular type).	Includes anotia and atypical microtia where the ear remnant is markedly displaced without components that can be used to reconstruct the ear in the correct location. Almost always associated with a low hairline.

Fig. 10.1 Microtia classifications

Table 10.1 Options for addressing a low hairline in patients with microtia

Management	Advantage(s)	Disadvantage(s)
Laser epilation	Less invasive, does not require additional surgery Safe, without evidence of damage to the skin or cartilage [15] More successful in patients with very light skin and very dark hair May improve elasticity and texture of the skin May be performed preoperatively when the skin is more uniform, requiring less treatments [16]	Time-consuming, up to 1 year with multiple sessions (4–7) [15, 16] Thins and decreases terminal hairs, but does not completely eradicate them Does not change the skin thickness of hair-bearing skin [15] Different lasers may have different efficacies and settings (i.e., nm, J/cm^2), dependent on Fitzgerald skin type Pain Rare complications include erythema and blisters Insurance coverage may be variable
Place cartilage framework slightly into the hairline	Hair on the superior helix may hide well in patients with long hair Post-surgical epilation options are still available	Not ideal for patients with extremely low hairlines, greater than 15% covering the auricle [17]
Place the framework slightly anterior to the hairline	Small changes may not be noticeable	Poor position placement on the lateral view
Create a slightly smaller auricle below the hairline	Better suited for bilateral microtia May be advantageous in moderate to severe hemifacial microsomia [18]	Poor symmetry on the frontal view May need to reduce the size of the contralateral ear
Raise an ultra-delicate split-thickness skin graft, and excise the underlying hair follicles during the second stage of autologous reconstruction [4]	Good color match contiguous with helical rim skin Allows for correct positioning of the auricle	Variable skin graft quality [19] Time-consuming and difficult to raise Not ideal for patients with extremely low hairlines, greater than 15% covering the auricle [17]
Excise hair-bearing skin, and cover the framework with fascia and a skin graft during the first stage of autologous reconstruction	Allows for correct position placement even with an extremely low hairline	Variable skin graft quality Donor site morbidity Increased risk for cartilage atrophy

Table 10.1 (continued)

Management	Advantage(s)	Disadvantage(s)
Use a tissue expander to expand non-hair-bearing skin	One stage reconstruction, two surgical procedures Provides sufficient non-hair-bearing skin for draping over anterior ear Excellent color match No additional scars Ideal for patients with a small auricle and cranioauricular angle [20]	Hematoma (0.9–6.2%) [20–24] Infection (0.9–1.1%) [23, 24] Tissue expander exposure (2.8%) [25] Flap necrosis (0.9%) [25] Formation of a fibrous capsule that may influence skin contouring over the framework [23] Flap edema present for months postoperatively [22] Inappropriate in patients with scar tissue from previous surgery
Reconstruct using a porous implant and skin grafts	See Table 10.2	

Table 10.2 Advantages and disadvantages of different reconstruction options in patients with congenital microtia

Treatment	Age (years)	Advantage(s)	Disadvantage(s)
Observation	Any	No risk	Cosmesis Difficult visual aid retention (i.e., glasses) Psychosocial factors
Prosthesis	≥3–5	Predictable outcome Manufactured as a mirrored replica of the opposite side No donor site morbidity Rescue procedure in failed reconstructions	Daily maintenance/cleaning/removal/reattachment Discoloration and aging of materials over time (UV/environmental factors/cigarette exposure) Lifelong renewal (every 2–3 years) May not be amenable to contact sports/swimming Cost varies substantially by healthcare system and/or providers (US $2000–$7000) [26]
Adhesive-retained prosthesis		Non-invasive Does not preclude further reconstruction Interim solution	Less reliable positioning and retention Oily skin and excessive hair may compromise retention May not be tolerated by younger patients Adhesive decreases the longevity of prosthesis More challenging adhesion with larger remnants Allergic reaction to adhesive

(continued)

Table 10.2 (continued)

Treatment	Age (years)	Advantage(s)	Disadvantage(s)
Implant-retained prosthesis	>2–4 [27] > 5 in the USA	Longer prosthetic lifespan compared with adhesive retainment Ease of and precise positioning More reliable retention Improved aesthetics with thinner margin at fitting surface Patient adoption of prosthesis via possible "osseoperception" [28] Retention is less influenced by environmental factors	Scars may preclude further reconstruction Skin irritation and infection (9.1–39%) [27] May require revision surgery due to growth of temporal bone (22%) [27] Loss of implant (1.7–5.8%) [27, 29–32] Cortical bone width must be more than 2.5–3 mm Daily home hygiene needs Lifetime replacement of prostheses Retentive suprastructure, i.e., magnets or bar, may require removal for MRI imaging
Porous polyethylene alloplastic implant (Medpor, Su-por)	≥3	More standardized outcomes among surgeons Single stage Less donor site morbidity Less variability in carving Ideal for younger patients Excellent biocompatibility, stability, tissue integration, and resistance to infection	Scars may preclude further reconstruction Difficult to remove Lifetime risk of exposure Lifetime risk of implant fracture (3–25%) [33] Complication rate (4%) [34] Complete loss of framework (<1%) [35] Technically unforgiving with a high learning curve Rarely taught in training programs/fellowships [36]
Autologous costal cartilage reconstruction	[a]	Well established for over 50 years Growth of costal cartilage framework [37] Preferred over osseointegrated implant (88%) [38] Withstands trauma [2] Suitable for all microtia types with modifications [4]	Scars may preclude further reconstruction Donor site complications (pneumothorax, atelectasis, and scarring) Chest wall contour deformity, mitigated by replacing cartilage off-cuts into the perichondrial sleeve [39] Outcomes depend on surgeons' artistic and spatial expertise
Two-stage (Nagata and Firmin) technique	≥7–10	Requires multiple surgeries, two stages	Cartilage resorption from infection (1.6%) [40] Blunted contours (4.8%) [40] Hypertrophic scar (2.4–6%) [40, 41] Complications requiring reoperation (8.9–22%) [24, 42] Variable posterior partial flap necrosis (0.1–13.9%) [41, 43]
Tissue expander		See Table 10.1	

[a]Determined by the amount of cartilage needed. Nagata recommends a 60-cm rib circumference at the xiphoid and age 10 years old [4]

appropriate expertise. Even in the most skilled hands, this procedure can take an entire day to complete, and most experienced teams involve two surgeons. For example, one surgeon may harvest cartilage, while the second surgeon removes vestigial cartilage, elevates a skin flap, carves, and sets the framework. The steps with surgical pearls (*) are as follows:

Preoperative Steps

1. Position the patient for a long procedure.
   * Pad or suspend pressure points including the heels, scapula, and hips.
2. Shave, braid, or tie hair away from the surgical area.
   * Minimal hair removal is preferred by our patient population.
3. Determine and mark the location for the reconstructed ear.
   * The angle of the ear should be 15–20 degrees back for bilateral cases and should match the contralateral ear for unilateral cases.
   * Measure the following contralateral ear landmarks: lateral orbital rim to helical root, nasal ala to tragus and oral commissure to anterior lobule insertion prior to taping the endotracheal tube.
   * The Frankfort horizontal line and zygomatic root should cross just above the planned tragus.
   * The angle of the nasal dorsum can serve as a reference.
   * Create a positioning template using the contralateral ear position with cutouts for the ear, lateral brow, commissure of the eye, nasal ala, and oral commissure using radiographic film, and sterilize per institutional guideline. The positioning template and contralateral anteroposterior measurements are used to verify the correct location, size, and angulation of the ear [17, 38].
   * The outer edge of the planned ear position may be tattooed on the skin at the beginning of the case using methylene blue and a 25-gauge needle.
   * The top of the planned microtia reconstruction should be even with the contralateral ear and usually at the level of the lateral eyebrow unless the opposite ear is low set. The sideburn to helical root distance is usually 1.5 cm.
   * In more severe forms of hemifacial microsomia, the position may need to be slightly more anterior and slightly smaller than the contralateral ear, but the sideburn measurement should be respected [11, 18].
4. Create and sterilize a carving template based on the cartilage to be reconstructed (see Fig. 10.2).
   * Measure the height and width of the contralateral ear. For bilateral microtia, the patient may choose the size; generally, a smaller size is preferable.
   * The contralateral ear can be used to create the carving template using radiographic film. Dr. Nagata uses sized preprinted templates [4].
   * 3D templates have also been described using various methods and materials and may improve patient satisfaction while decreasing surgical time [47, 48].
5. Plan costal cartilage harvest incision.

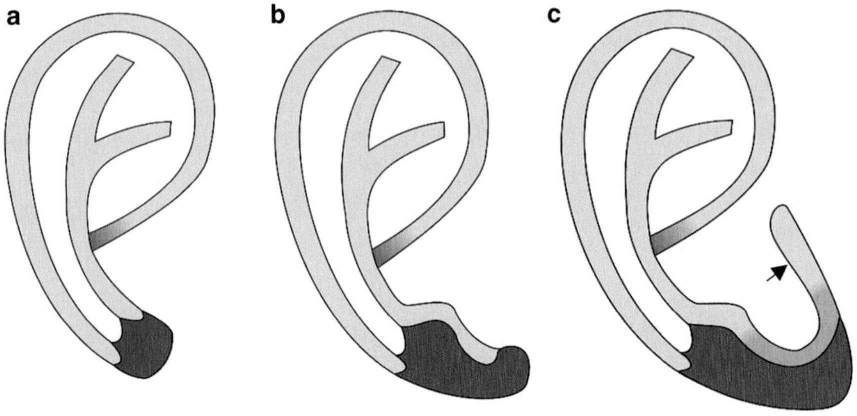

Fig. 10.2 Carving template examples for (**a**) grade IIa, (**b**) grade IIb, and (**c**) grade III–IV microtia where the lighter segments represent the stacked portions of the cartilage graft. The grade III–IV template should have the tragus 3 mm anterior (arrow) compared to the opposite ear to help create a deep conchal bowl

   * Identify ribs 6–9 on the ipsilateral side to the microtia ear. Contralateral costal cartilage can be used, but for the carving technique in this chapter, the ipsilateral cartilage is described.

   * Mark a 4-cm oblique or horizontal chest incision near the inferior border of the seventh rib. Oblique incisions improve access, while horizontal incisions correspond with relaxed skin tension lines.

   * The incision may need to be extended in obese patients but may be as small as 2 cm in non-obese patients [46].

6. Prepare and drape the patient with the opposite ear in the operative field for ease in confirming accurate placement.

   * Be mindful of fire risks with some sterilizing solutions particularly if hair is exposed.

   * Most patients with microtia have aural atresia (76%). However, if an ear canal is present, then prepare the ear canal with 5% betadine [49].

   * In patients with an ear canal, antibiotic otic drops for 1 week prior to surgery has been described [3].

Auricular Reconstruction Site Preparation

1. Plan and mark the lobule transposition incision. The incision and subcutaneous vascular pedicle sites are marked based on microtia classification and location of the remnant auricle (see Fig. 10.3). For grade IV reconstruction, see Figs. 10.4 and 10.5.

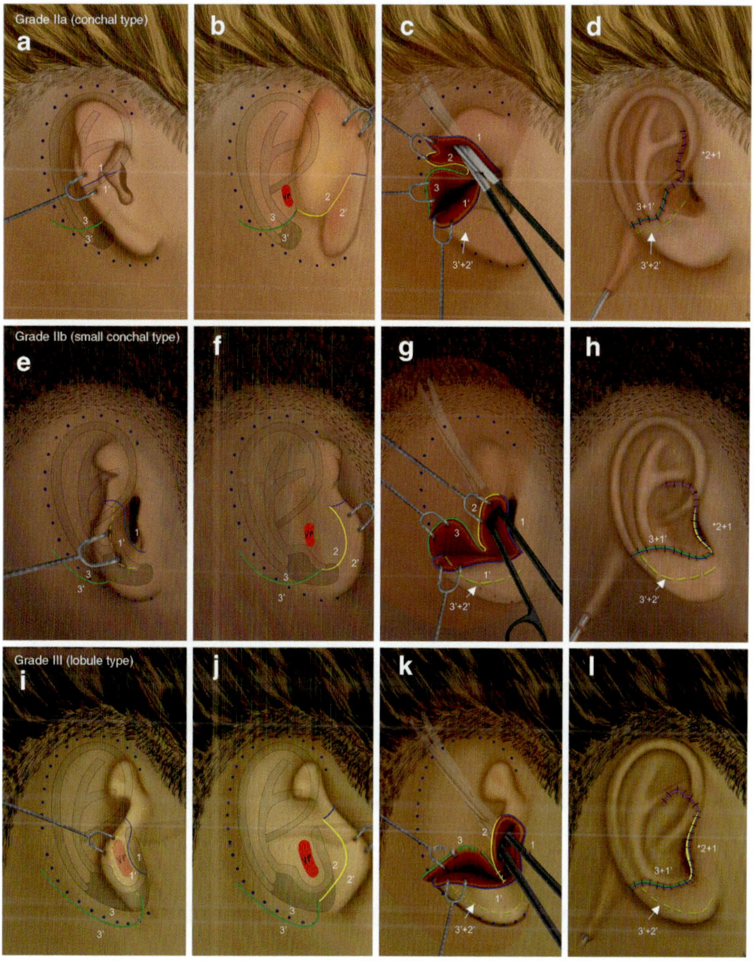

Fig. 10.3 Lobule transposition incisions and flap elevation for microtia reconstruction; methylene blue dots mark the correct position for the reconstructed ear, and the carving template is shown for reference. The skin at the vascular pedicle (vp) site is not elevated. (**Grade IIa – a**, **b**) The anterior ear incision 1/1′ crosses the conchal bowl and extends above the antitragus around the ear to the posterior ear incision 2/2′ allowing access for removal of irregular microtia cartilage and rotation of the inferior ear into the desired position, and the mastoid incision 3/3′ allows for elevation of the skin flap to cover the cartilage framework, (**c**) subdermal dissection extends 1–2 cm beyond the marked cartilage graft position (shaded area), and (**d**) closed incisions after removing redundant skin (*2 + 1 is variable and must be tailored to each patient), which is aided by placing a small suction catheter. (**Grade IIb – e**, **f**) Incision 1/1′ crosses above the vertically oriented lobule, and incision 2/2′ extends posteriorly slightly lower than for grade IIa splitting the lobule. Incision 3/3′ creates a larger mastoid flap to help cover the larger cartilage framework, which includes the anti-tragus in the framework, **g** shows the elevated flaps, and **h** closed incisions. (**Grade III – i**, **j**) Incision 1/1′ creates a small anteriorly based flap to cover the tragus (1) and allows the anterior lobule flap (1′) to rotate inferiorly, and incision 2/2′ and 3/3′ extend posteriorly lower than for Grade IIb also splitting the lobule and creating a larger flap to cover the cartilage framework that includes reconstruction of the tragus and intertragal notch; **k**, **l** show the area to be elevated and the closed incisions after removing redundant skin

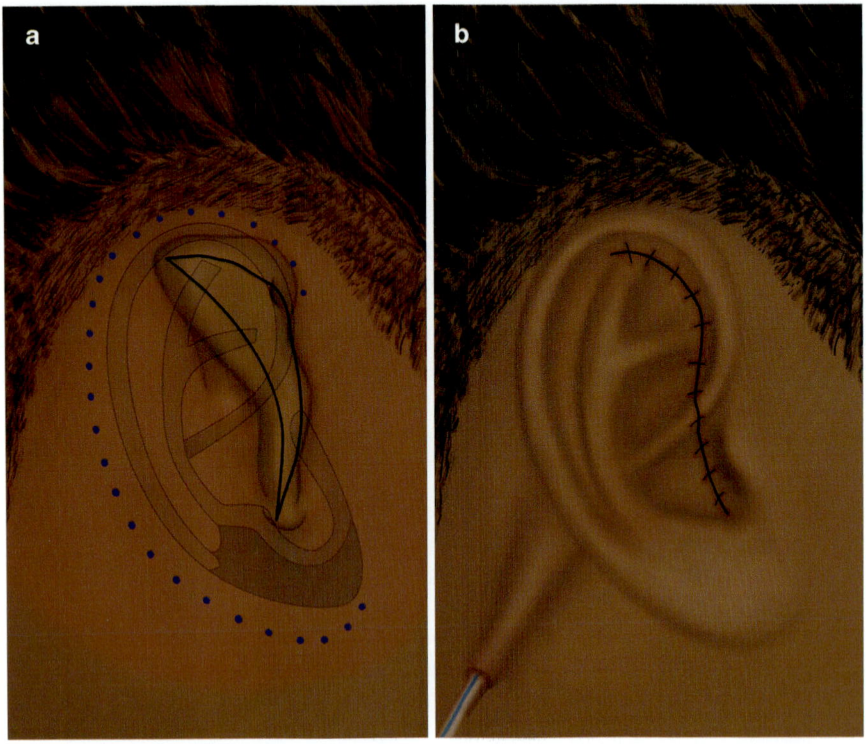

Fig. 10.4 *Grade IV* (without low hairline): (**a**) incision placed to allow access for removal of irregular cartilage and redundant skin. Skin flap elevated widely for placement of the cartilage framework, and (**b**) shows cartilage in place and incision closed

* In some patients with grade IIa (conchal type) microtia, the incision does not need to extend around into the postauricular sulcus if the ear is not significantly over projected, e.g., Fig. 10.6.

* The vascular pedicle should be at the normal location of the external auditory canal, which is just below the root of the zygomatic arch, and can be confirmed using the carving template. The pedicle improves the blood supply to the skin flap, deepens the conchal bowl, and tethers the skin down to create a depression that mimics the external auditory canal and accentuates the tragus, e.g., Fig. 10.7 [50].

* In lobular-type microtia, ample skin from the posterior lobule and mastoid should be elevated to line a deep conchal bowl.

* If possible, the anterior surface of the tragal cartilage should be covered with the skin contiguous with the cheek to avoid a more visible scar.

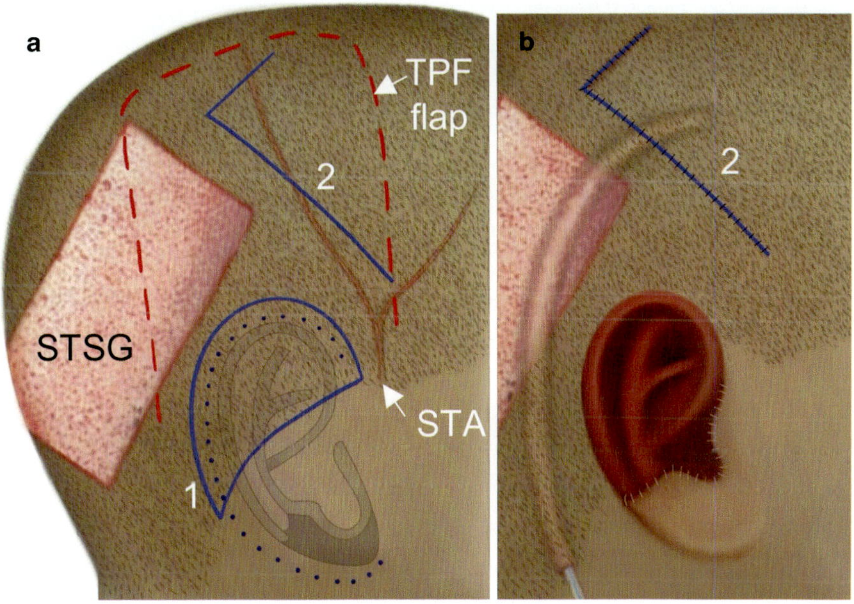

Fig. 10.5 *Grade IV* (with low hairline): (**a**) incision (1) allows for excision of unwanted hair-bearing skin and placement of the cartilage framework. Optional incision (2) allows easy access for TPF harvest in these patients who are more likely to have an aberrant or tenuous blood supply. Optional scalp STSG site also shown. (**b**) shows the cartilage framework in place with the TPF flap folded over the framework and sutured in place. The TPF is then covered with a skin graft

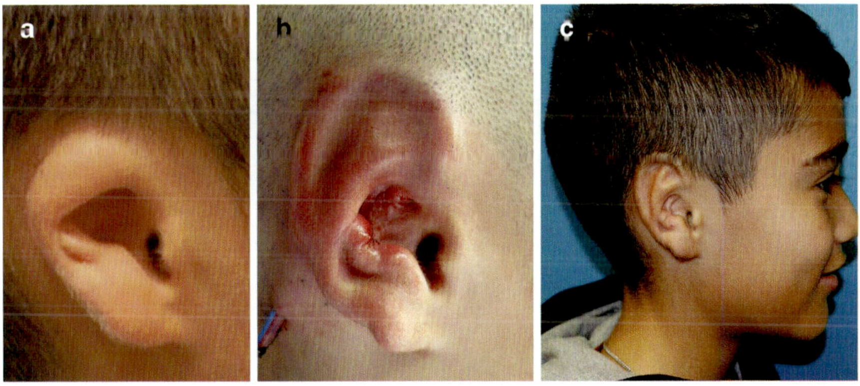

Fig. 10.6 (**a**) Grade IIa microtia with normal projection. (**b**) Intraoperative image with incision in the neo-cymba concha. (**c**) Postoperative stage 1 reconstruction

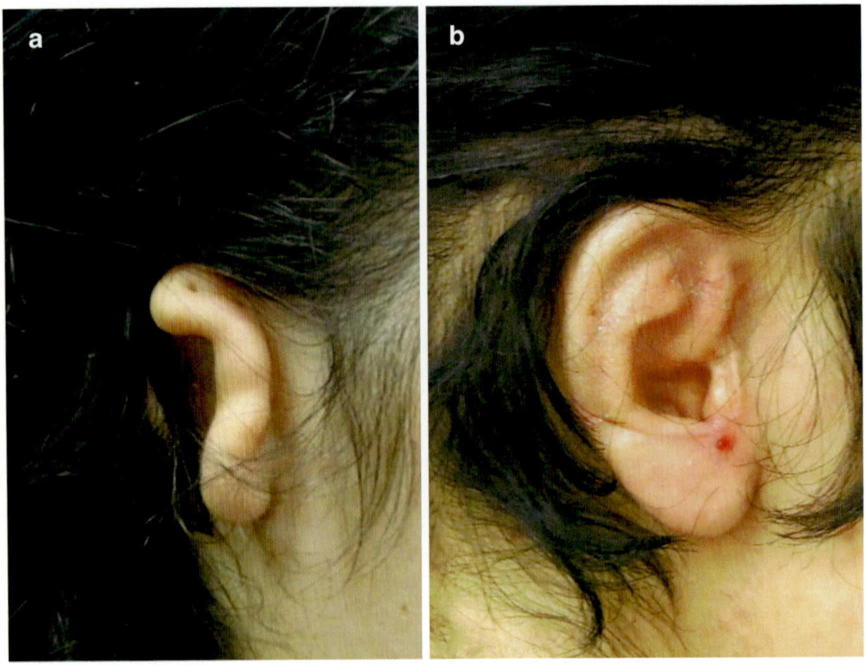

Fig. 10.7 (**a**) Grade III (lobule type) microtia with aural atresia. (**b**) Post two-stage auricular reconstruction. The subcutaneous vascular pedicle helps deepen the conchal bowl and creates a shadow at the normal site for the external auditory canal in patients with aural atresia

* If there is a significantly low-lying hairline (>15%) (usually grade III or IV), then a temporoparietal fascial (TPF) flap and skin graft may be necessary to cover the framework where the hair-bearing skin must be excised (see TPF harvest description in stage 2). A separate fascial flap will be necessary for stage 2 in these cases.

2. Remove the vestigial auricular cartilage; leave the tragus and antitragus if present.

   * Straight tenotomy scissors, 15-blade, q-tip, and cottle, are helpful for skin elevation.

   * If present, removing the vestigial conchal bowl cartilage improves the depth of the neo-conchal bowl.

3. Create a subcutaneous temporal pocket, which should be elevated at least 2 cm past the marked framework position while maintaining a vascular pedicle.

   * Elevate a uniform flap to allow the skin to drape evenly over the framework. If the skin flap is too thin, then the risk of skin necrosis, cartilage atrophy, and exposure of the cartilage framework increases. If the skin flap is too thick, the auricular contours will be less pronounced.

   * Maintain the subdermal plexus by elevating just over fascia. The mastoid fascia, which contains the posterior auricular muscles, is continuous with the

TPF cranially and the superficial cervical fascia caudally [51]. The subcutaneous layer thins over the mastoid tip, and care should be taken to maintain a sufficiently thick subcutaneous flap to avoid a skin thickness mismatch with the lobular transposition flap. Maintaining intact fascia also protects venous outflow from the TPF.

Costal Cartilage Harvest

1. Consider options for decreasing postoperative pain using an intercostal block, paravertebral regional block, or pain pump.
2. Make the preplanned incision down through the subcutaneous tissue, and create a suprafascial pocket overlying costal cartilages 6–9.
3. Elevate the rectus and external oblique muscle from the perichondrium to widely expose ribs 6–9.
   * Muscle transection may be minimized by lateralizing these muscle groups.
4. Divide the anterior perichondrium of the sixth and seventh ribs with care to avoid injuring the underlying cartilage. The rib anatomy is variable, but these ribs usually have a synchondrosis.
   * Use a flat paddle Bovie tip on a low setting or a 15-blade scalpel.
   * Elevate the perichondrium superiorly and inferiorly with a freer or osteotome.
5. Once the costochondral joint is exposed, divide at the bony cartilaginous junction using a molt or malleable to protect the pleura, leaving a small beveled rim of cartilage on the bone.
6. Elevate the costal cartilage off the posterior perichondrium from lateral to medial. Divide the medial attachment at the sternochondral joint.
   * If possible, maintain the synchondrosis for stability of the base framework.
   * Finger dissection under the rib can aid in elevation.
7. Harvest the eighth and possibly the ninth rib.
   * Free the medial attachments, and elevate each rib laterally with care not to overbend and fracture the rib, leaving the perichondrium on the harvested rib [3].
   * Conchal-type microtia reconstruction may not require the ninth costal cartilage, but enough cartilage should be harvested to bank for the second-stage projection graft if a second stage is required.
8. Place the harvested costal cartilage in antibiotic saline solution (e.g., gentamicin 50 mg/500 mL).
9. Check for a pleural tear and repair if present.
10. Close the sixth and seventh rib perichondrial sleeve leaving a small opening for replacing the cartilage off-cuts.
11. Close the chest incision after carving the framework so that cartilage off-cuts can be replaced prior to closure.

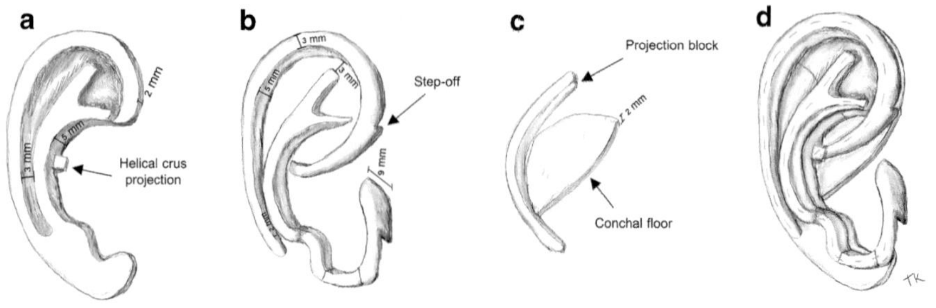

Fig. 10.8 Creating the cartilage framework. (**a**) The base framework is carved from the sixth and seventh rib synchondrosis. The scapha and triangular fossa are deepened. The conchal bowl is removed except for a small projection for attachment of helical crus. (**b**) The helical rim is attached first at the projection piece. A step-off is carved on the undersurface at the root where the helix transitions onto the base framework. The antihelix, antitragus, and tragus are carved as needed from different off-cuts of cartilage and secured to the base framework. (**c**) The conchal floor graft and sometimes a projection block (for single stage) are secured under the base framework and helical crus to create a deep conchal bowl. (**d**) The three-layered costal cartilage graft

Creating the Cartilage Framework (See Fig. 10.8)

Microtia reconstruction surgery requires meticulous attention to detail, and carving the framework requires spatial expertise in ear anatomy to create an optimal 3D structure. Care should be taken when handling cartilage and should be treated as a living sculpture. For lobular-type microtia (grade III) and anotia (grade IV), the full cartilage framework will need to be created as described below. For conchal-type microtia (grade II), the tragus and sometimes the antitragus do not need to be reconstructed if they are well-formed, e.g., Fig. 10.9. Older patients may have calcified costal cartilage, and a drill may be necessary to create portions of the framework. Use a 5.0 double-armed steel suture (or 40 gauge) for efficient attachment of cartilage components. Permanent clear suture (e.g., 4.0 or 5.0 Nylon) may also be used if steel suture is not available.

Base Framework

1. The ipsilateral sixth and seventh costal cartilages are flipped over so that the inner surface of the costal cartilage in situ becomes the lateral surface of the ear framework, taking advantage of the natural curve (see Fig. 10.10).

   * The surgeon carving the framework should sit on the same side as the microtia to help avoid mistakenly carving the wrong side.

   * The synchondrosis may need suture reinforcement if the attachment is loose. If the location of the synchondrosis has a notch or does not fit the template correctly, then the sixth and seventh rib should be separated and reattached.

   * Use a 15-blade, gouge, or biopsy punch for carving [46].

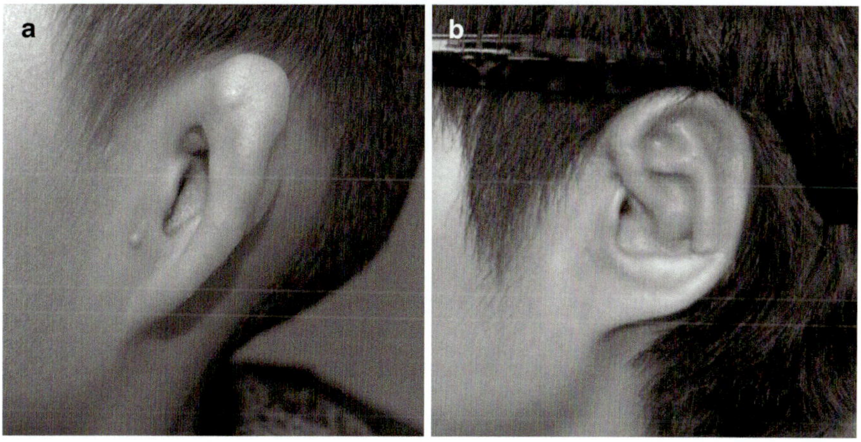

Fig. 10.9 (**a**) Preoperative and (**b**) postoperative grade IIa (conchal type) microtia requiring reconstruction of the upper ear only

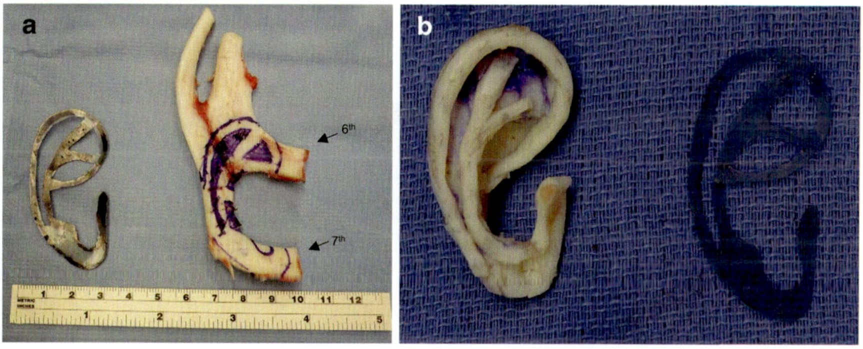

Fig. 10.10 (**a**) Create the base framework by placing the carving template over the synchondrosis such that it will support the stacked helix and antihelix. (**b**) Completed cartilage framework

Helix, Antihelix, Antitragus, Intertragal Notch, and Tragus (Fig. 10.10b)

2. Divide the eighth rib to create the helical rim, which is generally ~3 mm wide.
   * Thin the cartilage until it will bend without breaking. If possible, leave the perichondrium intact on the outer edge.
3. Attach the helical rim to the base framework.
   * A small incision in the cartilage allows the steel suture to recess into the cartilage as it is tightened, which helps prevent suture extrusion. Suture extrusion thins the skin and can lead to cartilage atrophy or exposure.
   * Begin by attaching the helical rim cartilage to the base framework at the projection where the helical crus crosses the conchal bowl.

* The helical rim wraps around the base framework to the level of the antitragus. If the eighth costal cartilage graft is short (<10 cm), then a second piece may need to be added to prevent an unnatural notch at the transition between the bottom of the helix and lobule.

4. Carve the antihelix from one of the following pieces: an off-cut from the sixth, seventh, or eighth rib (after creating the base framework and helix, respectively), or the ninth rib.

   * The inferior crus is usually thinner than the more broad superior crus.

   * The antihelix is often more projected than the helix in the mid portion of the ear on the frontal view and should mirror the contralateral ear.

   * The antitragus can be created from an extension of the antihelix, but there should be a change in the angle at the transition from the antihelix to the antitragus.

5. Carve out the tragal attachment from an off-cut of the sixth or seventh rib.

   * Some surgeons carve the tragus, antitragus, and intertragal notch from a single piece of cartilage [3].

6. Attach a thin piece of cartilage (conchal floor graft) under the base framework and helical crus to create a deep conchal bowl leaving a space for the vascular pedicle.
7. A projection block may also be added under the framework to improve projection if considering a single-stage reconstruction [42].
8. Close the chest incision after replacing the remaining off-cuts into the sixth and seventh rib perichondrial sleeves.

   * Placing off-cuts into the perichondrial sleeve allows for regeneration of more structurally sound costal cartilage and prevents a chest wall deformity [39].

   * If a second stage is required for projection of the framework, then bank a piece of cartilage in the subcutaneous fat to be used as a projection block for the next stage.

Cartilage Graft Placement, Dressing, and Postoperative Care

9. Ensure hemostasis and insert a drain into the temporal pocket.
10. Place a permanent tacking suture on the deep side of the framework at the level of the anterior triangular fossa, and pass the same suture through the deep fascia at the correct level prior to placing the framework into the temporal pocket while access is optimal. This suture will secure the framework and prevent migration.

    * Take care to avoid injuring the superficial temporal artery (STA).

11. Place the cartilage framework by rotating it counterclockwise into place around the vascular pedicle.

    * Use the positioning template, preoperative measurements, and direct comparison to the contralateral ear to confirm the correct position and angle.

* Check the capillary refill along the helical rim when the framework is in place and suction is activated. If the skin does not drape easily over the framework or blanches significantly, the pocket size should be enlarged.

12. Once the correct position is confirmed, tie the tacking suture.
13. Transpose the lobule and mastoid flaps into the correct position, and close the skin.

    * Excise redundant skin with care to avoid devascularization of the skin flap.

    * Small z-plasties at the transverse closure across the antihelix and helix may help hide the incision.

    * Placing a deep permanent suture between the tragus and helical root once the framework is in place helps maintain the shape of the cartilage framework.

    * If a TPF is necessary to cover the cartilage framework due to a severely low-lying hairline (common in grade IV), then the cartilage framework is placed, and the TPF flap is folded over the top of the framework, sutured in place, and covered with a skin graft.

    * Close the incisions with 6.0 permanent or 5.0 fast-absorbing sutures.
14. Dressing and postoperative care.

    * Cover the reconstructed ear with antibiotic ointment, and suture a bolster in place for 5–7 days using Xeroform sterile non-adherent petrolatum gauze secured with 3.0 Prolene sutures or similar material.

    * Place a mastoid dressing with care to ensure the dressing is not too tight using fluffs and Kling gauze.

    Negative pressure without a bolster has also been described [41].

    * Remove sutures on postoperative day 10.

Second-Stage Auricular Reconstruction Using Autologous Costal Cartilage

The second stage is often necessary to achieve adequate projection in order to match the contralateral ear. In this stage a cartilage graft is placed in the postauricular sulcus to elevate the framework. The cartilage projection graft is then covered with fascia and a skin graft. This stage is generally performed 6 months after the first stage. Some patients do not require a second stage as shown by Drs. Kasrai and Fisher [42]. See Fig. 10.11 for an example of a single-stage bilateral reconstruction.

Preoperative Steps

1. Measure and record the superior, middle, and inferior projection distances of the contralateral and reconstructed ear.

   * Minor adjustments in the position and angle of the ear can be made if needed once the ear is elevated.

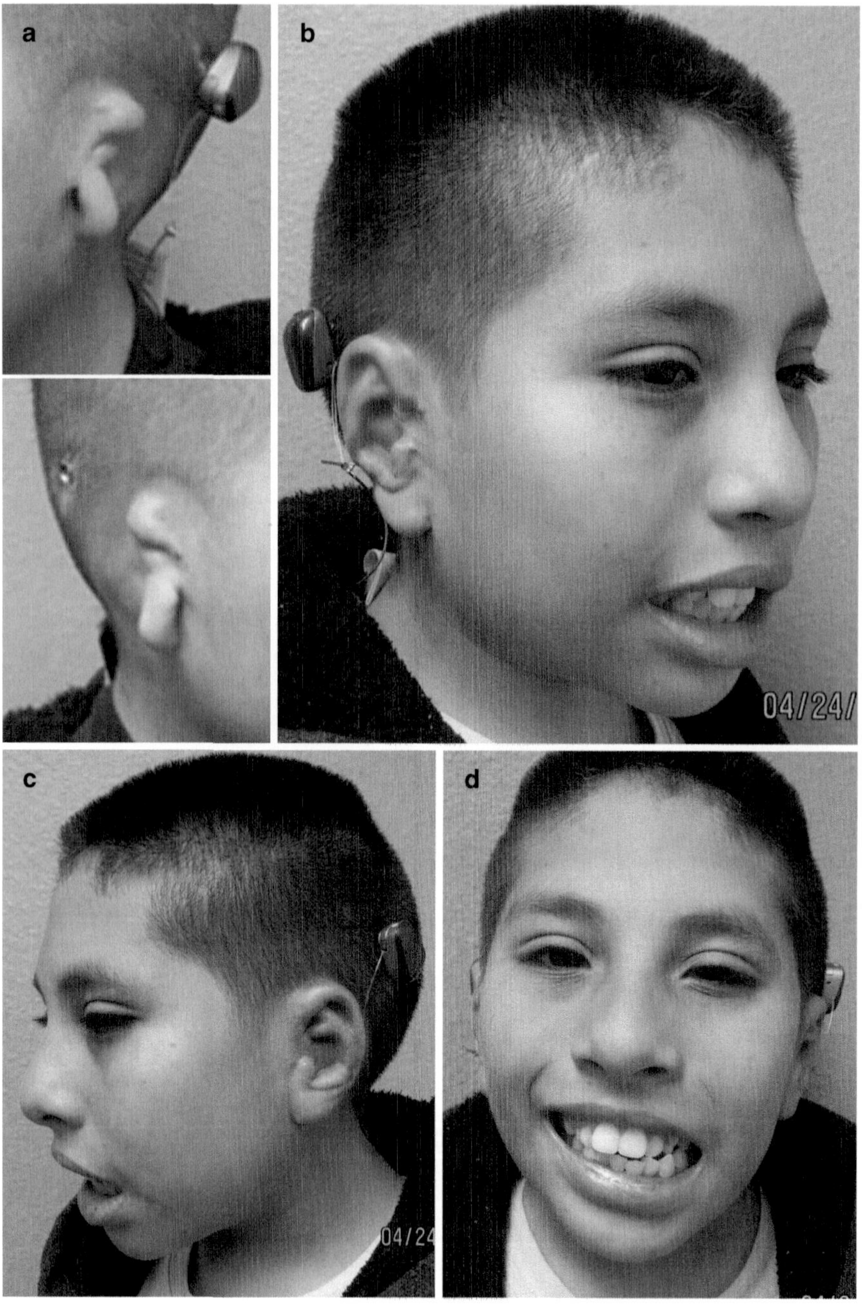

Fig. 10.11 Single-stage microtia reconstruction in a patient with bilateral microtia and aural atresia: (**a**) preoperative right and left lateral, (**b**) postoperative right lateral, (**c**) postoperative left lateral, and (**d**) postoperative frontal view

2. Create and sterilize a projection template using radiographic film (see Fig. 10.12).
3. Mark the incisions and skin graft harvest site (see Fig. 10.13).

   * The postauricular incision is 6–10 mm from the edge of the framework superiorly and then tapers inferiorly into the sulcus incision at transition to the lobule.

   * If hair is overlying the superior framework, then plan to elevate an inferiorly based ultra-delicate split-thickness skin graft (UDSTSG) over the unwanted hair follicles so that they can be excised.

   * The advantages and disadvantages of different skin harvest sites to cover the postauricular sulcus are reviewed in Table 10.3.

   * The skin graft may need to be as long 10 cm and as wide as 4 cm.

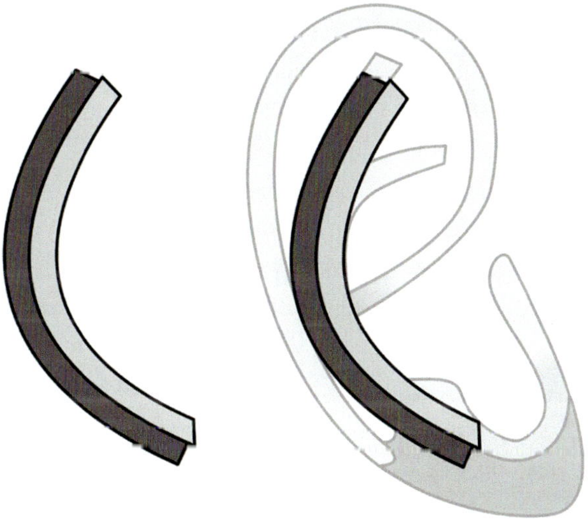

Fig. 10.12 Projection block template. The cartilage graft for projection extends from the level of the triangular fossa to the antitragus. Lighter portion represents the stacked portion of the template

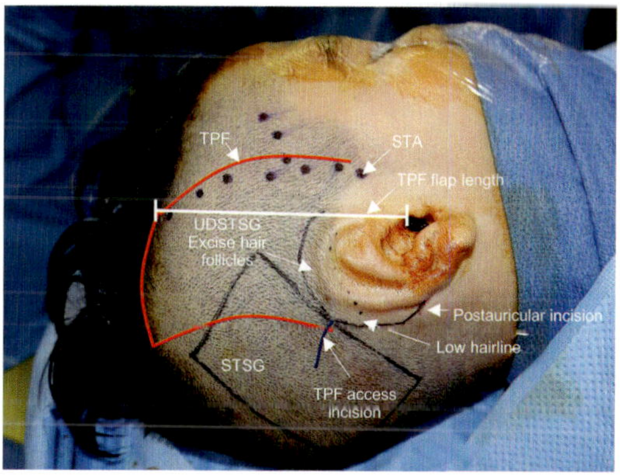

Fig. 10.13 TPF outline, STA, ultra-delicate STSG elevation area, planned incisions. The TPF flap may need to be 13 cm in length, measured from the external auditory canal toward the vertex of the scalp to fully cover a well-projected ear

Table 10.3 Advantages and disadvantages of different skin graft harvest sites for microtia reconstruction

Skin graft	Location	Advantage(s)	Disadvantage(s)
UDSTS/ STSG	Scalp	Better color match Same operative field No additional scar Dermatome may be used Hair follicle located 1–1.8 mm deep, so ideal to cut at depth less than 0.8–0.9 mm [52] May be raised with dermatome at 0.3 mm or free hand [19, 53]	Risk for alopecia (1%) [19] Variable healing and possible wound contracture (7.5%) [19] Need to shave more hair to obtain an adequate graft Challenging technique that takes practice if done free hand Donor site morbidity by secondary intention healing, chronic folliculitis
FTSG [46]	Contralateral postauricular	Slight deprojection of the opposite ear if needed Good skin color match Smooth contour Scar hides in retroauricular sulcus	Size may be insufficient Contralateral ear distortion
FTSG	Supraclavicular	Same operative field	Visible scar Must be aggressively thinned [6]
FTSG	Chest	May use previous chest incision Hides in breast line incision for a woman	Hypertrophic scar Distortion of the nipple Graft may develop hair growth with age
FTSG	Inner arm	Relatively hidden scar	Limited in size Separate surgical site Noticeable scar with arm raised Prone to keloid
FTSG	Low lateral abdomen	Easily hidden scar if at the beltline Same operative field as banked costal cartilage harvest Generally non-hair-bearing	Poor color match Visible scar
FTSG	Groin	Easily hidden scar	Poor color match Graft may grow pubic hair Donor incision breakdown (2%) [19]

FTSG full-thickness skin graft, *STSG* split-thickness skin graft, *UDSTS* ultra-delicate split-thickness scalp skin

* A scalp split-thickness skin graft (STSG) is preferred by some patients as the harvest site is well hidden and the skin color match is good, e.g., Fig. 10.14. Other patients may prefer to avoid the extensive hair removal needed for harvesting a scalp STSG. For these patients, the scar associated with a low lateral abdomen full-thickness skin graft (FTSG) hides well, and the graft is generally non-hair-bearing.

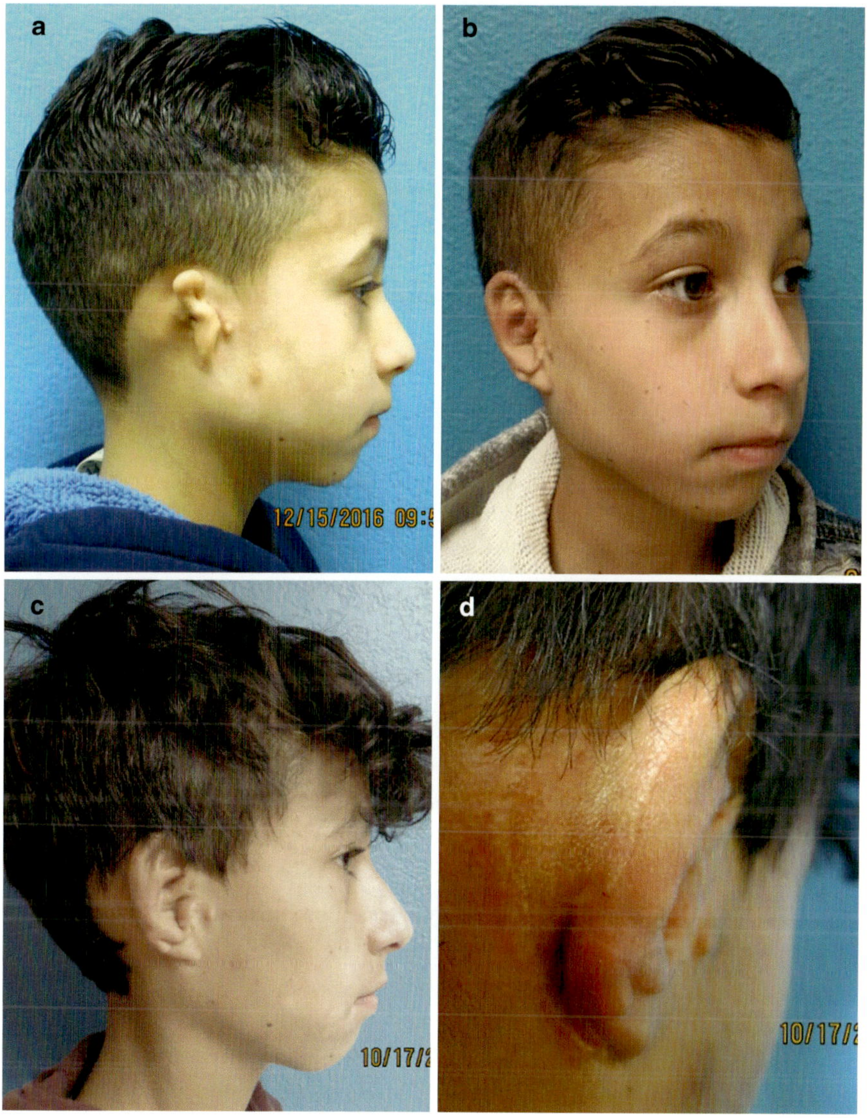

Fig. 10.14 (**a**) Preoperative. (**b**, **c**) Post second-stage reconstruction. (**d**) Postauricular sulcus using scalp STSG harvested with dermatome (5.1 × 9 cm at depth of 0.45 mm)

4. Mark the incision for raising a vascularized fascial flap to cover the cartilage for projection. Table 10.4 reviews the advantages and disadvantages of the different fascial flaps that may be utilized in microtia reconstruction.

   * The TPF flap is commonly used and can be harvested via the same postauricular incision used to elevate the framework with a short posterior extension to improve access. If the TPF was used in the first stage, then a deep temporal fascial flap or other fascial flaps will be needed.

Table 10.4 Fascial flaps described in microtia auricular reconstruction

Fascial flaps[a]	Advantage(s)	Disadvantage(s)
Temporoparietal fascia (TPF) [4, 54] Inferiorly based containing TPF and branches of the superficial temporal artery Dimensions: Vary based on reconstruction needs For porous polyethylene coverage: 10 × 13 cm [46, 55], 6–7 × 10 cm	Large and robust flap that can be used to cover both lateral and medial surfaces of the auricular framework Reliable blood supply and described for over 50 years	Potential large scalp incision, though minimal incisions and endoscopic approaches reduce this morbidity [56] Alopecia (28.6%) [37] Scalp numbness (17.4%) [37] Objection to visible scar (25% in male patients) [37] Partial flap necrosis (2%) [57] Risk of damage to the frontal branch of the facial nerve (<1%) [57]
Deep temporal fascia (DTF) [58] Inferiorly based pericranial flap containing periosteum, temporalis muscle, and deep temporal fascia with middle temporal artery. Harvested via the same incision as TPF. Dimensions: 10 × 10 cm [58], 6 × 10 cm [59]	Useful when TPF has already been utilized Harvested via the same incision Useful for salvage surgery Large enough to cover both lateral and medial surfaces of the auricular framework	Can only be used if TPF has been previously harvested Similar disadvantages as TPF harvest with donor site morbidity Circulation is less reliable particularly in the setting of previously failed TPF due to similar blood supply Partial necrosis (33%) [58]
Mastoid fascia (MF)[b] [22, 60–63] Anteriorly based mastoid fascia with vascular supply from branches of the posterior auricular artery. The mastoid periosteum is kept intact Dimensions: 2.5–3 × 4 cm or 4.5 × 7 cm [22], covers posterior auricular sulcus and the margin of the helix Width to length ratio 2:2 to 3:2 [41] 5 cm above, 3 cm below Frankfurt horizontal and 6 cm posteriorly [64]	No additional incision required May harvest a larger superior flap by modifying the incision, which has a smaller profile than the typical TPF skin incision [61] TPF is still available for salvage surgery Ideal for patients with low-lying hairline [61] May be used as salvage to treat small areas of framework exposure, especially in the superior aspect [59] Neurovascular flap that allows for sensation to light touch, pinprick, and temperature if the lesser occipital nerve remains intact [22]	Unable to drape the entire framework with a well-vascularized flap, especially the inferior auricle. May be better suited for Conchal-type rather than lobular-type microtia [57] May not be feasible in patients with bone-anchored hearing devices Major bleeding may occur from mastoid emissary vein Variable degree of reported partial skin necrosis (0–43.3%) [41, 60]
Occipital fascia [65] Anterior transposition of an inferiorly based occipital artery fascia flap. Skin incision along the course of occipital artery dimensions: 9 × 13–15 cm (may be more narrow at pivot)	Option if TPF is not available Reliable flap with wide arch rotation (90–180 degrees) and able to drape the entire framework	Large skin incision with associated morbidity Framework exposure requiring revision surgery (10%) [65] Partial flap necrosis (1%) [65]

[a]Fascia flap should be raised 20% larger than required for coverage [33]
[b]Also described as a postauricular or retroauricular fascial flap in the literature

* Some severe forms of craniofacial microsomia may have a small or aberrant STA necessitating the use of a different fascial flap [44, 45].

5. Position and prepare the patient as previously described.

Banked Costal Cartilage and Skin Graft Harvest

1. Harvest banked costal cartilage from stage 1.
   * Further costal cartilage may need to be harvested if insufficient cartilage was harvested during the first stage.
   * Some surgeons use a custom-designed polyethylene wedge [66].
2. Harvest the skin graft for postauricular coverage.

Incisions for Ear Elevation and TPF Flap Harvest to Cover the Postauricular Cartilage Graft and Helical Rim

3. Make the initial postauricular incision into the dermis, and elevate an ultra-delicate split-thickness skin graft anteriorly over the unwanted hair follicles on the helical rim.
4. Excise the subcutaneous tissue containing the unwanted hair follicles under the UDSTSG.
5. Complete the postauricular incision down to the TPF superiorly and mastoid fascia inferiorly.
   * Making a small TPF access incision into the scalp helps with visualization for TPF elevation and avoids a larger scalp incision. This is also where a dog ear generally forms once the postauricular scalp is elevated and advanced.
6. TPF flap elevation.
   * Elevate a suprafascial flap posterior to the ear (3–4 cm) and superior (9–10 cm) to the helical rim. This will allow the scalp to advance forward for closure and provide access for harvesting the TPF. The plane is just under the subcutaneous fat where dermal fibrous attachments are carefully divided to elevate the flap.
   * An extended Colorado® microdissection monopolar cautery, long retractor, and Andrews suction are useful for elevating the skin flap off the fascia.
   * The flap width (generally 6–7 cm) should allow for coverage of the cartilage projection graft, helical rim, and extend down to the level of the lobule for grade III (lobular-type) microtia. The TPF helps reduce helical rim cartilage atrophy by improving blood supply to the cartilage.
   * Once the skin has been adequately elevated over the TPF, incise the anterior edge of the planned flap at least 2 cm anterior to the dominant STA branch above the level of the inferior temporal septum (ITS), which is approximated by the hairline. Below the ITS, the loose areolar tissue becomes a fibrofatty layer that is more difficult to dissect; this also helps avoid the temporal branch of the facial nerve [67]. The anterior branch of the STA is generally divided to improve mobility of the flap.

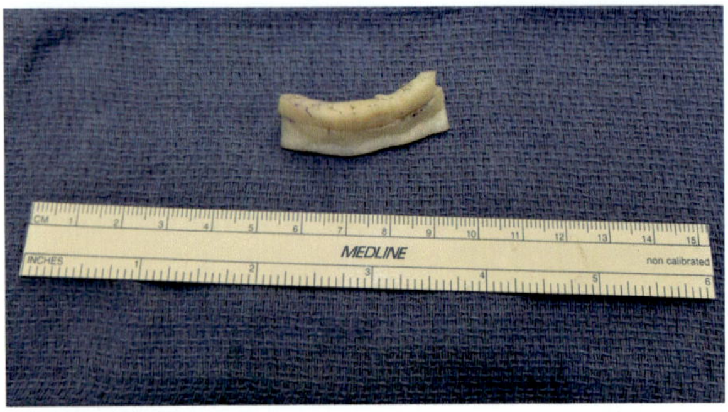

Fig. 10.15 Cartilage projection block

* Incise the posterior edge of the planned TPF flap followed by the superior edge.

* Elevate the deep side of the TPF in the loose areolar tissue plane superficial to the periosteum and deep temporal fascia in a cranial to caudal direction using a Kittner, blunt right angle forceps, and scissors.

* Some advocate including the loose areolar fascial tissue in the harvested TPF flap to improve vascular supply and allow the skin to slide over the cartilage [33].

* Keep the flap hydrated and in its anatomical position until it is ready to be sutured in place.

7. Carve the projection block using the template (see Fig. 10.15).

   * The height of the projection block should be based on the superior, middle, and inferior measurements from the contralateral ear minus the height of the reconstructed framework (usually 6–8 mm). Cartilage may need to be stacked to achieve the correct height and secured using a 5.0 steel or a permanent suture.
8. Elevate under the cartilage framework over the underlying fascia, and place the projection graft to achieve symmetry with the contralateral ear.

   * Secure the projection graft to the framework and the underlying soft tissue with a permanent suture to prevent migration.
9. Place a 10 French channel suction under the elevated scalp to prevent hematoma.
10. Fold the TPF over the helical rim and postauricular sulcus, and secure the flap to the cartilage with fine suture such as 5.0 Monocryl.
11. Advance and secure the postauricular scalp flap with deep tacking sutures.

    * Avoid advancing the superior hair-bearing scalp into the superior auricular sulcus, which will be lined with a skin graft.

    * Excise and close the dog-ear deformity at the TPF access incision.
12. Place the harvested skin graft, and suture in place with a 6.0 permanent or absorbable suture.
13. Place a bolster over the skin graft sutured in place to the cartilage framework and postauricular scalp, and place a dressing as described in stage 1.
14. Remove bolster on postoperative day 5–7 and sutures on postoperative day 10.

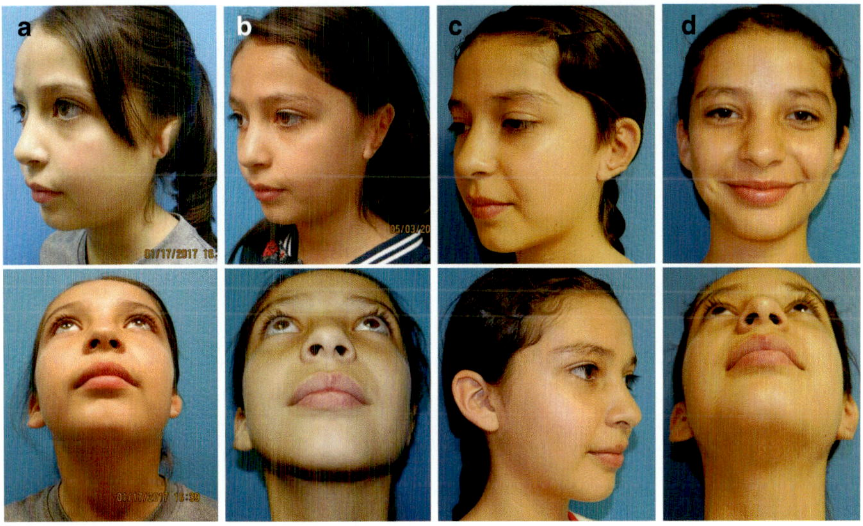

Fig. 10.16 (**a**) Preoperative, (**b**) post stage 1, and (**c**, **d**) post stage 2

Postoperative swelling improves over 3–6 weeks after each stage. Patients are asked to avoid activities that could injure the reconstructed ear for 3 months after each surgery. An example is shown in Fig. 10.16 demonstrating the results before and after stage 1 and stage 2 autologous cartilage auricular reconstruction.

Porous Implant Ear Reconstruction (PIER)

Porous Implant Ear Reconstruction (PIER), first described in 1982 by Dr. Alexander Berghaus, has become an accepted alternative to autologous costal cartilage ear reconstruction for the treatment of microtia [5, 35, 68–71]. Much like the rib cartilage technique, reconstructions using porous polyethylene have a steep learning curve and are technically challenging. Far fewer surgeons use the PIER technique as compared to rib cartilage, which is likely due in part to less exposure to this technique during training [36].

Surgery may be performed as young as 3 years old and is ideally completed before a child enters kindergarten. There is a psychological advantage to patients who get early reconstruction (3–6 years) [72]. The author's youngest age for surgery was increased to 4 years old in October 2015, after the release of a consensus statement on the use of anesthetic and sedative drugs in infants and toddlers that recommended waiting until 4 years of age before performing elective surgery longer than 3 hours.

Certain anatomic conditions predict a more difficult ear reconstruction (e.g., hemifacial microsomia, presence of a surgical canal, an inferiorly positioned native canal, anteriorly displaced microtia remnant). This section will discuss the author's protocol for single-stage total ear reconstruction using porous polyethylene implants. The description below will focus on the most typical anatomy encountered, grade III microtia with aural atresia.

Preoperative Surgical Planning

1. The patient is positioned 180° from anesthesia with appropriate padding.
   * A shoulder roll is placed at the beginning of surgery to aid with visualization during TPF flap harvest and then removed once the flap dissection is completed.
   * Extremities are moved every 2 hours to avoid pressure ulcers.
   * The anesthesiologist is informed not to use any paralytics so stimulation of the frontal branch of the facial nerve will be evident during the flap dissection.
2. The hairline is shaved 2 cm around the microtic ear.
3. Create a positioning template of the unaffected ear on clear film.
   * The positioning template should include the ear, hairline, sideburn, eyebrow, eyelid, and the position of the midline at the radix.
4. Determine and mark the appropriate size and position of the ear.
   * When operating on young children, surgeons must be aware of the growth patterns of the ear over time in order to estimate the adult size of the unaffected ear [73].
   * In symmetric patients, the position template is reversed, and the position of the ear is marked. The author uses a 3D-printed mirror image model of the unaffected ear to confirm the position.
   * For patients with hemifacial microsomia, the implant should be placed closer to the midline than the opposite ear depending on the degree of asymmetry.
   * If the orbit on the side of the microtia is smaller and more inferior, the eyelid and eyebrow on the positioning template must be adjusted to account for the bony asymmetry.
   * Inclination of the ear is referenced against the angle of the nasal dorsum.
   * Although some utilize precise measurements to determine ear position, the author relies heavily on past experience, and therefore implant position is ultimately a subjective one determined during surgery.
   * Care must be taken to keep a boundary of hairless skin around the reconstructed ear symmetric to the unaffected side.
   * There will almost always be some area of hair-bearing scalp superiorly that must be resected and discarded.

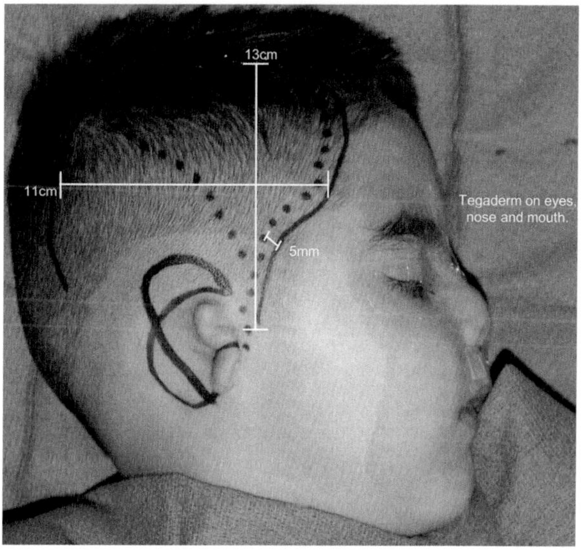

Fig. 10.17 Surgical markings depicting anterior and posterior branches of the STA, auricular position, and incisions for the TPF, lobule transposition, and anteriorly based auricular flap

5. Mark out the TPF flap and its blood supply (see Fig. 10.17).

   * Starting at the level of the microtic remnant, the STA, which is usually located just anterior or sometimes underneath the remnant, is palpated and marked. If the latter occurs, extreme care must be taken when excising the cartilaginous remnant to avoid injuring the vascular pedicle.

   * The surgeon should note the position of the postauricular artery (to avoid injury) and the anterior branch of the occipital artery (to preserve in the event a salvage reconstruction is required).

   * Mark the boundary of the TPF flap.

   * If the anterior branch is very close to the lateral eyebrow (<1 cm), an alternate flap is designed utilizing the posterior branch of the STA and the anterior branch of the occipital artery to avoid injury to the frontal branch of the facial nerve.

   * In cases where the anterior branch courses too close to the facial nerve, there may be small branches that take off more inferiorly that can be safely incorporated into the flap to augment the blood supply.
6. Mark an inferiorly based lobule flap leaving a 1.5-cm pedicle.
7. Mark an anteriorly based auricular skin flap incorporating all of the hairless skin around the microtia remnant.

   * The auricular skin is used either as an anteriorly based flap or a full-thickness skin graft depending on the patient's anatomy.
8. Prepare and drape the patient.

   * The non-sterile positioning template is trimmed and placed between two sterile Tegaderms onto the operative field.

Implant Preparation

There are two main implant manufacturers [Medpor (Stryker), Su-Por (Poriferous LLC)] that make two-piece porous polyethylene implants consisting of a helical rim and an antihelical base that are soldered together to create the ear. The two-piece implant is the most prevalent option at this time and therefore will be described below. However, the author currently uses one-piece implants of her own design based on a 3D scan of the patient's opposite ear (see Fig. 10.18).

9. Carve the antihelical base to create a more realistic shape based on the patient's unaffected ear.

   * Thin and shape the inferior crura, and create a more realistic curvature to the conchal bowl.

   * Remove the tragus and intertragal incisura as they are preferably reconstructed with cartilage from the microtia remnant.
10. Solder the inferior helical rim to the antihelical base along all aspects including the superior and inferior crura using a high-temperature fine-tip battery-powered cautery.

    * The positioning template of the unaffected ear, projected to adult size based on the child's age, is used to guide the length and shape of the helical rim.

    * If there is no canal, the rim is brought into the notch of the antihelical base to form the helical crus.

    * A smoke evacuator is used during the soldering process to the reduce fume inhalation.

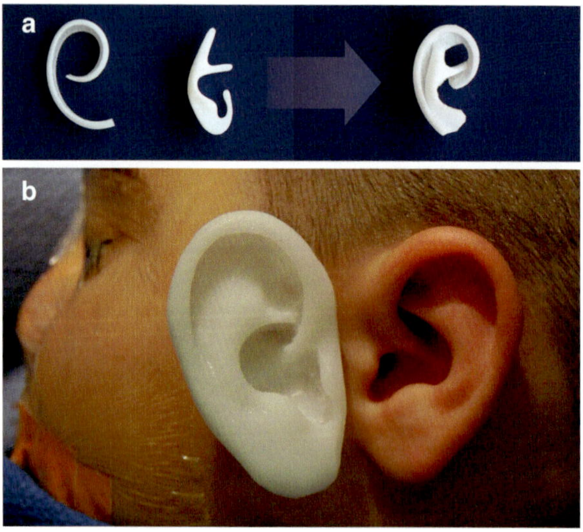

Fig. 10.18 (**a**) Two-piece porous implant (Su-Por) and (**b**) 3D Lewin ear implant (Su-Por)

11. Strengthen the two-piece implant.
    * Extra pieces of polyethylene are soldered between the open spaces of the rim and the base at all sites except the triangular fossa. One of these pieces is used to create a more broad and subtle shape of the superior crura.
    * This step is required to minimize the risk of implant fracture.
12. The base of the implant is altered to create symmetric projection and angulation of the implant.
    * The implant is kept in saline until ready for use.
    * It is important to ensure there are no sharp edges on the implant, especially when carving detail into the thin inferior crura.

Dissection of Microtia Remnant and Auricular Skin

13. Incise the lobule transposition flap.
    * The lobule of the microtia is usually too anterior and too superior. The dissection should allow for a posterior and inferior rotation that will match the opposite earlobe.
    * In the case of a lobule remnant that is much lower than the unaffected earlobe, the lobule may be rotated posteriorly on a superior pedicle to achieve better symmetry if the anatomy is appropriate.
14. Raise the anteriorly based auricular flap between the subcutaneous tissue and the superficial TPF to include all hairless skin around the microtic ear (see Fig. 10.19).

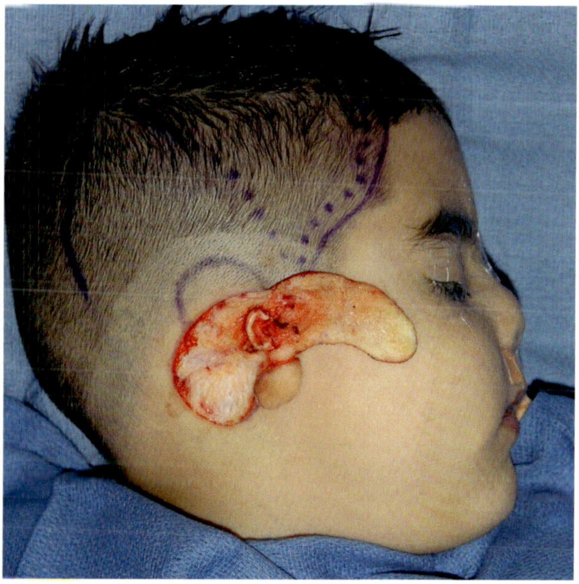

Fig. 10.19 Lobule transposition and anteriorly based auricular flap

* Colorado-tip cautery is used for precise dissection.

* The flap is defatted to remove all of the subcutaneous tissue. The skin flap is left attached until the implant and fascia are in place, at which point it is laid onto the anterior surface of the reconstructed ear. If the skin orientation is compromised by the limitations of the anterior attachment, the skin is removed and used as a full-thickness skin graft.

15. The vestigial cartilage remnant is then dissected free of the surrounding soft tissues, removed, and kept in saline until ready for use in the tragal reconstruction.

    * All vascular structures near the remnant are noted and protected during cartilage excision. When the cartilage is in close proximity to a vessel, only the portion above the plane of the surrounding fascia is removed.

Fascial Flap Dissection (See Fig. 10.20)

The TPF flap is the most critical aspect of PIER surgery [33, 74]. In 2006, the author developed a technique to harvest the TPF flap with no scars in the scalp using a lighted retractor through a periauricular incision. However, until one is completely comfortable with this flap dissection, a zig-zag or horizontal scalp incision will allow for better visualization.

16. Dissect the superficial surface of the TPF.

    * The blood supply to the flap is within the fascia proximally and becomes more superficial distally. In some patients, the distal vessels must be pulled down from the subcutaneous tissue. In order to avoid injuring these small vessels, the author uses the tip of a Yankauer suction to push on the subcutaneous fat upward in order to create enough tension to visualize the plane just above the vessel.

Fig. 10.20 TPF flap

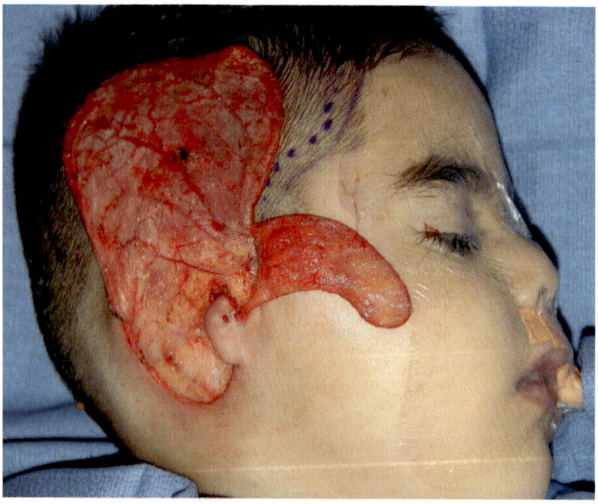

* Bovie dissection with a fine Colorado tip (3-inch length with 1-cm 45-degree tip) is used at the lowest effective cautery settings (cutting 12, coagulation 10) to avoid injuring the hair follicles. In older patients, these settings must be raised.

* Surgicel may be used for minor bleeding to preserve the flap vascularity.

17. Dissect the deep surface of the TPF.

* Start near the pedicle of the STA.

* The correct depth of dissection, which is below the subgaleal fascia, is identified using tenotomy scissors.

* Dissection should continue just above the characteristic whitish-blue color of the deep temporal fascia along the anterior, superior, and then posterior borders.

* Take care to coagulate both the anterior and posterior branches where they cross the flap perimeter to avoid bleeding from these larger vessels postoperatively.

* Blunt dissection with cherry dissector sponges is used to dissect the deep surface of the superficial TPF along with its underlying subgaleal fascia. Including the subgaleal fascia creates a bilaminar flap that aids with skin mobility over the implant, improving durability. This is especially critical in young children since their tissue is so thin.

* Stimulation of the frontal nerve should be noted when dissecting close to the eyebrow. If excessive movement is seen, the anterior branch of the STA should be cut more proximally. Alternatively, the posterior branch of the STA and the anterior branch of the occipital artery may be used to supply the flap.

* In older patients, the surgeon may prefer to leave the subgaleal fascia behind in order to get a thinner flap.

* The deep surface of the flap becomes more adherent inferiorly, so it may be more effective to switch to tenotomies for the last 2–3 cm of dissection.

* The inferior border of the flap should stop at the superior margin of the final implant position.

* If the flap seems too small to completely cover the implant, extra length can be gained by releasing along the STA pedicle inferiorly. If this vessel is not easily seen in the field of view, the flap is transilluminated from below.

18. Irrigate copiously and ensure hemostasis of the scalp and the flap.

* No drain is used for the scalp unless the patient was noted to bleed more than a typical amount during the flap harvest.

* The TPF flap should always be placed under the scalp until ready for use.

Covering the Implant with the Fascial Flap (See Fig. 10.21)

19. Secure the porous implant to the deep fascia.

* The implant is placed into the proper position and inclination as determined by the template and visual assessment of symmetry.

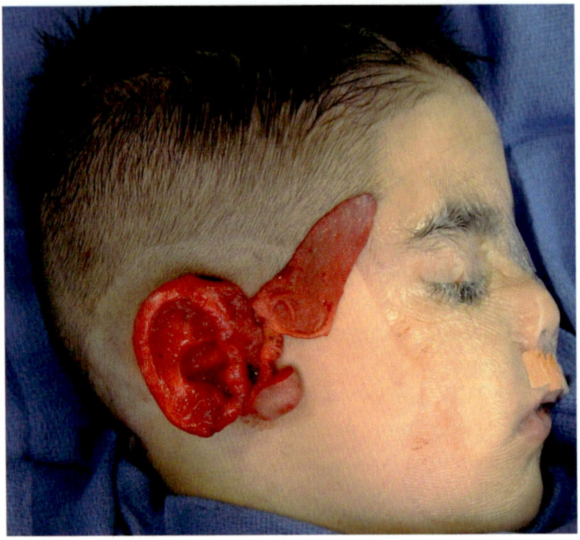

Fig. 10.21 TPF flap folded over the 3D implant

* 3–0 PDS sutures are used to hold the implant in place, taking care not to injure any vessel within the fascia.

* A 10 French round channel drain is placed through the posterior hairline and laid against the back surface of the implant.

20. Wrap the TPF flap around the implant and apply suction.

* If necessary, a 5–0 Monocryl is sutured around the periphery to achieve satisfactory adherence of the flap to the implant.

* Care must be taken that 100% of the implant is covered by the flap. The flap should be generous enough in size to conform to all the interstices of the implant without tenting over any concavities, especially the helical rim.

* If the flap is still too small after all options for dissection have been completed, the implant will need to be altered by carving down the inferior aspect and/or removing some of the base so that it projects less.

* If a patient has a particularly large ear, an extra centimeter of flap should be designed at the beginning of the surgery.

Skin Coverage (See Fig. 10.22)

21. Use auricular skin on the front of the ear whenever possible to have the best color match.

* All of the non-hair-bearing skin around the microtia is used as either a flap or a full-thickness skin graft.

22. Harvest full-thickness skin graft from behind the unaffected ear.

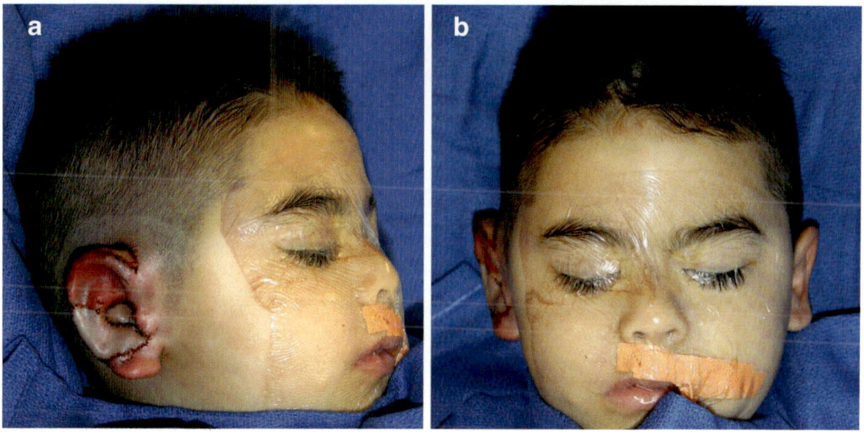

Fig. 10.22 Skin grafts over flap: (**a**) lateral and (**b**) frontal view

* Approximately 6 cm × 2 cm of the skin may be taken and used in conjunction with the skin from the microtia side to cover the majority of the front of the ear.

* In order to avoid altering the projection of the unaffected ear, a postauricular scalp flap is advanced anteriorly and sutured near the postauricular sulcus. This will move the postauricular hairline about 1 cm anteriorly but will still leave enough of a skin perimeter around the back of the ear to look appropriate.

* In rare cases when a larger skin graft is required, the skin from the entire posterior aspect of the unaffected ear may be used and replaced with the skin from another site such as the abdomen. In this case, a sponge bolster tie-over dressing is recommended.

* If there is not enough auricular skin to cover the entire front of the ear, the conchal bowl and the deep aspect of the tragus and intertragal incisura should be covered with abdominal skin graft.

23. If there is not enough hairless auricular skin to use on the front of the ear, harvest full-thickness skin graft from the upper inner arm.

    * This occurs most commonly in patients with bilateral microtia, a low hairline, significant hemifacial microsomia, prior atresia repair, or prior failed microtia surgery.

    * An ellipse of 10–12 cm length by 3 cm wide may be taken from the arm without undue tension on the closure.

    * The arm scar has a tendency to widen and should be managed with silicone tape. If possible, avoid using arm skin in patients prone to thickened scars or keloids.

24. Harvest full-thickness skin graft from the lower lateral abdomen avoiding the central hair-bearing area to cover the posterior aspect of the ear reconstruction.

25. Place the final scar between the anterior skin grafts and the posterior skin graft along the apex of the helical rim so the scar will be less conspicuous.
    * All grafts are sutured in place with interrupted 5–0 and 6–0 chromic suture.

Tragal Reconstruction

26. Carve the remnant cartilage into a neo-tragus using the template to match the shape of the tragus on the unaffected ear.
27. An anteriorly based cheek flap is raised just under the subcutaneous fat in order to advance the skin posteriorly to cover the tragus. The flap is folded over both above and below the cartilage and secured to the deeper tissues to hold the position.
    * It is best to incorporate some auricular skin with the cheek skin to ensure full coverage of the cartilage graft.
    * It can be challenging to reconstruct the tragus in a symmetric position because it is essentially suspended in front of the canal.

Dressing and Postoperative Care

28. Cover all skin grafts with antibiotic ointment.
29. Pack Vaseline gauze into the bowl, the helical rim, and the postauricular sulcus.
30. Place a non-adherent dressing around the ear against the scalp and face.
31. A two-component silicone-based ear impression material (Azoft, Oticon Germany) is placed over the entire ear (see Fig. 10.23).

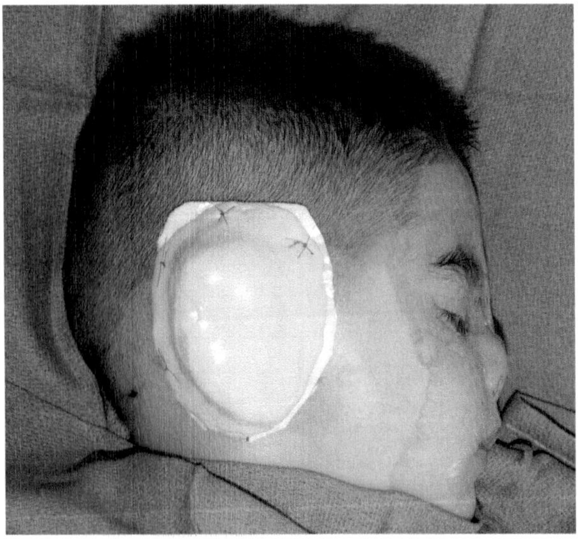

Fig. 10.23 PIER dressing

* 3–0 Prolene is used to secure the Azoft mold to the scalp.

* Attention must be given to avoid placing sutures at areas of the ear where the flap could be injured.

32. Remove the drain.
33. Wrap the head and ears with gauze using Hypafix tape around the face.

    * 3–0 Prolene is sutured at the top of the scalp to keep the gauze from migrating.

    * Cover with a Velcro headband and a protective ear cup (Romo-Guard).
34. The dressing is removed 5–8 days after surgery.
35. Daily cleaning and application of ointments are initiated.

The PIER will be mostly healed by 6 months after surgery, although scars and the color of skin grafts can continue to change over a year. Postoperative results of a patient with a two-piece implant (Fig. 10.24) and a 3D implant (Fig. 10.25). Note that in both patients, the PIER ear is intentionally larger than the unaffected side, which has not yet reached adult size.

Prosthetic Ear Reconstruction of the Pinna

External prosthetic reconstruction of the pinna using artificial materials, e.g., medical grade silicone, is a well-demonstrated treatment option for the patient with congenital microtia [75, 76]. Historically, proponents of surgical versus prosthetic ear reconstruction may have viewed these as competing treatment options; however, the well-informed and experienced practitioner recognizes the value of a patient-centered approach in presenting these complementary treatments [29, 46, 71, 77].

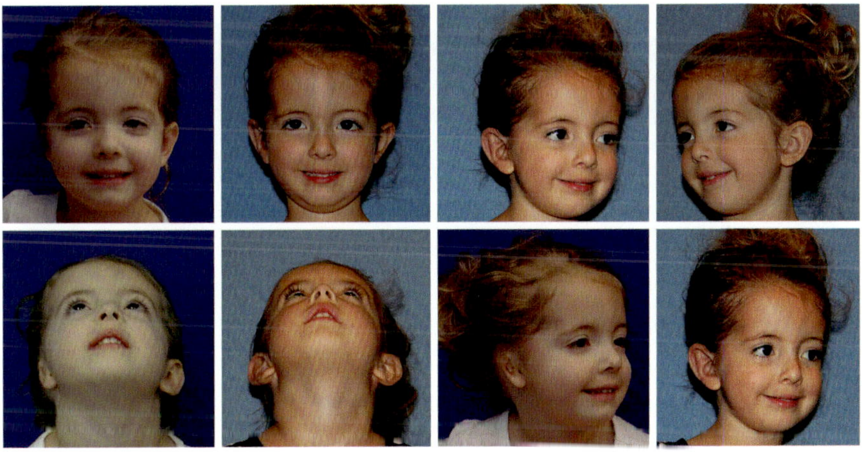

Fig. 10.24 Preoperative and 6 months postoperative PIER patient (two-piece Su-Por implant)

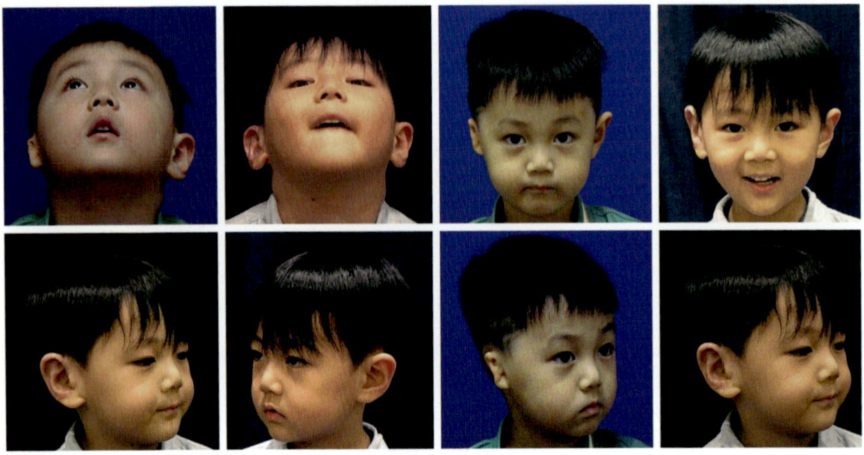

Fig. 10.25 Preoperative and 3.5 months postoperative PIER patient (3D Lewin ear implant by Su-Por)

The patient is best served when treatment potential is presented in a comprehensive and collaborative manner – the purpose of this chapter.

The function of facial prosthetics is to improve an individual's quality of life [78]. Aside from restored facial and auricular symmetry, the prosthetically reconstructed ear enables the individual to wear devices designed to fit in, on, or around the external ear such as eyeglasses (sun, safety, reading, or other corrective lenses). One example specific to healthcare providers is the ability to use a stethoscope in a customary manner.

When considering prosthetic ear reconstruction, the patient can elect either a surgical or non-surgical approach. The consulting practitioner must have a sound understanding of the fundamentals of prosthetic rehabilitation and associated options such that they can appropriately and accurately educate the patient and family and subsequently that the patient fully understands their commitment to a respective treatment choice. This section will review the fundamentals of facial prosthetic rehabilitation; explain non-surgical and surgical treatment approaches, and address aspects of prosthetic rehabilitation related to function, psychological considerations, quality of life, and lifetime maintenance.

Consultation and Education

Patient education is critical to achieving successful outcomes. Appropriate education about prosthetic reconstruction helps establish the patient's and family's expectations from the beginning. All too often patients are introduced to unachievable expectations, which lead to disappointment and possibly even depression. When patient expectations are managed carefully from the start, they possess the greatest potential for treatment success and full rehabilitation [79].

Facial Prosthetic Rehabilitation: The Basics

An ear prosthesis, or epithesis, is an external removable device made of *alloplastic* materials – typically a medical-grade silicone elastomer (see Fig. 10.26). Prostheses are designed to be removed daily for cleaning and skin hygiene and to maintain a healthy tissue bed. Facial prostheses are typically made by a skilled anaplastologist (or other prosthetic specialists), who manages the patient's treatment from consultation through device design, fitting, delivery, and lifetime maintenance. Ideally, the anaplastologist is part of a multidisciplinary team of specialized practitioners dedicated to the comprehensive surgical, reconstructive, and rehabilitative care of the patient with microtia and/or craniofacial microsomia. Silicone prosthetic devices are relatively short-lived, lasting on average 18–36 months. Reasons for replacement of prostheses are discoloration, material degradation, fungal growth in the silicone leading to adverse skin reactions, and changes in the tissue bed contour as a result of developmental growth or surgery. The type of retention used to secure the prosthesis also influences the lifespan [80, 81].

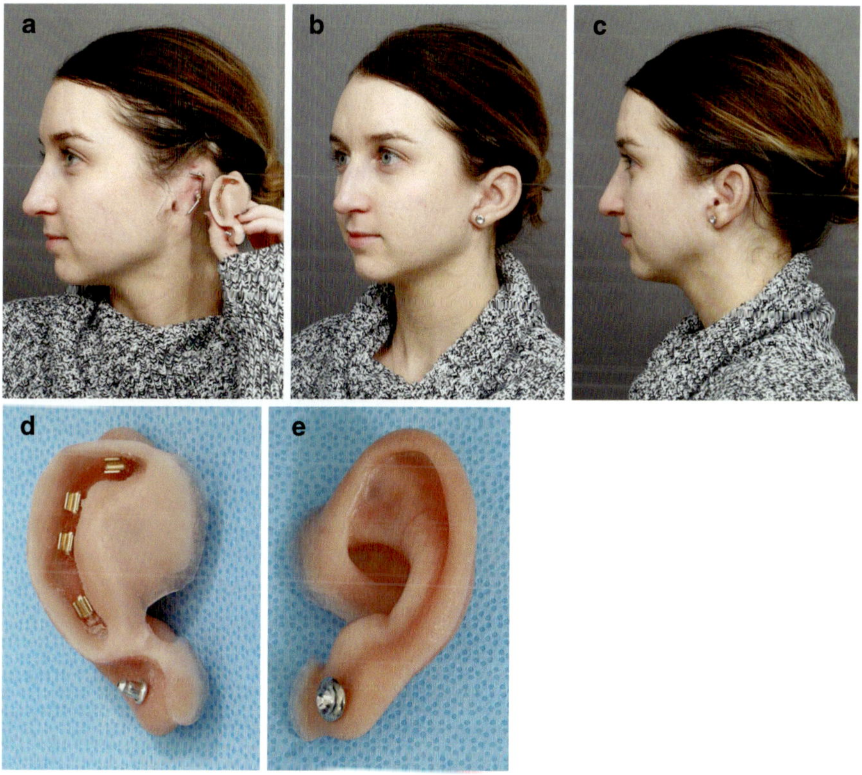

Fig. 10.26 (**a**–**c**) Patient fitted with implant-retained prosthetic ear following removal of failed autologous reconstruction post-trauma. (**d**) Fitting surface of prosthesis with four clips for bar retention. (**e**) External surface of prosthesis with patient-selected earring adornment

The Process of Prosthesis Fabrication

Prosthetic devices are fashioned based on the patient's existing anatomy or borrowed from a donor form. A digital database of anatomic forms may also be utilized, particularly for patients with bilateral microtia [82].

Patient Records

1. A full series of clinical photographs are recorded for the pre-treatment record at the initial clinic visit (see Fig. 10.27).

   * Position the head in the Frankfurt horizontal position for reference consistency [83].

   * Clinical and technical standards for patient photography and other data acquisition methodologies should be maintained for reliable treatment records and planning [84].
2. A 3D form of the patient's existing anatomy is created for treatment planning and design fabrication. This can be achieved by conventional means of a direct impression (or moulage) of the patient in clinic or by digital means with 3D surface scanning, photography (photogrammetry), or CT/cone-beam CT (CBCT) radiographic imaging [85, 86].

   * Patient positioning and technical props are carefully considered when capturing digital data to ensure that facial anatomy is adequately captured, to accurately mimic the patient's position during daily activity and function with a donned prosthetic device, and to not obscure relevant anatomical information. Figure 10.28 demonstrates that the chin prop contributes to image integrity by stabilizing the head position but may compromise usefulness of the virtual model for facial analysis purposes. In this instance, the chin prop did not compromise effective design of the prosthetic ear.

Design

The restored anatomical deficiency is designed by the anaplastologist with feedback from the patient, family, and treating practitioners. Conventionally, this is done in wax or clay; however, digital techniques using 3D modeling software and computer-aided design/manufacturing (CAD/CAM) methods have become routine and are quickly becoming the standard of care (see Fig. 10.29).

* Design should address the functional needs and goals of the patient.
* and allow for anything the patient might wear *in*, *on*, or *around* the restored prosthetic pinna, i.e., eyeglasses, earrings, earbuds, headphones, hearing device, stethoscope, etc.

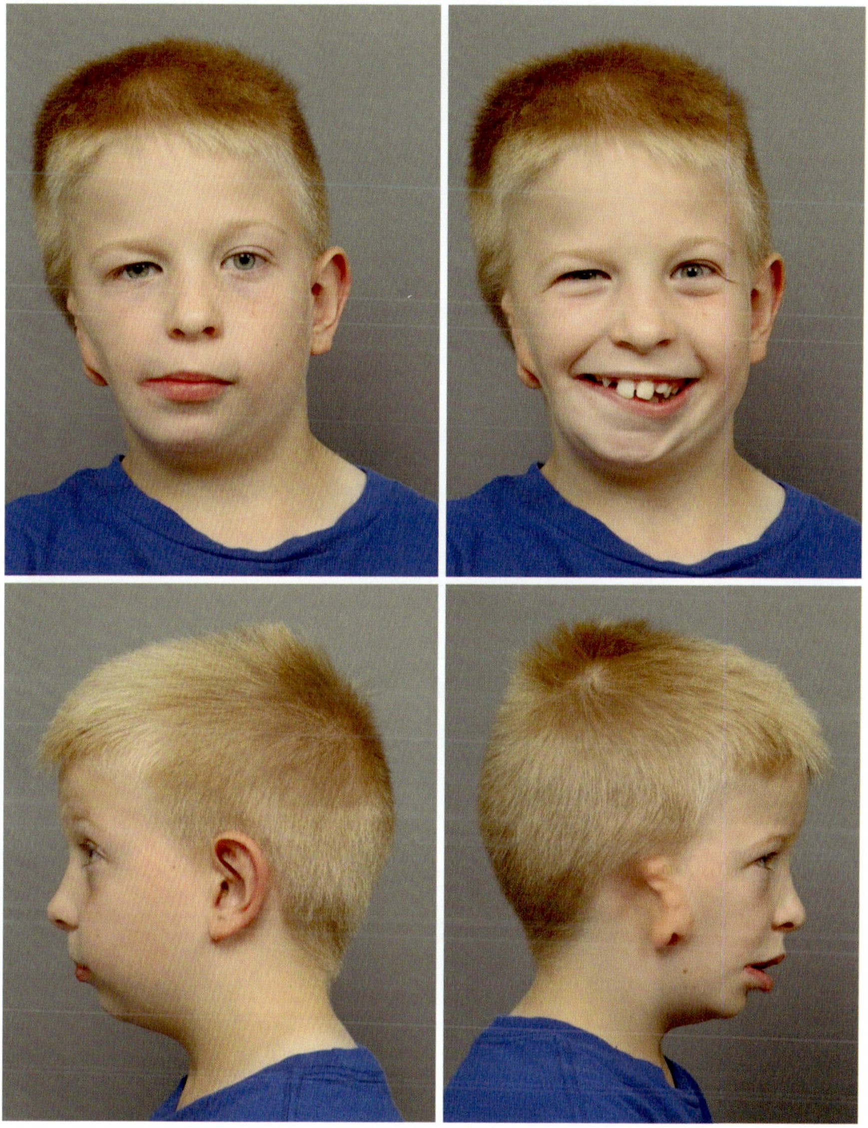

Fig. 10.27 Two-dimensional photographic record from initial consultation of patient's pre-treatment, presenting condition in frontal and lateral views

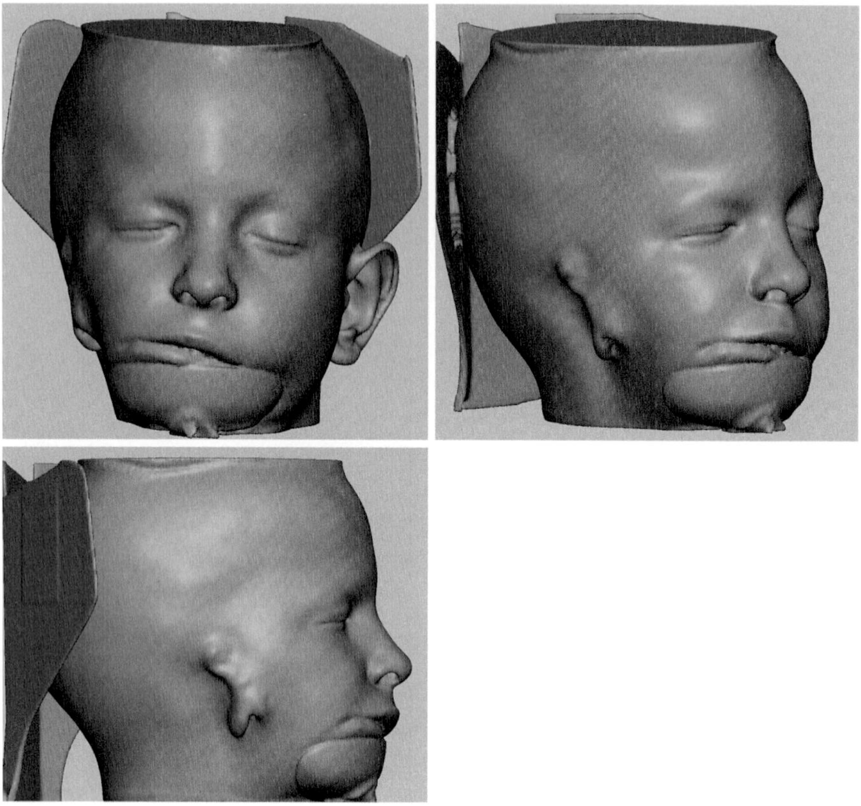

Fig. 10.28 CBCT imaging used to capture patient's soft tissue anatomy. Note both pinnae are fully imaged; however, chin prop limits the ability to visualize full facial anatomy to assess asymmetry

* Design prototype is evaluated in situ on a patient in the clinic from all head positions and with dynamic movement such as chewing and smiling as this may impact fit.
* Careful attention to the patient's overall facial *gestalt* of appearance should be considered when designing the size, shape, and projection. With marked facial asymmetry, "visual symmetry" is often achieved with parts unidentical in size, shape, and projection. Exact mirrored anatomical replicas often look unnatural, oversized, and malpositioned when viewed in situ in the patient with facial asymmetry.

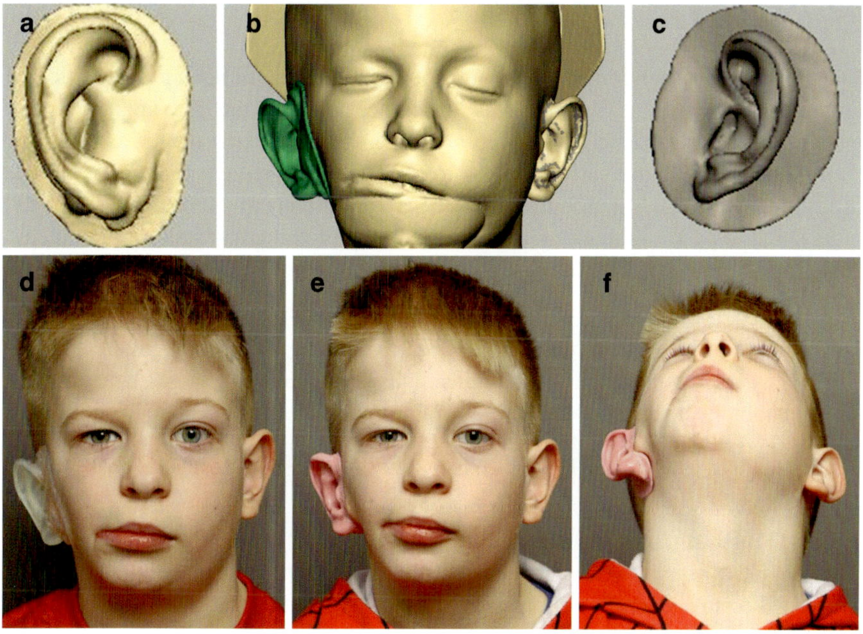

Fig. 10.29 (**a–c**) Virtual design of prosthetic right ear based upon the mirrored contralateral side derived from CBCT imaging. (**d**) CAD model of prosthetic ear fabricated by 3D printing designed to fit over the remaining microtic remnant evaluated on patient. (**e**, **f**) Duplicated in a workable clinical wax for the final design modification and fitting

Casting

Once approved, the final prosthetic form is cast in silicone from a mold. Conventionally, the wax prototype is literally "cast in stone," i.e., dental stone or gypsum using a "lost-wax" technique common in dentistry. Contemporary digital methods are working toward direct printing of silicone prosthetic devices, though precise methodologies are still in development [87, 88].

* The patient and family must fully understand and appreciate that once a wax prototype is approved, no further changes can be made in shape, size, or fit. Patients and families who do not fully appreciate this are often disappointed when changes cannot be made to shape or size when the technical process has passed the design prototype stage. Digital methods may offer greater flexibility in making design changes.

Color Matching

Color matching of silicone to the skin is an essential step requiring an artistic eye grounded in scientific knowledge of color science and materials. A convincing color match to the skin is critical to a successful prosthetic outcome (see Fig. 10.30). A poor color match to the surrounding skin results in a more conspicuous prosthetic restoration. Skin color matching can be done subjectively "by eye" or with the aid of a skin color measurement device like a colorimeter or spectrophotometer. Artistically trained anaplastologists often rely on subjective "by eye" color matching techniques [89].

* A combination of both subjective and objective methods offers the greatest potential for managing prosthetic outcomes and maintenance while saving time through a repeatable and predictable process, providing greater reassurance to the patient and clinician [89, 90].

Fitting, Finishing, and Delivery

The prosthesis is generally processed by heat curing methods in a laboratory, which requires several hours. Faster processing is possible with appropriate selection of silicone; however, this can compromise the final outcome and ultimate mechanical properties of the cured silicone, which can lend to a shorter prosthetic lifespan. The prosthesis must then be carefully trimmed and fitted to the patient.

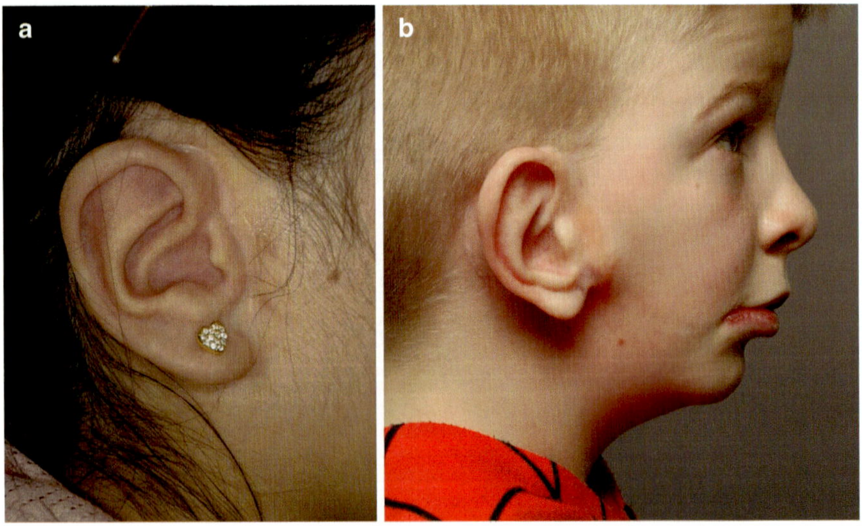

Fig. 10.30 (**a**) Implant-retained. (**b**) Adhesive-retained prosthetic ears with convincing color match of silicone to surrounding skin. Color was matched using a combined technique of using spectrophotometery and computerized color formulation to establish the "base" color and "by eye" technique for remaining colors and their respective distribution in the mold

* It is essential that during trimming the retentive complex is not altered, disturbed, or compromised. Care should be taken to avoid scratches to the titanium surface of magnets (which protects the magnet from corrosion) or separation of the silicone from the acrylic retentive substructure for bar-clip retention systems.
* Secure seating of the retentive components and fit against the skin along aesthetic margins must be ensured with the prosthesis in situ.
* Silicone should be relieved in areas of excessive pressure. Pressure sores easily develop if excess silicone is present in bulky areas of the prosthesis. Keep in mind that the prosthesis may be worn daily for up to 18 hours per day.
* Comfort and fit should be assessed on the patient with the prosthetic ear in situ, during dynamic behaviors such as chewing, speaking, yawning, with extended neck and head movements, and with donning and doffing of "ear accessories," i.e., headphones, sunglasses, and stethoscope, e.g., Fig. 10.31.
* Additional coloring on the exterior of the prosthesis may be necessary if the "intrinsic" color match seems inadequate. This should be primarily driven by the patient's interests and feedback rather than the clinician; the skilled practitioner will *always* find "something to fix," which is not always in the patient's best interest.
* Patients should be instructed to "ramp" up the amount of time wearing the prosthesis daily, in the same manner that one might break in a new pair of leather shoes. This will provide time for silicone-skin adaptation in areas previously left uncovered.

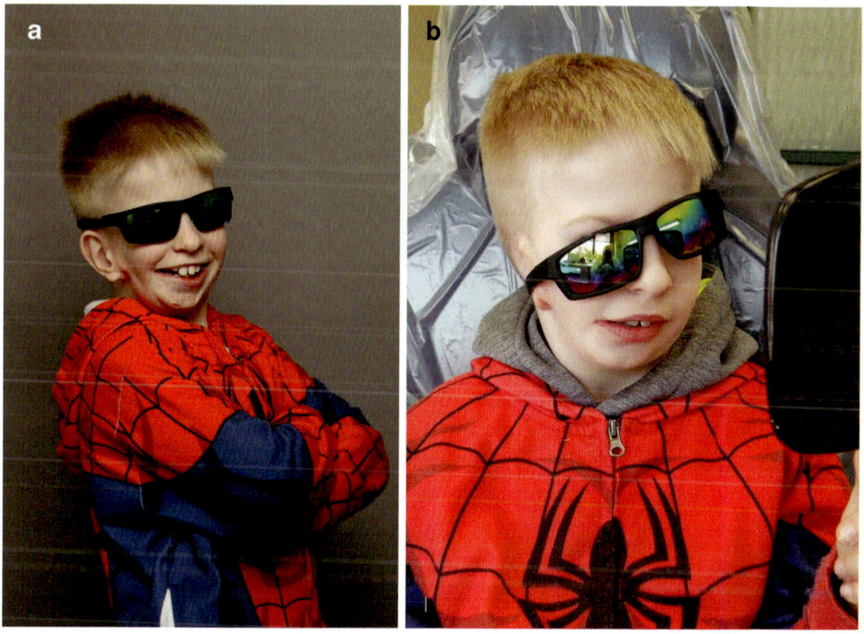

Fig. 10.31 (**a**) Successful prosthetic result (**b**) Preoperative photograph showing difficulty wearing sunglasses

* Re-educating the patient on daily care and maintenance of the prosthesis and managing the skin-fitting surface (including the periabutment tissue) are essential.
* Providing time for the patient to practice placement and removal of the prosthesis (in the clinic with supervision) helps ensure smooth adaptability.
* The "delivery" visit is a critical moment when the patient will leave donning their newly fitted prosthetic device. This can be a substantial adjustment for the patient and family alike. A positive, supportive environment should be provided to enable this unveiling and the patient's renewed becoming [91].

Non-surgical Prosthetic Options

For biological, psychological, or social reasons, not all patients are good surgical candidates. Developmental age, personal preference, and inability to commit due to time, cost, or travel constraints are a few potential considerations. If a patient elects not to pursue surgery for any reason, a prosthetic solution may be available. This has provided a good option for some children who are undecided about whether surgical reconstruction is the right choice [92].

When surgery is not involved, a prosthetic device can be worn with the use of adhesives, by engaging portions of existing anatomy or by mechanism of external retention, like eyeglasses. While these alternative options are possible and may seem simple as they do not require surgery, they are not always ideal and have variable reliability for comfort and retention. Among the non-surgical options, the use of adhesives has provided the most historically reliable solution [78].

Regardless of the type of retention, a prosthetic device should be removed daily to allow for cleaning and aeration of the tissue bed. When using adhesives, the prosthesis must be carefully relieved of all adhesive upon doffing before cleaning with soap and water. Adhesive is applied anew each time the prosthesis is donned. The length of time a prosthesis will stay in place varies among patients and with the type of adhesive. Environmental factors such as humidity can impact the wear time and retentiveness of adhesives, particularly for water-based products.

* The patient must demonstrate good manual dexterity to manage the daily tasks of adhesive application and removal.
* The optimal tissue bed for adhesive use is the skin that is flat, tight, immobile, and non-hair-bearing.
* An adhesive-retained prosthesis is typically designed over and around the existing anatomy and tissue tags or remnants. Because of this, fabricating an exact mirrored replica of the contralateral ear is not always possible.
* A low hairline can interfere with adhesive retention, and accumulation of adhesive in the hair can become a nuisance for the patient. This has been identified as a contributing factor in patients' subsequent decision to pursue surgery either to place implants for prosthetic retention or for auricular reconstruction.

* Prosthetic adhesives are available in variable bond strengths; both water-based and acetate- or silicone-based adhesives are available. The type of adhesive an individual patient uses should be determined by the anaplastologist and the patient, and typically is identified through a trial-and-error period following delivery. Some adhesives require a solvent for removal.
* Adverse skin responses should be carefully monitored through multiple follow-up visits post-delivery.
* Prostheses should be replaced on a regular basis to minimize fungal or bacterial colonization in the silicone and development of a skin infection.
* Skin products, e.g., Skin Prep, can be applied to aid in retention and to protect the skin from adverse reactions. Adhesive is generally applied to the silicone-fitting surface of the prosthesis and not the patient's skin.
* An adhesive-retained prosthesis can be provided as an interim prosthetic solution, while the patient considers more definitive surgery, either surgical ear reconstruction or the placement of implants to retain a prosthetic ear [29].

Surgery for the Prosthetic Patient

Surgery can complement prosthetic treatment to ensure optimal outcomes but must be carefully coordinated with the anaplastologist and in keeping with the patient's goals [29, 77].

Pre-prosthetic Surgery

Surgery to optimize the tissue bed is often required to ensure the best prosthetic outcome. Contouring the soft tissues is necessary to accommodate a prosthesis and may be necessary to remove an extruding implant or cartilaginous framework, manage infection, remove skin tags or remnant cartilage, or for scar revision. The tissue bed must be well healed before the prosthesis can be definitively fitted. Soft tissue contouring can be performed before or after placing surgical implants. This decision is based on the patient's needs and the tissue to be addressed, e.g., some patients use their existing microtia to assist with wearing glasses. Compared to autologous or alloplastic surgical ear reconstruction, surgical placement of implants to retain a prosthetic ear is less complex. However, it requires diligence by the surgeon to ensure good implant stability with precise technical execution [32].

* Create a flat, immobile, and hairless tissue bed that accommodates the prosthesis. Surgical modification of the hairline can also contribute to greater ease with retention and prosthetic management over the patient's lifetime.
* Flaccid, mobile tissue tags without cartilaginous or bony structural support generally should be removed, though patient-specific conditions should be first discussed with the anaplastologist.

* Periodically, incorporation of existing anatomy into the prosthetic restoration is possible and should be discussed with the anaplastologist and patient. It may also be necessary to move tissue to achieve natural proportions and position. Surgical repositioning of the tragus, for example, may improve the final prosthetic result.
* The patient and family should be well educated on what needs to be removed and why.
* If there are psychological concerns related to the removal of the patient's existing and natural anatomy, then consultation with a psychologist is recommended. The anaplastologist can explore design options to work around these issues. Patients born with congenital microtia have described emotional and mental attachment to their "special ear," so any plans to remove any part of the ear should be carefully presented and managed.

Implant Placement and Osseointegration

Osseointegration was introduced by P.I. Branemark in the late 1970s. It describes the situation whereby bone grows in close proximity to commercially pure titanium. By means of osteogenesis, bone can anchor a screw in the skull and thus allows for rehabilitation with "bone-anchored" devices for hearing and prostheses [93]. Osseointegrated implants were first used to retain a bone conduction hearing device and a prosthetic ear via percutaneous abutments in 1977 and 1979, respectively [94, 95]. Implant-retained prostheses represent the most reliable retention method for patients seeking facial prosthetic treatment and are considered the gold standard [78, 96].

Placement of implants to retain a facial prosthesis requires collaboration between the surgeon and anaplastologist. The anaplastologist must be consulted before implants are placed so that accurate positioning of the implants can be preplanned. Implants are placed into available bone in the vicinity of the prosthetic reconstruction and allowed to "osseointegrate." The amount of time allowed for osseointegration can vary substantially based upon patient-specific conditions and comorbidities ranging from 3 to 12 months. Shorter healing times have been described in the literature for bone-anchored hearing devices in healthy adults [97, 98].

For pediatric patients with microtia or adults with compromised bone quality, the implant is frequently placed as a two-staged surgical procedure. The titanium implant is placed first and allowed to osseointegrate for a minimum of 3 months. The second stage attaches the abutment/bar-clip or magnet retention system to the implant. Patients with congenital conditions such as hemifacial microsomia, Treacher-Collins syndrome, or Goldenhar syndrome may present with anomalous anatomy in the craniofacial skeleton. Therefore, bone volume and quality should be carefully evaluated to ensure availability of adequate bone. A single-staged surgical procedure may be considered in healthy adults with good temporal cortical bone [32, 95].

Connection of the percutaneous abutments (the "second stage") puts a load on the implant in the bone, and therefore timing of this connection should be carefully considered [99, 100]. When an extensive healing period is expected for osseointegration, often a temporary prosthesis can be fabricated to assist the patient during this time.

Preoperative Planning

Precise implant positioning must be guided by the anaplastologist so that the optimal aesthetic result can be achieved. Virtual surgical planning (VSP) can be performed to specifically indicate implant positions, and soft tissue or bone-fitting guides can be fabricated by 3D printing to clearly indicate the recommended positions for implant placement (Figs. 10.32 and 10.33). Alternate implant positions and "sleeper implants" should be included in the VSP to provide options for the surgeon if the bone quality at primary implant sites is suboptimal. VSP is possible when relevant patient data is captured by scanning methodologies that enable the creation of a patient specific virtual 3D model.

* Surgeons interested in patient-specific 3D-printed guides or models should first investigate recommendations related to data acquisition of patient information. Scanning protocols specific to 3D printing are commonly required [101, 102].
* Accuracy and integrity of data capture are often dictated by the intended clinical application. It is best to consult with the anaplastologist (engineer or other technicians) who may provide 3D-printed model(s) or guides for planned surgical procedures.
* Bone-fitting guides designed with CBCT data have demonstrated less reliability in exact seating compared to bone-fitting guides designed from medical CT data. Material choice for fabrication often contributes to this, as acrylic guides may "slip" more easily over the bone surface and/or periosteum compared to, for instance, 3D-printed guides fabricated in metal, i.e., stainless steel by selective laser sintering (SLS) technology.
* If medical grade CT is used, imaging the area of interest using a bone algorithm and a slice distance of <1 mm is recommended [103, 104]. No cushions or straps should be used that may compress, distort, or contort the ears (both the treatment side and the non-treatment side). This provides a greater value in using the data not only for surgical planning but for prosthetic design and fabrication as well.
* Request that the imaging protocol includes the entire pinnae bilaterally in both the anterior-posterior and superior-inferior directions. When planning for the placement of implants into bone, it is easy to forget about the importance of capturing accurate soft tissue anatomy.
* If CBCT imaging is utilized, a field of view sufficient to capture as much of the full head as possible is recommended (23cmD × 17cmH "V17" for iCAT FLX, Henry Schein, USA) [102].
* Communicate clearly to the anaplastologist (or other VSP technicians) timelines related to surgery to ensure that necessary imaging, guide design, and 3D printing of guides can be completed with sufficient time to allow for test-fitting, cleaning, and sterilization of guides before surgery, typically a minimum of 2–3 weeks.

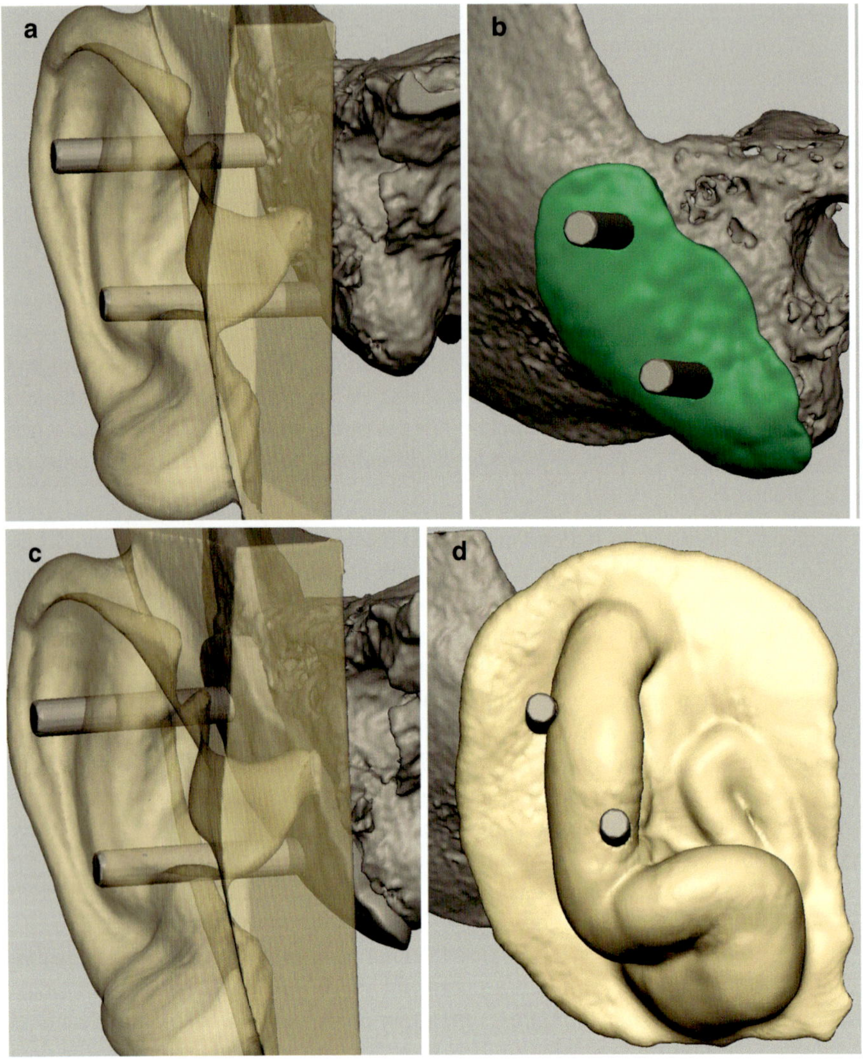

Fig. 10.32 Virtual (CAD) planning using mirrored contralateral ear as a reference with data derived from a CBCT scan: (**a**) implant position, (**b**, **c**) design of bone-fitting and soft tissue-fitting, (**d**) surgical guide with remnant ear for reference (Implant cylinder length are for simulation and design purposes only; they do not reflect *actual* implant geometry)

* Refer to manufacturers' recommendation for sterilization of surgical guides, which is often dictated by the material used for guide fabrication.
* Surgical navigation can also be used for accurate placement of craniofacial implants when VSP for navigation has been appropriately executed by the anaplastologist [105, 106].

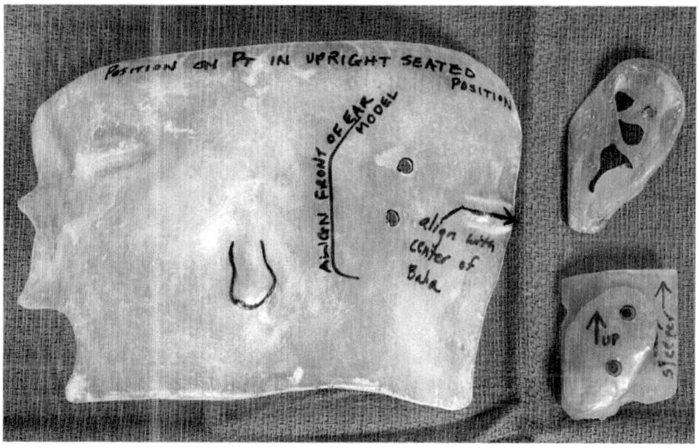

Fig. 10.33 3D-printed soft tissue-fitting and bone-fitting surgical guides with 3D-printed ear reference to assist in understanding relationship of implants to planned prosthetic restoration. Note the smallness of bone-fitting guide (lower right) and notations made to assist with accurate positioning of guides on the patient. Guides are often designed to extend over the dorsum of the nose for more reliable placement. Fit of guides will differ based upon the position of the patient during initial data capture – patients are seated upright for CBCT and reclined or in supine position for medical CT. Therefore, guides should be used in a similar fashion in the OR. This should be clearly communicated and appreciated by collaborating designer and surgeon

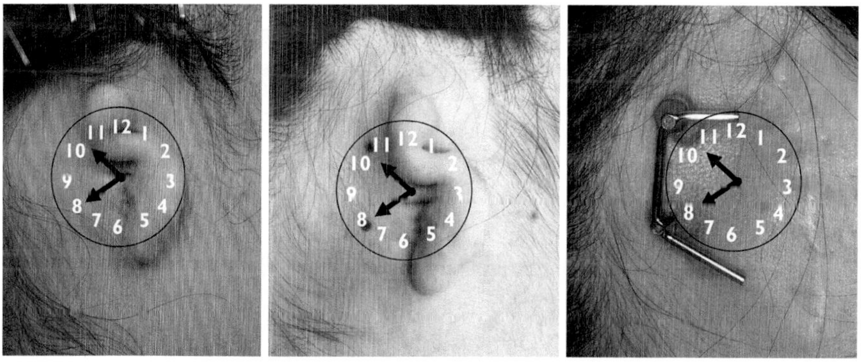

Fig. 10.34 Implant locations for right-side ear reconstruction are indicated at the 8:00 and 10:30 o'clock positions

Implant Placement (First Stage)

Two implants are required for bar-clip retention for the ear. For the right side, the implants are placed at the 8:00 and 10:30 o'clock positions relative to the external auditory meatus (EAM) (Fig. 10.34) or expected location of the EAM for patients with aural atresia and 1:30 and 4:00 o'clock for the left side. The implants are placed approximately 20 mm from the native EAM or expected EAM. The implants should be placed 12–15 mm apart measured from outer perimeter to outer perimeter. This is not always possible, especially with implant manufacturers introducing implant designs with larger diameters. While greater implant circumference may provide greater surface area for osseointegration, it also contributes to design challenges for the anaplastologist. For magnet retention, three triangulated implants are recommended. Additional "sleeper" implants may be necessary in the pediatric population or for patients with known compromised bone. Implants should be parallel to one another and perpendicular to the bone and skin surface to facilitate design of retentive structures for the prosthesis, assist with patient home hygiene, and provide greater ease for placing and removing the prosthesis. Often a "perpendiculator" appliance is available in the surgical set to assist in visualizing the correct angle.

1. Mark the implant sites using the prepared surgical guide (Fig. 10.35).
   * Soft tissue-fitting guides and implant positions must be determined *prior* to the injection of local anesthetic. Local anesthetic may prevent full seating of soft tissue guides and distort the perceived position of planned implant locations.
   * Implant positions are first marked on the soft tissue and then transferred down to the bone using methylene blue and a 25-gauge needle.
   * The anaplastologist can often be available in the OR to assist with accurate surgical guide positioning so that VSP can be efficiently and accurately executed.
2. A "C"-shaped incision is typically made 10–15 mm posterior to the position of the implants and carried down through the periosteum.
3. Elevate and reflect a flap in the sub-periosteal plane.
4. Verify implant positions.
   * If bone-fitting guides are used, seating of the guide onto the bone surface should demonstrate reliable positioning by engaging unique landmarks on the bone surface.

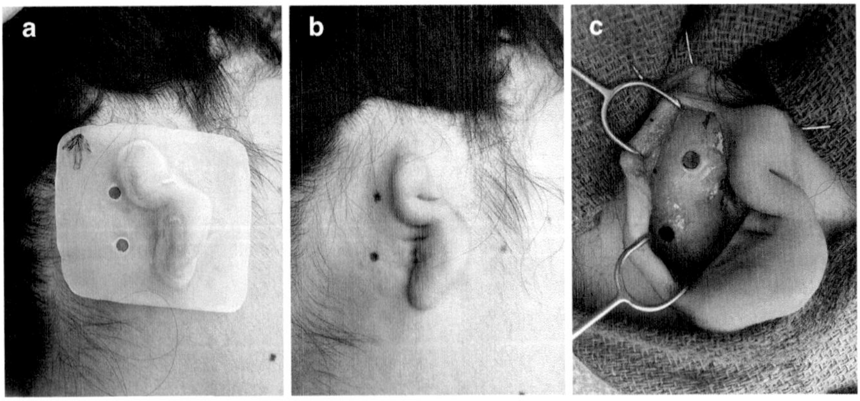

Fig. 10.35 (**a**) Placement of soft tissue-fitting guide, (**b**) marked implant positions, and (**c**) position verified with bone-fitting guide

5. Use the guide drill at 2000 rpm to drill pilot holes using continuous irrigation.
   * The inferiorly positioned implant should be placed first. This allows greater flexibility to identify alternate sites superiorly should the initial planned site prove unusable.
   * Irrigation is essential to prevent injury to the bone from excessive heat; osteocyte death can occur at 42 °C [107].
   * Move the guide drill up and down and with the slight widening motion to allow irrigation to reach the tip of the guide drill [107].
   * Drill perpendicular to the bone surface using the 3-mm stop on the guide drill first; then if sufficient bone remains with probing, proceed to 4 mm depth with the guide drill.
   * If less than 4 mm of bone depth is achieved, the shorter 3 mm implant should be used.
   * Drilling to the full depth of planned implant length with the guide drill is important for reliable full seating of the implant.
6. Use the widening drill to widen the pilot hole to enable subsequent placement of the implant also at 2000 rpms with continuous irrigation (Fig. 10.36).
   * Use the appropriate length widening drill to match the depth of the drilled pilot hole.
   * Continue with the widening drill to create a slight countersink (0.5 mm) around the circumference of the hole.
   * *Do not overwiden* when using the widening drill. Movement of the drill should be limited to strict up and down movement with no lateral movement. There are no "rescue implants" for craniofacial applications, so overwidening the hole intended for implant placement can mean complete loss of "bone real estate" in that area.
7. The implant is picked up directly from its ampule using the implant inserter in the drill hand piece.
   * Implants are made of commercially pure titanium, and the surface of the implant should never be touched by anything other than the bone into which it

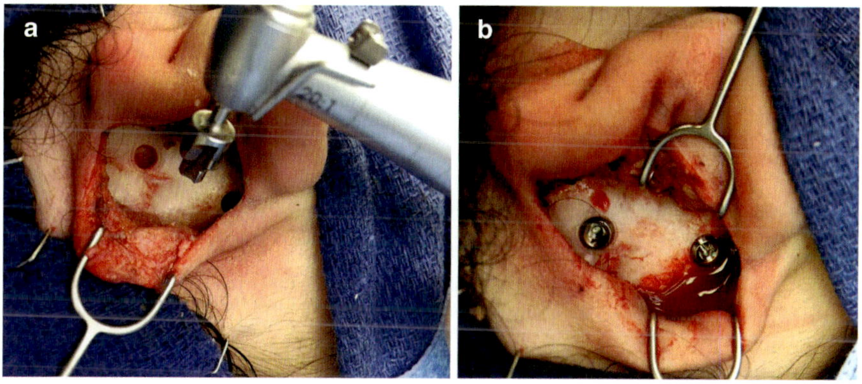

Fig. 10.36 (**a**) Widened pilot hole with countersink and (**b**) two implants in place

is placed. Contamination of the implant surface can compromise osseointegration.

* Surgical implant kits are designed to enable careful handling of implant-containing vessels, and surgical teams should be well trained in the handling of implant components and instrumentation.

8. Carefully position the implant perpendicularly into the widened hole; the implant should be inserted by two full rotations before irrigation begins. Irrigation continues until the implant is fully seated; the drill will stop when the implant reaches the set torque.

   * Implants are placed with a torque setting appropriate to the softness or hardness of the bone. The recommended setting for hard, compact bone is 40–50 NcM. For soft or compromised bone, recommended torque setting is 20–30 NcM.
9. Carefully remove the implant inserter from the top of the implant, avoiding any levering motion that may loosen the implant.
10. If a two-staged approach is elected, cover screws are placed into the implants, and the surgical site is closed including the periosteum.

Abutment Placement Surgery (Second Stage)

The second stage of surgery involves the connection of skin-penetrating abutments and reduction of the subcutaneous tissue in the area of the planned prosthesis such that the overlying skin can be sutured directly to the periosteum lending to flat, immobile, periabutment tissue. Mobile tissue around the abutment is believed to contribute to soft tissue responses that can be difficult to manage [108]. The second-stage surgery is also the recommended time for the removal of residual microtia remnant:

1. An incision is designed to remove any unwanted soft tissue and access the implants for abutment placement (Fig. 10.37).
2. Cover screws are removed, and either healing abutments or standard definitive abutments are connected to the implants.
3. Abutments are placed using a uni-grip or external hex screwdriver and then torqued to 25 NcM using a torque wrench or drill hand-piece.
4. Subcutaneous tissue is removed to allow for direct adhesion of the skin to the bone surface.

   * Removal of subcutaneous tissue may require extending and ramping the soft tissue reduction outward from the area directly around the implant/abutment complex to minimize "stair-stepping" or an abrupt drop-off of the subcutaneous tissue.
5. Abutments are brought through the skin using a biopsy punch or cruciform incision.

   * Suture (or tack) the incision made for removal of the remnant ear once the implant sites have been visualized, so that the skin incision for the abutment is made in the correct position over the implant.

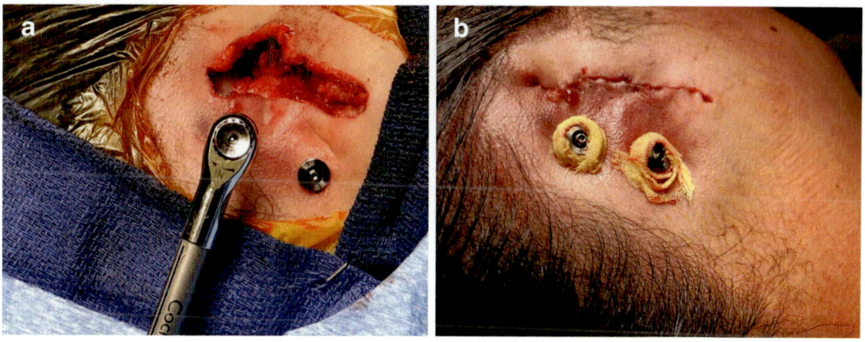

Fig. 10.37 (**a**) Incision for remnant removal and access to implants for abutment placement using a torque wrench and (**b**) closed incision with appropriate soft tissue reduction showing abutments wrapped with Xeroform dressing

* Xeroform gauze is wrapped around the full circumference of each abutment and should remain for 10–14 days to assist in the skin healing flat and tight against the bone surface.

* If definitive standard abutments are connected during second-stage surgery, then the exact length should be determined in consultation with the anaplastologist who likely has a design plan in mind using specific abutments.

* In the absence of a plan, definitive abutment length should be selected such that the external abutment surface is exposed above the skin surface 1–2 mm at a minimum (3–4 mm is preferred by this author) to facilitate home hygiene protocols and minimize the potential for skin overgrowth. Abutment lengths vary and generally range from 3.5 mm to 7.5 mm for facial prosthetic applications. Custom abutments can also be designed in special circumstances [109].

* Healing abutments may be preferred to allow healing of the surgical site before definitive abutment length is determined.

Combined Prosthetic Ear and Hearing Device Implant Placement

Congenital microtia is commonly associated with aural atresia and hearing loss, which can be rehabilitated using an implant-retained bone-anchored hearing device (Fig. 10.38). In this situation, careful consideration should be made regarding the placement of implants. The implant to retain the hearing device should be well out of the field of any planned surgical or prosthetic ear reconstruction, so as to not interfere with necessary surgical procedures, flaps, or vascular supply. Additionally, the planned ear reconstruction should not come into contact with the hearing processor as this can cause unwanted and audio feedback. Hearing concerns are at times addressed earlier than external ear reconstruction, particularly for children with bilateral microtia and aural atresia. For this reason, placement of an implant to address hearing loss should take into account the patient's potential interest in future external ear reconstruction.

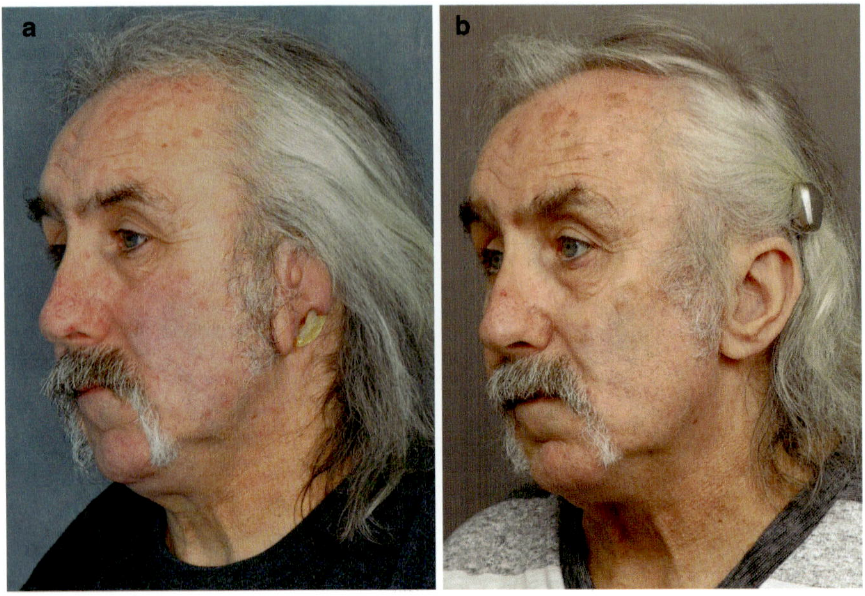

Fig. 10.38 (**a**) Exposed porous implant and (**b**) implant-retained prosthesis and bone-anchored hearing device

Lifetime Maintenance

The "delivery" visit in many ways may seem like the "finish line" with the completion of what for many patients has been a very long journey. It may very well represent the end of one journey, but it is also a new "starting point." The patient having received their finished and fitted prosthesis will then embark on a lifetime of prosthetic maintenance. For this reason alone, surgical reconstructive options should be considered as a "best first" option. Prosthetic restorations are always a possibility to complement surgical reconstruction or as a "backup plan" when surgical outcomes do not meet the defined treatment goals.

* For ongoing prosthetic maintenance, patients should have reliable access to skilled and experienced anaplastology services.

* Annual visits recommended for lifetime maintenance with at least two to three visits in the first year.

Conclusion

Microtia reconstruction is challenging and ideally involves an interdisciplinary team. Explaining the advantages and disadvantages of reconstruction are key to informed decision-making and consent. Every effort should be made to explain the different options to avoid surgical regret due to uninformed decisions or unrealistic expectations. One major challenge is obtaining assent in this frequently young population. A single-stage reconstructive surgery is possible, more commonly with porous polyethylene reconstruction. This technique is also advantageous in that it can be performed at an earlier age, avoids harvesting costal cartilage, and addresses the frequently low hairline. Autologous cartilage reconstruction has evolved dramatically over decades and avoids the use of alloplastic material, which has a higher rate of infection, and the skin quality overlying the framework may be less variable. Prosthetic reconstruction is also a good option, particularly for those preferring a simpler surgical procedure (for implant-retained) or those wanting to avoid surgery all together (for adhesive-retained). Prosthetic reconstruction is also an option for patients who have less than optimal autologous or alloplastic reconstruction. The disadvantages and surgical outcomes are heavily dependent on experience. The psychological impact of a poor reconstruction can be long-standing, and the need for revision surgery should be avoided in all manners possible as the results are less favorable. Long-term complications such as autologous cartilage atrophy or alloplastic implant exposure decades after repair are not well understood. For prosthetic reconstruction there is an ongoing need for replacements due to damage or fading and potential skin problems surrounding implants. Ultimately, specialists devoted to caring for patients with this unique condition should tailor the technique to the goals and unique characteristics of each patient.

Acknowledgments Special thanks to graphic artist Alinna Brigitte Diaz-Porro for her careful drawings demonstrating the approach to different grades of microtia for autologous auricular reconstruction.

References

1. Tanzer RC. Total reconstruction of the auricle: the evolution of a plan of treatment. Plast Reconstr Surg. 1971;47(6):523–33.
2. Brent BMD. Technical advances in ear reconstruction with autogenous rib cartilage grafts: personal experience with 1200 cases. Plast Reconstr Surg. 1999;104(2):319–34.
3. Firmin F, Dusseldorp J, Marchac A. Auricular reconstruction. New York: Thieme Medical Publishers; 2017.
4. Nagata S. Auricular reconstruction: congenital auricular defects-Microtia. In: Plastic surgery: indications and practice. Philadelphia: Saunders Elsevier; 2008. p. 671–99.
5. Reinisch JF, Lewin S. Ear reconstruction using a porous polyethylene framework and temporoparietal fascia flap. Facial Plast Surg. 2009;25(03):181–9.
6. Park SS, Hood RJ. Auricular reconstruction. Otolaryngol Clin N Am. 2001;34(4):713–38.
7. Marx H. Die Missbildungen des ohres. Denker-Kahlersche Handbuch der Hals, Nasen und ohrenheilk. Gehororganl. 1926;131–69.
8. Meurman Y. Congenital microtia and meatal atresia: observations and aspects of treatment. AMA Arch Otolaryngol. 1957;66(4):443–63.
9. Tanzer RC, RC T. Microtia. 1978.
10. Weerda H. Classification of congenital deformities of the auricle. Facial Plast Surg. 1988;5(05):385–8.

11. Firmin F, Marchac A. A novel algorithm for autologous ear reconstruction. Semin Plast Surg. 2011;25(4):257–64.
12. Park C, Park JY. Classification and algorithmic management of constricted ears: a 22-year experience. Plast Reconstr Surg. 2016;137(5):1523–38.
13. Campo AA, Victor-Baldin A, Contreras-Mérida SM. Surgical-based classification for microtia. J Craniofac Surg. 2018;29(6):1651–4.
14. Park C. Upper auricular adhesion malformation: definition, classification, and treatment. Plast Reconstr Surg. 2009;123(4):1302–12.
15. Takase M, Hashimoto I, Nakanishi H, Tanaka S, Matsumoto K, Matsuo S. Reconstruction of microtia with laser hair removal before transplantation of costal cartilage. J Plast Reconstr Aesthet Surg. 2008;61:S86–91.
16. Guo Y, Shan J, Zhang T. Clinical application of intense pulsed light depilation technology in total auricular reconstruction. Lasers Med Sci. 2017;32(6):1367–73.
17. Yamada A. Autologous rib microtia construction: Nagata technique. Facial Plast Surg Clin North Am. 2018;26(1):41–55.
18. Park JY, Park C. Microtia reconstruction in hemifacial microsomia patients: three framework coverage techniques. Plast Reconstr Surg. 2018;142(6):1558–70.
19. Li D, Zhang R, Zhang Q, Xu Z, Xu F, Li Y, et al. Clinical results of ear elevations in patients with microtia using skin grafts from three donor sites: a retrospective study. Aesthet Plast Surg. 2020;44(5):1545–52.
20. Yang M, Jiang H, Zhang Y, Pan B. A new method using tissue expander makes auricular reconstruction easier. Clin Otolaryngol. 2019;44(3):437–42.
21. Pan B, Jiang H, Guo D, Huang C, Hu S, Zhuang H. Microtia: ear reconstruction using tissue expander and autogenous costal cartilage. J Plast Reconstr Aesthet Surg. 2008;61:S98–103.
22. Wang Y, Zhuang X, Jiang H, Yang Q, Zhao Y, Han J, et al. The anatomy and application of the postauricular fascia flap in auricular reconstruction for congenital microtia. J Plast Reconstr Aesthet Surg. 2008;61:S70–6.
23. Xing W, Wang Y, Qian J, Wang B, Zhou X, Liu T, et al. Simultaneous bilateral Microtia reconstruction using single-expanded postauricular flap without skin grafting. Ann Plast Surg. 2018;81(6):669–74.
24. Tripathee S, Xiong M, Zhang J. Microtia ear reconstruction using tissue expander and autologous costal cartilage: our experience and comparing two age groups. World J Plast Surg. 2019;8(3):324.
25. Chen Q, Zhang J, Wang B, Wang Y, Kang C, Zhang Q. Total auricular reconstruction using a single extended postauricular flap without skin grafting in two stages: experiences of 106 cases. Aesthet Plast Surg. Switzerland, 2019;44(2):365–72.
26. Thorne CH, Brecht LE, Bradley JP, Levine JP, Hammerschlag P, Longaker MT. Auricular reconstruction: indications for autogenous and prosthetic techniques. Plast Reconstr Surg. 2001;107(5):1241–52.
27. Granström G, Bergström K, Odersjö M, Tjellström A. Osseointegrated implants in children: experience from our first 100 patients. Otolaryngol Head Neck Surg. 2001;125(1):85.
28. Klineberg I. Introduction: from osseointegration to osseoperception. The functional translation. Clin Exp Pharmacol Physiol. 2005;32(1–2):97–9.
29. Federspil PA. Auricular prostheses in microtia. Facial Plast Surg Clin North Am. 2018;26(1):97–104.
30. Tolman DE, Taylor PF. Bone-anchored craniofacial prosthesis study. Int J Oral Maxillofac Implants. 1996;11(2):159–68.
31. Parel SM, Tjellströ A. The United States and Swedish experience with osseointegration and facial prostheses. Int J Oral Maxillofac Implants. 1991;6(1):75.
32. Wolfaardt JF, Wilkes GH, Parel SM, Tjellström A. Craniofacial osseointegration: the Canadian experience. Int J Oral Maxillofac Implants. 1993;8(2):197.
33. Lewin S. Complications after total porous implant ear reconstruction and their management. Facial Plast Surg. 2015;31(06):617–25.

34. Romo T, Presti PM, Yalamanchili HR. Medpor alternative for microtia repair. Facial Plast Surg Clin North Am. 2006;14(2):129–36.
35. Romo T, Reitzen SD. Aesthetic microtia reconstruction with Medpor. Facial Plast Surg. 2008;24(01):120–8.
36. Im DD, Paskhover B, Staffenberg DA, Jarrahy R. Current management of microtia: a national survey. Aesthet Plast Surg. 2013;37(2):402–8.
37. Brent B. Auricular repair with autogenous rib cartilage grafts: two decades of experience with 600 cases. Plast Reconstr Surg. 1992;90(3):355–74; discussion 375–6.
38. Cabin JA, Bassiri-Tehrani M, Sclafani AP. Microtia reconstruction: autologous rib and alloplast techniques. Facial Plast Surg Clin North Am. 2014;22(4):623–38.
39. Kawanabe Y, Nagata S. A new method of costal cartilage harvest for total auricular reconstruction: part I. Avoidance and prevention of intraoperative and postoperative complications and problems. Plast Reconstr Surg. 2006;117(6):2011–8.
40. Cho BC, Kim JY, Byun JS. Two-stage reconstruction of the auricle in congenital microtia using autogenous costal cartilage. J Plast Reconstr Aesthet Surg. 2007;60(9):998–1006.
41. Zhang Q, Zhang R, Xu F, Jin P, Cao Y. Auricular reconstruction for microtia: personal 6-year experience based on 350 microtia ear reconstructions in China. Plast Reconstr Surg. 2009;123(3):849–58.
42. Kasrai L, Snyder-Warwick AK, Fisher DM. Single stage autologous ear reconstruction for microtia. Plast Reconstr Surg. 2014;133(3):652–62.
43. Firmin F. Ear reconstruction in cases of typical microtia. Personal experience based on 352 microtic ear corrections. Scand J Plast Reconstr Surg Hand Surg. 1998;32(1):35–47.
44. Márquez-Gutiérrez EA, Gutiérrez-Gómez Del Hierro C, Rodríguez-Quintero JH, Pereyra-Arzate JE, Rivera-Martínez R. Descriptive analysis of the arterial supply to the auricle in patients with unilateral microtia. Plast Reconstr Surg Glob Open. 2017;5(12):e1594.
45. Olcott CM, Simon PE, Romo T III, Louie W. Anatomy of the superficial temporal artery in patients with unilateral microtia. J Plast Reconstr Aesthet Surg. 2019;72(1):114–8.
46. Bly RA, Bhrany AD, Murakami CS, Sie KC. Microtia reconstruction. Facial Plast Surg Clin North Am. 2016;24(4):577–91.
47. Mussi E, Furferi R, Volpe Y, Facchini F, McGreevy KS, Uccheddu F. Ear reconstruction simulation: from handcrafting to 3D printing. Bioengineering. 2019;6(1):14.
48. Fan X, Niu X, Wang Y, Chen Y, Fan Y, Wang J, et al. Comparison of three-dimensional and two-dimensional templates on auricle reconstruction in patients with unilateral microtia. Am J Transl Res. 2019;11(6):3771.
49. van Nunen DP, Kolodzynski MN, van den Boogaard M-JH, Kon M, Breugem CC. Microtia in the Netherlands: clinical characteristics and associated anomalies. Int J Pediatr Otorhinolaryngol. 2014;78(6):954–9.
50. Ishikura N, Kawakami S, Yoshida J, Shimada K. Vascular supply of the subcutaneous pedicle of Nagata's method in microtia reconstruction. Br J Plast Surg. 2004;57(8):780–4.
51. Hongo T, Komune N, Shimamoto R, Nakagawa T. The surgical anatomy of soft tissue layers in the mastoid region. Laryngoscope Investig Otolaryngol. 2019;4(3):359–64.
52. Jimenez F, Izeta A, Poblet E. Morphometric analysis of the human scalp hair follicle: practical implications for the hair transplant surgeon and hair regeneration studies. Dermatol Surg. 2011;37(1):58–64.
53. Goldsztein H, Ort S, Roberson JB Jr, Reinisch J. Scalp as split thickness skin graft donor site for congenital atresia repair. Laryngoscope. 2013;123(2):496–8.
54. Davidge KM, van Furth WR, Agur A, Cusimano M. Naming the soft tissue layers of the temporoparietal region: unifying anatomic terminology across surgical disciplines. Operative Neurosurgery. 2010;67(3):ons120–3.
55. Stephan S, Reinisch J. Auricular reconstruction using porous polyethylene implant technique. Facial Plast Surg Clin North Am. 2018;26(1):69–85.
56. Helling ER, Okoro S, George Kim II, Wang PT. Endoscope-assisted temporoparietal fascia harvest for auricular reconstruction. Plast Reconstr Surg. 2008;121(5):1598–605.

57. Park C, Lew D-H, Yoo W-M. An analysis of 123 temporoparietal fascial flaps: anatomic and clinical considerations in total auricular reconstruction. Plast Reconstr Surg. 1999;104(5):1295–306.
58. Kim YS, Yun IS, Chung S. Salvage of ear framework exposure in total auricular reconstruction. Ann Plast Surg. 2017;78(2):178–83.
59. Hirase Y, Kojima T, Hirakawa M. Secondary ear reconstruction using deep temporal fascia after temporoparietal fascial reconstruction in microtia. Ann Plast Surg. 1990;25(1):53–7.
60. Li Y, Zhang R, Zhang Q, Xu Z, Xu F, Li D. An alternative posterosuperior auricular fascia flap for ear elevation during microtia reconstruction. Aesthet Plast Surg. 2017;41(1):47–55.
61. Maeda T, Oyama A, Funayama E, Yamamoto Y. Reconstruction of low hairline microtia of Treacher Collins syndrome with a hinged mastoid fascial flap. Int J Oral Maxillofac Surg. 2016;45(6):731–4.
62. Ou L-F, Yan R-S, Tang Y-W. Firm elevation of the auricle in reconstruction of microtia with a retroauricular fascial flap wrapping an autogenous cartilage wedge. Br J Plast Surg. 2001;54(7):573–80.
63. Yoshimura K, Nakatsuka T, Ichioka S, Kaji N, Harii K. One-stage reconstruction of an upper part defect of the auricle. Aesthet Plast Surg. 1998;22(5):352–5.
64. Lohasammakul S, Turbpaiboon C, Chompoopong S, Ratanalekha R, Aojanepong C. Vascular nature and existence of anastomoses of extrinsic postauricular fascia: application for staged auricular reconstruction. Ann Plast Surg. 2017;78(6):723–7.
65. Reinisch JF, Tahiri Y, Yao CA. The occipital artery–based fascial flap for ear reconstruction. Plast Reconstr Surg. 2019;143(3):592e–601e.
66. Bonilla A. Pediatric microtia reconstruction with autologous rib: personal experience and technique with 1000 pediatric patients with microtia. Facial Plast Surg Clin North Am. 2018;26(1):57–68.
67. O'Brien JX, Ashton MW, Rozen WM, Ross R, Mendelson BC. New perspectives on the surgical anatomy and nomenclature of the temporal region: literature review and dissection study. Plast Reconstr Surg. 2013;131(3):510–22.
68. Berghaus A, Toplak F. Surgical concepts for reconstruction of the auricle: history and current state of the art. Arch Otolaryngol Head Neck Surg. 1986;112(4):388–97.
69. Zhao Y, Wang Y, Zhuang H, Jiang H, Jiang W, Hu X, et al. Clinical evaluation of three total ear reconstruction methods. J Plast Reconstr Aesthet Surg. 2009;62(12):1550–4.
70. Zhang T, Bulstrode N, Chang KW, Cho Y-S, Frenzel H, Jiang D, et al. International consensus recommendations on microtia, aural atresia and functional ear reconstruction. J Int Adv Otol. 2019;15(2):204.
71. Baluch N, Nagata S, Park C, Wilkes GH, Reinisch J, Kasrai L, et al. Auricular reconstruction for microtia: a review of available methods. Plast Surg (Oakv). 2014;22(1):39–43.
72. Johns AL, Lucash RE, Im DD, Lewin SL. Pre and post-operative psychological functioning in younger and older children with microtia. J Plast Reconstr Aesthet Surg. 2015;68(4):492–7.
73. Adamson JE, Hortox CE, Crawford HH. The growth pattern of the external ear. Plast Reconstr Surg. 1965;36(4):466–70.
74. Reinisch J, Tahiri Y. Polyethylene ear reconstruction: a state-of-the-art surgical journey. Plast Reconstr Surg. 2018;141(2):461–70.
75. Louis PJ, Aponte-Wesson RA, Fernandes RP, Clemow J. Autogenous and prosthetic reconstruction of the ear. Oral Maxillofac Surg Clin North Am. 2013;25(2):271–86.
76. Korus LJ, Wong JN, Wilkes GH. Long-term follow-up of osseointegrated auricular reconstruction. Plast Reconstr Surg. 2011;127(2):630–6.
77. Wolfaardt J, Gehl G, Farmand M, Wilkes G. Indications and methods of care for aspects of extraoral osseointegration. Int J Oral Maxillofac Surg. 2003;32(2):124–31.
78. Chang T-L, Garrett N, Roumanas E, Beumer J III. Treatment satisfaction with facial prostheses. J Prosthet Dent. 2005;94(3):275–80.
79. Littlefield PD, Tolisano AM, Sabol JV, Herberg ME, Coppit GL III. Total auricular rehabilitation: combined cosmetic and functional lateral temporal bone reconstruction. J Craniofac Surg. 2015;26(5):1467–70.

80. Visser A, Raghoebar GM, van Oort RP, Vissink A. Fate of implant-retained craniofacial prostheses: life span and aftercare. Int J Oral Maxillofac Implants. 2008;23(1):89.
81. Hatamleh MM, Haylock C, Watson J, Watts DC. Maxillofacial prosthetic rehabilitation in the UK: a survey of maxillofacial prosthetists' and technologists' attitudes and opinions. Int J Oral Maxillofac Surg. 2010;39(12):1186–92.
82. Reitemeier B, Götzel B, Schöne C, Stockmann F, Müller R, Lexmann J, et al. Creation and utilization of a digital database for nasal prosthesis models. Oncol Res Treat. 2013;36(1–2):7–11.
83. Capon T. Standardised anatomical alignment of the head in a clinical photography studio. A comparison between the Frankfort Horizontal and the natural head position. J Vis Commun Med. 2016;39(3–4):105–11.
84. Rhee SC. A simple method for international standardization of photographic documentation for aesthetic plastic surgery. Aesthet Plast Surg. 2017;41(2):461–5.
85. Salazar-Gamarra R, Seelaus R, da Silva JVL, da Silva AM, Dib LL. Monoscopic photogrammetry to obtain 3D models by a mobile device: a method for making facial prostheses. J Otolaryngol Head Neck Surg. 2016;45(1):1–13.
86. Deli R, Galantucci LM, Laino A, D'Alessio R, Di Gioia E, Savastano C, et al. Three-dimensional methodology for photogrammetric acquisition of the soft tissues of the face: a new clinical-instrumental protocol. Prog Orthod. 2013;14(1):32.
87. Unkovskiy A, Spintzyk S, Brom J, Huettig F, Keutel C. Direct 3D printing of silicone facial prostheses: a preliminary experience in digital workflow. J Prosthet Dent. 2018;120(2):303–8.
88. Nuseir A, Hatamleh MM, Alnazzawi A, Al-Rabab'ah M, Kamel B, Jaradat E. Direct 3D printing of flexible nasal prosthesis: optimized digital workflow from scan to fit. J Prosthodont. 2019;28(1):10–4.
89. Coward TJ, Seelaus R, Li SY. Computerized color formulation for African-Canadian people requiring facial prostheses: a pilot study. J Prosthodont. 2008;17(4):327–35.
90. Seelaus R, Coward TJ, Li S. Coloration of silicone prostheses: technology versus clinical perception. Is there a difference? Part 2, clinical evaluation of a pilot study. J Prosthodont. 2011;20(1):67–73.
91. Steffen A, Klaiber S, Katzbach R, Nitsch S, König IR, Frenzel H. The psychosocial consequences of reconstruction of severe ear defects or third-degree microtia with rib cartilage. Aesthet Surg J. 2008;28(4):404–11.
92. Steffen A, Wollenberg B, König IR, Frenzel H. A prospective evaluation of psychosocial outcomes following ear reconstruction with rib cartilage in microtia. J Plast Reconstr Aesthet Surg. 2010;63(9):1466–73.
93. Albrektsson T, Johansson C. Osteoinduction, osteoconduction and osseointegration. Eur Spine J. 2001;10(2):S96–101.
94. Granström G. Craniofacial osseointegration. Oral Dis. 2007;13(3):261–9.
95. Wolfaardt JF, Wilkes GH. Craniofacial osseointegration. J Can Dent Assoc. 1994;60(9):805–9.
96. Schoen PJ, Raghoebar GM, van Oort RP, Reintsema H, van der Laan BF, Burlage FR, et al. Treatment outcome of bone-anchored craniofacial prostheses after tumor surgery. Cancer. 2001;92(12):3045–50.
97. Kruyt IJ, Nelissen RC, Mylanus EA, Hol MK. Three-year outcomes of a randomized controlled trial comparing a 4.5-mm-wide to a 3.75-mm-wide titanium implant for bone conduction hearing. Otol Neurotol. 2018;39(5):609.
98. Nelissen RC, den Besten CA, Faber HT, Dun CA, Mylanus EA, Hol MK. Loading of osseointegrated implants for bone conduction hearing at 3 weeks: 3-year stability, survival, and tolerability. Eur Arch Otorhinolaryngol. 2016;273(7):1731–7.
99. Miller KL, Faulkner G, Wolfaardt JF. Misfit and functional loading of craniofacial implants. Int J Prosthodont. 2004;17(3):267.
100. Faulkner G, Wolfaardt J, del Valle V. Console abutment loading in craniofacial osseointegration. Int J Oral Maxillofac Implants. 1998;13(2):245–52.
101. Jacobs R, Salmon B, Codari M, Hassan B, Bornstein MM. Cone beam computed tomography in implant dentistry: recommendations for clinical use. BMC Oral Health. 2018;18(1):1–16.

102. Hatamleh M, Turner C, Bhamrah G, Mack G, Osher J. Improved virtual planning for bimaxillary orthognathic surgery. J Craniofac Surg. 2016;27(6):e568–73.
103. Chepelev L, Wake N, Ryan J, Althobaity W, Gupta A, Arribas E, et al. Radiological Society of North America (RSNA) 3D printing Special Interest Group (SIG): guidelines for medical 3D printing and appropriateness for clinical scenarios. 3D Print Med. 2018;4(1):1–38.
104. Giannopoulos AA, Pietila T. Post-processing of DICOM images. In: 3D printing in medicine. Cham, Switzerland: Springer; 2017. p. 23–34.
105. Verma S, Gonzalez M, Schow SR, Triplett RG. Virtual preoperative planning and intraoperative navigation in facial prosthetic reconstruction: a technical note. Int J Oral Maxillofac Implants. 2017;32(2):e77.
106. Verma SN, Schow SR, Stone BH, Triplett RG. Applications of surgical navigational systems for craniofacial bone-anchored implant placement. Int J Oral Maxillofac Implants. 2010;25(3):582.
107. Tjellström A, Stalfors J, Bergström K. Cochlear vistafix, treatment and surgery guide [Internet]. 2012.; Available from: www.CochlearAmericas.com.
108. Rebol J. Soft tissue reactions in patients with bone anchored hearing aids. Ir J Med Sci (1971-). 2015;184(2):487–91.
109. Kincade C, McHutchion L, Wolfaardt J. Digital design of patient-specific abutments for the retention of implant-retained facial prostheses. J Prosthet Dent. 2018;120(2):309–12.

Chapter 11
Correction of the Soft Tissue Deformities Associated with Craniofacial Microsomia: Facial Reanimation and Soft Tissue Grafting Techniques

Farooq Shahzad

Manuscript

Craniofacial microsomia is a spectrum of deformities that occur due to abnormal development of structures derived from the first and second branchial arches (Table 11.1). The involved territory is represented by Tessier # 6, 7, and 8 facial clefts [1]. There is bilateral involvement in approximately 15 to 24% of cases which is usually asymmetric [2, 3]. The SAT and OMENS classification systems include soft tissue deficiencies in their scheme (Table 11.2). The SAT system is modeled after the TNM classification of tumors [4]. The OMENS system is more comprehensive, with a later modification including extra-craniofacial involvement with a plus (+) [3, 5].

The first step in management is an assessment of all structural and functional abnormalities so that a plan and timeline for reconstruction can be made. Involvement of multiple structures implies that several reconstructive procedures will be needed. These operations need to be properly sequenced for optimal long-term aesthetic and functional outcomes (Fig. 11.1).

Soft Tissue Reconstruction

The soft tissue involvement in craniofacial microsomia is highly variable. There can be deficiency of all types of soft tissue components including the skin, subcutaneous tissue, muscles of mastication, and parotid gland. Ear abnormalities comprise a spectrum of severity from accessory tragi to microtia or anotia. Middle ear

F. Shahzad (✉)
Division of Plastic & Reconstructive Surgery, Memorial Sloan-Kettering Cancer Center, Weill Medical College of Cornell University, New York, NY, USA
e-mail: shahzadf@mskcc.org

D. M. Yates, M. R. Markiewicz (eds.), *Craniofacial Microsomia and Treacher Collins Syndrome*, https://doi.org/10.1007/978-3-030-84733-3_11

Table 11.1 Important structures derived from the first and second branchial arches

	First branchial arch	Second branchial arch
Skeletal	Maxilla Mandible Zygoma Palatine bone Squamous part of temporal bone Spine of sphenoid bone	Styloid process Hyoid bone (lesser cornu and upper part of the body)
Muscle	Muscles of mastication (masseter, temporalis, lateral, and medial pterygoids) Tensor veli palatini Tensor tympani Anterior belly of digastric Mylohyoid	Muscles of facial expression Platysma Occipitofrontalis Stylohyoid muscle Stapedius Posterior belly of digastric
Ear	Anterior ear (helical root, superior helix, tragus) Malleus, incus Eustachian tube	Posterior ear (helix, antihelix, tragus, lobule) Stapes
Nerve	Maxillary (V2) and mandibular (V3) divisions of trigeminal nerve (CN V)	Facial nerve (CN VII)

Table 11.2 Classification systems for hemifacial microsomia

SAT system	
Skeletal	
S_1	Small mandible with normal shape
S_2	Condyle, ramus, and sigmoid notch grossly distorted but identifiable
S_3	Poorly identifiable ramal components to complete agenesis of ramus
S_4	S_3 plus posterior displacement of inferior and lateral orbital rims
S_5	S_4 plus orbital dystopia
Auricle	
A_0	Normal
A_1	Small, malformed auricle maintaining characteristic features
A_2	Rudimentary auricle with hook at cranial end corresponding to the helix
A_3	Malformed lobule with the rest of the pinna absent
Soft tissue	
T_1	Minimal contour defect with no cranial nerve involvement
T_2	Moderate defect
T_3	Major defect with obvious facial scoliosis, possibly severe hypoplasia of cranial nerves, parotid gland, and muscles of mastication; eye involvement; and clefts of the face or lips
OMENS system	
Orbit	
O_0	Normal orbital size and position
O_1	Abnormal orbital size
$O_{2\uparrow}$	Abnormal orbital position (superior displacement)
$O_{2\downarrow}$	Abnormal orbital position (inferior displacement)
O_3	Abnormal orbital size and position

Table 11.2 (continued)

Mandible	
M_0	Normal mandible
M_1	Small mandible and glenoid fossa
M_{2A}	Short and abnormally shaped ramus. Glenoid fossa in anatomically acceptable position
M_{2B}	Short and abnormally shaped ramus. Hypoplastic condyle. Temporomandibular joint is inferiorly, medially, and anteriorly displaced
M_3	Absence of ramus and glenoid fossa
Ear	
E_0	Normal ear
E_1	Mild hypoplasia and cupping, but all structures present
E_2	Absence of external auditory canal with hypoplasia of concha
E_3	Absence of auricle with malpositioned lobule
Nerve	
N_0	No facial nerve involvement
N_1	Upper facial nerve involvement (temporal, zygomatic)
N_2	Lower facial nerve involvement (buccal, mandibular, cervical)
N_3	All branches affected
Soft tissue	
S_0	No soft tissue deficiency
S_1	Minimal soft tissue deficiency
S_2	Moderate soft tissue deficiency
S_3	Severe soft tissue deficiency

hypoplasia may also occur, leading to conductive hearing loss. The eye may be involved, resulting in microphthalmia or anophthalmia. Eyelid abnormalities can include lateral canthal displacement, colobomas, and missing lashes. Transverse facial clefting from the oral commissure may occur leading to macrostomia of variable degrees. Hypoplasia of muscles of mastication may contribute to occlusal abnormalities and chin point deviation toward the hypoplastic side. Hypoplasia of the palatal muscles may also occur leading to palatal deviation and velopharyngeal dysfunction. The degree of soft tissue deficiency has been shown to be positively correlated with the degree of mandible, orbit and facial nerve abnormalities, and the presence of macrostomia [2].

Management of facial asymmetry has traditionally consisted of correction of skeletal abnormalities followed by volume augmentation with soft tissue flaps [6]. This results in creation of a stable skeletal base allowing a more precise assessment of soft tissue deficiency for accurate volume correction. The advent of structural fat grafting has changed this paradigm. Fat grafting does not provide as much volume in a single operation as a soft tissue flap but is a much less invasive operation. Fat injections can be started at an earlier age and even combined with other reconstructive procedures. Alloplastic implants are a useful method for targeted and precise volume correction with the least donor site morbidity. A comparison of these techniques is outlined in Table 11.3.

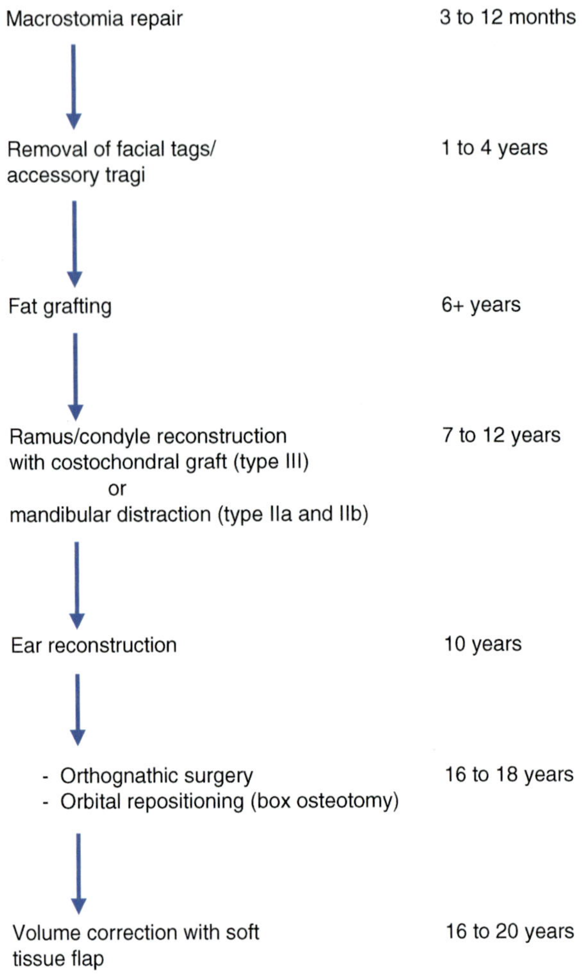

Fig. 11.1 General time line of commonly performed soft tissue and bone reconstruction procedures in patients with craniofacial microsomia

Flaps

Soft tissue flaps provide a large volume of autologous tissue. They are a good choice in severe deformities where a considerable amount of soft tissue may be needed for volume correction. Volume restoration can be performed in a single operation. Bone can also be incorporated in the flap for simultaneously mandible or midface reconstruction. The main disadvantage of flaps is donor site morbidity like scarring, pain, contour deformity, and possible functional deficits. Flaps sag with time due to gravity, and therefore secondary operations are typically needed for flap resuspension and soft tissue contouring [7]. Both pedicled flaps and free flaps can be used, based on soft tissue requirements.

Table 11.3 Comparison of various techniques of soft tissue volume correction

	Flaps	Fat grafting	Alloplasts
Extent of procedure	Most invasive	Least	Moderately invasive
Donor morbidity	Most	Minimal	None
Volume correction	Most (frequently overcorrection)	Small volume correction usually achieved	Accurate volume correction, especially with custom implants
Need for repeat procedures	Usually requires second operation for flap debulking, resuspension, and contour refinement	Usually requires repeat procedures for adequate volume correction	Precise volume correction can be achieved with a single operation
Timing	At or near skeletal maturity, after bony procedures	Can be done at any age Frequently performed in conjunction with other reconstructive procedures	At or near skeletal maturity, after bony procedures
Complications	Partial or total flap loss Donor site morbidity Complication rate 27.1% [9]	Resorption of fat Fat necrosis, oil cysts Pain and hematoma at donor site Complication rate 4.2% [9]	Malposition Infection Extrusion

Free Flaps

Free tissue transfer provides an almost unlimited supply of soft tissue for volume repletion. It also allows greater flexibility of flap inset, allowing customized flap design. Any type of fasciocutaneous or adipofacial flap can be used, depending on volume requirements and available donor sites. Pure muscle flaps are not generally used as they atrophy unpredictably over time. Soft tissue flaps almost always require a revision procedure for resuspension, contouring, or volume redistribution. The most common complications of free flaps are hematoma, wound dehiscence, infections, and flap loss [8].

The most commonly reported flap for craniofacial microsomia reconstruction is the parascapular flap and its variant, the inframammary extended circumflex scapular (IMECS) flap [9, 10]. Other reported flaps are the gracilis, rectus abdominis, anterolateral thigh, latissimus dorsi, omentum, deep inferior epigastric perforator (DIEP), superficial inferior epigastric artery (SIEA), superficial circumflex iliac (SCIA), and groin flaps. The most commonly used recipient vessels are the superficial temporal vessels, followed by the facial vessels.

Each flap has its own advantages and drawbacks. The scapular/parascapular flap is popular because it provides a large amount of soft tissue with low donor site morbidity. If a very large flap is required, tissue expansion of the donor site be performed for primary donor site closure [8]. The inframammary extended circumflex scapular (IMECS) flap is a variant of the parascapular flap in which the incision is slightly more anteriorly placed and curves to the inframammary fold [10]. This allows harvest in an oblique position obviating a position change and allowing simultaneous face recipient site and flap dissection. A larger volume of tissue can be harvested with a more aesthetically placed scar. A chimeric flap based on the subscapular system can be harvested comprising bone (lateral scapular border) and soft tissue (scapular/parascapular flaps) for simultaneous soft tissue and skeletal reconstruction [11, 12].

The latissimus dorsi flap is a good choice when a very large volume of tissue is required [13, 14]. The thoracodorsal artery perforator flap spares muscle and minimized donor site morbidity [15]. Chimeric flaps based on the thoracodorsal vessels can be designed for simultaneous soft tissue and bone reconstruction. The soft tissue latissimus flap is used for soft tissue augmentation, and the serratus/costochondral flap is used for ramus and condyle reconstruction [16].

Groin-based flaps like the SCIA and SIEA flaps provide a moderate amount of soft tissue with low donor site morbidity [17]. The scar is in a relatively hidden location. The deep circumflex iliac artery osteocutaneous flap can be used for simultaneous ramus reconstruction and volume augmentation. The rectus abdominis myocutaneous flap provides a large volume of tissue [18]. The deep inferior epigastric artery perforator flap decreases donor site morbidity and increases volume predictability by eliminating the issue of post-operative muscle atrophy [19]. The anterolateral thigh flap and superior gluteal artery-based flaps can also be utilized in the appropriate candidate [20, 21]. The omentum flap provides a large volume of pliable tissue that allows freedom of inset into different areas of volume deficiency of the face [22]. A major disadvantage of the flap is that it requires a laparotomy.

Surgical technique:

- The patient is marked preoperatively in the upright position. The areas of volume deficiency are marked in a topographic fashion with areas of thicker and thinner tissue needs identified.
- Intubation is performed orotracheally. The endotracheal tube is secured to the premolar teeth with silk suture or wire.
- A template of the defect is made, marking the areas of thicker and thinner soft tissue needs.
- Local anesthetic containing epinephrine is injected widely in the face. A preauricular incision is made. If exposure is not sufficient, the incision can be extended retro-auricularly or into the neck (modified Blair incision). The incision should not compromise future ear reconstruction, if planned.
- The cheek skin flap is elevated in a plane just above the superficial musculoaponeurotic system (SMAS). Dissection is carried out about a centimeter beyond the area of deficiency.
- The recipient vessels are dissected out and prepared. The superficial temporal vessels are most commonly used. If future ear reconstruction is anticipated, these vessels are preserved as they will be needed for supplying the temporoparietal fascia flap. Alternatively, the neck vessels (facial, superior thyroid, lingual, occipital) can be used.

- The template is placed on the donor site. The flap pedicle position with respect to the recipient vessels in the face/neck is considered while positioning the template on the donor site. The template is centered on the main axis of the flap, with the area of the thickest tissue needs on this central axis. Flap skin paddle depends on the ability to close donor site and size of soft tissue required. If larger flap is needed than the skin paddle, it is harvested in SQ plane so that donor skin can be closed. The position of the template can also be adjusted later once the location of the perforators and main pedicle are visualized.
- The harvested flap is temporarily secured to the face. Microvascular anastomoses are performed.
- Flap inset is then performed meticulously. The flap is usually completely buried. If overlying skin is deficient and closure may cause pedicle compression, a skin paddle is left in the preauricular area, and the remainder of the flap is de-epithelialized. The flap is secured to the periosteum of the zygoma and inferior orbital rim. If needed, fixation to the piriform aperture can be performed via an intraoral incision. A lateral upper eyelid incision can be useful for fixation of the flap high on the lateral orbital rim [23]. Facial extensions of the flap can be used to augment areas around the lips, chin nose, and eyes. If there is depression of the alar base or ear, these structures can be released, and the flap placed under to build up their base support. The edges of the flap are beveled to create a smooth contour. The distal parts of the flap are suspended to the overlying skin via trans-dermal sutures tied to petrolatum gauze bolsters. Quilting sutures are performed from the flap to parotid fascia. Patient is sat up after inset for assessment, and any necessary fine-tuning is performed.
- Patients are placed on prophylaxis dose low-molecular-weight heparin while they are in the hospital and on aspirin for 1 week. Flap monitoring is performed via implantable Doppler, every hour for the first 2 days, then every 2 hours for the next 2 days, and then every 4 hours. Patients are discharged after 3 to 5 days. Transcutaneous bolsters are removed in 1 week. A case example is illustrated in Fig. 11.2.

Microsurgical considerations:

1. Blood vessels should be handled with extreme care in children. The vessels are small and tend to spasm when injured or handled roughly.
2. The superficial temporal artery vessels may be small in patients with craniofacial microsomia [21, 24]. More proximal dissection of these vessels in the substance of the parotid gland will yield vessels of larger size [25]. Alternatively, the facial vessels can be dissected in the area of the sub-mandibular gland. Neck vessels may also be used.
3. Neck vessels may be diminutive or displaced from their normal position, e.g., the facial vessels have been reported be absent or malpositioned in children with craniofacial microsomia [26].

Flap Revisions

Additional procedures are required in the majority of patients for flap resuspension and/or fat contouring. Revisions are performed after 6 to 12 months. If there are minor contour problems, liposuction is performed for areas of volume excess, and

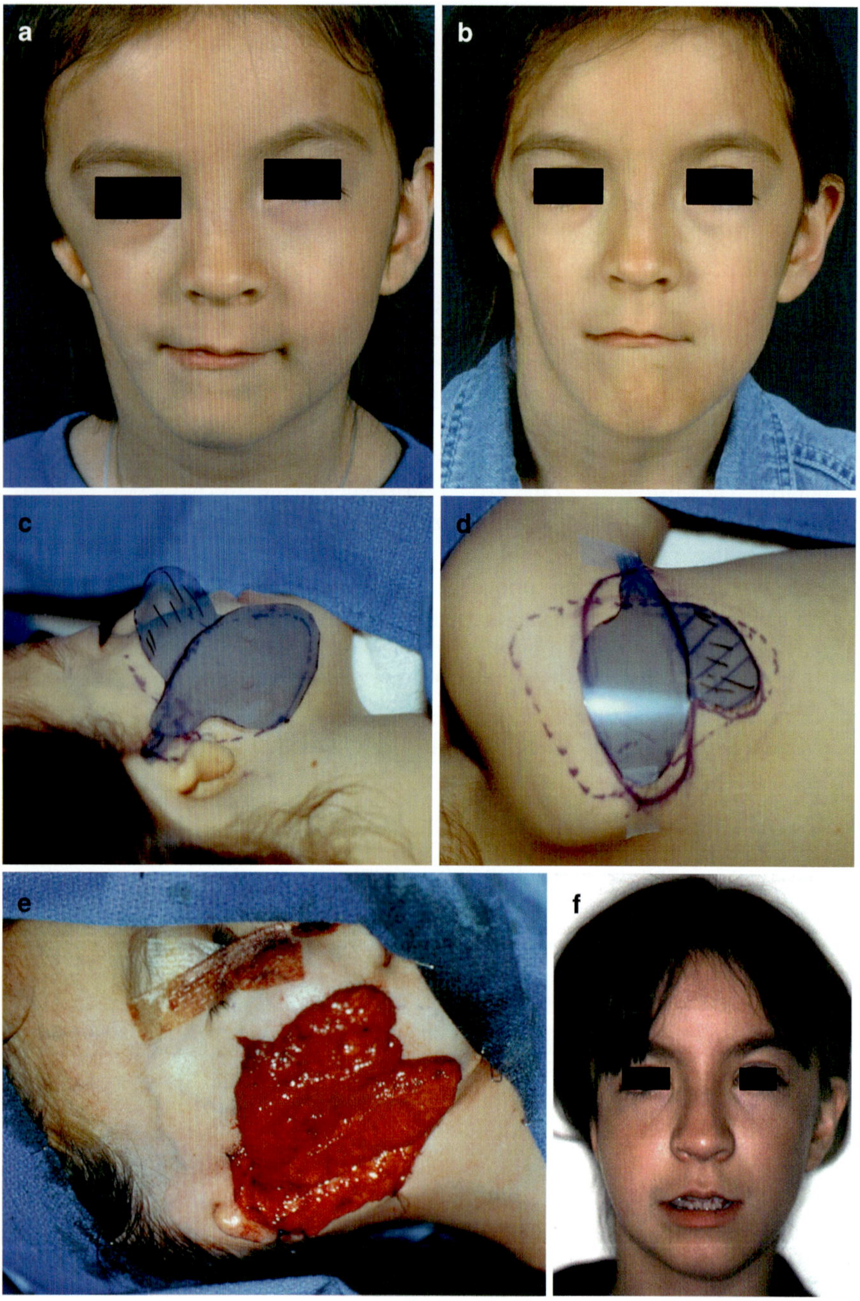

fat grafting is performed for areas of volume deficiency. However, in most patients, direct flap contouring is needed. The preauricular incision is opened up, and a skin flap is developed in the subcutaneous plane. The flap is re-elevated and suspended. Soft tissue is excised in areas of excess [27]. Usually there is tissue excess in the lower face at the area of the jaw line which needs contouring and tissue deficiency in the upper face which needs fat augmentation.

Pedicled Flaps

Regional pedicled flaps have the advantage of obviating the need for microsurgery. They are, however, limited by available soft tissue and their arc of rotation. Various flaps have been described. With the ubiquitous and routine use of free tissue transfer, the use of pedicled flaps for management of craniofacial microsomia has become very infrequent. However, they are useful in situations where microsurgery facilities are not available.

The submental flap can be used for volume replacement of the lower and midface [28]. The main drawback of this flap is a scar in the neck. The temporoparietal fascia flap in itself does not have a sufficient bulk to correct the typical volume deficits in craniofacial microsomia. Temporoparietal fascia flap can be combined with dermis-fat grafts to increase bulk [29].

Composite soft tissue and bone flaps have also been used for simultaneous correction of bone and soft tissue deficits. A chimeric flap based on the thoracodorsal pedicle has been described. The serratus/costochondral segment is used for ramus/condyle reconstruction, and the de-epithelialized skin paddle of the latissimus segment is used for soft tissue augmentation [16]. A composite temporoparietal fascia and parietal bone flap has also been described for simultaneous mandibular reconstruction and soft tissue augmentation [30].

Grafts

Structural Fat Grafting

Structural fat grafting has become the most popular technique for volume replacement in patients with facial contour abnormalities like craniofacial microsomia and Romberg's disease. Its major advantage is that it is a short, minimally invasive

Fig. 11.2 Case demonstrating soft tissue reconstruction. (**a**) A 5-year-old girl with right-sided craniofacial microsomia. (**b**) She underwent right mandibular distraction for Pruzansky 2A mandibular hypoplasia, which resulted in correction of mandibular asymmetry and chin point but did not address the soft tissue deficiency. (**c**) Due to the severity of soft tissue deficiency, correction with a scapular fasciocutaneous free flap was undertaken. A template of the soft tissue defect was created. (**d**) This template was transposed on the scapular donor site for planning of the incisions and flap harvest. (**e**) Flap tailored to the soft tissue deficiency. Microvascular anastomosis was performed to the facial vessels. A fat grafting procedure was subsequently performed a few years later to correct localized areas of deficiency. (**f**) Follow-up at 8 years demonstrated durability of the procedure. (Case courtesy of Arun Gosain MD, FACS) outpatient procedure without the donor site morbidity of a free flap. By obviating the need for extensive facial dissection, facial suspensory ligaments and dermal attachments are preserved. Volume correction can be targeted to areas of deficiency. Fat grafting can be undertaken at any age, and procedures can be staged through childhood at times convenient for the patient. Fat grafting can also be performed at the time of other reconstructive procedures that these patients may need, thus decreasing the total number of operations. The major disadvantage of fat grafting is that fat take is unpredictable. Approximately 50 to 60% of the injected fat survives [31]. Therefore several sessions of grafting are typically needed for optimal volume correction. A systematic review showed that the mean number of fat grafting sessions in patients with craniofacial microsomia is 2.7 with a range of one to six sessions [9]. Operations are spaced at a minimum of 1 year apart. Enrichment of fat grafts with adipose-derived stromal cells may increase fat graft take [32].

Fat grafting can be performed prior to school age so that better facial symmetry is achieved prior to child's interaction with their peers [33]. Fat grafting improves the quality of the overlying skin due to regenerative effects of adipose-derived stem cells. One point that should be kept in mind is that the injected fat retains the characteristics of the donor site. Therefore, as the patient gains weight, the transplanted fat hypertrophies more than the native facial fat [34]. Fat grafting is a safe procedure, with a recent systematic review reporting an overall complication rate of less than 5% [31]. The most commonly reported complications are infections, hematomas, and contour irregularities.

Technique:

- The areas of volume deficiency are marked preoperatively with the patient upright. Topographic markings are made according to the amount of volume deficiency.
- The donor sites are assessed. Most common donor sites are the lower abdomen and flanks. In young kids or thin individuals, the medial thighs or buttocks are used. Topographic markings are performed that identify harvest areas.
- Tumescent solution containing normal saline, lidocaine, and epinephrine is injected at the donor sites. The maximum amount of lidocaine that can be administered via tumescent solution is 35 mg/kg.
- Hand suction of fat is performed using a 3-mm (2.5-mm) blunt cannula connected to a 30-mL Luer-Lok syringe. Pulling back on the plunger generated negative pressure for suction. It is important to harvest from the wide area so as not to create a donor site contour deformity (Fig. 11.3).
- The suction cannula is taken off the syringe and replaced with a cap. The fat-filled syringe is placed vertically on a stand for 10 minutes. With gravity, injected fluid and blood separate at the bottom. This layer is removed by opening the plug. The fat is then placed in Telfa gauze, which absorbs the oil. This purified fat is loaded into 1 mL syringes.
- Access incisions of 2 mm are made depending on areas to be injected. Common locations are the oral commissure and the preauricular side burn.

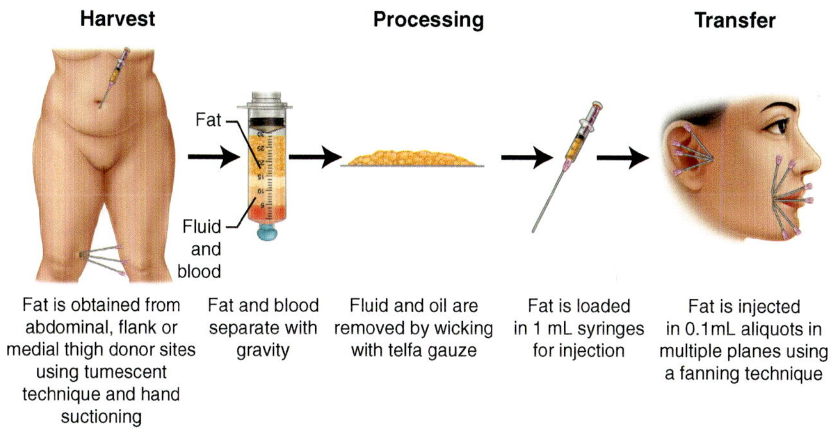

Fig. 11.3 The main steps in structural fat grafting

- The fat is injected with a 17-G one-hole Coleman cannula in very small aliquots. Approximately 0.1 mL are injected per pass as the cannula is withdrawn. A fanning technique is used to distribute the fat. Fat is deposited in multiple tissue planes, e.g., subdermal, subcutaneous, intramuscular, and supraperiosteal [35]. The goal is to achieve slight overcorrection.
- The injected areas should not be massaged post-operatively. Patients are advised to refrain from contact sports and strenuous activities for a few weeks so as to prevent trauma or migration of the fat.

Dermal Fat Grafting

The efficacy, safety, and versatility of structural fat grafting have relegated dermal fat grafting to a secondary role in facial volume augmentation. However, it is useful for targeted correction of contour abnormalities and mild volume augmentation [36]. Its drawbacks are unpredictable graft resorption and donor site scar.

When used for volume correction of the hemiface, the procedure is similar to a vascularized flap but without the microsurgical component. The areas of deficiency are marked, a template of the defect is made, and access to the face is obtained via a preauricular incision. The groin is the most common donor site, although any available site can be used. De-epithelialization is performed in situ, and the graft is harvested with a thin layer of fat. Inset is performed very precisely suturing to the underlying periosteum and deep fascia.

A useful application for dermal fat grafts is lip volume augmentation. Mobile areas such as lips have poor long-term retention of fat grafts [37]. Dermal fat grafting has been used successfully for correction of vermillion deficiencies [38]. Whether dermal fat grafting is more effective than fat injections in these areas is not known. However, it may allow more precise placement of fat.

Alloplastic Implants

Alloplasts allow precise correction of contour abnormality by augmenting the skeleton in localized areas of deficiency without any donor site morbidity. Furthermore, the result is predictable as there is no resorption as is seen with fat, bone, and cartilage grafts. Areas that are commonly corrected with implants are the malar areas [7], mandibular angle [39], chin [40], and temple [41] (Fig. 11.4). The implants are typically placed in the subperiosteal plane and secured to the facial skeleton with screws. Access can be obtained by standard extraoral or intraoral incisions. These procedures are performed after completion of skeletal growth.

Implant materials that have been used include silicone [7], porous polyethylene (PPE) [39, 42], ceramics [40], polyetheretherketone (PEEK) [43], expanded polytetrafluoroethylene (ePTFE) [41], and hydroxyapatite [44]. Each material has its benefits and drawbacks. The most common complications of alloplasts are infection, displacement, and extrusion.

Porous polyethylene (PPE) is a popular choice for skeletal augmentation. PPE has a porous structure which allows fibrovascular ingrowth allowing tissue incorporation, thus preventing implant migration and providing resistance to infections. PPE comes in different shapes and sizes, which can then be trimmed with a scalpel to the desired configuration. The implants can be screwed in place. Their ease of use, versatility, and good safety profile have made PPE one of the most popular choices for facial skeletal augmentation [45].

Hydroxyapatite cement can be used for augmenting localized areas of skeletal deficiency. The power is mixed with liquid to form a putty that can be placed over the bone at the area of deficiency and molded to the desired shape. Hardening occurs over a few minutes. Hydroxyapatite is osteoconductive, allowing ingrowth of bone

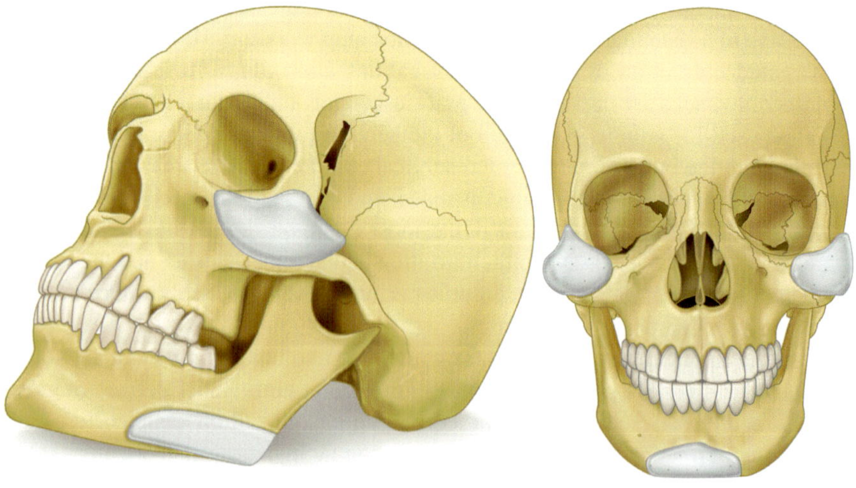

Fig. 11.4 Common areas of facial contour correction with alloplastic implants

and thus tissue integration. It is useful for augmenting localized areas of skeletal deficiency like the paranasal areas, malar area, mandibular angle, and forehead [44].

The most accurate method of skeletal contour correction is by custom-made implants created by virtual surgical planning [43]. A three-dimensional computer tomographic scan of the face is obtained which is used for computer-aided design (CAD) and computer-aided manufacturing (CAM) of custom implants [46]. The implant is thus of ideal size, shape, and volume for correcting the deformity. The biggest limitation to CAD-CAM at this time is high cost. As 3D printing and computer-assisted technology become cheaper and more widely available, custom implants will likely become the technique of choice for skeletal augmentation.

Facial Reanimation

Facial nerve palsies are present in 10–45% of patients with craniofacial microsomia [3, 47]. There is a wide spectrum of facial nerve involvement ranging from mild weakness to complete paralysis and involving a single branch to the entire facial nerve. The etiology is thought to be abnormal development of the temporal bone which houses the facial canal through which the facial nerve runs [47]. Multiple facial nerve abnormalities have been described, including anomalous course through the middle ear, posterior displacement, bifurcation, and complete absence [48]. Hypoplasia or absence of facial musculature may also occur [48, 49]. A meta-analysis by Kline et al. showed that partial nerve involvement (63%) is more common than paralysis of all branches of the facial nerve (37%) [48]. Of the partial involvement, paralysis of lower divisions is twice as common as that of the upper divisions. There has been shown to be a positive correlation between the degree of the facial nerve involvement and ear abnormalities [2]. The association with mandibular abnormalities is not as strong as that with the ear [48].

Facial asymmetry usually becomes evident soon after birth when the child cries. It is important to distinguish between traumatic and developmental facial palsies (Fig. 11.5) [50]. Traumatic facial palsy typically improves over time, while developmental does not. Evidence of birth trauma includes prolonged labor, use of forceps, bruising/marks over the mastoid, and hemotympanum. Facial asymmetry or dysmorphic features may indicate developmental facial palsy associated with craniofacial microsomia or a syndrome (Mobius, CHARGE, etc.).

Electrophysiologic studies can help determine the cause of facial palsy if the clinical picture is not clear. Electroneurography (ENoG) measures the compound muscle action potential of facial muscles. This test consists of transcutaneous stimulation of the facial nerve at the stylomastoid foramen and then recording the action potentials at various facial nerve branch locations [51]. Since it takes up to 48–72 hours for Wallerian degeneration to occur, ENoG is normal in traumatic facial palsy if performed during this time. In traumatic palsy, it can be repeated every 3–5 days to assess the degree of nerve degeneration which predicts prognosis for recovery. The study is not useful after 3 weeks, since by that time Wallerian

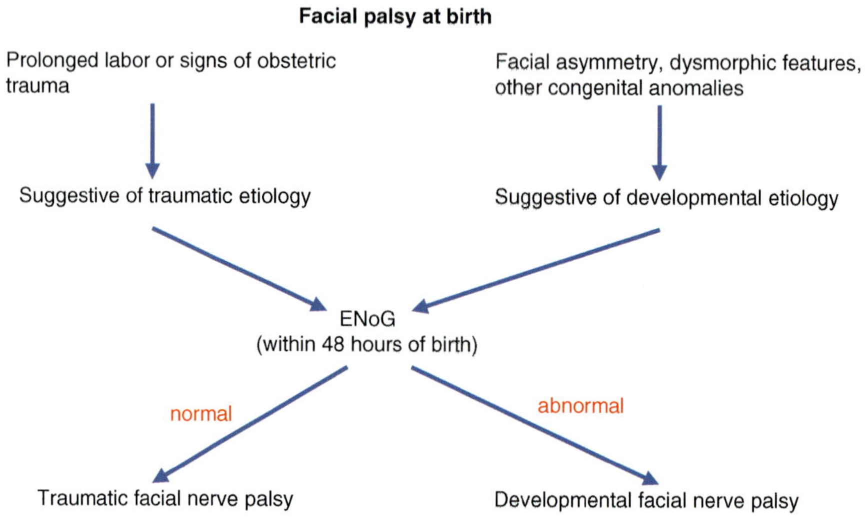

Fig. 11.5 Evaluation of congenital facial palsy

degeneration is complete. Electromyography (EMG) consists of direct stimulation of muscles with a surface electrode or needle to record their motor unit action potential (MUAP). The amplitude and duration of MUAPs are proportional to the number of innervated muscle fibers; decrease or absence of MUAPs indicates hypoplasia or absence of facial nerve or facial muscles. EMG is a useful test in traumatic palsy after 3 weeks of the insult. Fibrillation potentials indicate facial nerve degeneration, and polyphasic reinnervation potentials indicate facial nerve regeneration [52].

Hearing evaluation should be performed in all babies with facial nerve palsy and craniofacial microsomia, since ear abnormalities and hearing loss are associated with craniofacial microsomia. Auditory brainstem response (ABR) is used for screening of hearing loss. A computed tomographic scan of the temporal bones can assess for abnormalities of the facial canal and middle and inner ear.

Clinical assessment of facial nerve function is performed by facial nerve grading scales. The most commonly used instrument is the House-Brackmann scale (Table 11.4) [53]. Its popularity lies in the fact that it is simple and easy to use. Its major criticism is that it is very subjective and does not detect subtle changes after treatment [54]. The Sunnybrook scale is a more objective system that assigns points to different facial regions (Table 11.5). Assessments are made for resting symmetry, movement, and synkinesis. This scale has good inter- and intraobserver reliability and is more sensitive in measuring changes. These scales are not accurate in bilateral facial paralysis as there is no normal side for comparison.

The timing for surgical management should take into account functional and psychological development of the child. Periocular operations are usually not needed in infancy as adequate corneal protection can be achieved with non-surgical methods. We perform facial reanimation surgery at around 5 years of age, as younger

Table 11.4 House-Brackmann scale

Grade	Physical findings		
	Rest	*Movement*	*Synkinesis*
I. Normal	Symmetry	Normal	None
II. Mild dysfunction	Symmetry	Slight weakness	None
III. Moderate dysfunction	Symmetry	Obvious weakness	Obvious
IV. Moderately severe dysfunction	Symmetry	Disfiguring weakness	Disfiguring
V. Severe dysfunction	Possible asymmetry	Barely perceptible	Absent
VI. Total paralysis	Asymmetry	Absent	Absent

Table 11.5 Sunnybrook scale

Rest					
Eye	Normal Narrow Wide Eyelid surgery	0 1 1 1			
Cheek	Normal Absent Less pronounced More pronounced	0 2 1 1			
Mouth	Normal Corner drooped Corner pulled up/ out	0 1 1			
Movement					
	None	*Slight*	*Mid excursion*	*Almost complete*	*Complete*
Forehead wrinkle	1	2	3	4	5
Gentle eye closure	1	2	3	4	5
Open-mouth smile	1	2	3	4	5
Snarl	1	2	3	4	5
Lip pucker	1	2	3	4	5
Synkinesis					
	None	*Slight*	*Obvious*	*Disfiguring*	
Forehead wrinkle	0	1	2	3	
Gentle eye closure	0	1	2	3	
Open-mouth smile	0	1	2	3	
Snarl	0	1	2	3	
Lip pucker	0	1	2	3	

Total score (0–100) = (movement × 4) – (resting × 5) – synkinesis

children may not have sufficient length of sural nerve available for multiple nerve grafts. Cross-face nerve grafting is our treatment of choice for developmental facial paralysis as it restores spontaneous and synchronous facial movements.

Facial rehabilitation procedures can be static or dynamic. Static procedures improve facial symmetry at rest, while dynamic procedures recreate the function of the paralyzed muscles. Dynamic procedures are of two types: (1) reinnervation of native facial muscle via direct neurotization and (2) substitution of paretic muscles via regional or free muscle flaps. Direct muscle neurotization can augment the function of paretic muscles in incomplete facial palsy. A needle EMG can help determine viability of facial muscles. If EMG shows viable muscles (fibrillations, positive sharp waves), direct muscle neurotization can be performed. If after waiting for a suitable period of time (9–12 months), muscle reanimation does not occur or is insufficient, muscle substitution is performed to which this nerve is coapted. If the initial EMG shows electro silence, muscle substitution is performed.

For the purposes of facial paralysis management, the face can be divided into three: the upper face (periorbital region), midface (lip elevation), and lower face (lip depression).

Upper Face

Paralysis of the orbicularis oculi results in lagophthalmos (upper lid) and ectropion (lower lid). Incomplete eye closure causes corneal dryness which can lead to ulceration and eventual blindness. Corneal protection is therefore the top priority in management of facial paralysis. Epiphora occurs because of lid ectropion resulting in eversion of the lacrimal punctum, dysfunction of lacrimal pump due to orbicularis paralysis, and reflex increase in tear production because of corneal dryness.

All patients with facial paralysis should be evaluated by an ophthalmologist. The width of the palpebral fissures is compared between both eyes. The position of the upper and lower eyelids is assessed at rest and with blink. The marginal reflex distance (MRD 1, distance of corneal eye reflex to upper lid margin; MRD 2, distance of corneal eye reflex to lower lid margin) is measured and compared to the non-paralyzed eye. Bell's phenomenon (oculogyric reflex) is reflex vertical rotation of the globe on eye closure. Patients with absent Bell's reflex are at risk for exposure keratopathy, especially when they are in the supine position.

Patients are immediately started on a corneal protection regimen consisting of lubricating eye drops every 2–3 hours during daytime and corneal ointment at night. Eye patching and lid taping can be done at night. Tarsorrhaphy are rarely performed in children. They are short-term temporizing measures in patients who present with corneal ulceration, and there is concern about non-compliance with eyelid protection regimen. In infants, occlusion of the visual axis, even for a short period of time, leads to deprivation amblyopia which can result in permanent deterioration of vision.

Brow

Brow asymmetry typically does not manifest till adulthood. Brow asymmetry in young patients can be corrected with botulinum toxin injection to paralyze the normal side. Brow lift can be performed via endoscopic or direct excision techniques (Fig. 11.6).

Endoscopic Brow Lift

Endoscopic brow lift has the advantage of having small concealed scars in the hairline. It is useful if a small amount of elevation is needed.

Direct Brow Lift

Direct excision allows correction to a large degree with longer-lasting results. Excision can be performed just above the brow hairline (supraciliary lift), at the midbrow (midbrow lift), or at the hairline (coronal lift). We prefer the supraciliary lift for its predictability. The patient is marked preoperatively in the sitting position. The incision is made at the upper edge of the brow hairline. The amount of desired elevation at midbrow and at fixed points medially and laterally is marked. In the operating room, the marked ellipse of the skin is removed leaving the frontalis intact, thus preserving the supraorbital and supratrochlear nerves. The brow is then fixed into position by tacking its deep surface to the frontalis at four to five spots. The skin is then closed in layers. The scar usually heals very well as there is minimal stress on the incision due to absent frontalis muscle action.

Upper Eyelid

Lagophthalmos occurs due to paralysis of the orbicularis oculi and unopposed action of the levator palpebrae superioris and Muller's muscle. Passive techniques to correct lagophthalmos consist of active or passive counteraction of the upper lid elevators. Eye opening then entails an active effort of levator contraction.

Lid Loading

Upper eyelid loading by placement of weights counteracts the effect of the lid elevators, allowing the lid to close passively with gravity (Fig. 11.6). Gold is inert and malleable and has high density allowing a small volume of implant to be placed. Problems with gold weights are visibility, migration, capsule formation, infection, extrusion, entropion, and gold allergy. The long-term extrusion rate is approximately 10% [55].

Weights are most commonly placed in the pretarsal location. The appropriate weight is selected by taping the weight on the upper lid which results in adequate eye closure with minimal ptosis. Most commonly used weights are in the range of 0.6–1.4 g. An incision is made in the eyelid crease at the peak of the upper lid. The skin and orbicularis are elevated off the anterior surface of the tarsus, creating a pocket centered over the medial corneal limbus and staying at least 2 mm above the lid margin. The weight is secured in place with 60 silk sutures' partial thickness through the tarsus and then through the positioning holes of the weight. The superior hole is aligned with the superior tarsal border. The orbicularis and skin are closed in layers.

The weight can also be placed in the post-septal location. The orbital septum is opened, postseptal fat is retracted, and the implant is fixed to the levator aponeurosis just superior to the upper tarsal border. Another technique is to recess the levator off the tarsal plate and place the implant between the upper border of the tarsus and lower edge of the levator aponeurosis. The postseptal location decreases the risk of visibility, astigmatism, extrusion, and entropion. However, sizing is more difficult. and typically a heavier weight is required (0.2 g heavier on average), since this is a mechanically less favorable position [56]. This is also a useful technique in revision procedures for complications of pretarsal weights.

Platinum is denser than gold, and therefore platinum weights have a thinner profile. Platinum weights have shown to have a lower rate of extrusion [57]. Platinum chain implants contour better to the shape of the tarsus than platinum weights. This results in better cosmesis and less chance of corneal astigmatism. Multiple fixation holes also allow more points of fixation, thus potentially decreasing the risk of implant migration. Platinum segment chains are even more versatile as the individual segments can be added or removed if adjustments are needed [58].

Autologous conchal cartilage has also been used for lid loading [59]. It obviates the complications associated with synthetic materials. It is a less precise technique, and therefore correction may not be complete. However, it is a useful technique if gold or platinum weights are not available.

Palpebral Springs

Palpebral springs actively close the upper lid [60]. The central coil of the spring is fixed to the lateral orbital rim, the superior arm to the superior orbital rim, and the inferior arm to the tarsus (Fig. 11.6). Springs produce a brisker blink. However, they have a higher rate of extrusions than upper lid weights and need more frequent adjustments. They are also technically challenging procedures and thus have a steep learning curve. Their best indication is for motivated patients who desire a more dynamic blink and understand the need for revision procedures. Patients who do not have satisfactory corneal protection with eyelid weights (especially in supine position) may also be candidates for conversion to palpebral springs [61].

Levator Lengthening

Levator lengthening consists of recession of the levator aponeurosis and interposition of graft material (fascia or cartilage) between the tarsus and levator aponeurosis [62]. This lengthens and weakens the levator, thus decreasing the lagophthalmos. However, correction is usually not complete, and residual lagophthalmos remains. It is a useful technique in patients who have complications of eyelid weights or springs.

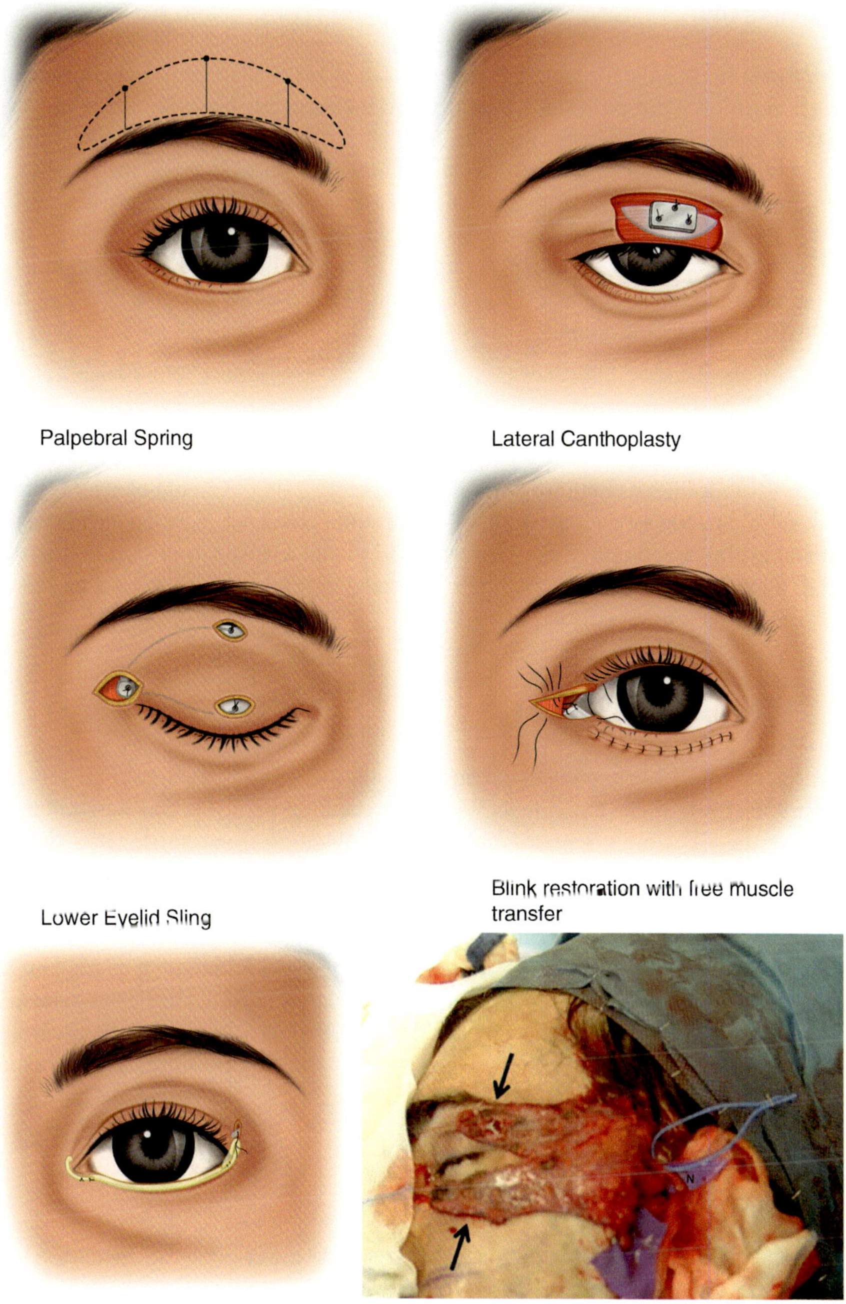

Fig. 11.6 Periorbital rehabilitation

Lower Eyelid

The lower lid is typically not affected in children because of good eyelid tone and cheek position. Ectropion starts laterally and then spreads medially over time. The normal position of the lower lid is at the level of the lower limbus of the cornea. Malposition of the lower lid leads to inadequate globe protection and inefficient tear film maintenance. The projection of the globe is a very important consideration in lower lid surgery; eyelid elevation procedures are more difficult in patients with proptotic eyes (negative vector). Treatment of the midface paralysis, via static or dynamic procedures, supports the lower lid and increases the effectiveness and longevity of lower lid elevation [63].

Lateral Canthopexy

Fixation of the lateral canthus is useful in correcting a small amount of scleral show. It is useful in younger patients with mild ectropion. However, it does not address the medial eyelid. Canthopexy can be performed via an anterior or posterior (transorbital) approach [64]. The transorbital canthopexy procedure can correct a more significant degree of lid laxity.

Lateral Canthoplasty

The lateral canthal strip procedure causes lid elevation and tightening (Fig. 11.6). It is very useful in older individuals with long-standing paralysis and horizontal lid laxity. A lateral canthotomy and inferior cantholysis are performed. The skin and mucosa are removed from the lateral edge of the tarsus. This lateral strip of tarsus is then sutured to the periosteum just inside the lateral orbital wall, thus creating a superoposterior vector of fixation of the lower lid. A slight overcorrection is achieved by fixing the canthal position a little higher. A sharp lateral canthal angle is created by approximating the grey lines. Orbicularis and skin are closed in layers. This procedure does not address medial lid, and therefore there may be recurrent eyelid droop over time. Furthermore, it may worsen the position of the medial canthus.

Lower Lid Cartilage Graft

A conchal cartilage graft can be placed between the lower border of the tarsus and the inferior orbital rim to better support the lower lid. A lateral tarsal strip procedure is also performed. The drawbacks of this technique are a visible bulge in the lower lid and risk of visual field restriction in downgaze.

Tendon Sling

Elevation of the entire lid can be effectively performed by a lower lid sling (Fig. 11.6). The palmaris longus tendon or a strip of fascia lata is used. The palmaris tendon is harvested from the non-dominant forearm. A subciliary tunnel is created from lateral to medial canthus, protecting the lacrimal system with a probe. The tendon graft is anchored at the medial canthal tendon. It is then tensioned in a superoposterior vector and fixed at the desired position at lateral orbital rim with a suture anchor, opposing the lid to the globe and producing a slight overcorrection of lid position.

Blink

Restoration of spontaneous blink is one of the most challenging undertakings in facial reanimation. Although it is difficult to obtain complete eye closure with dynamic techniques, a combination of dynamic with static techniques can result in full eye closure with excellent functional and aesthetic outcomes [65]. The addition of dynamic procedures has been shown to confer better corneal protection compared with static procedures alone [66].

The only way to achieve spontaneous blink is via cross-face nerve grafting from contralateral facial nerve branches responsible for eye closure. The best results are obtained via direct muscle neurotization of the orbicularis oculi [67]. Younger age at neurotization may result in better outcomes [67]. A needle EMG can be used to see if any viable muscles (fibrillations, positive sharp waves) are present. If there is evidence of muscle activity (incomplete facial palsy), cross-face nerve graft with direct muscle neurotization is performed. If there is insufficient return of orbicularis function after waiting for 9–12 months, muscle substitution with free muscle transfer is performed to which the cross face nerve grafts are connected. If there is no muscle activity on the initial EMG (complete facial palsy), a stage cross-face nerve graft is performed following 9–12 months later by muscle substitution (Fig. 11.6). Gracilis and platysma free muscle flaps can be used for muscle substitution [68]. Terzis has also described cross-face nerve graft neurotized to pedicled frontalis muscle [67].

The pectoralis minor muscle can be used for both lip elevation and blink restoration, as described by Terzis [69]. The multiple slips more closely mimic the muscles of facial expression. The uppermost slips have separate innervation (lateral pectoral nerve) from the remainder of the muscle (medial pectoral nerve) and thus can be neurotized separately to cross-face nerve grafts, thus providing independent blink function. This is however a technically challenging operation due to inconsistent neurovascular anatomy of the pectoralis minor muscle.

The pedicled temporalis muscle can be transferred for eye sphincter closure. This is a one-stage operation that obviates the need for microsurgery. However, the patient has to bite down to activate the muscle. Chewing produced eye movements, and aesthetically the eyes have a slit-like appearance. This is a good operation in elderly patients in whom nerve regeneration is not as robust and a multistage technique is not desired.

Midface

The majority of work in facial reanimation has focused on upper lip animation. Smile has been categorized into three patterns: the Mona Lisa smile (corners of mouth pulled up to show upper teeth), canine smile (levator labii superioris activated to show canines), and full denture smile (upper lip elevators and lower lip depressors simultaneously activated to show all the teeth) [70]. In children, static procedures are rarely performed as every attempt is made to perform dynamic smile reconstruction (Fig. 11.7). Children demonstrate better outcomes with dynamic procedures due to superior nerve regeneration and cortical plasticity.

Two-Stage Free Muscle Flap with Cross-Face Nerve Grafting

Spontaneous smile that is synchronous with the other side can be obtained by muscle substitution by a free muscle flap with neural input provided by contralateral facial buccal branches via cross-face nerve grafts (Fig. 11.7). Muscle flaps that have been used and described include gracilis, pectoralis minor, and latissimus dorsi [69, 71, 72]. The gracilis has emerged as the muscle of choice for the majority of surgeons due to its consistent neurovascular anatomy, ability to trim the muscle, low donor site morbidity, and location in the lower extremity permitting a two-team approach.

In the first stage, facial nerve dissection is performed on the normal side via a preauricular incision. The branches for lip elevation are stimulated, and the appropriate branch is chosen. If eye sphincter or lower lip animation is also planned, the appropriate facial nerve branches are stimulated and identified. Sural nerve grafts are then coapted to these nerve branches in an epineural manner. The nerve grafts are then tunneled to the contralateral side: the graft for lip elevation across the upper lip, lip depression across the lower lip, and periocular area across the forehead.

Regeneration of axons across the nerve graft is clinically documented by an advancing Tinel sign. When axonal growth across the graft is judged to be complete, a process that takes 6 to 12 months, the second stage is performed.

The nasolabial fold, oral commissure, and vector of smile are marked preoperatively. A two-team approach is used, one for facial preparation and the other for muscle flap harvest. A preauricular incision is made on the paralyzed side, and the

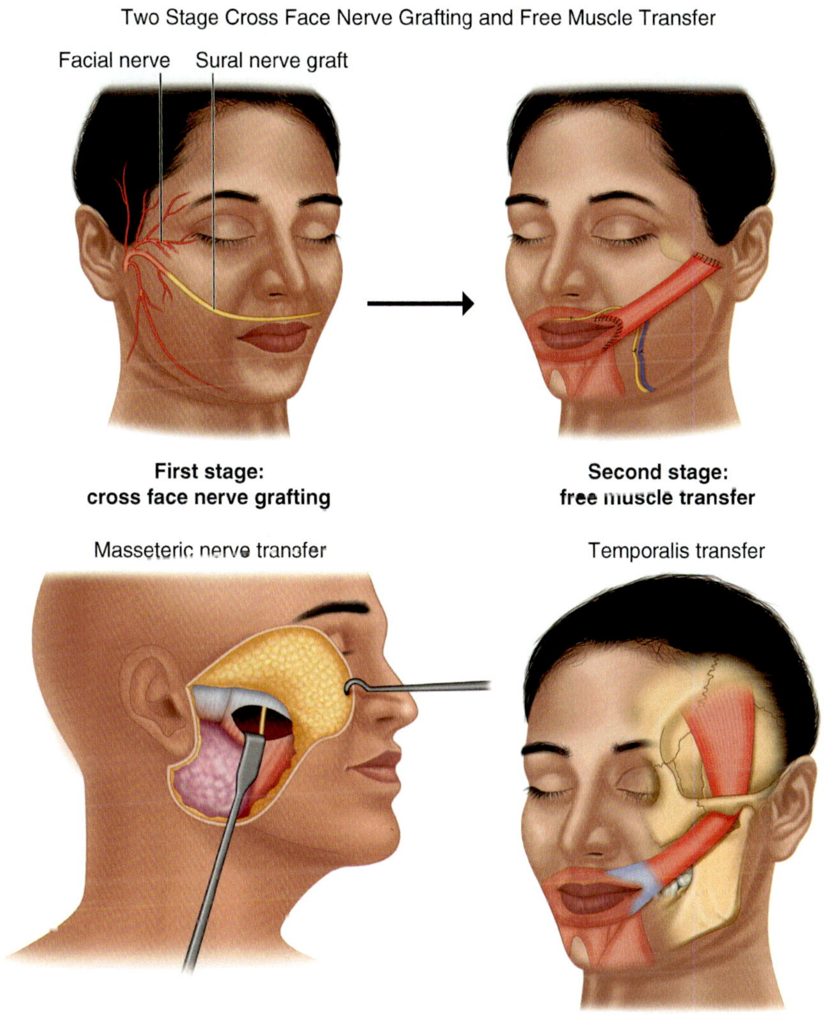

Fig. 11.7 Rehabilitation of lip elevation

dissection is carried out in a supra-SMAS plane. The end of the cross-face nerve graft can be biopsied to confirm viable axons. A segment of the gracilis muscle (usually 1/3 width) is harvested that shows powerful contraction on stimulation of the anterior obturator nerve. The muscle is first inset medially to the marked sites at the nasolabial fold and oral commissure. Microvascular and neural anastomoses are then completed. The lateral inset is performed to the temporal and parotid fascia, setting the appropriate tension so that the oral commissure is in a slightly overcorrected position.

Post-operatively, patients are referred for therapy, although this is difficult in children. Movement of the muscle is seen around 3 months. Revisions may be needed for debulking a thick flap or reinsetting a malpositioned flap. If eventual smile excursion is suboptimal, additional procedures like a mini-temporalis transfer can be performed for smile augmentation [73].

One-Stage Free Muscle Flap with Masseteric Nerve Transfer

An effective one-stage reconstruction can be achieved by free muscle flap to which the masseteric motor branch of the trigeminal nerve is coapted. The masseteric nerve provides more powerful neural input than a cross-face nerve graft. The masseteric nerve is located deep in the masseter at the area of the sigmoid notch, approximately 3 cm anterior to the tragus and 1 cm inferior to the zygomatic arch (Fig. 11.7) [74]. The fibers of the masseter are spread, and the nerve is located with the aid of a nerve stimulator. The descending branch is dissected for approximately 2 cm, transected, and then brought up for end-to-end coaptation to the motor nerve of the muscle flap. The procedure is useful if a single-stage operation is desired or if contralateral facial nerve donors are not available (bilateral facial palsy). Patients practice smiling by biting down. The age of surgery is thus an important consideration as patients need to able to participate in post-operative therapy. Studies have shown that in a significant proportion of patients, the smile eventually becomes spontaneous [75].

Dual innervation of a free muscle flap by both a cross-face nerve graft and masseteric nerve transfer has recently become popular [76]. The masseteric nerve provides more power as there are a larger number of axons, while the cross-face graft provides spontaneity. The goal is to enable faster muscle recovery with a spontaneous smile that is stronger and thus more symmetric with the contralateral side. A case example is illustrated in Fig. 11.8.

Temporalis Transfer

Local muscle transfers are infrequently performed in children as outcomes with free tissue transfer are superior. Their advantage is that they are a single-stage procedure that does not require microsurgical expertise. They may be useful if contralateral

Fig. 11.8 A case demonstrating dynamic smile reanimation. (**a**) A young girl with right-sided facial paralysis. (**b, c**) She underwent first-stage cross-face nerve grafting. Facial nerve branches were stimulated, and a suitable branch responsible for lip elevation was coapted to sural nerve graft in an end-to-end epineural manner. (**d**) A second-stage free gracilis muscle transfer was performed 9 months later. The red vessel loop is encircling the medial circumflex vessels, and the blue vessel loop is encircling the obturator nerve. (**e**) the masseteric branch of CN V is dissected out for dual innervation to the gracilis muscle. (**f**) The gracilis flap has been inset in place. Microvascular anastomosis was performed to the facial vessels and neural coaptation to cross-face nerve graft and the masseteric branch of CN V. (**g**) Post-operative smile excursion. (Case courtesy of Arun Gosain MD, FACS. Photos by Paul Berg, Lurie Children's Hospital)

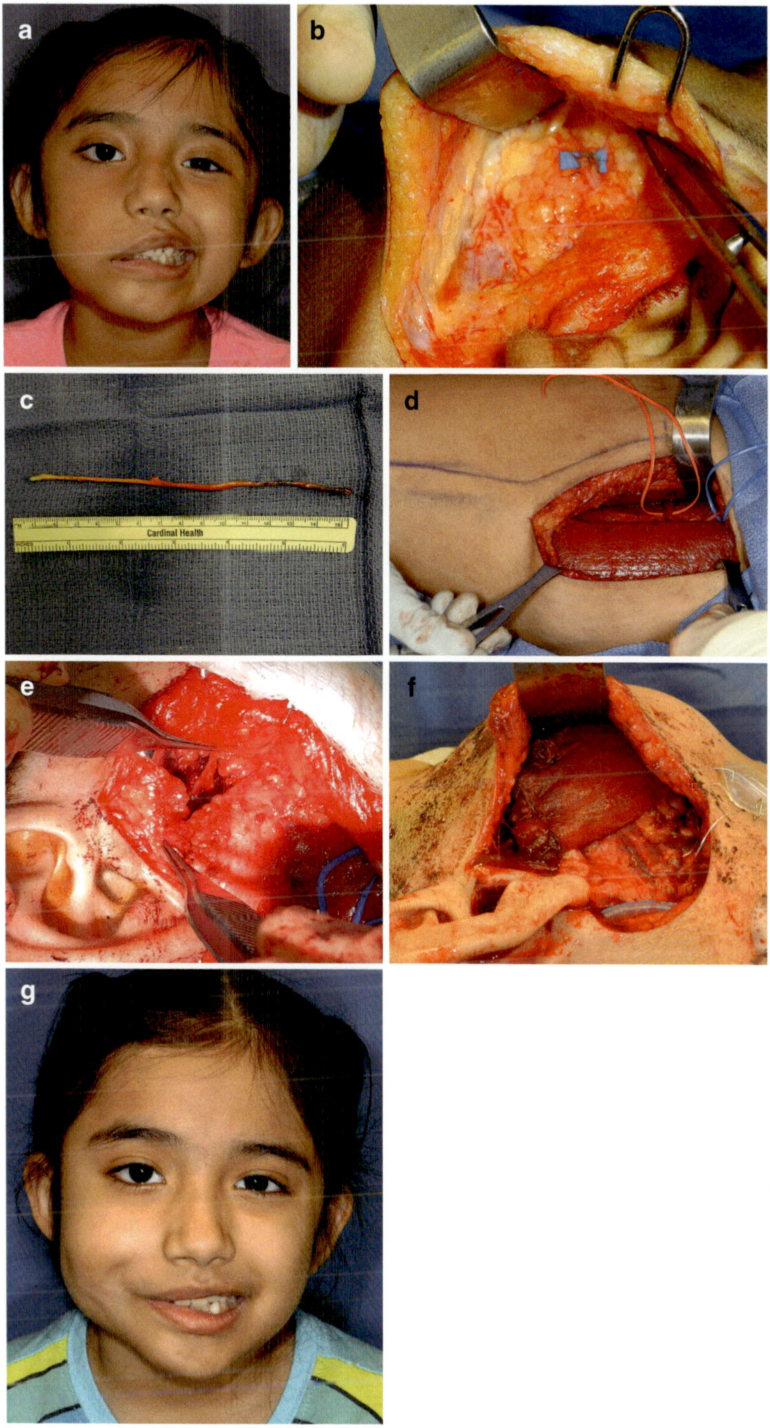
a
b
c
Cardinal Health
d
e
f
g

facial nerve donor is not available, e.g., in bilateral paralysis or to improve smile excursion if outcome of previous free tissue transfer has not been satisfactory [73]. Labbe demonstrated good functional outcomes of lengthening temporalis myoplasty in children with the attainment of spontaneous smile (Fig. 11.7) [77]. Patients need to train to smile by activating the temporalis muscle and thus need to be old enough to participate in post-procedure therapy.

Lower Face

Isolated lip depressor paresis is one of the most common phenotypes of facial paralysis in craniofacial microsomia. Paralysis of lip depressors precludes a full-denture smile and causes asymmetry on lip animation. Techniques that attempt to create lower lip symmetry are of two types: procedures that paralyze the contralateral normal lip and those that animate the paralyzed ipsilateral lower lip.

Contralateral Lip Paralysis

Lip symmetry can be achieved by paralyzing the depressors of the normal lip. Paralysis can be obtained by botulinum toxin injection into the depressor complex. Fifteen units are injected in the depressor muscles, staying 1 cm below the vermillion border to avoid the orbicularis. The injections need to be repeated every 4 to 6 months. If patients are happy with the aesthetic and functional outcome and desire permanent paralysis, depressor myomectomy or marginal mandibular neurectomy can be performed [78, 79]. These procedures are technically simple with minimal additionally donor site morbidity. However, they result in lip closure weakening which may impair oral continence. Furthermore, they are permanent and preclude future dynamic procedures.

Ipsilateral Lip Depression

Fascial Slings

A “semi-dynamic” method of reconstruction was described by Watanabe et al. (Fig. 11.9) [80]. A fascia lata graft is placed along the length of the paralyzed lip, extending a bit to the normal side. A second fascia graft is placed from the midpoint of the lip graft to the lower mandibular border. This maintains the distance of the lower lip from the mandibular border, thus maintaining a symmetric lip position on animation. This technique is also useful for upgrading an unsatisfactory result of a dynamic lower lip animation procedure.

Digastric Muscle Transfer

The digastric muscle may be absent in up to 40% of patients with craniofacial microsomia and up to 55% patients with marginal mandibular nerve palsy [81]. Imaging, such as ultrasound, can be useful to evaluate for the presence of muscle. The anterior belly of digastric is supplied by the facial artery and the mylohyoid branch of the trigeminal nerve. After division of the posterior belly, the anterior belly and intermediate tendon are transferred to the lower lip via a subcutaneous tunnel (Fig. 11.9). The neurovascular bundle, which lies posterior to the muscle, is carefully preserved. The tendon is longitudinally split into four strips and sutured to the lower lip orbicularis, via an incision just posterior to the junction of wet and dry vermillion. The mandibular origin of the muscle may be transected and reinset to create a vector of pull that matches the contralateral side. This operation restrains the lower lip down, thus resulting in more symmetric lip animation [82]. Active lip depression that is synchronous with the contralateral side can be obtained by coapting a cross-face nerve graft to the motor nerve of the transferred digastric muscle.

Cross-Face Nerve Grafting

Synchronous lower lip movements can be achieved with cross-face nerve grafting from the contralateral marginal mandibular nerve branches. If there is partial facial nerve palsy, as indicated by clinical examination and needle EMG, direct depressor muscle neurotization of the cross-face nerve graft may be performed. If after 9 to 12 months, restoration of lip depression is unsatisfactory, muscle substitution can be performed to which the cross-face nerve graft is coapted. If there is complete depressor palsy with no evidence of muscle viability on EMG, a two-stage procedure of cross-face nerve grafting followed by muscle substitution is performed.

The muscles most commonly used for lower lip depressor substitution are the anterior belly of digastric and the platysma. The platysma may be absent in craniofacial microsomia, and therefore imaging should be performed to conform its presence [83]. The platysma is supplied by the facial artery and cervical branch of the facial nerve. The lateral 2/3 of the muscle can be harvested carefully protecting its neurovascular pedicle, tunneled to the lower lip, and sutured to lower lip via several slips. The cross-face nerve graft is neurotized to the cervical branch of the facial nerve. If the digastric and platysma are absent or not available, a free muscle flap, e.g., gracilis, can be coapted to the cross-face nerve graft (Fig. 11.9).

Mini-hypoglossal Nerve Transfer

The mini-hypoglossal nerve transfer to the facial nerve was described by Terzis as a "baby sitter" operation to maintain viability of the facial muscles while waiting for a cross-face nerve graft to regenerate [84]. In incomplete lower lip

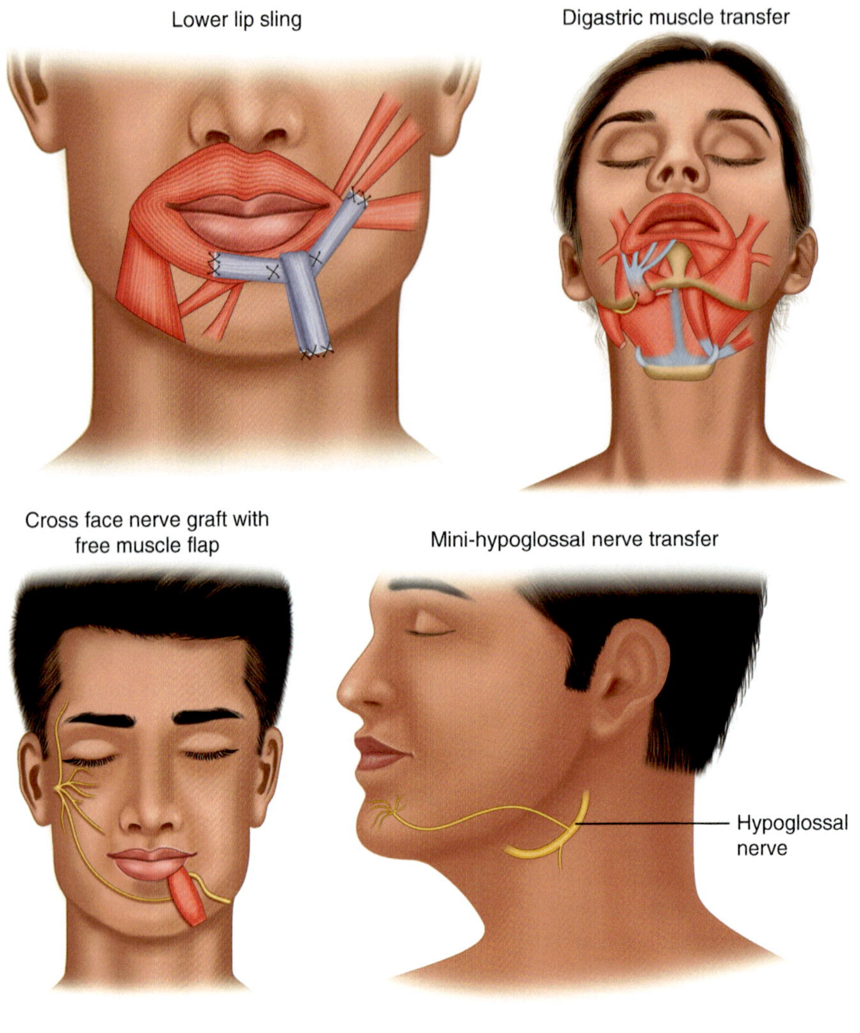

Fig. 11.9 Rehabilitation of lip depression

palsy, the function of lower lip depressors can be upgraded by direct depressor muscle neurotization from the hypoglossal nerve with a nerve graft (Fig. 11.9) [85]. The hypoglossal nerve can also provide neural input to muscle flaps in patients with bilateral paralysis where facial nerve donors are not present. Patients are trained to activate the nerve by pushing the tongue against the teeth. In young children, spontaneous lip depression usually develops because of cortical plasticity [85].

References

1. Tessier P. Anatomical classification facial, cranio-facial and latero-facial clefts. J Maxillofac Surg. 1976;4(2):69–92.
2. Tuin AJ, Tahiri Y, Paine KM, Paliga JT, Taylor JA, Bartlett SP. Clarifying the relationships among the different features of the OMENS+ classification in craniofacial microsomia. Plast Reconstr Surg. 2015;135(1):149e–56e.
3. Vento AR, LaBrie RA, Mulliken JB. The O.M.E.N.S. classification ofhemifacial microsomia. Cleft Palate Craniofac J. 1991;28(1):68–76; discussion 77
4. David DJ, Mahatumarat C, Cooter RD. Hemifaciall microsomia: a multisystem classification. Plast Reconstr Surg. 1987;80(4):525–35.
5. Horgan JE, Padwa BL, LaBrie RA, Mulliken JB. OMENS-plus: analysis of craniofacial and extracraniofacial anomalies in hemifacial microsomia. Cleft Palate Craniofac J. 1995;32(5):405–12.
6. Brandstetter KA, Patel KG. Craniofacial microsomia. Facial Plast Surg Clin North Am. 2016;24(4):495–515.
7. Upton J, Albin RE, Mulliken JB, Murray JE. The use of scapular and parascapular flaps for cheek reconstruction. Plast Reconstr Surg. 1992;90(6):959–71.
8. Siebert JW, Anson G, Longaker MT. Microsurgical correction of facial asymmetry in 60 consecutive cases. Plast Reconstr Surg. 1996;97(2):354–63.
9. Sinclair N, Gharb BB, Papay F, Rampazzo A. Soft tissue reconstruction in patients with hemifacial microsomia: a systematic review of the literature. J Craniofac Surg. 2019;30(3):879–87.
10. Siebert JW, Longaker MT, Angrigiani C. The inframammary extended circumflex scapular flap: an aesthetic improvement of the parascapular flap. Plast Reconstr Surg. 1997;99(1):70–7.
11. Longaker MT, Siebert JW. Microsurgical correction of facial contour in congenital craniofacial malformations: the marriage of hard and soft tissue. Plast Reconstr Surg. 1996;98(6):942–50.
12. Warren SM, Borud LJ, Brecht LE, Longaker MT, Siebert JW. Microvascular reconstruction of the pediatric mandible. Plast Reconstr Surg. 2007;119(2):649–61.
13. Inigo F, Jimenez-Murat Y, Arroyo O, Fernandez M, Ysunza A. Restoration of facial contour in Romberg's disease and hemifacialmicrosomia: experience with 118 cases. Microsurgery. 2000;20(4):167–72.
14. de la Fuente A, Jimenez A. Latissimus dorsi free flap for restoration of facial contour defects. Ann Plast Surg. 1989;22(1):1–8.
15. Kim EJ, Lee KT, Lim SY, et al. Reconstructing facial contour deformities using stereoscopic thoracodorsal artery perforator adipofascial flaps. Microsurgery. 2017;37(4):300–6.
16. Poole MD. A composite flap for early treatment of hemifacial microsomia. Br J Plast Surg. 1989;42(2):163–72.
17. Koshima I. Short pedicle superficial inferior epigastric artery adiposal flap: new anatomical findings and the use of this flap for reconstruction of facial contour. Plast Reconstr Surg. 2005;116(4):1091–7.
18. Fisher J, Jackson IT. Microvascular surgery as an adjunct to craniomaxillofacial reconstruction. Br J Plast Surg. 1989;42(2):146–54.
19. Koshima I, Inagawa K, Urushibara K, Ohtsuki M, Moriguchi T. Deep inferior epigastric perforator dermal-fat or adiposal flap for correction of craniofacial contour deformities. Plast Reconstr Surg. 2000;106(1):10–5.
20. Abdullaev KF, Orlova EV, Yadav MK, Vasilyev EA, Mokhirev MA, Gileva KS. Preoperative planning for advanced modelling of anterolateral thigh flaps in the treatment of severe haemifacial atrophy in Parry-Romberg and Goldenhar syndrome. JPRAS Open. 2018;16:36–49.
21. La Rossa D, Whitaker L, Dabb R, Mellissinos E. The use of microvascular free flaps for soft tissue augmentation of the face in children with hemifacial microsomia. Cleft Palate J. 1980;17(2):138–43.

22. Jurkiewicz MJ, Nahai F. The omentum: its use as a free vascularized graft for reconstruction of the head and neck. Ann Surg. 1982;195(6):756–65.
23. Haddock NT, Saadeh PB, Siebert JW. Achieving aesthetic results in facial reconstructive microsurgery: planning and executing secondary refinements. Plast Reconstr Surg. 2012;130(6):1236–45.
24. Hemmer KM, Marsh JL, Clement RW. Pediatric facial free flaps. J Reconstr Microsurg. 1987;3(3):221–9. 231
25. Venkatesh V, Fracol M, Turin S, Ellis M, Alghoul M. Utilization of intraparotid segments of superficial temporal vessels for head and scalp free flap microanastomosis: a clinical, histological, and cadaveric study. J Reconstr Microsurg. 2020;36(4):253–60.
26. Huntsman WT, Lineaweaver W, Ousterhout DK, Buncke HJ, Alpert BS. Recipient vessels for microvascular transplants in patients with hemifacial microsomia. J Craniofac Surg. 1992;3(4):187–9.
27. Spector JA, Warren SM, Singh SP, McCarthy JG, Siebert JW. Marriage of hard and soft tissues of the face revisited: when distraction meets microsurgery. Ann Plast Surg. 2007;59(1):1–5; discussion 5
28. Tan O, Atik B, Parmaksizoglu D. Soft-tissue augmentation of the middle and lower face using the deepithelialized submental flap. Plast Reconstr Surg. 2007;119(3):873–9.
29. Zhang Y, Jin R, Shi Y, Sun B, Zhang Y, Qian Y. Pedicled superficial temporal fascia sandwich flap for reconstruction of severe facial depression. J Craniofac Surg. 2009;20(2):505–8.
30. Choung PH, Nam IW, Kim KS. Vascularized cranial bone grafts for mandibular and maxillary reconstruction. The parietal osteofascial flap. J Craniomaxillofac Surg. 1991;19(6):235–42.
31. Krastev TK, Beugels J, Hommes J, Piatkowski A, Mathijssen I, van der Hulst R. Efficacy and safety of autologous fat transfer in facial reconstructive surgery: a systematic review and meta-analysis. JAMA Facial Plast Surg. 2018;20(5):351–60.
32. Tanikawa DY, Aguena M, Bueno DF, Passos-Bueno MR, Alonso N. Fat grafts supplemented with adipose-derived stromal cells in the rehabilitation of patients with craniofacial microsomia. Plast Reconstr Surg. 2013;132(1):141–52.
33. Denadai R, Raposo-Amaral CA, Buzzo CL, Raposo-Amaral CE. Isolated fat grafting for reconstruction of lower face volumetric asymmetry in skeletally immature patients: a clinical outcome study. Ann Plast Surg. 2019;83(5):529–37.
34. Rajan S, Ajayakumar K, Sasidharanpillai S, George B. Autologous fat graft for soft tissue camouflage in craniofacial microsomia. J Cutan Aesthet Surg. 2019;12(4):223–6.
35. Coleman SR. Structural fat grafting: more than a permanent filler. Plast Reconstr Surg. 2006;118(3 Suppl):108S–20S.
36. Abduch LSF, Rocha PBD, Nasser IJG, Ono MCC, Freitas RDS. Dermal-fat graft for facial contouring in patients with craniofacial Microsomia. J Craniofac Surg. 2019;30(7):2134–7.
37. Eremia S, Newman N. Long-term follow-up after autologous fat grafting: analysis of results from 116 patients followed at least 12 months after receiving the last of a minimum of two treatments. Dermatol Surg. 2000;26(12):1150–8.
38. Staebel C, Verheyden CN. The use of dermal fat grafts for the correction of secondary cleft lip deformities. Plast Reconstr Surg. 2009;123(4):151e–2e.
39. Masden D, Baker S. A novel approach for correcting mandibular asymmetry with a combination of autologous fat and alloplastic implants. Aesthet Surg J. 2010;30(4):513–5.
40. Duskova M, Kozak JI, Mazanek JI, Smahel ZK, Vohradnik M. Bioceramics as an option in correction of facial skeleton deformities. J Craniofac Surg. 2000;11(5):470–9.
41. Liu X, Zhang Y, Wang S, Lei Z, Li X, Fan D. The use of expanded polytetrafluoroethylene in depressed deformities of the face. Exp Ther Med. 2016;12(5):3151–4.
42. Andrade NN, Raikwar K. Medpor in maxillofacial deformities: report of three cases. J Maxillofac Oral Surg. 2009;8(2):192–5.
43. Day KM, Gabrick KS, Sargent LA. Applications of computer technology in complex craniofacial reconstruction. Plast Reconstr Surg Glob Open. 2018;6(3):e1655.
44. Lee DW, Kim JY, Lew DH. Use of rapidly hardening hydroxyapatite cement for facial contouring surgery. J Craniofac Surg. 2010;21(4):1084–8.

45. Rai A, Datarkar A, Arora A, Adwani DG. Utility of high density porous polyethylene implants in maxillofacial surgery. J Maxillofac Oral Surg. 2014;13(1):42–6.
46. Staal F, Pluijmers B, Wolvius E, Koudstaal M. Patient-specific implant for residual facial asymmetry following orthognathic surgery in unilateral craniofacial microsomia. Craniomaxillofac Trauma Reconstr. 2016;9(3):264–7.
47. Gorlin RJ, Cohen M, Levin LS. Syndromes of the head and neck. 3rd ed. New York: Oxford University Press; 1990.
48. Cline JM, Hicks KE, Patel KG. Characterization of facial paresis in hemifacial microsomia. Otolaryngol Head Neck Surg. 2014;150(2):188–93.
49. Nada Y, Sasaki K, Nozaki M, Soejima K. Congenital partial absence of the facial muscles. Br J Plast Surg. 1998;51(2):138–41.
50. Terzis JK, Anesti K. Developmental facial paralysis: a review. J Plast Reconstr Aesthet Surg. 2011;64(10):1318–33.
51. Lee DH. Clinical efficacy of electroneurography in acute facial paralysis. J Audiol Otol. 2016;20(1):8–12.
52. Guntinas-Lichius O, Volk GF, Olsen KD, et al. Facial nerve electrodiagnostics for patients with facial palsy: a clinical practice guideline. Eur Arch Otorhinolaryngol. 2020;277(7):1855–74.
53. House JW, Brackmann DE. Facial nerve grading system. Otolaryngol Head Neck Surg. 1985;93(2):146–7.
54. Fattah AY, Gurusinghe AD, Gavilan J, et al. Facial nerve grading instruments: systematic review of the literature and suggestion for uniformity. Plast Reconstr Surg. 2015;135(2):569–79.
55. Rofagha S, Seiff SR. Long-term results for the use of gold eyelid load weights in the management of facial paralysis. Plast Reconstr Surg. 2010;125(1):142–9.
56. Rozen S, Lehrman C. Upper eyelid postseptal weight placement for treatment of paralytic lagophthalmos. Plast Reconstr Surg. 2013;131(6):1253–65.
57. Silver AL, Lindsay RW, Cheney ML, Hadlock TA. Thin-profile platinum eyelid weighting: a superior option in the paralyzed eye. Plast Reconstr Surg. 2009;123(6):1697–703.
58. Malhotra R, Ziahosseini K, Poitelea C, Litwin A, Sagili S. Platinum segments: a new platinum chain for adjustable upper eyelid loading. Br J Ophthalmol. 2015;99(12):1680–5.
59. Abenavoli FM, De Gregorio A, Corelli R. Upper eye lid loading with autologous cartilage in paralytic lagophthalmos. Plast Reconstr Surg. 2006;117(7):2511–2.
60. Morel-Fatio D, Lalardrie JP. Palliative surgical treatment of facial paralysis. The Palpebral Spring. Plast Reconstr Surg. 1964;33:446–56.
61. Salloum G, Carruth BP, Hill RH 3rd, Czyz CN, Bersani TA. Transitioning from a gold weight to an "enhanced" palpebral spring in the management of paralytic lagophthalmos secondary to facial nerve palsy. Orbit. 2019;38(2):119–23.
62. Hayashi A, Yoshizawa H, Natori Y, Senda D, Tanaka R, Mizuno H. Levator lengthening technique using cartilage or fascia graft for paralytic lagophthalmos in facial paralysis. J Plast Reconstr Aesthet Surg. 2016;69(5):679–86.
63. Lisman RD, Smith B, Baker D, Arthurs B. Efficacy of surgical treatment for paralytic ectropion. Ophthalmology. 1987;94(6):671–81.
64. Moe KS, Linder T. The lateral transorbital canthopexy for correction and prevention of ectropion: report of a procedure, grading system, and outcome study. Arch Facial Plast Surg. 2000;2(1):9–15.
65. Terzis JK, Bruno W. Outcomes with eye reanimation microsurgery. Facial Plast Surg. 2002;18(2):101–12.
66. Mohanty AJ, Perez JL, Hembd A, Thrikutam NP, Bartley J, Rozen SM. Orbicularis oculi muscle reinnervation confers corneal protective advantages over static interventions alone in the subacute facial palsy patient. Plast Reconstr Surg. 2020;145(3):791–801.
67. Terzis JK, Karypidis D. The outcomes of dynamic procedures for blink restoration in pediatric facial paralysis. Plast Reconstr Surg. 2010;125(2):629–44.
68. Guelinckx PJ. Blink restoration in long-standing facial paralysis: use of free neurovascular platysma transfer. Plast Reconstr Surg Glob Open. 2018;6(10):e1939.

69. Terzis JK. Pectoralis minor: a unique muscle for correction of facial palsy. Plast Reconstr Surg. 1989;83(5):767–76.
70. Rubin LR. The anatomy of a smile: its importance in the treatment of facial paralysis. Plast Reconstr Surg. 1974;53(4):384–7.
71. Takushima A, Harii K, Asato H, Yamada A. Neurovascular free-muscle transfer to treat facial paralysis associated with hemifacial microsomia. Plast Reconstr Surg. 2002;109(4):1219–27.
72. Sharma PR, Zuker RM, Borschel GH. Gracilis free muscle transfer in the treatment of pediatric facial paralysis. Facial Plast Surg. 2016;32(2):199–208.
73. Terzis JK, Olivares FS. Use of mini-temporalis transposition to improve free muscle outcomes for smile. Plast Reconstr Surg. 2008;122(6):1723–32.
74. Mundschenk MB, Sachanandani NS, Borschel GH, Zuker RM, Snyder-Warwick AK. Motor nerve to the masseter: a pediatric anatomic study and the "3:1 rule". J Plast Reconstr Aesthet Surg. 2018;71(1):54–6.
75. Manktelow RT, Tomat LR, Zuker RM, Chang M. Smile reconstruction in adults with free muscle transfer innervated by the masseter motor nerve: effectiveness and cerebral adaptation. Plast Reconstr Surg. 2006;118(4):885–99.
76. Boonipat T, Robertson CE, Meaike JD, Vyas KS, Asaad M, Mardini S. Dual innervation of free gracilis muscle for facial reanimation: what we know so far. J Plast Reconstr Aesthet Surg. 2020;
77. Veyssiere A, Labbe D, Benateau H. Lengthening temporalis myoplasty and facial paralysis from birth. J Plast Reconstr Aesthet Surg. 2015;68(3):312–20.
78. Hussain G, Manktelow RT, Tomat LR. Depressor labii inferioris resection: an effective treatment for marginal mandibular nerve paralysis. Br J Plast Surg. 2004;57(6):502–10.
79. Breslow GD, Cabiling D, Kanchwala S, Bartlett SP. Selective marginal mandibular neurectomy for treatment of the marginal mandibular lip deformity in patients with chronic unilateral facial palsies. Plast Reconstr Surg. 2005;116(5):1223–32.
80. Watanabe Y, Sasaki R, Agawa K, Akizuki T. Bidirectional/double fascia grafting for simple and semi-dynamic reconstruction of lower lip deformity in facial paralysis. J Plast Reconstr Aesthet Surg. 2015;68(3):321–8.
81. MacQuillan A, Biarda FU, Grobbelaar A. The incidence of anterior belly of digastric agenesis in patients with hemifacial microsomia. Plast Reconstr Surg. 2010;126(4):1285–90.
82. Conley J, Baker DC, Selfe RW. Paralysis of the mandibular branch of the facial nerve. Plast Reconstr Surg. 1982;70(5):569–77.
83. MacQuillan A, Vesely M, Harrison D, Grobbelaar A. Reanimation options in patients with hemifacial microsomia and marginal mandibular nerve palsy. Plast Reconstr Surg. 2003;112(7):1962–3.
84. Terzis JK, Tzafetta K. "babysitter" procedure with concomitant muscle transfer in facial paralysis. Plast Reconstr Surg. 2009;124(4):1142–56.
85. Terzis JK, Tzafetta K. Outcomes of mini-hypoglossal nerve transfer and direct muscle neurotization for restoration of lower lip function in facial palsy. Plast Reconstr Surg. 2009;124(6):1891–904.

Chapter 12
An Overview of Treatment and Recommendations for the Craniofacial Microsomia Patient

Michael Miloro, Alexis Olsson, and Michael R. Markiewicz

Introduction

Craniofacial microsomia (CFM), also known as hemifacial microsomia, described by Gorlin and Pindborg in 1964, has been called oculoauriculovertebral syndrome due to the affected areas of clinical involvement [1, 2] (Figs. 12.1 and 12.2). This entity has been referred to as one of the first and second branchial arch syndromes due to involvement of the derivatives of these branchial arches. The first, or mandibular, branchial arch gives rise to the muscles of mastication; stylohyoid, anterior belly of the digastric, tensor tympani, and tensor veli palatini muscles; and the malleus, incus, and Meckel's cartilage, as well as the third division of the trigeminal nerve (V3). The second, or hyoid, branchial arch provides the muscles of facial expression, stapedius, stylohyoid, and posterior belly of the digastric muscle, as well as the stapes, styloid cartilage, lesser cornu of the hyoid bone, and Reichert's cartilage, and the facial (VII) nerve. From an epidemiologic standpoint, CFM occurs in 1:5000 live births (range: 1:3500–1:5600) making it the second most common facial anomaly after cleft lip and palate [3].

M. Miloro (✉)
Department of Oral and Maxillofacial Surgery, University of Illinois, Chicago, IL, USA
e-mail: mmiloro@uic.edu

A. Olsson
Oral and Maxillofacial Surgery, Northwestern University Feinberg School of Medicine, Northwestern Memorial Hospital, Chicago, IL, USA
e-mail: aolsson@nm.org

M. R. Markiewicz
Department of Oral and Maxillofacial Surgery, University at Buffalo, Buffalo, NY, USA
e-mail: mrm25@buffalo.edu

D. M. Yates, M. R. Markiewicz (eds.), *Craniofacial Microsomia and Treacher Collins Syndrome*, https://doi.org/10.1007/978-3-030-84733-3_12

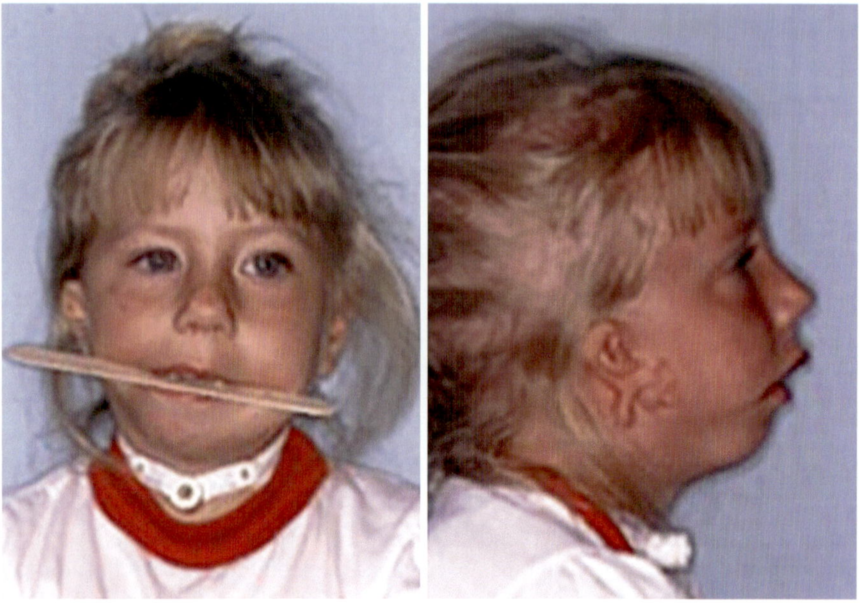

Fig. 12.1 Child with right craniofacial microsomia Type III showing an occlusal cant, orbital dystopia, and airway issues (left image). Also, macrostomia and a deformed and low-set ear on the affected side (right image)

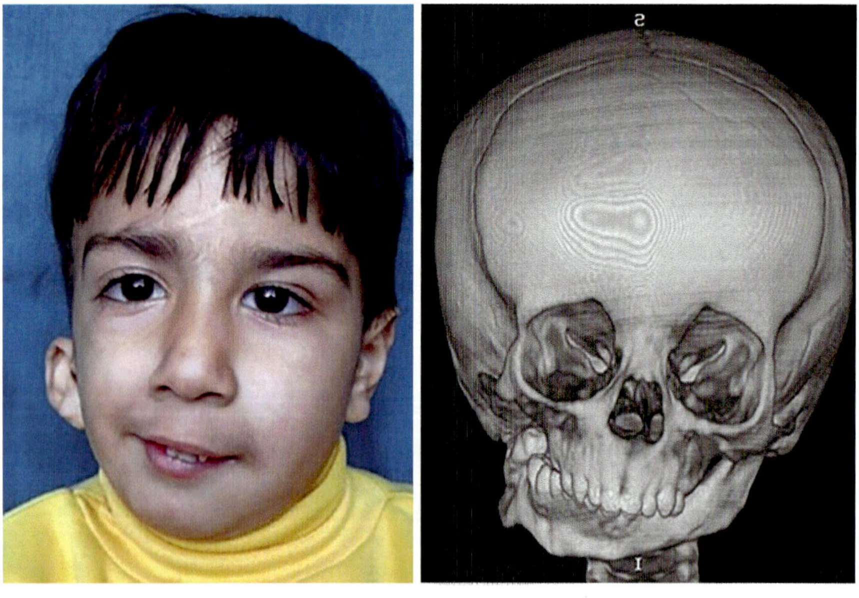

Fig. 12.2 Child with right craniofacial microsomia Type IIB showing an occlusal cant, low-set ear, orbital dystopia, and macrostomia (left image). 3D CT scan showing the skeletal features of CFM in including mandibular deviation, hypoplasia of the right ramus and condyle with medial rotation, zygomatic arch, and orbital asymmetry (right image)

Etiology and Pathogenesis

While the precise etiology is unknown, involvement of any mechanism that may interfere with the development of the first and second branchial arches during the first 4–6 weeks gestation is considered a possible causative factor in the pathogenesis of CFM, resulting in unilateral hypoplasia or underdevelopment of the facial skeleton and associated soft tissues. CFM occurs in 1:3000–1:5000 live births. There is a sporadic inheritance pattern, although reports of successive generation genetic inheritance exist as well [4]. A male predilection exists (male-female = 3:2), and the right side is more commonly involved than the left side (ratio 3:2) [5]. Risk factors for CFM include low socioeconomic status and delayed recognition of pregnancy (> 9 weeks) [4, 5]. Since the exact etiology of CFM is not known, various theories have been proposed. In 1973, Poswillo proposed that CFM was vascular in origin (sheep study) resulting from a focal in utero expanding hematoma of the stapedial artery that supplies first and second branchial arch development on, or about, day 33 of gestation. Another support for this theory includes an increase in CFM that has been shown to occur in children of mothers who used vasoactive medications (pseudoephedrine), especially with smoking (1–10 cigarettes/day), in the first trimester and had a 4.2 times higher risk [4, 6]. The exact size of the hematoma or magnitude of vasoconstriction and resultant tissue involvement may explain the variable clinical presentation of CFM. Other theories involve neural crest cell deficiencies with presumed failure of migration to the first and second branchial arches and decreased levels of vascular endothelial growth factor (VEGF) that promote the growth of Meckel's cartilage [3]. Animal studies have shown that the introduction of retinoic acid during early pregnancy results in neural crest cell death, with offspring that are phenotypically very similar to CFM. The etiology is most likely multifactorial and heterogeneous and includes maternal conditions such as diabetes mellitus, maternal teratogens such as thalidomide and retinoic acid, intrauterine fetal compression, and over-ripeness ovopathy among other factors (Table 12.1) [3]. Even though most cases are sporadic in nature, chromosomal defects including an autosomal dominant pattern (involving chromosome 14) and autosomal recessive pattern with reduced penetrance are possible. Twin studies have shown concordance for both monozygotic and dizygotic twins. Specific chromosomal alterations include chromosome 5p deletion, 7q duplication, 22q11.2

Table 12.1 Pathogenic factors (Chap. 1)

Extrinsic factors	Intrinsic factors
Thalidomide	Diabetes
Pseudoephedrine	Multiple gestation
Retinoic acid	Bleeding during second trimester
Triazene	Autosomal dominance
Alcohol consumption	

deletion, and trisomy 7, 8, and 9 mosaicism [3]. For a thorough discussion on this topic, please refer to Chap. 1.

Clinical Findings

There is a variable and complex phenotypic expression of the unilateral clinical findings involving the mandible, craniofacial hard and soft tissues, orbits, external and middle ear, and nerves. Mandibular hypoplasia results in maxillary growth restriction with facial asymmetry and an occlusal cant. There may be a "scissors-bite" or complete crossbite of the occlusion. There is orbital asymmetry and dystopia, as well as ear deformities. Goldenhar syndrome, or oculoauriculovertebral dysplasia, is a more severe variant of CFM comprising approximately 10% of the total [4]. Goldenhar syndrome presents with hemifacial hypoplasia, epibulbar or conjunctival lipodermoids, accessory auricular appendages, and vertebral anomalies including fusions, hemivertebrae, and scoliosis. The facial skeletal defects seen in CFM include variable forms of bony hypoplasia of the zygoma, zygomatic arch, orbit, frontal bone, pterygoid process of the sphenoid bone, mastoid and tympanic processes of the temporal bone, ear ossicles and bony external auditory canal, as well as maxillary involvement, with cleft palate seen in 10% of CFM cases. Regarding the mandible, involvement may be the earliest skeletal manifestation of CFM and, again, may have variable degrees of severity ranging from a small or flattened condyle to complete agenesis of the condyle, ascending ramus, and glenoid fossa [7]. There is impaired vertical and horizontal mandibular growth that inhibits ipsilateral vertical maxillary and midface growth resulting in an occlusal cant and ipsilateral mandibular deviation upon mouth opening. In the mandible, there is no correlation between the magnitude of the bony hypoplasia and the degree of associated muscular atrophy. The dentition may have dental crowding and crossbites, and the anterior teeth may be inclined toward the affected side [8]. There may be hypodontia in 25% of individuals, particularly in the mandible, and delayed tooth development and enamel hypoplasia on the affected side. Also, there may be mandibular midline and chin deviation toward the affected side. Mandibular protrusion may deviate toward the affected side, and ipsilateral lateral excursive movements of the mandible may be limited [9]. In addition, there are variable facial soft tissue defects with decreased mass of subcutaneous tissues involving the eyes, parotid gland, and muscles of mastication and muscles of facial expression. As opposed to the mandible, the degree of facial soft tissue hypoplasia is usually correlated with the degree of facial bony involvement. There may be macrostomia (asymmetric toward the involved side), and soft tissue tags, or appendages. Ear deformities are notable in CFM, and the ipsilateral ear may be low-set with microtia of the lobule, or occasionally complete anotia, as well as underdevelopment of the ear ossicles and external auditory meatus. A detailed review of the correction of the Associated Ear Deformities in the Craniofacial Microsomia Patient can be found in Chap. 10. There may be associated hearing loss and chronic otitis media in some affected individuals. Neurologic issues may include facial nerve palsy in 22–45% of cases, with the marginal mandibular branch being most often affected. A review of management of hearing Loss in patients with Treacher Collins syndrome and hemifacial microsomia can be found in Chap. 9. There may also be palatal deviation toward the affected side. Nerve issues correlate with ear deformity severity and not skeletal severity. Finally, extracranial issues are present in up to 55% of cases and include cardiac anomalies (atrial or ventricular septal defects), renal agenesis, and vertebral fusions (L3-L4-S1) which are not only seen in Goldenhar syndrome but may be present in over 10% of CFM cases as well [5]. A full review of extracranial manifestations of microsomia is provided in Chap. 4. There are certainly also psychosocial issues in these patients due to their appearance including denial, decreased self-confidence, and social withdrawal [10]. There may be breathing difficulties, sleep disorders, and speech impairment due to the presence of a cleft palate with velopharyngeal insufficiency and unilateral hearing loss. For a thorough discussion on the initial evaluation of the craniofacial microsomia patient, refer to Chap. 2.

Diagnosis and Classification Systems

Patient assessment and diagnosis is best managed in a multidisciplinary team setting (including an orthodontist, pediatric dentist, craniofacial surgeon (oral and maxillofacial surgery, otolaryngology, or plastic surgery), prosthodontist, speech therapist, audiologist, psychologist, and geneticist) with an appropriate history, clinical examination, radiographs (panoramic, 3D CT scan, MRI, lateral cephalography, chest radiograph, abdominal ultrasound, others), hearing and speech evaluation, laryngoscopic exam, and focused neurologic, cardiac, renal, and psychological evaluations. A multitude of anatomical and surgical classification systems have been proposed over the years including those by Gorlin, Poswillo, Prusansky, Kaban, Lauritzen, David, Vento, and Epker. Some have focused more on the mandibular and temporomandibular joint (TMJ) deformities (Pruzansky, Kaban), while others have included the spectrum of anomalies (Vento, Mulliken). The SAT system includes Skeletal, Auricular, and soft Tissue deformities. The OMENS system includes Orbital, Mandibular, Ear, Nerve, and Soft tissue deformities, while the OMENS+ classification also includes extracranial anomalies. These classification systems were reviewed extensively in previous chapters (Table 12.2). The Pruzansky and Kaban classifications include Types I, IIA, IIB, and III with progressive hypoplasia of the mandible and articular structures. In Type I, the condyle is present and normal in shape but small in size. Type IIA has a condyle that is small and abnormal in shape but with normal TMJ function. The differentiating factor between Types IIA and IIB is the abnormal function in IIB with significant medial displacement of the small and abnormally shaped condyle with minimal or no condyle-fossa articulation resulting in abnormal TMJ function. In Type III, there is complete absence of the condyle and ramus of the mandible [4, 7]. This particular classification scheme therefore guides the treatments that may be indicated for mandibular reconstruction.

Table 12.2 OMENS classification

Orbit
O0: Normal size and position
O1: Abnormal size
O2: Abnormal orbital position (arrow depicts whether superior or inferior)
O3: Abnormal size and position
Mandible
M0: Normal mandible
M1: Mandible and glenoid fossa are small with shortened ramus
M2: Mandibular ramus is short and abnormally shaped
M2A: Glenoid fossa is in relatively normal position compared with contralateral side
M2B: Temporomandibular joint is inferior, medial, and anteriorly displaced with hypoplastic condyle
M3: Complete absence of ramus, glenoid fossa, temporomandibular joint
Ear
E0: Normal ear
E1: Mild hypoplasia and cupping with all structures present
E2: Absence of external auditory canal with variable hypoplasia of concha
E3: Malpositioned lobule (usually inferior and anterior) with absent auricle
Facial nerve
N0: No facial nerve involvement
N1: Upper facial nerve involvement; temporal and zygomatic branches
N2: Lower facial nerve involvement; buccal, mandibular, and cervical branches
N3: All branches of facial nerve affected (Other nerves such as trigeminal and hypoglossal may be denoted with superscript, i.e., $N^{5}0$ or $N^{12}0$)
Soft tissue
S0: No soft tissue or muscle deficiency
S1: Minimal soft tissue or muscle deficiency
S2: Moderate soft tissue or muscle deficiency
S3: Severe soft tissue or muscle deficiency

The differential diagnosis of CFM may include idiopathic unilateral mandibular hypoplasia, Parry-Romberg syndrome, and other branchial arch disorders such as Treacher Collins syndrome, Nager syndrome, and Pierre-Robin Sequence [11]. Variants of craniofacial microsomia are listed in Table 12.3.

Overall Management

It is important to understand that treatment of CFM requires a multidisciplinary approach that is sequenced appropriately based upon the age of the patient. Of course, airway issues, if present, are paramount, and are of primary concern, as are issues associated with feeding difficulties and failure to thrive. Obstructive sleep apnea signs and symptoms warrant evaluation with polysomnography [5, 6]. For a thorough review of this topic, see Chap. 3. During the first year of life, excision of

Table 12.3 Variants of craniofacial microsomia

Hemifacial microsomia
First and second branchial arch syndrome
Oral-mandibular-auricular syndrome
Otomandibular dysostosis
Otomandibular dysmorphogenesis
Oculoauriculovertebral spectrum (OAVS), sequence, or dysplasia
Facioauriculovertebral sequence or syndrome
Lateral facial dysplasia
Auriculobranchiogenic dysplasia
Intrauterine facial necrosis
Hemignathia and microtia syndrome
Necrotic facial dysplasia
Mandibular laterognathism
Goldenhar syndrome

ear tags, macrostomia reconstruction, and cleft palate repair may be considered [12]. Within the first 2 years of life, severe plagiocephaly, if present, may be addressed [4]. At years 4–5 of life, neurologic dysfunction of the facial nerve may be corrected with microneurosurgical reconstruction or facial reanimation procedures. Next, in the 5–8 years of age range, with costochondral development, ear reconstruction may be considered using cartilage, as well as TMJ and ramus reconstruction with rib grafting for CFM Types IIB and III. Of course distraction osteogenesis may be an option for CFM Types I, IIA, and possibly IIB and III using transport distraction techniques in an attempt to create a new condyle [4]. At this time, consideration can be given for simultaneous correction of severe orbital dystopia. After age 12, other treatment options may include skeletal augmentation using autogenous (bone grafts) or alloplastic (e.g., porous polyethylene) materials and implants, and soft tissue augmentation using local, regional, or distant pedicled, non-vascularized, or vascularized tissue flaps [7, 13]. Upon growth cessation, maxillary, mandibular, and genial orthognathic surgical procedures are performed if indicated. Also, consideration may be given toward TMJ and glenoid fossa reconstruction with autogenous or alloplastic total joint replacement as described in previous chapters in this text. The use of 3D imaging allows a comprehensive assessment of the complexity geometry of the skeletal deformities and allows precision and accuracy in the diagnosis and virtual surgical planning (VSP) for each individual case [14].

Maxillofacial Treatment

Mandibular management is the keystone for facial reconstruction in CFM, and treatment protocols vary based upon age and stage of dental development. Variations of these treatment protocols have been described in this book. The specific surgical techniques, methods, and materials vary with the severity of the individual deformity and experience and preferences of the team but typically involve orthodontic intervention, orthognathic surgical procedures, distraction osteogenesis (DO), and TMJ reconstruction with costochondral grafting, vascularized flaps (e.g., fibula), or alloplastic joint replacement. Various treatment options are discussed in detail in Chaps. 5, 6, and 7. In general, in the primary dentition stage, consideration for mandibular surgery exists only for Type III cases with TMJ reconstruction. This allows the creation of an ipsilateral open bite with vertical elongation of the ramus and the use of an occlusal splint (functional appliance therapy) that is reduced sequentially to allow the mandibular occlusal plane to remain corrected while allowing the maxilla to grow normally without interference by the mandibular dentition [9]. In the mixed dentition stage, orthodontic activator appliances may be used effectively in Type I, and some IIA, deformities to improve function and possibly prevent continued asymmetric development of the hard and soft tissues. Types IIB and III are managed with ramus and condyle reconstruction as described with rib grafting and open bite creation with the expectation for continued maxillary/midface growth without mandibular restriction (Figs. 12.3, 12.4, and 12.5). Also, distraction osteogenesis is another option for management for Types IIA and IIB (Fig. 12.6), and DO in Type III cases is controversial since there is no condyle to physically distract, and this may not achieve the desired outcome and require additional surgery [15, 16] (Figs. 12.7, 12.8, 12.9, 12.10, 12.11, 12.12, and 12.13). In the event that the patient is evaluated first in the permanent dentition stage of dental

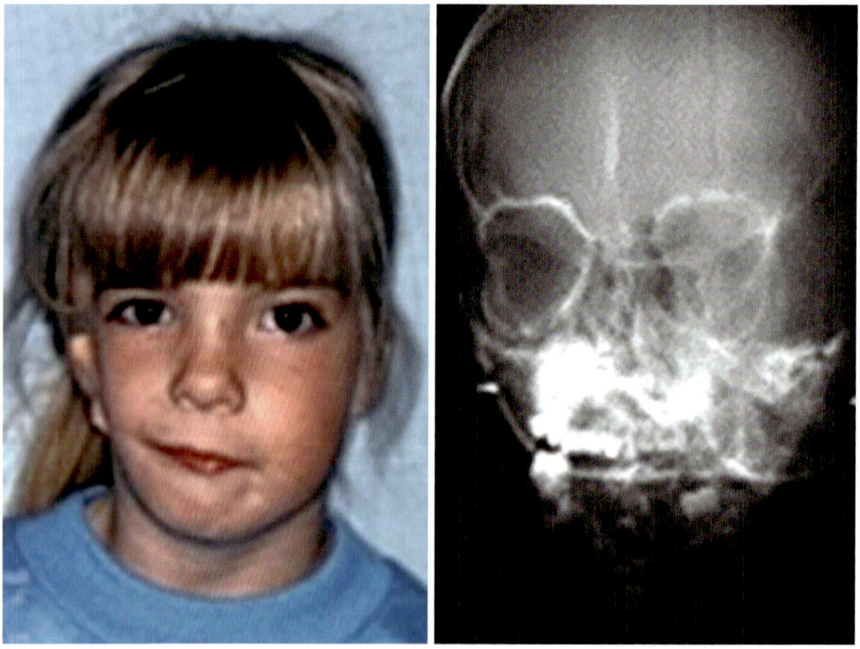

Fig. 12.3 7-year-old right CFM Type III patient in the mixed dentition stage (left image) with lack of a condyle and ramus (right image)

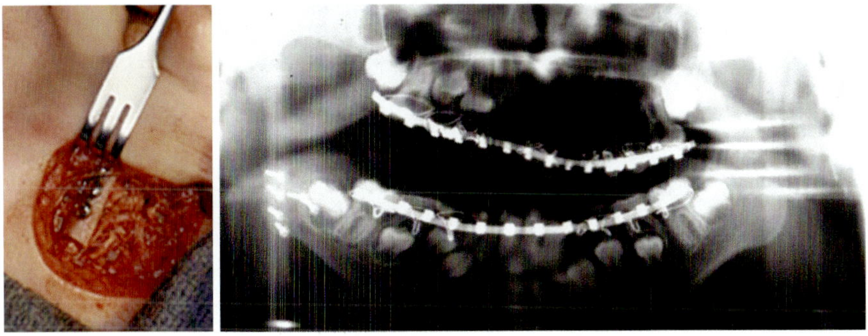

Fig. 12.4 CFM right Type III patient undergoes rib graft to right TMJ/ramus (left image) with postoperative panoramic radiograph (right image). Note open bite that is created on the affected side, and a splint is used to maintain the open bite

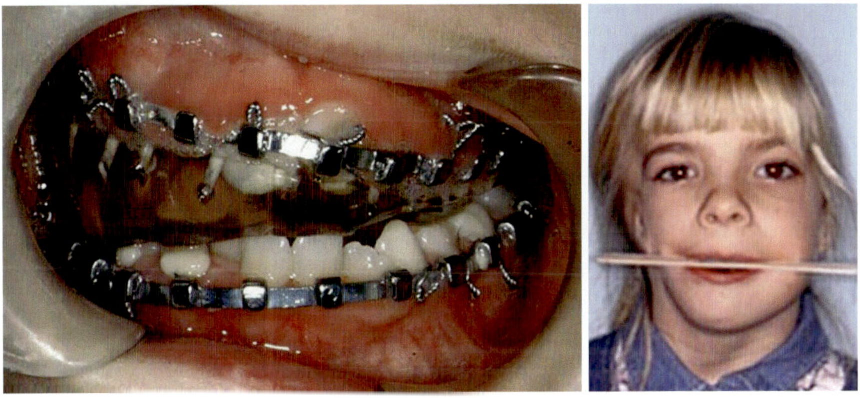

Fig. 12.5 Interocclusal splint used to maintain the open bite and allow maxillary growth (left image). The mandibular occlusal plane is maintained while the splint is reduced sequentially to allow maxillary growth (right image)

development, then conventional orthodontics and orthognathic surgical correction may be performed, and, again, consideration may be given toward distraction osteogenesis, as well as total alloplastic TMJ reconstruction, if indicated.

The principle of orthodontic therapy in patients with hemifacial microsomia is reviewed in detail in Chap. 8. Initially the occlusion can be modified with a functional appliance and provide support for the mandibular muscles to function with a more symmetrically positioned mandible in anticipation of completing surgery on the abnormal side of the mandible. Phase 1 orthodontic treatment is used to alleviate dental issues with a possible growth modification followed by a second phase of treatment when skeletal maturity is complete. The functional appliance must be designed to reposition the mandible downward, forward, and shifted to the unaffected side, producing a posterior open bite. The acrylic is progressively removed from the occlusal surface of the maxillary posterior teeth to allow overeruption for the purpose of leveling the occlusal plane. Goals of this approach as outlined in

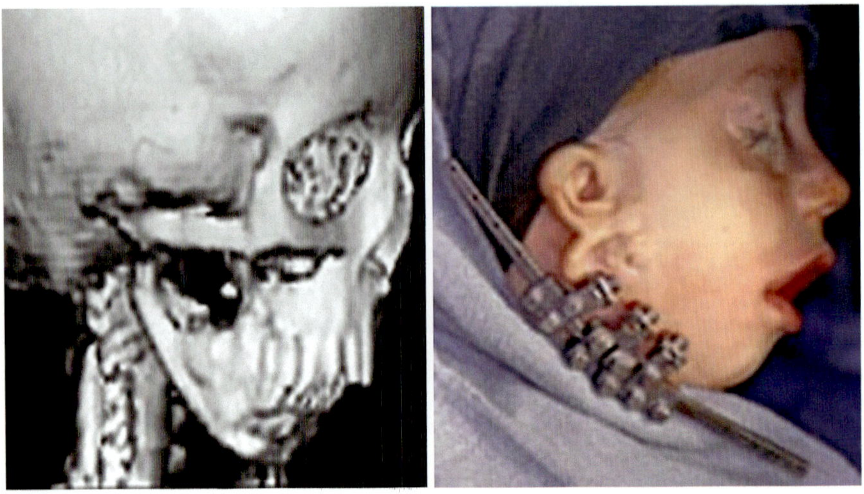

Fig. 12.6 An example of a CFM Type IIB case (left image) using external multivector trifocal distraction osteogenesis (right image)

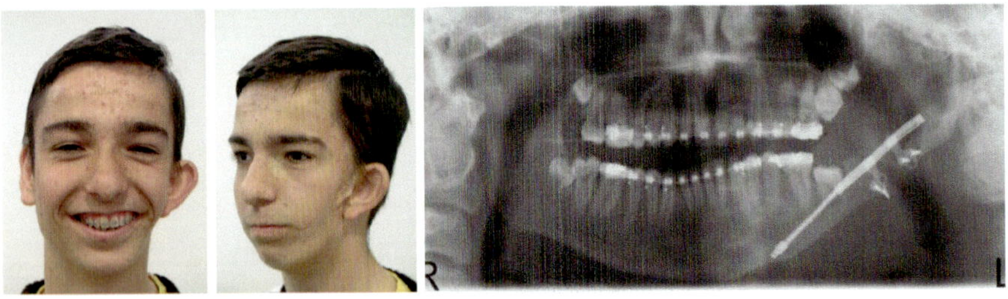

Fig. 12.7 An example of a left CFM Type III patient (left and middle images), who underwent standard DO without a successful outcome since there was no condyle or ramus to distract (right image)

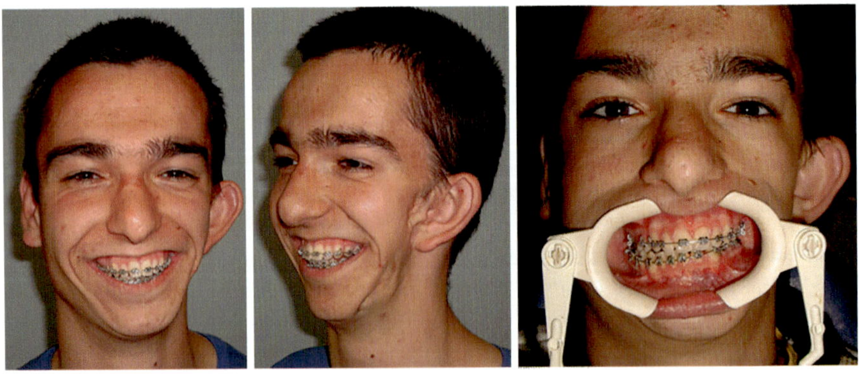

Fig. 12.8 Same CFM Type III patient after DO with persistent occlusal cant and facial asymmetry and lack of a condyle and glenoid fossa

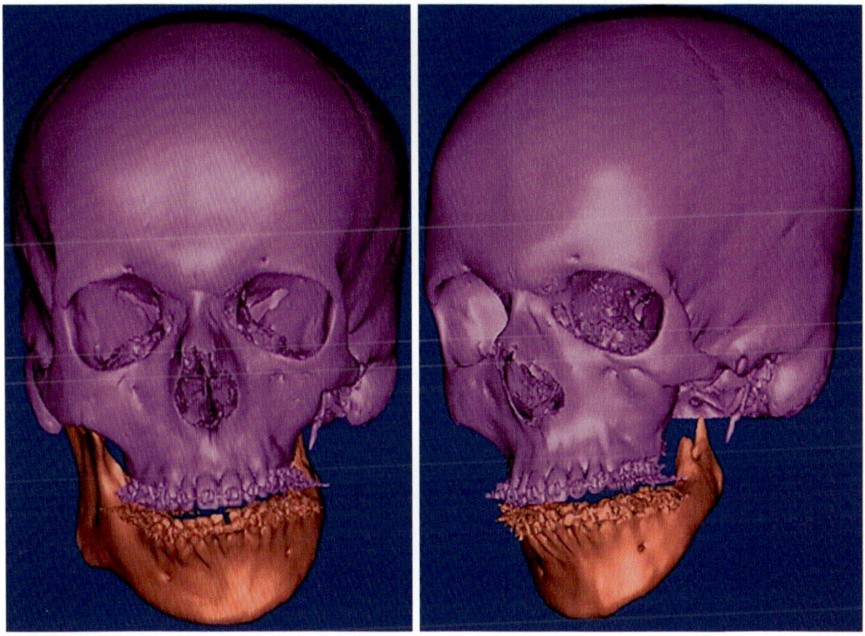

Fig. 12.9 Same CFM Type III patient showing 3D CT scan of the left facial skeletal problems and occlusal cant

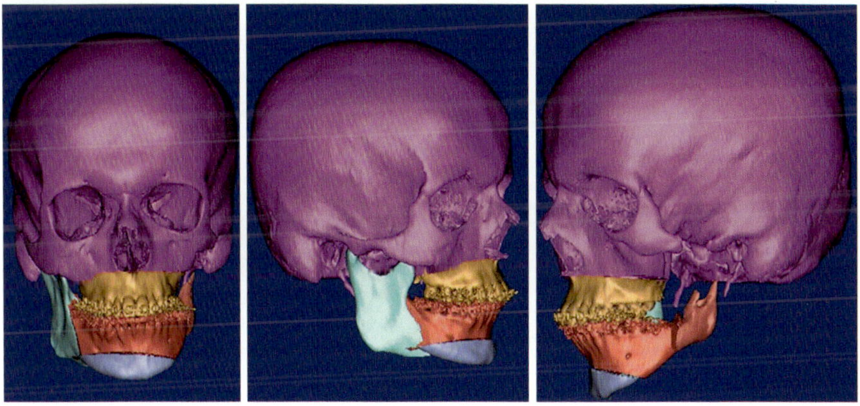

Fig. 12.10 VSP plan for LeFort I osteotomy, unilateral mandibular sagittal split osteotomy, right ramus, condyle, and glenoid fossa reconstruction, and asymmetric genioplasty

Chap. 8 include correcting of the mandibular deviation and maxillary cant occlusion, controlling the vertical growth pattern to prevent excessive mandibular clockwise rotation, monitoring proper permanent dentition development, and achieving an aesthetical, functional, and stable occlusion.

The use of VSP allows an assessment of the specific location of the skeletal issues and permits the surgeon to correct the individual problem, which includes the

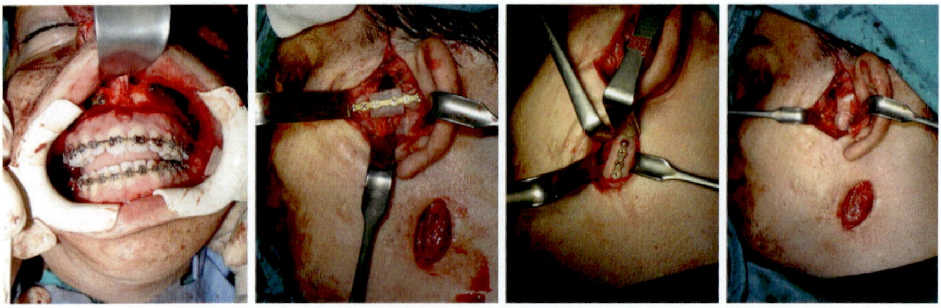

Fig. 12.11 Intraoperative reconstruction showing the LeFort maxillary osteotomy correction of the occlusal cant prior to mandibular reconstruction (left image) and glenoid fossa and condyle and ramus reconstruction with costochondral grafting (right three images)

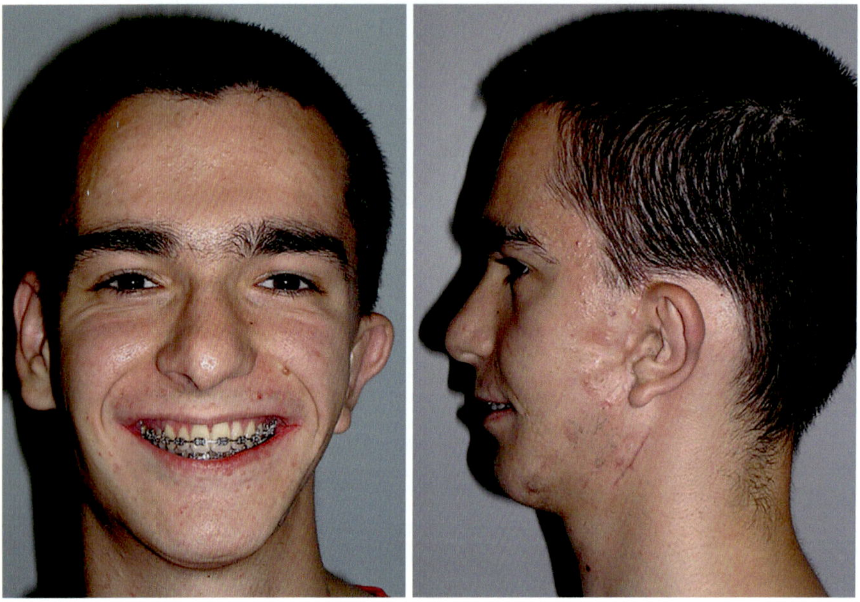

Fig. 12.12 Postoperative appearance showing improved maxillary and mandibular symmetry following reconstruction and otoplasty

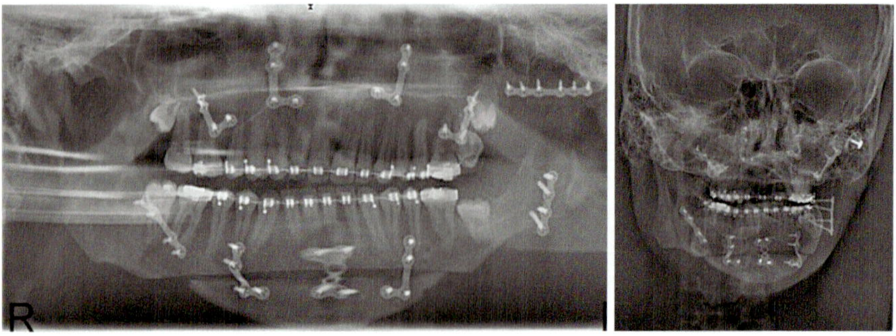

Fig. 12.13 Postoperative radiographs showing maxillary and mandibular reconstruction

need to determine the precise fulcrum of maxillomandibular movement in order to determine whether to vertically lengthen the involved (short) side, while simultaneously shortening the contralateral (long) side [5]. This involves the use of a LeFort I maxillary osteotomy, possibly segmental, with typically a mandibular bilateral sagittal split osteotomy, or unilateral vertical ramus osteotomy or inverted-L osteotomy with bone grafting for a severe asymmetry, as well as a genioplasty procedure. The use of distraction osteogenesis (DO) has been applied to all three CFM types in both pediatric and adult patients. DO for pediatric CFM cases that create an open bite also require the use of interocclusal splints for maxillary growth; however, another option is bimaxillary DO, or simultaneous maxillary-mandibular DO. In bimaxillary DO, a unilateral mandibular osteotomy is created with application of a DO device, while simultaneously a LeFort I osteotomy is performed, and maxillomandibular fixation (MMF) is used during the distraction period such that both the mandible and the maxilla are distracted simultaneously when activating the mandibular distraction device. This avoids the need to create an open bite on the involved side and unpredictable maxillary growth and poor occlusal control. Of course, the decision regarding treatment depends upon the recommendations of the multidisciplinary team, as well as the education, training, and skills of the surgeon. The outcomes and success of treatment are based upon many factors but include the magnitude, severity (e.g., degree of occlusal cant), and complexity of the individual case. It should be noted that despite the use of VSP, complete symmetrical correction of hard and soft tissue asymmetries may not be possible, and acceptable results may be preferred over ideal, or perfect results, and secondary or revision surgical procedures are not uncommon in complex facial asymmetry cases [17].

The associated soft tissue deformities and nerve abnormalities are significant to the patient with hemifacial microsomia and cannot be overlooked. They play a critical role in the quality of the life of the patient. Chap. 11 reviews in detail the correction of the soft tissue deformities associated with craniofacial microsomia and discussed facial reanimation and soft tissue grafting techniques. Briefly, soft tissue volume correction can be achieved with soft tissue flaps, fat grafting, and alloplastic implants. Various static and dynamic procedures can be implemented for the restoration of facial function and aesthetics with the ultimate goal is rehabilitation of spontaneous movement of facial musculature.

Conclusions

It must be recognized that there is no consensus on diagnosis or management of CFM and, therefore, evidence-based decisions are difficult based upon the existing low-level evidence [18]. There is certainly controversy about the preferred treatment for condyle and ramus reconstruction using either distraction osteogenesis (DO), rib grafts, vascularized fibula flaps, or alloplastic TMJ prostheses for the CFM Type III (and, even IIB) patient, and this certainly depends upon the severity of the complex maxillofacial issues and the age at the time of intervention [7]. Of course a team approach is the best, and an individualized sequenced treatment plan approach may be the most ideal. Despite these limitations, some progress has been made in an attempt to develop guidelines for CFM assessment and treatment by the Facial Asymmetry Collaborative for Interdisciplinary Assessment and Learning (FACIAL) group established in 2009 to support CFM research and collaboration, as well as the International Consortium for Health Outcome Metrics CFM Group to evaluate patient-centered health-related quality of life outcomes of the various forms of treatment for this complex condition [4].

References

1. Hopkins B, Dean K, Appachi S, Drake AF. Craniofacial interventions in children. Otolaryngol Clin N Am. 2019;52:903–22.
2. Gorlin RJ, Cohen MM, RCM H. Syndromes of the head and neck. Oxford England ; New York: Oxford University Press; 2001. p. xiv, 1283 p.
3. Chen Q, Zhao Y, Shen G, Dai J. Etiology and pathogenesis of Hemifacial Microsomia. J Dent Res. 2018;97:1297–305.
4. Birgfeld C, Heike C. Craniofacial Microsomia. Clin Plast Surg. 2019;46:207–21.
5. Vong A, Funamura J. Multidisciplinary management of oculo-auriculo-vertebral spectrum. Curr Opin Otolaryngol Head Neck Surg. 2018;26:234–41.
6. Ornoy A. Craniofacial malformations and their association with brain development: the importance of a multidisciplinary approach for treatment. Odontology. 2020;108:1–15.
7. Brandstetter KA, Patel KG. Craniofacial Microsomia. Facial Plast Surg Clin North Am. 2016;24:495–515.
8. Heike CL, Hing AV, Aspinall CA, et al. Clinical care in craniofacial microsomia: a review of current management recommendations and opportunities to advance research. Am J Med Genet C Semin Med Genet. 2013;163C:271–82.
9. Akram A, McKnight MM, Bellardie H, Beale V, Evans RD. Craniofacial malformations and the orthodontist. Br Dent J. 2015;218:129–41.
10. Tapia VJ, Epstein S, Tolmach OS, Hassan AS, Chung NN, Gosman AA. Health-related quality-of-life instruments for pediatric patients with diverse facial deformities: a systematic literature review. Plast Reconstr Surg. 2016;138:175–87.
11. Alfi D, Lam D, Gateno J. Branchial arch syndromes. Atlas Oral Maxillofac Surg Clin North Am. 2014;22:167–73.
12. McCarthy JG. Craniofacial microsomia. A primary or secondary surgical treatment program. Clin Plast Surg. 1997;24:459–74.
13. Sinclair N, Gharb BB, Papay F, Rampazzo A. Soft tissue reconstruction in patients with hemifacial microsomia: a systematic review of the literature. J Craniofac Surg. 2019;30:879–87.
14. Manara R, Schifano G, Brotto D, et al. Facial asymmetry quantitative evaluation in oculoauriculovertebral spectrum. Clin Oral Investig. 2016;20:219–25.
15. van de Lande LS, Pluijmers BI, Caron C, et al. Surgical correction of the midface in craniofacial microsomia. Part 1: a systematic review. J Craniomaxillofac Surg. 2018;46:1427–35.
16. Nagy K, Kuijpers-Jagtman AM, Mommaerts MY. No evidence for long-term effectiveness of early osteodistraction in hemifacial microsomia. Plast Reconstr Surg. 2009;124:2061–71.
17. Kobus K, Kobus-Zalesna K. The treatment of facial asymmetry: review. Adv Clin Exp Med. 2017;26:1301–11.
18. Bekisz JM, Fryml E, Flores RL. A review of randomized controlled trials in cleft and craniofacial surgery. J Craniofac Surg. 2018;29:293–301.

Part II
Treacher Collins Syndrome TCS

Chapter 13
Etiology and Anatomical Variation in Treacher Collins Syndrome

Francis Joel Smith

A Personal Perspective on Treacher Collins Syndrome by the Author

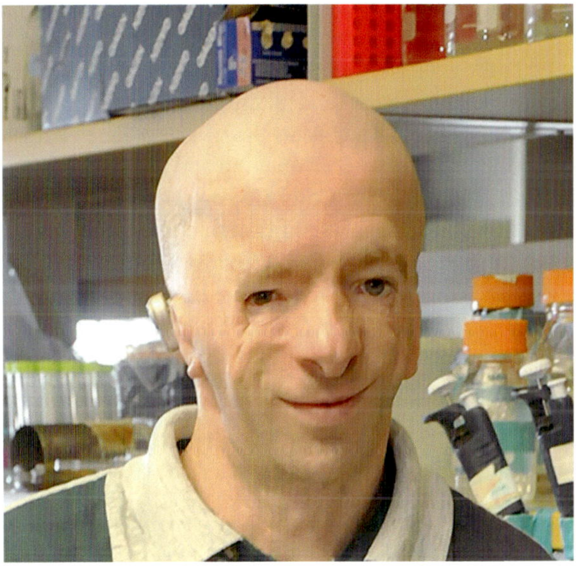

My life with Treacher Collins syndrome has led me into a unique career in craniofacial biology and craniofacial anomaly research and global public outreach for

F. J. Smith (✉)
Department of Cell & Developmental Biology, Modern Human Anatomy Program,
University of Colorado Anschutz Medical Campus, School of Medicine,
Aurora, CO, USA
e-mail: francis.smith@cuanschutz.edu

D. M. Yates, M. R. Markiewicz (eds.), *Craniofacial Microsomia and Treacher Collins Syndrome*, https://doi.org/10.1007/978-3-030-84733-3_13

awareness and research of craniofacial differences. I was born with severe Treacher Collins syndrome and needed a tracheostomy to save my life at birth. I have had over 20 facial reconstructive surgeries, speech therapy, and bone conduction hearing aids. My challenges were not only medical but also social and emotional. I faced years of bullying in school, along with stares and questions in public, and discrimination. Despite these challenges over my lifetime, my faith, my adoptive family, my friends, and my colleagues have all been an encouragement to me to persevere and pursue the unique goals of my life. After sensing the call to enter the craniofacial medical field while in high school, I studied biology at Purdue University for my bachelor and master of science degrees. After unsuccessful attempts at applying to medical school, I furthered my education in biomedical science at King's College London in the United Kingdom and received my first education and research experience in craniofacial embryology and genetics there. My mentors at King's College London saw potential in me as a craniofacial research scientist and encouraged me to pursue a PhD. This I achieved at the University of California San Francisco in 2012. My first postdoctoral fellowship, at the University of Calgary Faculty of Medicine, introduced me to the exciting field of three-dimensional (3-D) imaging and morphometrics (morphological or shape analysis) of the craniofacial region in animal models and in humans. My work in craniofacial 3-D imaging and morphometric analysis led to the majority of my published papers and subsequent opportunities in 3-D craniofacial imaging and analysis in clinical situations including airway imaging and volume assessment in Brazil and planned future collaborative research in craniofacial and airway 3-D imaging and analysis. My second postdoctoral fellowship, at the University of Colorado Anschutz Medical Campus, focused on craniofacial gene expression analysis. I continue to engage in public and educational outreach for craniofacial anomaly awareness and research, by speaking and guest-lecturing worldwide as well as through media interviews and even a recently published memoir, *Wonderfully Made: The Dr. Francis Joel Smith, PhD Story.*

Introduction to Treacher Collins Syndrome

Treacher Collins syndrome (mandibulofacial dysostosis, Treacher Collins-Franceschetti syndrome, Franceschetti-Zwahlen-Klein syndrome) (OMIM 154500) is a rare disorder of craniofacial development (1:50,000 live births), and 60% of cases arise as de novo mutations [1, 2]. The syndrome is named after nineteenth-century British surgeon and ophthalmologist Edward Treacher Collins, who first described the essential traits of the condition in 1900, particularly the outer notching of the eyelids and malar bone defects [3]. Genetically, it is of variable genotype and penetrance, and in terms of severity, it has a wide phenotypic variation from extremely mild to severe malformations. It is a disorder of development of the first and second branchial arches in the embryo. Defects of bone and tissues derived from these arches include malar and zygomatic hypoplasia, maxillary and mandibular defects including micrognathia and retrognathia, cleft palate, and ear defects including auditory canal stenosis or atresia, microtia or anotia, and incomplete or missing middle ear ossicles. External characteristics include not only the aforementioned outer ear defects (microtia or anotia) but also downward slanting of the eyes due to the incomplete orbital rims, sunken cheeks for lack of zygomatic arches, and retruded chin due to the micrognathia and retrognathia [1, 2]. Figure 13.1 shows the characteristic facial features of a severe manifestation of Treacher Collins syndrome. The inheritance pattern of Treacher Collins syndrome is autosomal dominant [1, 2].

Part I: Etiology of Treacher Collins Syndrome

TCOF1: *The Master Gene of Treacher Collins Syndrome*

The gene responsible for the majority of cases of Treacher Collins syndrome is *TCOF1*. Through studies of families with Treacher Collins syndrome, their pedigrees, and candidate gene analysis, Dixon and colleagues [1, 2] pinpointed the true chromosomal location of the gene. After eliminating other putative chromosomal sites for the gene [1], Dixon and colleagues further narrowed the candidate region to a region on the long arm of chromosome 5, at locus 5q31–34 [2]. The locus was eventually more precisely pinpointed to 5q32–33.1 [4].

To understand the potential function of the gene *TCOF1*, Dixon and colleagues [5] isolated the mouse homologue of *TCOF1*, designated as *tcofl*. *Tcofl*, on mouse chromosome 18, was found to encode a low-complexity protein 133 kDa in size and rich in the amino acids serine and alanine; this protein was found to have 61.5% identity with human and other species' homologues [5]. This protein is conserved among species especially in regions of amino acid repeats and signals for nucleolar localization [5]. The nucleolus, located within the cell's nucleus, is where

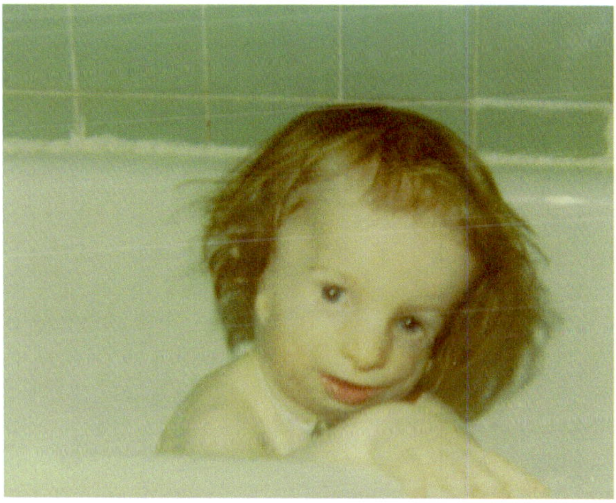

Fig. 13.1 The classic facial features of Treacher Collins syndrome, including microtia, downward slanting eyes, sunken cheeks, and micrognathia. Note tracheostomy tube. (Photo of author at age 2, from author's personal archive)

ribosomes (the protein machinery of translation of messenger RNA into proteins) are made, so the localization of the *tcof1* protein product to the nucleolus suggested to Dixon et al. [5] that this protein would be involved in ribosome biogenesis and nucleolar-cytoplasmic transport. *Tcof1* was shown to be expressed in a wide variety of mouse embryonic and adult tissues and regions, with peak expression in the embryonic neural folds immediately prior to fusion [5], and also in the developing branchial or pharyngeal arches at critical morphogenetic stages, all derived from the progenitor cell population known as the neural crest. Craniofacial tissues and structures are derived from cranial neural crest cells. Wise et al. [6] confirmed that human *TCOF1* encodes a nucleolar phosphoprotein (Treacle), and mutations within *TCOF1* (as seen in the families they studied) cause defects in this nucleolar trafficking and ribosomal biogenetic protein that is critical to craniofacial development. A study of the mutational spectrum of *TCOF1* in Treacher Collins syndrome by Edwards et al. [7] revealed a premature termination codon which leads to formation of a truncated Treacle protein; this malformed protein cannot carry out its ribosomal biogenetic and nucleolar trafficking functions; *TCOF1* mutations appear to be family-specific. Edwards and colleagues [7] concluded that Treacher Collins syndrome results from haploinsufficiency of *TCOF1* and, in turn, a defective Treacle protein. Marsh and colleagues [8] confirmed the requirement for Treacle to localize specifically to the nucleolus, via induced mutations that caused the defective Treacle to localize to random locations in the cell; these mutations deleted putative nucleolar localization signals in the gene. These findings supported the hypothesis that part of Treacle's function is shuttling between the nucleolus and cytoplasm [8]. Jones et al. [9] found that Treacle protein contains kinase phosphorylation sites in its sequence, which might be critical to its function; they found kinase activity in embryonic branchial arches 1 and 2 coinciding with expression of Treacle at its peak in these arches. Hot spots for mutations in *TCOF1* were found to be clustered in five exons (exons 10, 15, 16, 23, and 24), which are responsible for 50% of all pathogenic mutations [10]. In these hot spots, mutations in exons 10, 15, and 16 occur in a region of repetitive sequences that are normally phosphorylated by casein kinase II, and mutations in exons 23 and 24 occur in the nucleolar localization signal sequence [10] that demonstrate critical functions in Treacle involving nucleolar localization, shuttling, and kinase activity.

The function of Treacle was finally pinpointed in the mid to late 2000s. Treacle was found to have a critical function in transcription of ribosomal DNA (rDNA) by binding with upstream binding factor (UBF), in the process of ribosome biogenesis in the nucleolus [11]; Treacle and UBF were found to be co-localized in the nucleolus. Treacle and UBF interact together with rDNA chromatin during rDNA transcription; this was shown to be a critical interaction when Treacle expression was downregulated by the use of specific targeted short interfering RNA, preventing transcription of rDNA and cell growth [11]. Gonzales et al. [12] observed that Treacle, through its interaction with UBF and RNA polymerase I, controls transcription of the ribosomal DNA gene and methylates the pre-rRNA.

Further, since Treacle is most actively expressed in the embryonic neural crest and later on in the branchial arches (specifically arches 1 and 2), Dixon et al. [13]

discovered in the mouse model they created for *tcof1*/Treacher Collins syndrome via germline mutations that these mutations (and the resulting defective Treacle protein) lead to deficiency in formation and proliferation and, at the same time, mass apoptosis (death) of neural crest cells—those embryonic migratory progenitor cells that give rise to craniofacial bones, tissues, and structures—and result in craniofacial hypoplasia characteristic of Treacher Collins syndrome. This demonstrated the critical function of Treacle as a spatiotemporal regulator of mature ribosome biogenesis, and deficiency of Treacle results in disrupted neural crest cell formation and proliferation via mass apoptosis in the neural crest in response to deficient ribosome production [13]. However, these defects can be experimentally reversed, as Jones and colleagues [14] discovered through their targeted inhibition of p53 (a molecule involved in apoptosis) in neural crest cells, resulting in reduced neuroapoptosis (neural crest-specific mass apoptosis) and rescue of craniofacial defects in mouse embryos, a potential therapeutic avenue. Another role for Treacle is to protect the neuroepithelium and its daughter neural crest cells from reactive oxygen species (ROS), the oxygen radicals that cause metabolic oxidative stress that can be toxic to these cells and cause the neuroapoptosis leading to the craniofacial hypoplasia of Treacher Collins syndrome [15].

POLR1C and POLR1D Cause Rare Forms of Treacher Collins Syndrome

While mutations in *TCOF1* and defects in its protein product Treacle are responsible for most cases of Treacher Collins syndrome, there are two other genes more recently implicated in rarer forms of the syndrome including an autosomal recessive inherited form of TCS. These two additional genes, *POLR1C* and *POLR1D*, encode subunits of RNA polymerases I and III, which transcribe rRNA [16, 17]. Mutations in *POLR1C* cause an autosomal recessive form of Treacher Collins syndrome, while mutations in *POLR1D* can be either autosomal recessive or dominant [16–18]. In their zebrafish model for Treacher Collins syndrome, Watt and colleagues [17] observed that *Polr1c* and *Polr1d* are expressed spatiotemporally and dynamically at first ubiquitously throughout the embryo in the earliest stages, then more prevalently around the eyes and at the midbrain/hindbrain border, and especially in the craniofacial pharyngeal arches. Mutations in these two genes lead to craniofacial cartilage hypoplasia and cranioskeletal defects characteristic of Treacher Collins syndrome. On a mechanistic basis, these mutations cause a loss of function of the RNA polymerase I and III subunits, leading to a deficiency of mature ribosome production [17]. This in turn causes neuroepithelial cell death (neuroapoptosis) dependent on Tp53 and in turn a deficiency of migratory neural crest cells. Research on *TCOF1* and *POLR1C* and *POLR1D* demonstrates that Treacher Collins syndrome is both a ribosomopathy (disorder of ribosome production) and a neurocristopathy (deficiency of neural crest cells). Watt et al. [17] also found that the Tp53-dependent neuroapoptosis can be genetically inhibited, and this could be a potential avenue for prevention of Treacher Collins syndrome, as much as the research by Jones and colleagues [14] on *Tcof1* p53-dependent neuroapoptosis in mice shows that p53 can be inhibited leading to rescue of Treacher Collins syndrome anomalies. The research by Watt et al. [17] on mutations in *POLR1C* and *POLR1D* demonstrates the necessity for, and function of, these RNA polymerase I and III subunits in transcription of rRNA, mature ribosome biogenesis, proliferation of neural crest cells, and craniofacial development.

Part II: Anatomical Variation in Treacher Collins Syndrome

Treacher Collins Syndrome Is a Neurocristopathy

Craniofacial development begins in the neuroepithelium, the early embryonic tissue that gives rise to the neural crest. The neural crest forms when the neural plate invaginates to form parallel neural folds, which in turn close dorsally to form a tube (the neural tube) [19]. In the neural crest, neural crest cell formation is induced by signals from surrounding tissues, including Wnt signaling across the ectoderm-neural plate border, fibroblast growth factor (Fgf) signaling from the paraxial mesoderm surrounding the neural tube, and bone morphogenetic proteins (BMP) within the neural crest itself. During this process, neural crest cells are encouraged to begin migrating in a dorsoventral path away from the neural crest [19]. Induction of the neural crest is illustrated in Fig. 13.2.

Neural crest cells migrate along defined pathways leading from specific regions of the neural crest in the forebrain, midbrain, and hindbrain, and along the hindbrain there are rhombomeres r1 through r7 [20]. These pathways lead to particular destination regions including the anterior portions of the embryonic head as well as branchial arches (numbered 1–4). The craniofacial region of particular interest regarding Treacher Collins syndrome encompasses the region formed from arches 1 and 2 [20]. Neural crest cell migration along these defined pathways to particular destination regions is illustrated in Fig. 13.3.

The skull and its associated tissues originate from two progenitor populations—the paraxial mesoderm from somites and somitomeres and the neural crest. The frontal, nasal, zygomatic, lacrimal, ethmoid, sphenoid, anterior (squamous) temporal bones, maxilla, mandible, and hyoid originate from neural crest-derived cartilage, while the parietal, occipital, and posterior (petrosal) temporal bones originate from the paraxial mesoderm [21, 22]. The first arch neural crest-derived bones are the maxilla, mandible, zygoma, and the lower portion of the squamous temporal bone and, in the middle ear, the malleus and incus. Derived from the second arch are the hyoid and, in the middle ear, the stapes [21, 22]. Figure 13.4 illustrates the origins of skull bones from the paraxial mesoderm and neural crest.

However, as reviewed earlier, in Treacher Collins syndrome, faulty Treacle and RNA polymerase activity lead to metabolic oxidative stress, and this results in

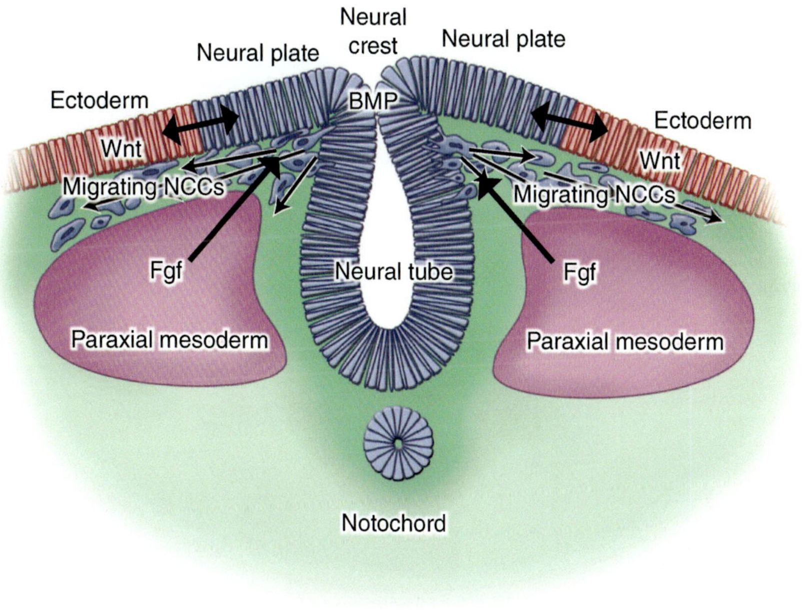

Fig. 13.2 Induction of the neural crest by morphogenetic signals from surrounding embryonic tissues and beginning of neural crest cell migration. Wnt signaling across the ectoderm-neural plate border, Fgf signaling from the paraxial mesoderm, and BMP signaling within the neural crest induce formation of neural crest cells, and these begin migrating away from the neural crest in a dorsoventral direction. (Hand-drawn by author)

massive neuroepithelial apoptosis, in turn causing a significant deficiency of neural crest cells. There are insufficient numbers of migrating neural crest cells available for complete formation of the cartilage and other tissues necessary to form the branchial arch 1 and 2 derivative craniofacial bones and tissues [13, 14].

Anatomy of Treacher Collins Syndrome: Craniofacial Malformations and Airway Obstruction

The anatomical abnormalities present in Treacher Collins syndrome are the result of hypoplasia of neural crest-derived branchial arch 1 and 2 cartilages which in turn cause hypoplastic cranioskeletal defects. These include hypoplasia or absence of the middle ear ossicles and stenosis or atresia of the auditory canals, as well as cleft palate, malar and maxillary hypoplasia, incomplete formation of the zygomatic arches and orbits, and mandibular defects including micrognathia (small mandible) and retrognathia (retruded mandible) and temporomandibular joint (TMJ) defects [1, 2]. Figure 13.5 illustrates the cranioskeletal defects of Treacher Collins syndrome.

Fig. 13.3 Migration of neural crest cells along specific defined pathways from specific forebrain, midbrain, and hindbrain regions (r1–r7 are hindbrain rhombomeres) to specific destinations in anterior head regions and branchial arches (BA1–4). (Hand-drawn by author)

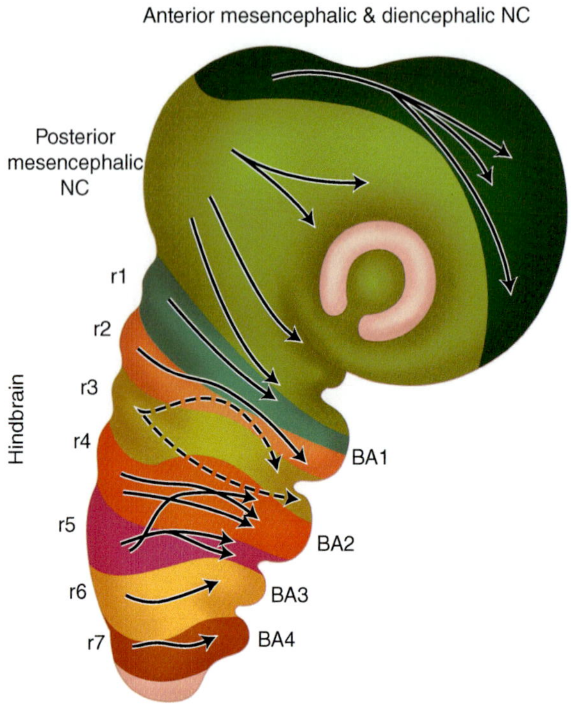

Fig. 13.4 Origins of skull bones from the paraxial mesoderm (red) and neural crest (blue). (Hand-drawn by author)

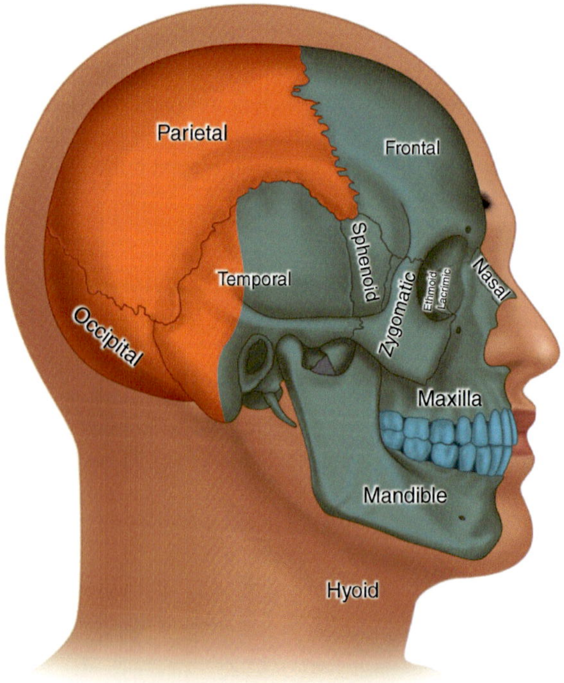

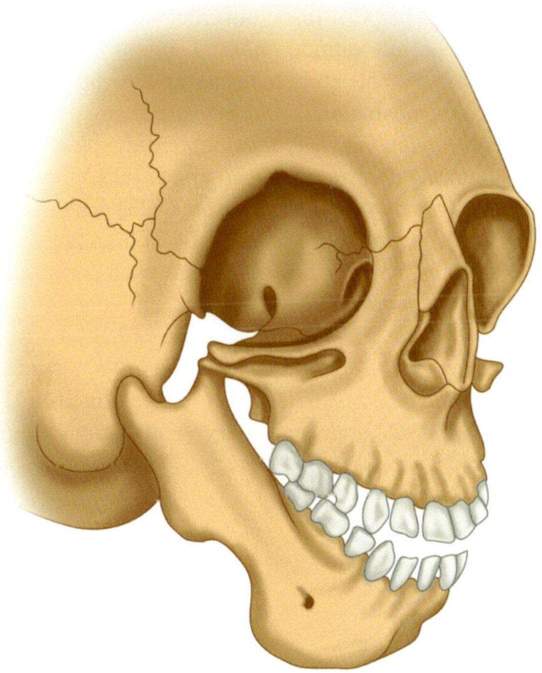

Fig. 13.5 The cranioskeletal defects characteristic of Treacher Collins syndrome. Mandibular micrognathia, retrognathia, maxillary and malar hypoplasia, absent TMJ, incomplete zygomatic arches and orbits. (Hand drawn by author, from personal medical history)

These cranioskeletal defects influence the development of overlying tissues and structures, previously illustrated in Fig. 13.1. The incomplete or absent zygomatic arches coupled with the open lower orbital rims give rise to a downward slanting of the eyes, colobomata of the eyelids, and a triangular appearance to the maxillary and malar region of the face (sunken cheeks). The mandibular micrognathia and retrognathia present themselves in a visible lack of a chin as well as an anterior open bite and lips widely parted at rest. The outer ear defects are either microtia (small outer ears) or anotia (total absence of outer ears), either with a visible stenotic ear canal opening or absent ear canal opening. These external defects vary with the severity of presentation of Treacher Collins syndrome.

Internal defects include a cleft palate (and even when repaired, short palate and velopharyngeal insufficiency) which can impair speech, as well as a stenosis or atresia of the auditory canals and incomplete or absent ossicles (malleus, incus, and stapes), which can cause conductive hearing loss or deafness. The nasal cavity and airway can be abnormally small, and in some severe cases, there is choanal atresia (blockage of the inferior openings of the nasal cavity, or choanae). The oral cavity is also abnormally small, with limited jaw opening and overcrowding of teeth due to the mandibular hypoplasia. The mandibular micrognathia and retrognathia also cause oropharyngeal airway obstruction, via glossoptosis (blockage of the oropharyngeal airway by the tongue forced posteriorly by mandibular hypoplasia). The jaw deformities, small mouth, cleft palate, and constricted throat create difficulties for mastication and swallowing, speech, and breathing.

Upper airway obstruction is the most serious, and potentially fatal, complication of Treacher Collins syndrome. Complications resulting from the upper airway obstruction include choking, impaired respiration, difficult intubation and airway placement, and sleep-disordered breathing and can lead to early death perinatally, postnatally, and any other time throughout life. Polysomnography (PSG), or sleep study, is a valuable diagnostic tool for sleep-disordered breathing including obstructive sleep apnea (OSA), which occurs with a higher prevalence in Treacher Collins syndrome [23]. Three-dimensional oronasopharyngeal imaging by computed tomography (CT) scanning for analysis of airway morphology and volume has also been used for studies on the oronasopharyngeal airway obstruction in Treacher Collins syndrome [24–26]. The studies by Ma et al. [24, 25] and Ribeiro et al. [26] have found reduced nasal, oral, and pharyngeal airway volume, which they have connected to skeletal dysmorphology in those regions including micrognathia, retrognathia, and skeletal hypoplasia in the nasal, oral, and pharyngeal regions. Figure 13.6 illustrates the upper

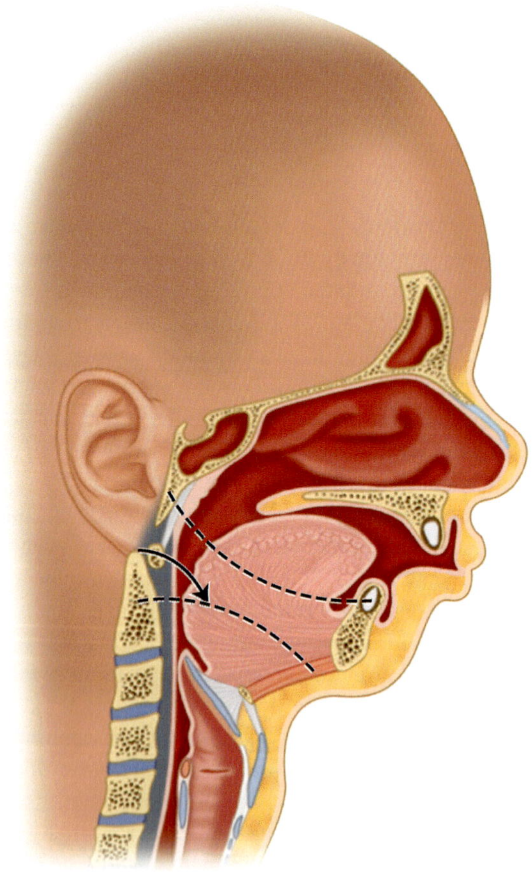

Fig. 13.6 Upper airway obstruction in Treacher Collins syndrome is caused by retrognathia (the mandibular border is drawn in dashed lines) pushing the tongue posteriorly into the oropharyngeal airway; this phenomenon is known as glossoptosis (Hand-drawn by author)

airway obstruction in Treacher Collins syndrome due to retrognathia that forces the tongue posteriorly into the oropharynx, occluding the airway (glossoptosis).

References

1. Dixon MJ, Haan E, Baker E, David D, McKenzie N, Williamson R, Mulley J, Farrall M, and Callen D. Association of Treacher Collins syndrome and translocation 6p21.31/16p13.11: exclusion of the locus from these candidate regions. *Am J Hum Genet* 1991a;48:274–80.
2. Dixon MJ, Read AP, Donnai D, Colley A, Dixon J, and Williamson R. The gene for Treacher Collins syndrome maps to the long arm of chromosome 5. *Am J Hum Genet* 1991b;49:17–22.
3. Collins ET. Cases with symmetrical congenital notches in the outer part of each lid and defective development of the malar bones. *Trans Ophthalmol Soc UK* 1900;20:190–92.
4. Dixon MJ, Dixon J, Houseal T, Bhatt M, Ward DC, Klinger K, and Landes GM. Narrowing the position of the Treacher Collins syndrome gene locus to a small interval between three new microsatellite markers at 5q32-33.1. *Am J Hum Genet* 1993;52:907–14.
5. Dixon J, Hovanes K, Shiang R, and Dixon MJ. Sequence analysis, identification of evolutionary conserved motifs and expression analysis of murine tcof1 provide further evidence for a potential function for the gene and its human homologue, TCOF1. *Hum Mol Genet* 1997;6(5):727–37.
6. Wise CA, Chiang LC, Paznekas WA, Sharma M, Musy MM, Ashley JA, Lovett M, and Jabs EW. *TCOF1* gene encodes a putative nucleolar phosphoprotein that exhibits mutations in Treacher Collins syndrome throughout its coding region. *PNAS* 1997;94:3110–115.
7. Edwards SJ, Gladwin AJ, and Dixon MJ. The mutational spectrum in Treacher Collins syndrome reveals a predominance of mutations that create a premature-termination codon. *Am J Hum Genet* 1997;60:515–24.
8. Marsh KL, Dixon J, and Dixon MJ. Mutations in the Treacher Collins syndrome gene lead to mislocalization of the nucleolar protein treacle. *Hum Mol Genet* 1998;7(11):1795–1800.
9. Jones NC, Farlie PG, Minichiello J, and Newgreen JF. Detection of an appropriate kinase activity in branchial arches I and II that coincides with peak expression of the Treacher Collins syndrome gene product, treacle. *Hum Mol Genet* 1999;8(12): 2239–2245.
10. Splendore A, Jabs EW, and Passos-Bueno MR. Screening of *TCOF1* in patients from different populations: confirmation of mutational hot spots and identification of a novel missense mutation that suggests an important functional domain in the protein treacle. *J Med Genet* 2002;39(7): 493 95.
11. Valdez BC, Henning D, So RB, Dixon J, and Dixon MJ. The Treacher Collins syndrome (*TCOF1*) gene product is involved in ribosomal DNA gene transcription by interacting with upstream binding factor. *PNAS* 2004;101(29):10709-10714.
12. Gonzales B, Henning D, So RB, Dixon J, Dixon MJ, Valdez BC. The Treacher Collins syndrome (*TCOF1*) gene product is involved in pre-rRNA methylation. Hum Mol Genet. 2005;14(14):2035–43.
13. Dixon J, Jones NC, Sandell LL, Jayasinghe SM, Crane J, Rey JP, Dixon MJ, and Trainor PA. Tcof1/Treacle is required for neural crest cell formation and proliferation deficiencies that cause craniofacial abnormalities. *PNAS* 2006;103:13403-13408.
14. Jones NC, Lynn ML, Gaudenz K, Sakai D, Aoto K, Rey JP, Glynn EF, Ellington L, Du C, Dixon J, Dixon MJ, Trainor PA. Prevention of the neurocristopathy Treacher Collins syndrome through inhibition of p53 function. Nat Med. 2008;14(2):125–33.
15. Sakai D, Trainor PA. Face off against ROS: Tcof1/Treacle safeguards neuroepithelial cells and progenitor neural crest cells from oxidative stress during craniofacial development. *Dev Growth Differ* 2016;58(7):577-85.

16. Dauwerse JG, Dixon J, Seland S, Ruivenkamp CA, van Haeringen A, Hoefsloot LH, Peters, DJ. Boers AC, Daumer-Haas C, Maiwald R, Zweier C, Kerr B, Cobo AM, Toral JF, Hoogeboom AJ, Lohmann DR, Hehr U, Dixon MJ, Breuning MH, and Wieczorek D. Mutations in genes encoding subunits of RNA polymerases I and III cause Treacher Collins syndrome. *Nat Genet* 2011;43(1):20–22.
17. Watt KEN, Achilleos A, Neben CL, Merrill AE, and Trainor PA. The roles of RNA polymerase I and III subunits Polr1c and Polr1d in craniofacial development and in zebrafish models of Treacher Collins syndrome. *PLOS Genet* 2016;12(7):e1006187.
18. Schaefer E, Collet C, Genevieve D, Vincent M, Lohmann DR, Sanchez E, Bolender C, Eliot MM, Nurnberg G, Passos-Bueno MR, Wieczorek D, van Maldergem L, and Doray B. Autosomal recessive POLR1D mutation with decrease of TCOF1 mRNA is responsible for Treacher Collins syndrome. *Genet Med* 2014;16(9):720–24.
19. Trainor PA. Specification and patterning of neural crest cells during craniofacial development. *Brain Behav Evol* 2005;66:266–80.
20. Creuzet S, Couly G, and LeDouarin NM. Patterning the neural crest derivatives during development of the vertebrate head: insights from avian studies. *J Anat* 2005;207:447–59.
21. Santagati F. and Rijli FM. Cranial neural crest and the building of the vertebrate head. *Nat Rev Neurosci* 2003;4(10):806–18.
22. Dubey A, Saint-Jeannet JP. Modeling human craniofacial disorders in Xenopus. *Curr Pathobiol Rep* 2017;5(1):79–92.
23. Akre H, Overland B, Asten P, Skogedal N, and Heimdal K. Obstructive sleep apnea in Treacher Collins syndrome. *Eur Arch Otorhinolaryngol* 2012;269:331–37.
24. Ma X, Forte AJ. Persing JA, Alonso N, Berlin NL, and Steinbacher DM. Reduced three-dimensional airway volume is a function of skeletal dysmorphology in Treacher Collins syndrome. *Plast Reconstr Surg* 2015a;135:382e–392e.
25. Ma X, Forte AJ, Berlin NL, Alonso N, Persing JA, and Steinbacher DM. Reduced three-dimensional nasal airway volume in Treacher Collins syndrome and its association with craniofacial morphology. *Plast Reconstr Surg* 2015b;135:885e–894e.
26. Ribeiro A.de A, Smith FJ, Filho HN, Trindade IEK, Tonello C, and Trindade-Suedam IK. Three-dimensional upper airway assessment in Treacher Collins syndrome. *Cleft Palate Craniofac J* 2020;57(3):371–77.

Chapter 14
Initial Evaluation of a Patient with Treacher Collins Syndrome

Paulo Zupelari Goncalves, Sean Peter Edwards, and Sharon Aronovich

Background

Treacher Collins syndrome-1 (TCS1) is a rare congenital craniofacial syndrome characterized by anomalies of structures arising from the first and second branchial arches. It is reported to have a birth incidence of 1 in 50,000 [1]. It was initially reported by a British ophthalmologist, Edward Treacher Collins, who described essential components of the syndrome. Later, Franceschetti and Klein coined the term mandibulofacial dysostosis (MFD1) to describe the same constellation of facial features and further characterized the disorder [2, 3]. It can arise as a de novo mutation or may be inherited in an autosomal dominant fashion. It is caused by a heterozygous mutation in TCOF1 on chromosome 5q32 which encodes the treacle gene (a nuclear phosphoprotein), which leads to neuroepithelial cell apoptosis and interferes with normal spatial and temporal regulation of ribosome biogenesis. This results in an insufficient number of neural crest cells and generalized craniofacial hypoplasia, dysplasia, or aplasia [4].

TCS exhibits genetic and phenotypic heterogeneity, with several other less common subtypes recognized such as TCS2 via mutation of POLR1D on chromosome 13q12, TCS3 via POLR1C on chromosome 6q21 and TCS4 via POLR1B on chromosome 2q14 [5].

P. Z. Goncalves
University of Michigan, Oral and Maxillofacial Surgery, Ann Arbor, MI, USA

University Center of Ourinhos, São Paulo, Brazil
e-mail: zupelari@med.umich.edu

S. P. Edwards · S. Aronovich (✉)
University of Michigan, Oral and Maxillofacial Surgery, Ann Arbor, MI, USA
e-mail: seanedwa@med.umich.edu; saronovi@med.umich.edu

D. M. Yates, M. R. Markiewicz (eds.), *Craniofacial Microsomia and Treacher Collins Syndrome*, https://doi.org/10.1007/978-3-030-84733-3_14

Clinical Features

The clinical features of TCS result from a hypoplasia of the orbits, midface, mandible, and ears. More specifically, orbitomalar/zygomatic arch hypoplasia is present in all patients with TCS. This results in a more inferior position of the lateral canthus and thereby the hallmark down-slanting of the palpebral fissures. Coloboma, a structural defect of the eyelid or the eye that appear as a cleft in the lid margin or the iris, while not present in every case, is highly specific for TCS. Lacrimal system anomalies are also common with atresia of the lacrimal puncta and canaliculi being typical. The mandible is also a prominent feature of the phenotype with a characteristic micrognathia that features marked antegonial notching and a steep mandibular plane. The TMJ may also be hypoplastic and/or dysplastic. The ears are typically bilaterally involved with microtia/anotia, atresia of the auditory canal, anomalous middle ear ossicles leading to a bilateral conductive hearing loss. Also common are preauricular skin tags and preauricular hair displacement. Less common features include cleft palate, maxillary hypoplasia, and an over-projected nasal dorsum (higher nasal root) [6]. Intelligence is usually normal in affected individuals.

Aside from craniofacial malformations, cardiac malformations such as patent ductus arteriosus and septal cardiac defects have also been reported in 12% of patients with TCS1. Anomalies of the kidneys, limbs, and calvarium (i.e., microcephaly) or brain are rare but have been reported [7].

These anatomical aberrations lead to a myriad of functional concerns, which must be considered during the initial evaluation of a newborn with suspected TCS. The micrognathia may result in airway obstruction and feeding and swallowing problems. The orbitomalar hypoplasia combined with colobomas of the eyelids may result in exposure keratopathy and visual disturbances. The auricular and ossicular anomalies typically lead to a bilateral conductive hearing loss which jeopardizes normal speech and language development. As the child grows, these functional concerns will need to be monitored and interventions timed and planned so as to minimize morbidity and treatment burden and maximize benefit. Long-term dependence on tracheostomies and gastrostomies are not infrequent and often the focus of these interventions. Speech and language development must be monitored along with hearing. Jaw function should be observed as well for the impact of malocclusions and limitations in mouth opening. Neuropsychological monitoring is essential to support psychological and mental development and identify any cognitive delays or deficits [8].

Prenatal Screening

Prenatal diagnosis of TCS may be accomplished during a second trimester ultrasound. Primary sonographic features identified include micrognathia and microtia [9]. Methods to identify micrognathia on prenatal 2D ultrasound include the mandible/maxilla ratio with values below 0.785 considered pathognomonic, the jaw index which incorporates the anterio-posterior and bigonial mandibular measurements to quantify a mandibular diameter/biparietal diameter x 100 [10] and the fronto-naso-mental angle [11]. These measures do little however to distinguish TCS from Robin sequence. The presence of additional features such as microtias and down-slanting palpebral fissures can help secure a diagnosis. As a result, 3D or 4D sonographic imaging or prenatal magnetic resonance imaging is more likely to aid in the identification of characteristic facial features [12]. Chorionic villus sampling may also be used to help with the diagnosis in at-risk families or suspected fetuses [13].

Specific aspects of the evaluation to prioritize in a patient with TCS can be divided into different time points in a child's development. These include the neonatal period and infancy, childhood, adolescence, and adulthood. Note that the treatment during these periods is not separated, and they merge one in another (Fig. 14.1) [6].

TCS in the Neonate and Infant

Airway

Recognition of micrognathia and airway obstruction are primary concerns in a newborn with TCS. Airway obstruction may be identified with labored breathing, cyanosis, frank apneas, stridor, desaturations, feeding difficulties, and hemodynamic alterations. Mild cases may be managed with positional changes or a nasopharyngeal airway placement, while severe cases may require emergent intubation or tracheostomy [8, 14]. If time permits, a polysomnogram (PSG) in a dedicated pediatric sleep laboratory can aid in the diagnosis of pediatric obstructive sleep apnea, while also identifying the presence of hypoventilation and central apnea. In addition to micrognathia, choanal atresia, adenotonsillar hypertrophy, glossoptosis, tracheomalacia, and laryngomalacia may contribute to airway obstruction [15].

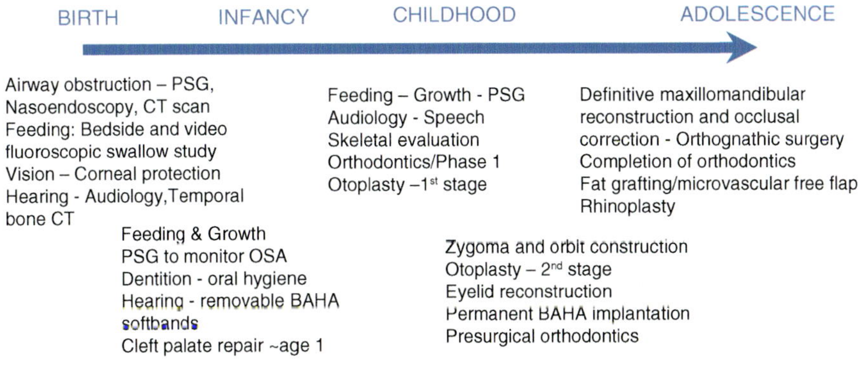

Fig. 14.1 Evaluation of patients with Treacher Collins syndrome at various stages of development

Choanal atresia, seen with a frequency of 14 to 28% in TCS, is stenosis or complete obstruction (atresia) at the nasal choana in the posterior nasal cavity. The obstructive tissue may be membranous and/or bony. This condition prevents the passage of air into the nasopharynx. Choanal atresia or stenosis may be unilateral or bilateral, with the former being more common as an isolated finding, whereas bilateral cases are more likely to be associated with a specific syndrome (i.e., CHARGE syndrome) and multiple other congenital anomalies [16]. A flexible nasoendoscopy, done awake or under intravenous sedation, should be considered to evaluate all sites of potential obstruction. A maxillofacial CT scan may help characterize the severity of choanal atresia and micrognathia and guide surgical treatment with computer-assisted planning or surgical navigation.

Feeding

Feeding difficulties, while often seen in the presence of airway obstruction, are compounded by the presence of a cleft palate. Infants are obligate nasal breathers, and the presence of choanal atresia may further hinder feeding. A bedside swallowing evaluation by an experienced member of the cleft and craniofacial team should be performed and should include an assessment of general tone, ability to latch, suck-swallow reflex, and oro-motor coordination. If a cleft palate is present, use of specialized bottles should be trialed under the guidance of a cleft palate feeding specialist. Caloric intake and weight changes should be monitored closely. Enteral feeding or a gastrostomy tube may be considered on an individual basis.

Ocular and Eyelid Anomalies

Eyelid abnormalities are often readily recognizable features of TCS. Patients may present with an eyelid coloboma, hypoplastic or missing eyelid appendages, downward slanting palpebral fissures, ectropion, excessive scleral show, and lagophthalmos. Exposure keratopathy may lead to corneal scarring, ulceration, and even blindness in severe cases and should be recognized and managed early. Ophthalmic ointments can be used in mild cases or as a temporizing measure in more severe instances. Early tarsorrhaphy may be considered in severe cases in consultation with a pediatric ophthalmologist or oculoplastic surgeon. Ophthalmological evaluation should be performed on a regular basis to assess vision and examine the cornea.

Hearing

Adequate hearing is a prerequisite for proper speech and language development and mandates early consultation and intervention. Most patients with TCS have at least a moderate conductive hearing loss, 58 dB loss on average, which correlates with the severity of external auditory canal and middle ear aberrations. The external auditory canal is often stenotic and may be atretic. Anomalies in the ossicular chain are common. The ossicles may be hypoplastic or ankylosed to the medial or lateral wall of the tympanic recess [17]. A pediatric otolaryngologist and audiologist must be part of the multidisciplinary team involved in the *initial* evaluation and provision of removable (i.e., removable bone conduction hearing aids (BAHA) headbands or softbands) and later implantable (i.e., permanent BAHA) hearing aids. Stenotic auditory canals need to be monitored for the development of cholesteatomas [6, 8, 18–20]. Patients with TCS should have serial audiological evaluations.

Speech

When cleft palate is present, special attention is given to determine the ideal timing for palatoplasty [6, 19, 21]. While there is data demonstrating that palatoplasty after 12 or 18 months of age increases the incidence of compensatory misarticulations, there are various factors that may delay timing of palate repair. Presence and severity of OSA, medical comorbidities, weight gain, cognitive development, and prelinguistic screening by a speech language pathologist may help guide the surgeon regarding timing of palatoplasty. Palatoplasty may worsen existing OSA or contribute to recurrent airway obstructions. Thus, a definite plan to manage and monitor the airway should be in place. Regular speech therapy appointments with a speech language pathologist on the cleft team are anticipated.

Genetics Counseling

Genetic consultation is typically sought to confirm the diagnosis of Treacher Collins syndrome (mandibulofacial dysostosis-1). Various genetic mutations have been identified that present with features of mandibulofacial dysostosis. These autosomal dominant types of mandibulofacial dysostosis include Guion-Almeida (MFDGA), Bauru, X-linked type Toriello, and Hedera-Toriello-Petty. Patients with CHARGE syndrome also present with auricular anomalies, choanal atresia, and hearing loss. While patients with oto-facial syndrome and those with a HOX2A gene mutations may present with deafness, microtia, and cleft palate.

Nager syndrome (NS) should be distinguished from Treacher Collins syndrome given the similarities in presentation. Nager syndrome usually presents more severe auricular deformation and limb defects that typically involve the anterior elements of the upper limbs and manifest as small or absent thumbs, triphalangeal thumbs, radial hypoplasia or aplasia, and radioulnar synostosis. Phocomelia of the upper limbs and, occasionally, lower limb defects have also been reported [22]. Regarding the affected genes, TCS is related to mutations of TCOF1, POL1B, POLR1C, and POLR1D genes, while NS is related to haploinsufficiency of SF3B4 gene (Table 14.1) [23].

Table 14.1 Clinical findings of main mandibulofacial dysostosis and its differential diagnosis

	Treacher Collins	Nager	CHARGE	HOXA 2 related	Oto-facial	Wieczorek et al. (2007)	OAVS	MD Toriello type	MD Toriello-Medera-Petty tyoe	MD Bauru type	MD Guion-Almeida type
Prenatal microcephaly	–	–	(–)	n.r.	+	+	(+)	+	–	–	+
Postnatal microcephaly	4%	–	(–)	n.r.	+	+	(+)	+	–	–	+
Global development delay	11%	–	>70%	n.r.	+	+	(+)	(+)	–	–	+
Craniofacial dysmorphism											
Palpebral fissures	Downslanting	Downslanting	Horizontal	n.r.	Upslanting	Upslanting	Horizontal	Downslanting	Downslanting	Upslanting	Upslanting
Lower eyelid coloboma	50%	+	–	n.r.	n.r.	–	–	–	–	–	–
Malar hypoplasia	100%	+	–	n.r.	n.r.	+	–	+	+	+	+
Microtia	78%	+	95–100%	+	+	+	+	+	+	+	+
Atresia/ stenosis of external auditory canal	27%	+	+	+	+	+	+	+	+	+	+
Preauricular tag	27%	+	+	–	n.r.	–	+	–	+	–	+
Buccal tag	–	n.r.	–	–	n.r.	–	+	–	–	–	–
Micrognathia	89%	+	+	n.r.	n.r.	+	+	+	+	+	+
Cleft palate	33%	+	15–20%	+	+	+	+	–	–	+	+
Choanal atresia	28%	+	35–65%	n.r.	n.r.	n.r.	+	–	–	–	–

Conductive hearing loss	88%	+	60–90%	+	+	+	+	+	+	–	–
Congenital heart defect	4%	+	50–85%	n.r.	n.r.	+	+	+	–	–	+
Limb anomalies	–	+	+	n.r.	+	+	–	–	–	–	+

‘+, present; – absent, n.r., not reported

The genetic counseling for a TCS patient and family consists in providing information related to the natural inheritance of the pathology and implications of the syndrome. It is advisable that individuals presenting at least two of the main phenotypic characteristics of the syndrome should undergo confirmative genetic testing [4–6, 23].

TCS in Childhood to Adulthood

As a child with TCS grows, general considerations include ongoing monitoring for vision and corneal protection, hearing assessments with audiology, speech, signs and symptoms of sleep disordered breathing, dental and jaw development, and psychosocial concerns. Among others, an orthodontist is typically involved in the care throughout childhood. Sleep disordered breathing should be monitored regularly and can be elicited verbally or assessed with screening instruments such as the PSQ (pediatric sleep questionnaire) [24].

Facial Skeletal Assessment

The maxillofacial assessment should include an evaluation of facial profile, symmetry, and proportions, as well as specific characterization of peri-ocular, zygomatic, nasal, auricular, and dental or occlusal abnormalities. Initial and follow-up facial and intra-oral photographs help document and track changes over time. Craniofacial features of TCS remain stable (non-progressive) over time, as demonstrated by similar facial proportions and extent of convexity between children and adults [25].

Two-dimensional cephalometric and panoramic radiographs help quantify the extent of maxillomandibular retrognathism relative to the neurocranium, airway narrowing, occlusion, and dental development. Furthermore, maxillomandibular growth and development can be followed with serial lateral cephalometric imaging. Three-dimensional imaging with computed tomography provides further detail to accurately characterize the severity of mandibular, temporal, and orbitomalar hypoplasia and dysmorphology.

Midface, Maxillary, and Oral Findings

Most patients with TCS have a prominent nasal dorsum with obtuse nasofrontal angle and a convex facial profile secondary to retro-micrognathia and normal nasomaxillary projection. Some patients present with a transversely hypoplastic maxilla, narrow palate, and increased buccal corridors on smile. In patients with a history of a cleft palate, maxillary hypoplasia may be present in all three planes of space. An anterior open bite with angle class 2 malocclusion is seen with increased frequency in TCS. The latter can be attributed to a hyperdivergent mandibular growth pattern and likely compensatory posterior vertical maxillary excess.

A standard occlusal and dental evaluation should be accomplished and include an assessment of oral hygiene, missing and impacted teeth, caries, and periodontal disease [26]. Dental anomalies such as tooth agenesis (33%), enamel opacities (20%), and ectopic eruption of the maxillary first molars (13%) are present in 60% of the individuals [7]. Patient with TCS requires care by a pediatric or general dentist, and age-appropriate orthodontic treatment and monitoring, and combined surgical orthodontics for future phases of care.

Mandible

The hyperdivergent facial form of patients with TCS is due to short posterior facial third, a steep mandibular and occlusal plane angle. Deep antegonial notching and a short chin throat length are characteristic features that result. These clinical findings have been confirmed with 2D cephalometric analyses of patients with TCS at various ages. These demonstrate a more acute skull base angle (B-S-N), an obtuse joint angle (S-Ar-Go), severely shortened ramus height (Ar-Go), a reduced mandibular corpus length (Go-Pg), increased lower anterior face height (ANS-Me), a very steep cranio-mandibular angle, a steep mandibular plane angle, and a retruded lower lip and chin [27].

In severe cases, the mandibular condyle and glenoid fossa of the temporomandibular joint (TMJ) may be severely hypoplastic and dysplasic, or absent. TMJ and myofascial dysfunction and ankylosis have all been reported. The latter may be iatrogenic as a complication of prior grafts or distraction osteogenesis surgery [28]. The masseter and temporalis muscles may be hypoplastic [29]. Clinical assessment should include a query about diet consistency tolerated, tenderness to palpation over the lateral TMJ capsule and muscle of mastication, TMJ noises with movement, maximal mouth opening, and protrusive and lateral excursive movements. The Jaw Functional Limitation Scale (JLFS) is a validated questionnaire that helps assess jaw function in patients with TMJ disorders and may be a helpful tool for any patient with syndromic TMJ abnormalities [30].

Zygoma and Orbit

Orbitomalar hypoplasia is a hallmark of TCS and involves both vertical and horizontal deficiencies, as well as asymmetries. Patients may also exhibit relative medial protrusion of the orbital walls, diminished length and projection of the lateral orbital rim, and greater than normal globe protrusion. Compared to controls, patients with

TCS have shorter zygomatic arch length, and smaller interzygomatic distances, as measured on axial CT scans [31]. Zygomatic dysmorphology and volume deficiency have been classified into three types, with type I being minor (all normal components with hypoplasia), type 2 being moderate (some normal components), and type 3 being severe (no normal components and inferior-lateral orbital cleft) [29].

Ocular

Hypoplasia and clefting of the lower eyelids, along with downward slanting of the palpebral fissures, are hallmarks of TCS. Depending on the severity of the lower lid retraction, and underlying bony support, definitive soft tissue reconstruction is usually better delayed until the bony orbitomalar reconstruction is completed.

Auricular

Microtia is a common feature of TCS, with the conchal type (grade 2 with external auditory stenosis) and lobular type (grade 3 with external auditory canal atresia) predominating. A smaller proportion of patients may have mild microtia (grade 1) with low-set ears. Rarely, anotia (grade 4) is seen. The severity of external auricular anomalies seems to correlate with the severity of ossicular anomalies and conductive hearing loss. Preauricular skin tags may also be present and are typically removed in infancy.

In addition to the soft tissue hypoplasia of peri-orbital and auricular structures, soft tissue hypoplasia or atrophy may be present in other parts of the face. A relative macrostomia is not unusual. A tightness of the soft tissue envelope, including the suprahyoid muscle attachments, may complicate surgical access and may limit the extent of bony advancement during orthognathic surgery.

Staging and Classifications

The OMENS classification has been previously described for Oculo-Auriculo-Vertebral Spectrum [32]. While not specific to TCS, it helps address some of the major findings of this syndrome when the zygomatic and peri-ocular findings are included. OMENS assigns a three-point grading scale to characterize hypoplasia, dysplasia, or aplasia or functional deficits involving the O – orbit; M, mandible; E, ears; N, nerve; and S, soft tissue.

Hayashi et al. described a grading system for patients with TCS that assigns a score for each of eight features of the syndrome, with increasing severity being given a higher number. The total cumulative score is then used to assign one of three grades. Features assessed included the malar bones, lower eyelids, mandible, ear, cleft palate, nasal root, other deformities, and mutation of TCOF1 [33].

Psychosocial Considerations

The identification and management of psychosocial disorders in patients with craniofacial differences is of critical importance. Low self-esteem, relationship difficulties, nonacceptance of his/her features, bullying, and prejudice are commonly reported by individuals with TCS [34].

A neuropsychologist or a psychologist familiar with craniofacial differences should be part of the craniofacial team to assess cognitive, emotional, and social development as well as assess family dynamics and available support. Diagnosable mental health disorders should be identified and managed. Psychological counseling and additional resources such as peer support groups can be offered to help build resilience and healthy coping skills and improve self-esteem and quality of life [6, 8, 35].

Patient Involvement in Decision-Making

Once a patient is mature enough, their active participation should be encouraged in treatment decisions. Time should be taken to help a patient understand their condition and the goals of various nonsurgical and surgical treatment options. Modifications to the treatment plan should be considered, once health conditions allow, based on the patient preference [33].

Conclusion

The initial assessment of a patient with TCS is critical to optimizing outcomes for affected individuals. Such a comprehensive assessment will confirm a diagnosis and evaluate the functional consequences of the anatomical features of the syndrome. From this point, a staged reconstruction can then be effectively planned prioritizing those impairments with the greatest impact on the health of the patient. Planning at this level of complexity is best accomplished in an interdisciplinary fashion with a team that comprises a pediatric otolaryngologist, ophthalmologist, geneticist, audiologist, a speech pathologist, cranio-maxillofacial surgeon, orthodontist, social worker, neuropsychologist, pediatric dentist, and care coordinator. Coordinating efficient and comprehensive care, while prioritizing patient and family needs, as well as quality of life, should be the guiding principles for all providers.

References

1. Gijn DR, Tucker AS, Cobourne MT. Craniofacial development: current concepts in the molecular basis of Treacher Collins syndrome. Brit J Oral and Maxillofac Surg. 2013;51:384–88. https://doi.org/10.1016/j.bjoms.2012.09.008.
2. Ravin JG. In the kingdom of the shah: Treacher Collins' persian adventure. Surv Ophthalmol. 1999;43:361–7. https://doi.org/10.1016/S0039-6257(98)00044-7.
3. Franceschetti A, Brocher JEW, Klein D. Dysostose mandibulo-faciale unilatérale avec déformations multiples du squelette (processus paramastoïde, synostose des vertèbres, sacralisation etc.) et torticolis clonique. Ophthalmologica. 1949;118:796–814. https://doi.org/10.1159/000300779.
4. Sakai D, Trainor PA. Treacher Collins syndrome: unmasking the role of Tcof1/treacle. Int J Biochem Cell Biol. 2009;41:1229–32. https://doi.org/10.1016/j.biocel.2008.10.026.
5. Kadakia S, Helman SN, Badhey AK, Saman M, Ducic Y. Treacher Collins syndrome: the genetics of a craniofacial disease. Int J Pediatr Otorhinolaryngol. 2014;78:893–8. https://doi.org/10.1016/j.ijporl.2014.03.006.
6. Chang CC, Steinbacher DM. Treacher Collins syndrome. Semin Plast Surg. 2012;26:83–90. https://doi.org/10.1055/s-0032-1320066.
7. Vincent M, Geneviève D, Ostertag A, Marlin S, Lacombe D, Martin-Coignard D, et al. Treacher Collins syndrome: a clinical and molecular study based on a large series of patients. Genet Med. 2016;18:49–56. https://doi.org/10.1038/gim.2015.29.
8. Posnick JC, Ruiz RL. Treacher Collins syndrome: current evaluation, treatment, and future directions. Cleft Palate-Craniofacial J. 2000;37:1–22. https://doi.org/10.1597/1545-1569_2000_037_0434_tcscet_2.0.co_2.
9. Crane JP, Beaver HA. Midtrimester sonographic diagnosis of mandibulofacial dysostosis. Am J Med Genet. 1986;25:251–5. https://doi.org/10.1002/ajmg.1320250209.
10. Paladini D, Morra T, Teodoro A, Lamberti A, Tremolaterra F, Martinelli P. Objective diagnosis of micrognathia in the fetus: the jaw index. Obstet Gynecol. 1999;93:382–6. https://doi.org/10.1016/S0029-7844(98)00414-1.
11. Palit G, Jacquemyn Y, Kerremans M. An objective measurement to diagnose micrognathia on prenatal ultrasound. Clin Exp Obstet Gynecol. 2008;35:121–3.
12. Kubo S, Horinouchi T, Kinoshita M, Yoshizato T, Kozuma Y, Shinagawa T, Ushijima K. Visual diagnosis in utero: Prenatal diagnosis of Treacher-Collins syndrome using a 3D/4D ultrasonography. Taiwan J Obstet Gynecol. 2019;58:566–9.
13. Edwards SJ, Fowlie A, Cust MP, Liu DTY, Young ID, Dixon MJ. Prenatal diagnosis in Treacher Collins syndrome using combined linkage analysis and ultrasound imaging. J Med Genet. 1996;33:603–6. https://doi.org/10.1136/jmg.33.7.603.
14. Plomp RG, Bredero-Boelhouwer HH, Joosten KFM, Wolvius EB, Hoeve HLJ, Poublon RML, et al. Obstructive sleep apnoea in Treacher Collins syndrome: prevalence, severity and cause. Int J Oral Maxillofac Surg. 2012;41:696–701. https://doi.org/10.1016/j.ijom.2012.01.018.
15. Perkins JA, Sie KCY, Milczuk H, Richardson MA. Airway management in children with craniofacial anomalies. Cleft Palate-Craniofacial J. 1997;34:135–40. https://doi.org/10.1597/1545-1569(1997)034<0135:AMICWC>2.3.CO;2.
16. Burrow TA, Saal HM, De Alarcon A, Martin LJ, Cotton RT, Hopkin RJ. Characterization of congenital anomalies in individuals with choanal atresia. Arch Otolaryngol Head Neck Surg. 2009;135:543–7. https://doi.org/10.1001/archoto.2009.53.
17. Pron G, Galloway C, Armstrong D, Posnick J. Ear malformation and hearing loss in patients with Treacher Collins syndrome. Cleft Palate-Craniofacial J. 1993;30:97–103. https://doi.org/10.1597/1545-1569(1993)030<0097:EMAHLI>2.3.CO;2.
18. Ma X, Forte AJ, Berlin NL, Alonso N, Persing JA, Steinbacher DM. Reduced Three-Dimensional Nasal Airway Volume in Treacher Collins Syndrome and Its Association with Craniofacial Morphology. Plast Reconstr Surg. 2015;135:885e–94e. https://doi.org/10.1097/PRS.0000000000001160.

19. Roberson JB, Goldsztein H, Balaker A, Schendel SA, Reinisch JF. HEAR MAPS a classification for congenital microtia/atresia based on the evaluation of 742 patients. Int J Pediatr Otorhinolaryngol. 2013;77:1551–4. https://doi.org/10.1016/j.ijporl.2013.07.002.
20. Marsella P, Scorpecci A, Pacifico C, Tieri L. Bone-anchored hearing aid (Baha) in patients with Treacher Collins syndrome: tips and pitfalls. Int J Pediatr Otorhinolaryngol. 2011;75:1308–12. https://doi.org/10.1016/j.ijporl.2011.07.020.
21. Heike CL, Wallace E, Speltz ML, Siebold B, Werler MM, Hing AV, et al. Characterizing facial features in individuals with craniofacial microsomia: a systematic approach for clinical research. Birth Defects Res Part A – Clin Mol Teratol. 2016;106:915–26. https://doi.org/10.1002/bdra.23560.
22. Stelnicki EJ, Lin WY, Lee C, Grayson BH, McCarthy JG. Long-term outcome study of bilateral mandibular distraction: a comparison of Treacher Collins and Nager syndromes to other types of micrognathia. Plast Reconstr Surg. 2002;109:1819–25. https://doi.org/10.1097/00006534-200205000-00006.
23. Bernier FP, Caluseriu O, Ng S, Schwartzentruber J, Buckingham KJ, Innes AM, et al. Haploinsufficiency of SF3B4, a component of the pre-mRNA spliceosomal complex, causes nager syndrome. Am J Hum Genet. 2012;90:925–33. https://doi.org/10.1016/j.ajhg.2012.04.004.
24. Chervin RD, Hedger K, Dillon JE, Pituch KJ. Pediatric sleep questionnaire (PSQ): validity and reliability of scales for sleep-disordered breathing, snoring, sleepiness, and behavioral problems. Sleep Med. 2000;1:21–32. https://doi.org/10.1016/S1389-9457(99)00009-X.
25. Roberts FG, Pruzansky S, Aduss H. An X-radiocephalometric study of mandibulofacial dysostosis in man. Arch Oral Biol. 1975;20:265–81. https://doi.org/10.1016/0003-9969(75)90124-7.
26. Magalhães MHCG. Barbosa da Silveira C, Moreira CR, Cavalcanti MGP. Clinical and imaging correlations of Treacher Collins syndrome: report of two cases. Oral surgery. Oral Med Oral Pathol Oral Radiol Endodontology. 2007;103:836–42. https://doi.org/10.1016/j.tripleo.2006.04.011.
27. Arvystas M, Shprintzen RJ. Craniofacial morphology in Treacher Collins syndrome. Cleft Palate-Craniofacial J. 1991;28:226–30. https://doi.org/10.1597/1545-1569(1991)028<0226:cmitcs>2.3.co;2.
28. Kaban LB, Moses MH, Mulliken JB. Surgical correction of hemifacial microsomia in the growing child. Plast Reconstr Surg. 1988;82:9–19. https://doi.org/10.1097/00006534-198882010-00003.
29. Wong KR, Pfaff MJ, Chang CC, Travieso R, Steinbacher DM. A range of malar and masseteric hypoplasia exists in Treacher Collins syndrome. J Plast Reconstr Aesthetic Surg. 2013;66:43–6. https://doi.org/10.1016/j.bjps.2012.07.028.
30. Ohrbach R, Larsson P, List T. The jaw functional limitation scale: development, reliability, and validity of 8-item and 20-item versions. J Orofac Pain. 2008;22:219–30.
31. Posnick JC, Al-Qattan MM, Moffat SM, Armstrong D. Cranio-orbito-zygomatic measurements from standard CT scans in unoperated Treacher Collins syndrome patients: comparison with normal controls. Cleft Palate-Craniofacial J. 1995;32:20–4. https://doi.org/10.1597/1545-1569(1995)032<0020:CMFSCS>2.3.CO;2.
32. Vento AR, LaBrie RA, Mulliken JB. The O.M.E.N.S. classification of hemifacial microsomia. Cleft Palate J. 1991;28:68–76. https://doi.org/10.1597/1545-1569(1991)028<0068:tomens>2.3.co;2.
33. Hayashi T, Sasaki S, Oyama A, Kawashima K, Horiuchi K, William M, et al. New grading system for patients with Treacher Collins syndrome. J Craniofac Surg. 2007;18:113–9. https://doi.org/10.1097/SCS.0b013e31802cf3ff.
34. Bemmels H, Biesecker B, Schmidt JL, Krokosky A, Guidotti R, Sutton EJ. Psychological and social factors in undergoing reconstructive surgery among individuals with craniofacial conditions: an exploratory study. Cleft Palate-Craniofacial J. 2013;50:158–67. https://doi.org/10.1597/11-127.
35. Beaune L, Forrest CR, Keith T. Adolescents' perspectives on living and growing up with Treacher Collins syndrome: a qualitative study. Cleft Palate-Craniofacial J. 2004;41:343–50. https://doi.org/10.1597/02-158.1.

Chapter 15
A Look at Breathing, Feeding, and Speech Problems in Patients with Treacher Collins Syndrome

Karin De La Fuente and Kevin E. Bright

The role of the speech pathologist in caring for patients diagnosed with Treacher Collins syndrome (TCS) is multifaceted and dynamic and requires interaction with multiple disciplines.

Collaboration with a strong interdisciplinary team helps to determine the services needed and clarify the treatment focus by integrating the expertise of all of the team members.

Treatment optimally starts during the prenatal period if the anatomic abnormalities are observed with prenatal ultrasound evaluation. Prenatal counseling can help the child's parents prepare for the birth of their child with special needs by familiarizing them with the sequence of evaluations and treatments which may be required and introducing them to members of the multidisciplinary team.

The earliest challenges which these children typically encounter are breathing and eating.

Breathing

At birth, breathing difficulties may be caused by mandibular hypoplasia and resultant hypopharyngeal obstruction. Temporomandibular joint anomalies, cleft palate, glossoptosis, and significant micrognathia combine to narrow the airway and can potentially result in acute respiratory distress.

K. D. L. Fuente
EL PASO SPEECH AND LANGUAGE SERVICE EXCELLENCE INC, El Paso, PA, USA
e-mail: kdelafuente@epslse.com

K. E. Bright (✉)
Department of Surgery, Texas Tech School of Medicine, Lubbock, TX, USA

El Paso Cleft Palate and Craniofacial Team, El Paso, PA, USA
e-mail: kbright@swent1.com

D. M. Yates, M. R. Markiewicz (eds.), *Craniofacial Microsomia and Treacher Collins Syndrome*, https://doi.org/10.1007/978-3-030-84733-3_15

Airway management may be necessary in the delivery suite, the newborn nursery, or the neonatal intensive care unit. If severe retrognathia is noted on prenatal ultrasound, a referral and prenatal evaluation by the craniofacial team is helpful in determining possible need for an EXIT procedure. The inferior facial angle is critical in measuring mandibular retrognathia and the need for a possible EXIT procedure prenatally. A decreased inferior facial angle (IFA) is a reliable predictor of retrognathia as measured on US. It is measured by taking the intersection of two lines: (1) a line perpendicular to the vertical part of the forehead, drawn at the level of the synostosis of the nasal and frontal bones, and (2) a line from the tip of the mentum and the anterior border of the more protrusive lip. An IFA of >2 standard deviations from normal (65.5°) corresponds with an angle of <50 degrees and is a reliable indicator for retrognathia (Figs. 15.1a–c and 15.2) [1]. Of neonates presenting with micrognathia, 54% require immediate airway support from simple positioning to tracheotomy [2, 3] (Figs. 15.1a–c and 15.2). If it is determined EXIT procedure is not needed, immediate helpful interventions may include prone positioning, placement of a nasal trumpet, or an oral airway with use of supplemental oxygen therapy. Should these interventions fail to provide relief, a tongue stitch or intubation may be required.

Securing an airway in these children is frequently challenging. Providers attempting to intubate these children should be familiar with the challenges associated with their unusual anatomy. When the child is stable from a respiratory perspective, the intubation attempt should be carefully planned. Different facilities have different

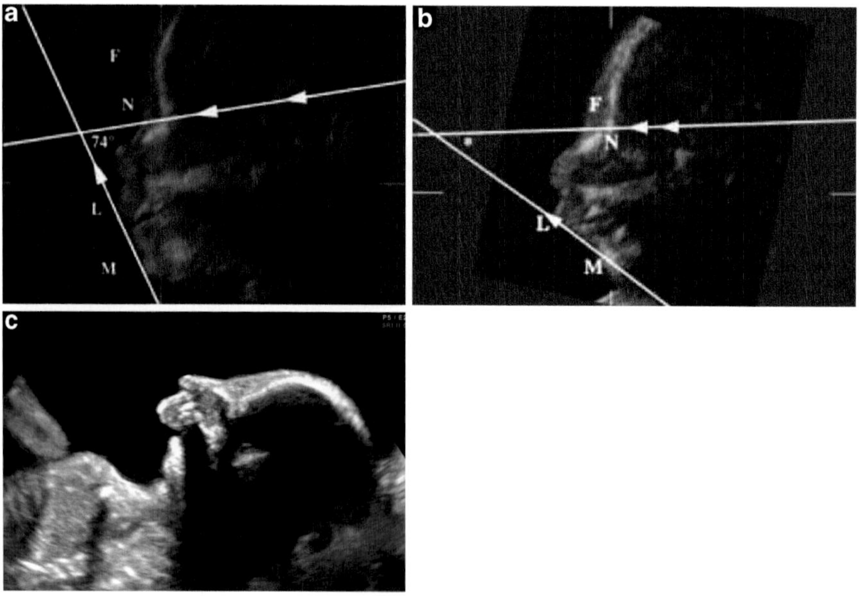

Fig. 15.1 (**a**) Normal mandible inferior facial angle. (**b**) Retrognathic mandible inferior facial angle. (**c**) Mid-sagittal view of prenatal ultrasound demonstrating severe micrognathia

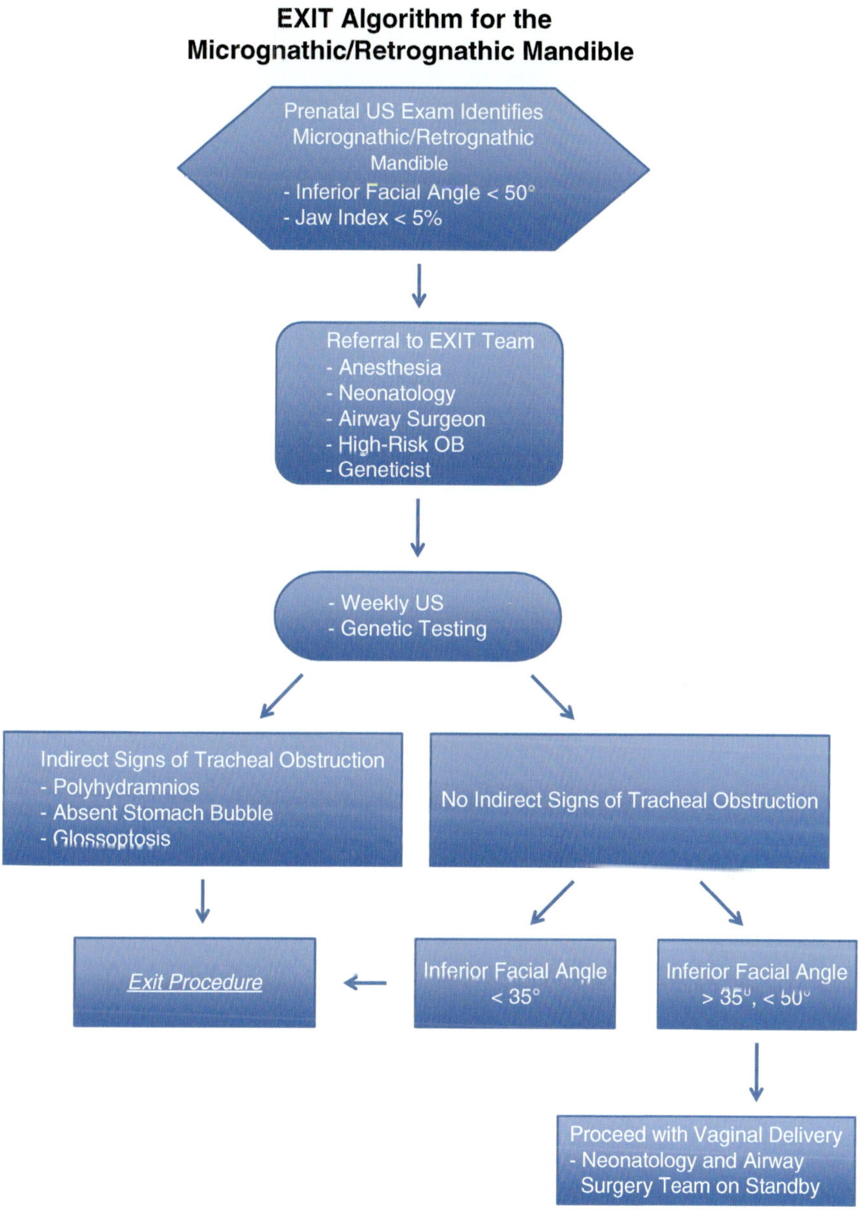

Fig. 15.2 EXIT algorithm

resources, so familiarity with the instrumentation available is essential. Anesthesia services and otolaryngology services may collaborate in the management of these difficult airways.

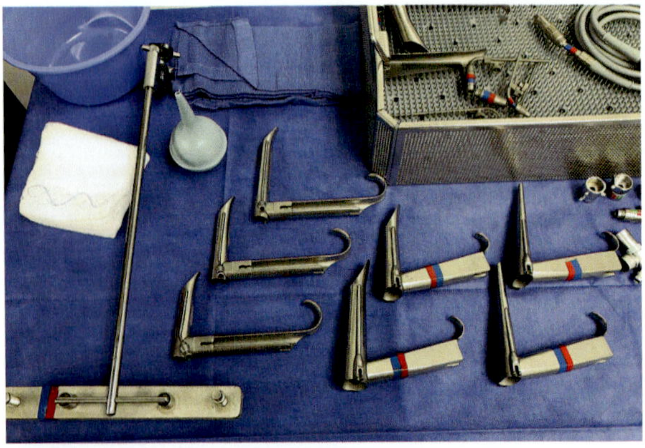

Fig. 15.3 Pediatric laryngoscopes

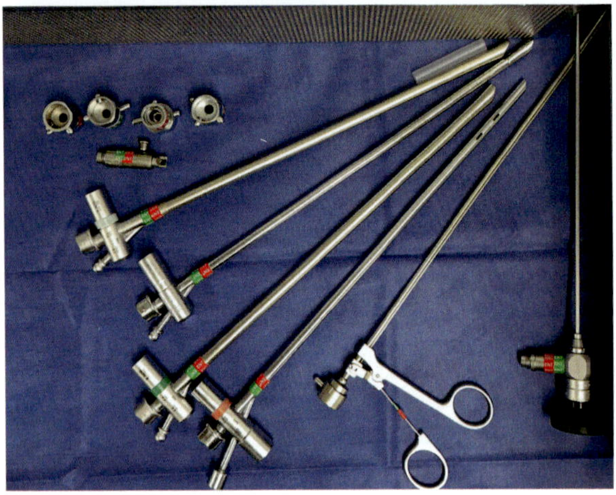

Fig. 15.4 Rigid ventilating bronchoscopes

Treacher Collins syndrome airways are especially challenging secondary to limited ability to open the mouth, crowding of the posterior oropharynx by the tongue, and a very anterior glottis. Some of these children may be successfully intubated using standard direct laryngoscopy with a McIntosh or Miller laryngoscope. Frequently a stylet in the endotracheal tube is helpful. When the glottis cannot be adequately visualized in a standard fashion, alternative techniques should be available. In some circumstances, a laryngeal mask airway (LMA) may fit and be a satisfactory way to ventilate the patient.

A Storz Parson's slotted neonatal/pediatric laryngoscope will frequently allow visualization of the very anteriorly located glottis and allow for intubation (Fig. 15.3). Visualization may also be accomplished in many cases using a rigid pediatric ventilating bronchoscope to place an endotracheal tube changing bougie and then sliding the tube over the bougie to intubate (Fig. 15.4). Glide scopes have become increasingly popular for managing difficult pediatric airways and frequently have a role in intubating these patients. There is a role particularly in older patients

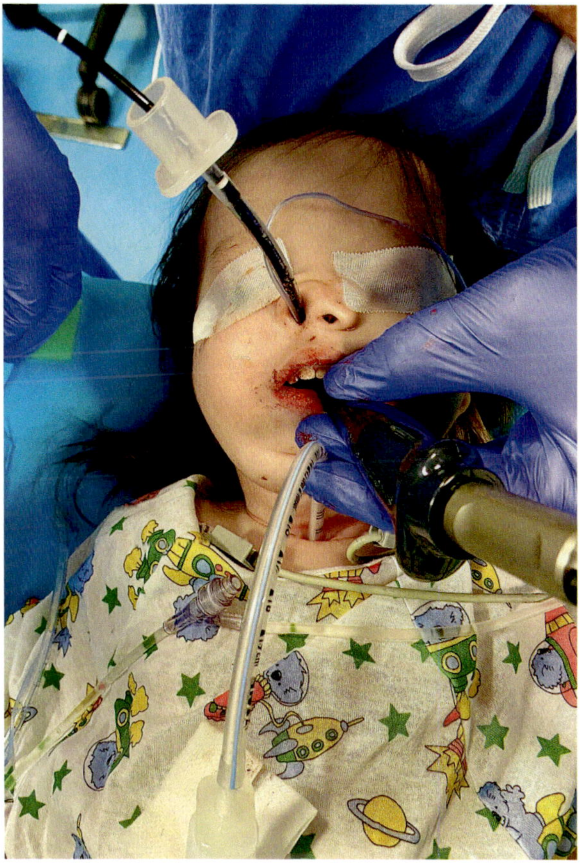

Fig. 15.5 Treacher Collins airway exam—flexible nasopharyngoscope with endotracheal tube per right nare; simultaneous use of glidescope to help identify vocal cords to aid in intubation from above

for flexible fiberoptic trans-nasal intubation of these patients (Fig. 15.5). Oral intubation of these children has also been accomplished in a retrograde fashion by placing a percutaneous guidewire through the skin of the neck into the trachea, bringing it out of the mouth or nose, and sliding the endotracheal tube over the wire to intubate.

Multiple attempts at oral intubation may cause significant swelling and further compromise the airway causing prolonged hypoxia and neurologic complications. Selecting the most skilled provider available to perform the intubation is generally advisable.

In children with the most severely abnormal airways, it is important to be prepared to perform an urgent tracheostomy at the time of the attempted oral or nasal intubation. The tracheostomy instrumentation should be completely set up and the surgeon fully prepared to surgically intervene.

For TCS children with less critically compromised airways who are failing to thrive, a discussion of early surgical interventions could include a lip tongue adhesion, tracheostomy, or early distraction osteogenesis with mandibular advancement.

The timing of any palate repair should also take into account the absence or presence of any ongoing airway obstruction.

A lip/tongue adhesion is a short-term intervention which can allow the mandible time to grow. It can be well tolerated; however it is of limited use in this population generally due to the degree of retrognathia. It will typically need to be taken down when the lower front teeth erupt.

A tracheostomy has been and remains the most dependable way to treat moderate to severe hypopharyngeal obstruction. It is not however without significant morbidity and risks. Children with tracheostomies require significantly greater resources. These includes prolonged hospitalization, parental training, possible need for ongoing skilled nursing, and expensive durable medical supplies. The mortality associated with a tracheostomy is said to be 1% for each year that the tracheostomy remains in place. The mortality and morbidity associated with a tracheostomy are multifactorial. It is associated with plugging, inadvertent decannulation, drowning, and infections. An additional disadvantage to tracheostomy in infants and young children is the adverse effect which the procedure may have on the development of speech and language.

Children with chronic hypopharyngeal obstruction frequently fail to thrive not only as a result of increased work of breathing and hypoxia but also because they have difficulty eating and breathing concurrently. Once they receive a tracheostomy, the patient frequently will be able to tolerate oral intake without difficulty. As a result, the tracheostomy procedure may help these children avoid placement of a gastrostomy tube. This can be greatly beneficial developmentally because it helps prevent the oral aversion that is frequently seen in children who are fed with a gastrostomy tube. Most TCS patients who require a tracheostomy are ultimately decannulated!

Maxillary and mandibular advancement when appropriate are also used to resolve upper airway obstruction and can help to avoid the need for a tracheostomy in some skeletally mature patients. This option will be discussed thoroughly in later chapters.

Tracheostomy Considerations for the SLP

Airway Assessment

The speech language pathologist needs to be familiar with the management of infants, children, and occasionally teens or young adult TCS patients with a tracheostomy. The issues which need to be addressed vary by age and the indication for the tracheostomy. This will be part of the evaluation process and the baseline for further assessments.

Communication with the neonatologist, pulmonologist, intensivist, otolaryngologist, nurse, and respiratory therapist may all be helpful in developing an appropriate SLP treatment plan.

Factors to consider in assessment:

1. Information about oxygenation, mode of ventilation, and tolerance.
2. Visual inspection of structures and missing anatomic components.
3. Tracheostomy type.
   (a) Cuffed, cuffless, inflated or deflated, oxygen support.
4. TCS patients with tracheostomy tubes may not want to have their tracheostomy removed because it provides them a sense of security.
5. Instruction on how to care for the tracheostomy may be provided by the surgeon, the nurse, and/or the speech language pathologist.

Treatment

The role of the speech language pathologist is to complete a dynamic assessment of airway tolerance and to coordinate the follow-up and support the pulmonologist's recommendations.

1. Decannulation can be considered or recommended when:
   (a) The upper airway is patent.
   (b) Oral and tracheal secretions are minimal.
   (c) Capping/plugging or use of a speaking valve is well tolerated.
   (d) The risk of aspiration has been assessed.
   (e) The patient can tolerate cuff deflation (if applicable).
   (f) The upper airway is being used for respiration, cough, throat clearing, and speech.

If the patient can manage their secretions, swallows safely, tolerates capping of the tube or prolonged use of a Passy Muir Valve, and does not need the tracheostomy to remain in place for pending surgical procedures, then decannulation may be considered and will likely be tolerated.

When patients do not meet the criteria for decannulation, the speech therapist's primary role is to assist them with communication and eating.

The structural abnormalities associated with TCS can contribute to sleep apnea. Breathing anomalies may not be evident at birth, but over time failure to thrive may become more evident due to increased work of breathing with hypoxia and/or hypercapnia. In these patients, a pediatric polysomnogram can determine the severity of the obstructive sleep apnea and determine whether supplemental oxygenation, nasal CPAP, oral pharyngeal surgery, or tracheostomy is necessary

Feeding

Respiratory complications may affect oral feeding at birth. Coordination of breathing and swallowing is primordial, and when affected, alternate modes of nutrition must be considered.

These babies present with flat or missing cheekbones, low-set ears with microtia and/or atresia, and micrognathia. They may also present with a cleft palate.

These abnormalities affect normal function:

1. Decreased intra-oral pressure (suck).
2. Increased risk of aspiration.
3. Difficulty coordinating breathing and swallowing.

Feeding Assessment

The evaluation starts with a thorough review of the case history, complications at birth, and initial craniofacial assessment by the physician. Initial assessment will focus on coordination of breathing and swallowing with careful observation of breathing with stress and movement, followed by an assessment of nutritive and nonnutritive sucking.

In some instances, delayed feeding problems may arise due to prematurity, long-term hospitalization, and an impaired sensory system.

If the breathing and swallowing are not coordinated, then an alternative mode of nutrition may become necessary. This problem may be short or long term. If oral feeding appears to be safe, determining a feeding method that will deliver adequate nutrition safely and in a timely basis is the next step.

Examination begins with a visual inspection of oral structures, primitive reflexes, sensory responses to touch, and movement. Non-nutritive sucking provides an impression of intraoral pressure and coordination and assesses fatigue and tolerance.

This portion of the assessment includes direct observation, monitoring of respiratory status, tolerance, positioning, and response to pacing. These observations provide a basis upon which recommendations can be made. After the initial assessment and formulation of a treatment plan, intermittent monitoring may be warranted.

When there are signs or symptoms of possible aspiration including rapid changes in breathing with movement, etc., SLP evaluation may be deferred until the child is stable. If there are overt signs or symptoms of possible aspiration, a modified barium swallow may be indicated to ensure that the feeding method chosen does not result in aspiration.

When a complete oral assessment has been completed and if the child is not meeting nutritional goals from breast or bottle, alternative feeding strategies will need to be considered. A feeding system which decreases the need for negative intraoral pressure particularly in those TCS children with cleft palates may need to be provided.

There are a wide array of feeders available that may allow the child to meet their nutritional needs. These vary in availability and cost. Feeding success is determined by trial and error. (Dr. Brown's Specialty Feeding System, SpecialNeeds Feeder by Medela®, Haberman Feeder, and Pigeon feeder with one-way valve are commonly used commercially available options.)

Posture, time to complete feeding, and patient/parent tolerance will need to be monitored simultaneously.

Most mothers will want to breastfeed or use their breast milk. Lactation consultants can be a valuable resource. Counseling and support for pumping and providing breast milk via bottle can be extremely beneficial.

Not all TCS children will tolerate oral feeds even with specialty feeders. In some instances, oral feeding may need to be augmented alternatively to reduce nutritional and/or respiratory compromise. When the nutritional requirements cannot be met with oral feeds, temporary feeding with a nasogastric tube, gavage feeds, or placement of a gastrostomy tube may need to be considered. As mentioned previously, children who undergo a tracheostomy will frequently be able to tolerate oral feedings shortly after surgery. Strong consideration should be given in any TCS child who requires tracheostomy tube placement to postponing gastrostomy tube placement until after a post-tracheostomy swallow evaluation has been completed.

Cultural Competence

The speech language pathologist and the craniofacial team as a whole need to be familiar with different cultural beliefs about craniofacial anomalies and breastfeeding and be able to determine the family's level of trust in the medical profession.

A culturally competent professional will be open minded and provide education accordingly.

The mother's need to be able to feed her child is incredibly important, and their input is important during the decision-making process.

Treatment Goals for the SLP

1. In the NICU, establishing a safe oral mode of nutrition while maintaining a safe airway and assisting with nutritional needs.
2. Reassessing, teaching, supporting, and communicating with key team members.
3. Change of nipples, modification of posture, reevaluation under fluoroscopy, and reeducation.
4. Troubleshooting different textures and identifying foods that cannot be part of the diet due to mastication difficulties.
5. Transition from alternative mode of nutrition to oral feeding.

Not all TCS patients will have feeding problems, but for those that do, the speech language pathologist's skills and timely interventions will prove invaluable.

Speech

The structural abnormalities associated with Treacher Collins syndrome have multiple effects on the development of speech and language. These patients have abnormal intraoral relationships. Their tongues are disproportionately large in relation to their oral cavity. They frequently have cleft palates. Their mandibles do not move normally. They typically have significant hearing loss associated with microtia and atresia. All these factors contribute to speech and language anomalies.

Speech Assessment

An interdisciplinary evaluation that provides information on hearing, musculoskeletal changes, maxillofacial abnormalities, and past and future surgeries is part of a thorough speech assessment. Information from the parents, teachers, caregivers, and from the patient help complete the evaluation.

The evaluation progresses as the patient ages, and their speech needs will evolve as they mature. A good sound inventory and speech intelligibility at both word and conversational level should be documented. Assessment of resonance and how it affects overall intelligibility is particularly valuable and should when possible be standardized and ideally recorded to determine responses to therapy and surgical interventions. When a cleft palate is present and timeline for closure is determined, the SLP will tailor the therapy to coordinate with the surgery.

Stimulability for correction, when possible, should be assessed. Identification of obligatory errors and compensatory errors with comparison to norms is part of the comprehensive evaluation.

Determination of whether direct therapy can improve articulation, resonance, or both and the design of a treatment plan may be dependent upon endoscopic evaluation of the nasopharyngeal and hypopharyngeal anatomic structures and their relationships. The timing of future maxillofacial surgeries and associated recovery periods should be considered when creating a speech and language treatment plan.

Successful assessment of communicative competence with language comprehension and expression, combined with appropriate SLP therapy, in conjunction with surgical repair of anatomic defects, can diminish the risk of social isolation and ensure that appropriate supports are in place.

Treatments

Integration of testing results, patient prognosis, and current and future patient's goals will allow design of a therapy plan that will have a major impact on communicative effectiveness. Some TCS patients have communication challenges that are so severe that they may need to develop nonverbal communication skills as well. Many of these patients will learn to sign.

Hearing loss can contribute significantly to their communication challenges. Most TCS patients will require amplification and/or otologic surgery to treat their hearing loss and allow them to communicate verbally. The SLP works closely with the audiologist and otolaryngologist tailoring the therapy plan based on the patient's ability to hear.

Co-articulation probing, modification of sound production, and dynamic changes to treatment throughout the surgical and reconstructive journey are necessary parts of successful treatment planning.

Open communication between parents, teachers, audiologists, and SLPs is needed to maximize progress.

Fine-tuning of the treatment plan involves addressing those sounds (determined through analysis) that will maximize speech intelligibility. Focusing on these will provide the most rapid improvement (pick the low-hanging fruit first).

Treatment is dynamic as surgeries can modify resonance and/or assist with articulation.

Tonsillectomy with or without adenoidectomy, palatoplasty, and jaw surgeries all may improve the impaired resonance in this population. Treatment plans may need to be modified before, during, and after these surgeries are completed. These procedures all alter the oral and nasal pharyngeal spaces which will affect breathing, sleep, resonance, and articulation.

The Role of the Speech Language Pathologist in the Medical Setting vs. the School Setting

Medical Setting

The primary focus is on establishing breathing and swallowing coordination while maintaining nutrition and preventing aspiration. Collaboration with the medical team, provision of education to the primary caregiver, and conducting dynamic assessments are the main responsibilities of the medical speech language pathologist. These interactions can be direct or indirect depending upon the unique needs of the individual.

Typical involvements would include:

1. Initial consultation.
2. Re-evaluation.
3. Parental training/instruction.
4. Frequent feeding sessions and establishing postural modifications.
5. Determination of the optimal nipple/feeder.
6. Providing supportive and informative education to the primary caregiver.

School Setting

The school speech language pathologist will typically:

1. Assess speech and language skills.
2. Follow up on hearing evaluation recommendations.
3. Develop a customized educational plan including therapy to help the student with TCS maximize their educational opportunities (TCS patients have normal intelligence!).

Prioritizing therapy and focus in the TCS patient requires knowledge and education. These patients will undergo multiple surgeries, which will affect resonance and articulation. Treatment modifications coordinated with the surgical team will help streamline services and allow the patient to improve to the best of their ability.

Evaluation for an alternative mode of communication may be necessary when speech intelligibility is severely affected. The selected system may be temporary or permanent but will need to be dynamically assessed as the patient develops language and their communication needs change.

The focus is to help the patient be understood by others outside of his immediate environment.

There are social factors that the school speech language pathologist can address. Children with TCS often live their lives with significant facial disfigurement. Their appearance puts them at high risk of bullying and victimization.

The school speech language pathologist can provide education about TCS to key staff prior to enrollment. Role playing to provide more tools for social communication may improve social competence and independence.

Referral to a counselor or psychologist can be initiated by any member of the team to help the patient manage social challenges and provide the tools needed to overcome them.

Velopharyngeal insufficiency (VPI) is a challenge in the school setting. Articulation may be intact, but VPI may dramatically diminish intelligibility. Evaluation methods and treatment modalities have improved in recent years. An endoscopic nasal examination can determine which surgical intervention is most appropriate and clarify the therapy goals for the SLP. Complete velopharyngeal competence is not always surgically or therapeutically attainable.

Speech Therapy Focuses for VPI

1. Placement.
2. Articulation.
3. Precision of strong consonants.
4. Using coarticulation to reduce velopharyngeal insufficiency.
5. A strong plan that fosters repetition and follow-up.

The mandibular deformities associated with TCS result in difficulty in opening and closing the jaw. This further affects their intelligibility. The school speech language pathologist can focus on strengthening voice projection and articulation precision to facilitate speech intelligibility.

The role of the speech language pathologist in caring for the Treacher Collins patient is multi-faceted, dynamic, and collaborative. The multidisciplinary craniofacial team approach to the evaluation, treatment, management, and education of TCS patients is considered the standard of care.

References

1. Rotten D, et al. The fetal mandible: a 2D and 3D sonographic approach to the diagnosis of retrognathia and micrognathia. Ultrasound Obstet Gynecol. 2002;19(2):122–30.
2. Morris LM, et al. Severe micrognathia: indications for EXIT-to-airway. Fetal Diagn Ther. 2009;26(3):162–6.
3. Vettraino IM, et al. Clinical outcome of fetuses with sonographic diagnosis of isolated micrognathia. Obstet Gynecol. 2003;102(4):801–5.

Chapter 16
Associated Systemic Health Conditions Associated with Treacher Collins Syndrome

Pat Ricalde and Imran Ahson

Treacher Collins syndrome (TCS) is a well-known condition that was named after Edward Treacher Collins, an English surgeon and ophthalmologist, who described its essential traits in 1900 [1]. There have been many publications since that time further analyzing and characterizing the features of the syndrome, discussing its etiology, genetic abnormalities, embryologic changes in the first and second branchial arches, as well as reports describing a myriad of treatment options. There is limited information, however, on the systemic manifestations associated with the syndrome. Since there is a wide spectrum of phenotypes, these manifestations may affect patients differently. A patient's craniofacial malformations should not be addressed in isolation. Rather, patients with Treacher Collins syndrome should be assessed with a holistic approach, taking into consideration how their syndrome may affect all body systems. The focus of this chapter is to review the literature and outline a review of systems that is appropriate to engage with patients with TCS. This list is by no means exhaustive, as the literature is heavily influenced by the unique craniofacial characteristics of this syndrome; we aim to redirect the focus to a patient-centric approach to management.

P. Ricalde (✉)
Florida Craniofacial Institute, University of South Florida, St. Joseph's Cleft & Craniofacial Center, Tampa, FL, USA
e-mail: ricalde@flcranio.com

I. Ahson
New Hampshire Oral and Maxillofacial Surgery, Nashua, NH, USA

D. M. Yates, M. R. Markiewicz (eds.), *Craniofacial Microsomia and Treacher Collins Syndrome*, https://doi.org/10.1007/978-3-030-84733-3_16

Nutrition

Patients with Treacher Collins syndrome can have difficulty feeding due to their craniofacial differences. Feeding difficulties may occur shortly after birth due to an associated cleft palate or micrognathia. There have been case reports describing infants with failure to thrive, need for nasogastric tube feeding, and even gastrostomy tube feeding. Typically, people with this syndrome have normal feeding reflexes and an appropriate swallowing mechanism. If they have a cleft palate, they cannot create negative pressure to allow transfer of milk from a breast or from a normal bottle into their mouth. Specialized bottle and nipples have been developed to allow for a mechanical form of milk expression, to allow for the infant tongue or alveolar ridges to compress the nipple to transfer milk. Or, they will allow the caregiver to compress the bottle or nipple to mechanically express milk into the infant's mouth. This can also be very important in infants with TCS who have mandibular retrognathia or glossoptosis, which can substantially increase their work of breathing. The increased work of breathing will make it more difficult to maintain an appropriate suck/swallow pattern while simultaneously maintaining their oxygen saturation. Often the amount of work to breathe may burn more calories than the feeding will provide, and the infant will not gain weight adequately. Increasing calories to their formula or breast milk may help, but it is most important to decrease the work of breathing by making the feeding process more efficient. Often feeding therapy by a certified speech and language therapist can help overcome difficulties to avoid surgical intervention. It is also important to assess for narrowing or obstruction of the nasal airways (choanal stenosis or atresia) [2]. This, too, will increase work of breathing as infants are obligate nasal breathers. Flexible endoscopy can help to evaluate for laryngomalacia as well, which may not be directly related to TCS but will certainly complicate feeding issues.

Difficulty feeding can also lead to abnormalities of bone mineral density and nutritional deficits. Specialized formula can be provided to offset these deficits but requires early nutritional intervention [3]. Patients with Treacher Collins syndrome should be followed closely to make sure they are feeding and gaining weight appropriately, and any deviation from normal should prompt early nutrition and/or gastroenterological evaluation. Feeding issues in infancy can be very stressful for caregivers and must be discussed and managed with calm, nurturing providers of care. Not all treatment options will be accepted by families in the same way. Consideration of the home environment, social support networks, and religious and cultural beliefs must all be made before finalizing the infant's feeding plan.

Head and Neck

People with Treacher Collins syndrome have a characteristic facial appearance, and the craniofacial manifestations of this syndrome will be more closely outlined elsewhere. However, the characteristic craniofacial appearance can create symptoms that affect the entirety of the child's development, and must therefore be addressed promptly, oftentimes before surgical intervention. For example, it may become evident during a review of systems that the patient has many ocular complaints, due to dry eyes, chronic tearing, chronic rubbing or eye redness, squinting, poor focusing or trouble following objects, or sensitive eyes. These may be the result of canthal dystopia, orbital lipodermoids, limbal dermoids, microphthalmos, anophthalmos, cataracts, lacrimal duct atresia, pupillary ectopia, uveal colobomas, paucity of eyelashes, or visual impairment [4]. Many symptoms may also be a result of surgical interventions to try and manage these conditions. Surgical scarring around the eyelids or complications from periorbital surgery can lead to entropion or ectropion, or abnormal lacrimal drainage systems [5]. The characteristic downward slanting palpebral fissures and adnexal hypoplasia/aplasia often leave a patient with Treacher Collins syndrome with a strong stigma of a person with facial differences, so both functional and aesthetic differences need to be considered during the review of systems.

Vision can be affected early in life, with many patients having amblyopia, anisometropia, refractive errors, strabismus, and visual loss [6]. Visual loss can lead to problems with learning as well as delays in all areas of development. In adults, it can lead to difficulty with daily activities, such as reading mail, watching television, paying bills, or walking up and down stairs. It can also affect psychosocial development and family relations and will require early therapy services.

All neonates with Treacher Collins syndrome need a formal otolaryngology and auditory assessment due to the common otologic manifestations. Patients typically present with external ear abnormalities including absent, small, or malformed ears, external auditory canal stenosis or atresia, as well as middle ear malformations. Otoscopy may be difficult or impossible. Up to 50% of patients will have associated conductive hearing loss. Children with hearing loss often can interact socially on equal terms with children without hearing impairment [7]. The child's ability to develop social skills will depend on their age, degree of hearing loss, time of diagnosis, treatment, and personality of the child and family dynamics. Hearing loss needs to be addressed early and aggressively because it can lead to speech delays, language delays, and social delays. Often children benefit from preferential classroom seating, and treatment, usually in the form of hearing aids. Early amplification is an important intervention, with band hearing aids for younger children and later bone-anchored hearing aids. Final rehabilitation usually involves fitting a BAHA with or without pinna epithesis and close audiology follow-up.

As mentioned above, nasal issues such as choanal stenosis/atresia can cause nasal breathing and feeding issues, which can affect nutrition, weight gain, and respiratory issues. These symptoms can occur throughout the patient's life and should be monitored closely by their craniofacial team.

Neurologic

Patients with Treacher Collins syndrome have normal intelligence. There can be various indirect effects on the neurologic system, however, as evidenced by secondary losses to cranial nerve function regarding visual deterioration and hearing loss.

It has also been reported that patients with TCS can have difficulty with balance and coordination requiring physiotherapy [8]. This is not from any direct effect on the vestibular system but may have some association with hearing loss. In general, hearing loss has been shown to be negatively associated with other neurologic systems as well. Hearing loss (whether bilateral or unilateral) may also be related to dementia in older adults [9]. Although intelligence is not affected in Treacher Collins syndrome, developmental delays are strongly associated with visual impairment and with hearing loss, both of which are common in this condition. Expectant management of cognition, especially in the developmental years, is much more effective than retroactive management.

Respiratory

When reviewing the respiratory system, one needs to focus questions based on patient age. Patients with Treacher Collins syndrome often have micrognathia or glossoptosis that will leave a neonate in distress immediately after birth. They may have periods of time when they are doing quite well but then may also deteriorate and have severe obstructive sleep apnea. Left untreated, chronic upper airway obstruction can lead to cor pulmonale and other apnea-associated conditions. Because they have decreased airflow through the upper airway, this can occur at any time, with varying degrees of severity. It is always important to ask about snoring but also to do sleep apnea-targeted screener questionnaires based on the patient's age [10]. There are many screeners available that have been evaluated for correlation with OSA in children. These can be used easily in the office setting, to help guide the clinician regarding proper timing for reevaluation with a polysomnogram. See below for one such example, the Pediatric Sleep Questionnaire (Fig. 16.1).

Taking into account the patient's age is important when evaluating for sleep apnea, as each age group will present differently. Neonates typically present with failure to thrive, whereas young children may present with small stature, hyperactivity, or bedwetting (in a previously potty-trained child). Other symptoms that are important to ask about include behavioral changes, poor attention, daytime drowsiness, or hyperactivity. Older children may describe shortness of breath and tachypnea or may report choking at night and difficulty staying asleep [10]. Older children may also present with the classic adult signs and symptoms of obstructive sleep apnea including difficulty concentrating, daytime somnolence, falling asleep easily doing quiet activities, and mood swings. Speaking with a child's teacher may also be helpful in diagnosing nonspecific symptoms, such as disruptive behavior in class. Chronic sleep deprivation in adults can lead to a myriad of other symptoms including sadness, decreased libido, irritability, etc.

The gold standard for evaluation of sleep is overnight polysomnography at a sleep laboratory or appropriately qualified facility. Recordings usually include four channel electroencephalogram (EEG), right and left electrooculogram (EOG), and submental electromyogram (EMG). Ribcage and abdominal wall movements are measured using respiratory inductance plethysmography. Pulse oximetry, EKG, and

	Yes	No	Don't Know
While sleeping does your child			
Snore more than half the time?			
Always snore?			
Snore loudky?			
Have "heavy" or loud breathing?			
Have trouble breathing or struggle to breathe?			
Have you ever...			
Seen your child stop breathing during the night?			
Does your child...			
Tend to breathe through the mouth during the day?			
Have a dry mouth on waking up in the morning?			
Occasionally wet the bed?			
Wake up feeling un-refreshed in the morning?			
Have a problem with sleepiness during the day?			
Has a teacher or other supervisor commented that your child appears sleepy during the day?			
Is it hard to wake your child up in the morning?			
Does your child wake up with headaches in the morning?			
Did your child stop growing at a normal rate at any time since birth?			
Is your child overweight?			
This child often...			
Does not seem to listen when spoken to directly			
Has difficulty organizing tasks			
Is easily distracted by extraneous stimuli			
Fidgets with hands or feet or squirms in seat			
Is "on the go" or often acts as if "driven by a motor"			
Interrupts or intrudes on others (e.g. butts into conversations or games)			

Total Number of "Yes" Responses ________________

If eight or more statements are answered "yes" , consider referring for sleep evaluation

Fig. 16.1 Pediatric sleep questionnaire (Chervin et al. [28])

body position are also usually recorded. Apnea hypopnea index (AHI) is usually defined as the number of apneas and hypopneas per hour of sleep, while oxygen desaturation index (ODI) was defined as the number of oxygen desaturations ≥3% per hour of sleep. Mild obstructive sleep apnea (OSA) is defined as AHI 5–15 in adults and AHI 1–5 in children, moderate OSA as AHI 15–30 in adults and AHI 5–10 in children, and severe OSA as AHI >30 in adults AHI >10 in children [10].

Obstructive sleep apnea is very common in patients with Treacher Collins, varying in prevalence from 46 to 100% [11]. Severity of apnea is independent from the severity of the phenotype, so close clinical follow-up is required, even in mildly affected patients. Many clinicians advise polysomnography to be repeated periodically throughout life when clinical suspicion arises. Repeating a sleep questionnaire over time allows the provider to perhaps notice changes in sleep that may benefit from further follow up.

Cardiovascular

There have been isolated reports of patients with Treacher Collins syndrome having cardiac malformations, although this is rare. In normal development, some neural crest cells migrate to form aspects of the aortopulmonary and conotruncal complex, as well as being involved in the formation of the semilunar valves. Ablation of these cells in experimental models has led to truncus arteriosus, transposition of the great vessels, double outlet right ventricle, tetralogy of Fallot, and the absence of various combinations of aortic arch arteries [12]. Theoretically, TCS could lead to any of these malformations. Isolated case reports in the literature include tetralogy of Fallot, transposition of the great vessels, and sinus of Valsalva aneurysm [13, 14]. Presenting symptoms in these isolated case reports included (in the case of tetralogy of Fallot and transposition of the great vessels) bluish coloration of the skin, poor weight gain, and shortness of breath during feeding. These two cases were found shortly after birth. Of note is that some of these abovementioned conditions are disorders of the connective tissue of the heart and its vessels, leading to issues later in life rather than in the patient's early years. In one case, a man suffered a sinus of Valsalva aneurysm; the only presenting symptom was shortness of breath at 48 years old. The aneurysm was found on clinical follow-up after vague symptoms including chest pain and coughing [14].

Congenital heart defects can be broadly divided into two types: cyanotic heart defects and acyanotic heart defects. These can be classically differentiated by the potential to turn blue or not based on shunting of the heart from the right side to the left side (cyanotic) versus left side to the right side (acyanotic) [15]. This classification is shown below in Fig. 16.2.

Cyanotic heart disease is usually diagnosed early in the child's life, due to bluish discoloration of the patient's skin and more immediate and obvious symptoms. These include episodes of syncope, squatting as a compensatory mechanism, and

Cyanotic Heart Disease	Acyanotic Heart Disease
Decreased Pulmonary Flow • Tetralogy of Fallot • Tricuspid Atresia • Other univentricular heart with pulmonary stenosis Increased Pulmonary Flow • Transposition of great arteries • Total anomalous pulmonary venous return	Left to Right Shunting of Flow • Ventricular Septal Defect • Atrial Septal Defect • Atrio-Ventricular Septal Defect • Patent Ductus Arteriosus Obstruction of Flow • Aortic Stenosis • Pulmonary valve stenosis • Coarctation of the Aorta

Fig. 16.2 Classification of congenital heart disease

fatigability. Digital clubbing may be a late presentation as well. Acyanotic heart disease does not include the bluish tinge to the skin but can cause the patient to be easily fatigued. These patients are usually diagnosed by heart murmur and can have respiratory symptoms such as coughing due to congestive heart failure. Long term, all patients with congenital heart defects can have growth retardation [16]. Close clinical follow-up with a cardiologist is recommended for any of these symptoms.

Another consideration are cardiovascular consequences of long-standing obstructive sleep apnea (OSA). Patients with TCS are at higher risk of relapse of OSA even after treatment. Therefore, if symptoms warrant it, a workup should commence to include repeat polysomnogram if needed.

Gastrointestinal

The altered craniofacial complex can lead to issues with oral feedings, failure to thrive, and nutritional deficits that can lead to distention, constipation, diarrhea, and belly pain. Children tend to be poor historians with lower GI symptoms, so patients' parents should be asked about feeding patterns and changes in mood. There should be a high index of suspicion for gastroesophageal reflux and regurgitation, which is common in patients with Treacher Collins syndrome. Classic symptoms such as sore throat and postnasal drip are most diagnostic but are often hard to elicit [17]. Vague symptoms such as excessive crying or colic, sleep disturbance, night coughing, or bad taste in the mouth should warrant referral to a GI specialist. Also, unexplained chronic rhinitis or sinusitis may be present. For those patients who are fed via gastrostomy tube, symptoms such as nausea and vomiting, constipation or diarrhea, and/or bloating or distention need to be monitored. These symptoms may be associated with an incorrect volume of tube feeds being delivered or could be due to reflux [18, 19].

In the same manner that neural crest cells may contribute to cardiac development, animal models have shown the role of the TCOF1 gene in ganglionic cell migration of the foregut. This can lead to colonic aganglionosis in mice, although the same results in humans have not been seen. Giabacini et al. reported a case of chronic intestinal pseudo-obstruction in a child with Treacher Collins syndrome [20]. These issues of the ganglionic cells failing to migrate can lead to a decrease in gastric motility. Although rare, intestinal motility issues such as these can lead to constipation or bloating and should be investigated.

Genitourinary

Cryptorchidism is the most common trait found in patients with TCS, although other rare conditions such as micropenis and anovaginal fistula have been reported [13]. Apart from a general evaluation of the genitourinary area, symptoms such as blood in the urine, painful urination, testicular pain, or an asymmetric or nonpalpable testis should be referred to a pediatric urologist immediately. Referral to a pediatric urologist is of paramount importance before the first year of life to manage the potential complications of cryptorchidism. These include infertility or subfertility, testicular cancer, testicular torsion, and inguinal hernia. Even after a surgical intervention (orchiopexy), the testis can still ascend and be susceptible to potential sequelae. Parents and children should be taught to examine and monitor this area themselves and report any suspicious findings, especially masses. Children with cryptorchidism are much more susceptible to testicular cancer, despite intervention [21].

Treatment can be hormonal, surgical, or both. Surgery is usually dependent on whether the testes are palpable and should occur between 6 months and 2 years of age. Delays in treatment can lead to lower surgical success, increased rates of testicular cancer, and probable impairment of spermatogenesis [22].

Dental

It is important to ask about masticatory dysfunction, tooth or jaw pain, and speech articulation disorders, as these issues may all be a consequence of the oral manifestations of Treacher Collins syndrome. Due to many variables, high levels of plaque and low effectiveness of tooth brushing have been described in patients with TCS. Many patients will also have Pierre Robin sequence, which includes micrognathia, a tongue that is displaced farther back in the mouth than normal (glossoptosis), and cleft palate. Even in patients where the palate fuses, it may remain high arched which can result in dental crowding and jaw malformation. These patients often present with jaw and dental abnormalities, such as teeth that are hypoplastic and/or misaligned (malocclusion) [23]. Tooth agenesis occurs in 60% of patients (most commonly lower second premolars) as well as occasional clouding or discoloration of the enamel of teeth (enamel opacity) and ectopic eruption of maxillary molars [24]. In addition, these patients may have decreased salivary flow, mouth breathing, and orthodontic crowding. These all can exacerbate oral disease such as gingivitis, periodontitis, and carious lesion formation. Salivary flow is known to increase caries index, and half of all TCS patients have some form of salivary gland dysplasia or aplasia. Despite decreased salivary flow, there are typically minimal complaints of salivary dryness [25]. Despite these predisposing conditions, patients with routine dental care can have normal oral health without high caries levels.

Psychiatric

Living with a craniofacial difference can be very challenging for children and adults and can lead to a number of psychiatric issues. Even in comparison to other children with craniofacial disorders, adults with TCS report higher levels of depression and lower levels of overall quality of life, well-being, and physical health-related quality of life [26]. To be clear, these children aren't born with depression or stress; it is their experiences with other people that lead to feelings of isolation and difficulty with socialization. TCS patients often report feeling isolated due to their facial appearance, which can lead to a lack of socialization and stress during social settings [27]. These outcomes can be expectantly managed, with excellent results shown with early and frequent pediatric psychiatric intervention. It is important for surgeons to be keenly aware of these issues and to be mindful when recommending procedures for "aesthetic" reasons, especially around the eyes and cheekbones, since these procedures often leave the patient with multiple interventions with little gain. The stigma of a facial difference in TCS is rarely corrected with surgery but rather with thought-provoking conversation and acceptance. It is more important to develop self-confidence and self-esteem during childhood, rather than subject these children to numerous ill-proven and minimally effective treatments and interventions trying to make them "look normal."

Conclusion

Although primarily a craniofacial syndrome, patients with Treacher Collins syndrome can have systemic involvement. Also, like many challenging craniofacial syndromes, patients with TCS are at risk for being lulled toward surgical "corrections" that will "normalize" their appearance. This thought process from well-meaning clinicians will usually lead to multiple failed or repeated interventions with little true gain for the patient and increased financial and psychological exhaustion. It is important as surgeons to consider holistic management with true multidisciplinary treatment for these patients.

Works Cited

1. Beighton G. The man behind the syndrome. London: Springer Science & Business Media; 2012. p. 173. ISBN 9781447114154.
2. Andrade EC, et al. Treacher collins syndrome with choanal atresia: a case report and review of disease features. Braz J Otorhinolaryngol. 2005;71(1):107–10. ScienceDirect,. https://doi.org/10.1016/S1808-8694(15)31296-9.
3. Durán GA, Castillo MÉB, Teja ÁE, et al. Problematic feeding in newborn patient, stomatological approach. Case report. Rev Odont Mex. 2012;16(4):285–93.
4. Hertle RW, Ziylan S, Katowitz JA. Ophthalmic features and visual prognosis in the Treacher-Collins syndrome. Br J Ophthalmol. 1993;77:642–5.
5. Bartley GB. Lacrimal drainage anomalies in mandibulofacial dysostosis. Am J Ophthalmol. 1990;109(5):571–4. ScienceDirect,. https://doi.org/10.1016/S0002-9394(14)70688-9.
6. Shete P, et al. Treacher collins syndrome. J Oral Maxillofac Pathol. 2011;15(3):348–51. PubMed Central. https://doi.org/10.4103/0973-029X.86722.

7. Wingfield A, Peelle JE. How does hearing loss affect the brain? Aging Health. 2012;8(2):107–9. PubMed Central. https://doi.org/10.2217/AHE.12.5.
8. da Rodrigues BGS, et al. Evolution of a child with treacher collins syndrome undergoing physiotherapeutic treatment. Fisioterapia Em Movimento. 2015;28(3):525–33. SciELO,. https://doi.org/10.1590/0103-5150.028.003.AO11.
9. Lin FR. Hearing loss and cognition among older adults in the United States. J Gerontol A Biol Sci Med Sci. 2011;66A(10):1131–6. PubMed Central,. https://doi.org/10.1093/gerona/glr115.
10. Chervin RD, et al. Pediatric sleep questionnaire (PSQ): validity and reliability of scales for sleep-disordered breathing, snoring, sleepiness, and behavioral problems. Sleep Med. 2000;1(1):21–32. ScienceDirect,. https://doi.org/10.1016/S1389-9457(99)00009-X.
11. Akre H, et al. Obstructive sleep apnea in treacher collins syndrome. Eur Arch Otorhinolaryngol. 2012;269(1):331–7. Springer Link. https://doi.org/10.1007/s00405-011-1649-0.
12. Walker MB, Trainor PA. Craniofacial malformations: intrinsic vs extrinsic neural crest cell defects in treacher collins and 22q11 deletion syndromes. Clin Genet. 2006;69(6):471–9. Wiley Online Library,. https://doi.org/10.1111/j.0009-9163.2006.00615.x.
13. Katsanis SH, Jabs EW. Treacher collins syndrome. In: GeneReviews®. Seattle: University of Washington; 1993.
14. Nikola D, et al. Treacher collins syndrome. Circulation. 2013;128(2):e12–3. ahajournals.org (Atypon). https://doi.org/10.1161/CIRCULATIONAHA.113.001588.
15. van der Linde D, et al. Birth prevalence of congenital heart disease worldwide: a systematic review and meta-analysis. J Am Coll Cardiol. 2011;58(21):2241–7. www.onlinejacc.org. https://doi.org/10.1016/j.jacc.2011.08.025.
16. Linde LM, et al. Growth in children with congenital heart disease. J Pediatr. 1967;70(3, Part 1):413–9. ScienceDirect,. https://doi.org/10.1016/S0022-3476(67)80139-2.
17. Shepherd RW, et al. Gastroesophageal reflux in children: clinical profile, course and outcome with active therapy in 126 cases. Clin Pediatr. 1987;26(2):55–60. DOI.org (Crossref),. https://doi.org/10.1177/000992288702600201.
18. Yi DY. Enteral Nutrition in Pediatric Patients. Pediatr Gastroenterol Hepatol Nutr. 2018;21(1):12–9. PubMed Central,. https://doi.org/10.5223/pghn.2018.21.1.12.
19. Singhal S, et al. Tube Feeding in Children. Pediatr Rev. 2017;38(1):23–34. pedsinreview.aappublications.org. https://doi.org/10.1542/pir.2016-0096.
20. Giabicani E, et al. Chronic intestinal pseudo-obstruction in a child with treacher collins syndrome. Arch Pediatr. 2017;24(10):1000–4. ScienceDirect,. https://doi.org/10.1016/j.arcped.2017.07.004.
21. Thorup J, et al. What is new in cryptorchidism and hypospadias—a critical review on the testicular dysgenesis hypothesis. J Pediatr Surg. 2010;45(10):2074–86. www.jpedsurg.org,. https://doi.org/10.1016/j.jpedsurg.2010.07.030.
22. Docimo SG, et al. The undescended testicle: diagnosis and management. Am Fam Physician. 2000;62(9):2037–44.
23. Åsten P, et al. Orofacial functions and oral health associated with treacher collins syndrome. Acta Odontol Scand. 2013;71(3–4):616–25. Taylor and Francis+NEJM. https://doi.org/10.3109/00016357.2012.700065.
24. Duque C, Cardoso IL. treacher collins syndrome and implications in the oral cavity. Clin Res Trials. 2019;5:1–5. bdigital.ufp.pt,. https://doi.org/10.15761/crt.1000278.
25. Østerhus IN, et al. Salivary gland pathology as a new finding in treacher collins syndrome. Am J Med Genet A. 2012;158A(6):1320–5. Wiley Online Library,. https://doi.org/10.1002/ajmg.a.35331.
26. Geirdal AØ, et al. Living with orofacial conditions: psychological distress and quality of life in adults affected with treacher collins syndrome, cherubism, or oligodontia/ectodermal dysplasia—a comparative study. Qual Life Res. 2015;24(4):927–35. Springer Link,. https://doi.org/10.1007/s11136-014-0826-1.

27. Lefebvre AM, Arndt EM. Working with facially disfigured children: a challenge in prevention. Can J Psychiatry. 1988;33(6):453–8. DOI.org (Crossref),. https://doi.org/10.1177/070674378803300605.
28. Chervin RD, et al. Pediatric sleep questionnaire: validity and reliability of scales for sleep disordered breathing, snoring, sleepiness, and behavioral problems. Sleep Med. 2000;1:21–32.

Chapter 17
Ophthalmologic Findings and Reconstruction of Soft Tissue Orbital Deformities: Coloboma and Eyelid Deformities

Ashish Francis, Shika Andhole, Raymond Harshbarger, Patrick Kelley, and Malena M. Amato

Clinical Findings

Orbital Features

The periorbital soft tissue dysmorphism seen in patients with Treacher Collins syndrome is greatly influenced by the skeletal malformation affecting the zygoma and the orbit. The normal cross-sectional anatomy of the orbit and lower eyelid is shown in Fig. 17.1. While a discussion regarding the midfacial bony deficiencies is discussed elsewhere in this text, a brief overview is worth highlighting given its impact on the overlying soft tissues. Tessier noted that the bilateral periorbital deformity seen in patients with Treacher Collins syndrome was a manifestation of clefts 6, 7,

A. Francis (✉)
Department of Surgery and Perioperative Care, The University of Texas at Austin Dell Medical School, Austin, TX, USA

Division of Craniofacial and Pediatric Plastic Surgery, Dell Children's Medical Center of Central Texas, Austin, TX, USA

Division of Craniofacial and Pediatric Plastic and Reconstructive Surgery, Akron Children's Hospital, Akron, OH, USA

S. Andhole
The University of Texas at Austin, Austin, TX, USA

R. Harshbarger · P. Kelley
Department of Surgery and Perioperative Care, The University of Texas at Austin Dell Medical School, Austin, TX, USA

Division of Craniofacial and Pediatric Plastic Surgery, Dell Children's Medical Center of Central Texas, Austin, TX, USA

M. M. Amato
Department of Ophthalmology, The University of Texas at Austin Dell Medical School, Austin, TX, USA

D. M. Yates, M. R. Markiewicz (eds.), *Craniofacial Microsomia and Treacher Collins Syndrome*, https://doi.org/10.1007/978-3-030-84733-3_17

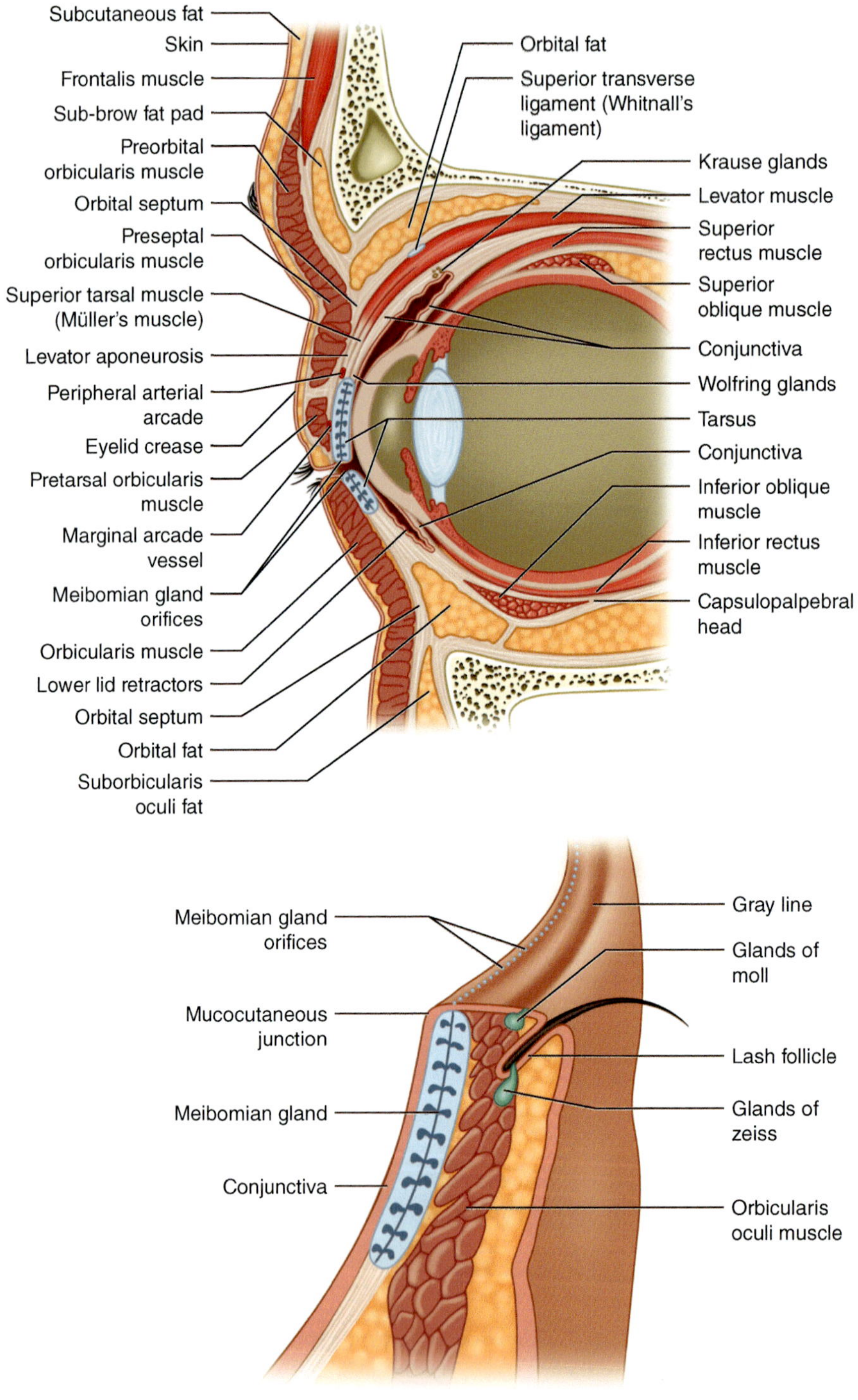

Fig. 17.1 Normal cross-sectional anatomy of the orbit (*above*) and lower eyelid (*below*). Note the bilamellar structure of the lower eyelid (anterior lamella consisting of skin and orbicular is oculi; posterior lamella consisting of tarsus and conjunctiva)

and 8 (Fig. 17.2) [1, 2]. The tissues affected in TCS arise early in embryonic development within the first and second branchial arches.

In combination, the clefts isolate the zygoma and produce malar deficiency. However, the degree of involvement resulting from the clefts is variable. For example, clinical forms of Treacher Collins syndrome have been described as complete, incomplete, abortive, unilateral, or atypical by Franceschetti and Klein [3]. The complete form presents with all features of the syndrome, whereas the incomplete form produces less severe malformations. The abortive form is largely confined to soft tissue abnormalities of the eyelid. Furthermore, the location of the deficiency on the zygoma can be medial, lateral, or a combination, presumably reflecting varying expression of the clefts.

The number 6 cleft accounts for the medial malar hypoplasia and extends toward the mandibular angle. The number 8 cleft affects the lateral orbital wall with deficiency at the zygomaticofrontal suture. Given the deficiency of the lateral orbital wall, the lateral canthal attachment can be attenuated or absent, creating the downward-slanting palpebral fissure. The zygomatic deficiency causes the orbit to become shallow with inferolateral rotation, thereby creating an elliptical orbital shape [4]. The hypoplastic orbito-zygomatic complex also creates a perception of enophthalmos due to the normal nasal and frontonasal development and size (Fig. 17.3) [5].

The contribution of these underlying bony periorbital anomalies to clinical findings has been confirmed radiographically with computed tomographic (CT) data [6]. The average orbital width, as measured between medial and lateral walls, is normal. However, when utilizing the lateral orbital rim as a reference, lateral orbital

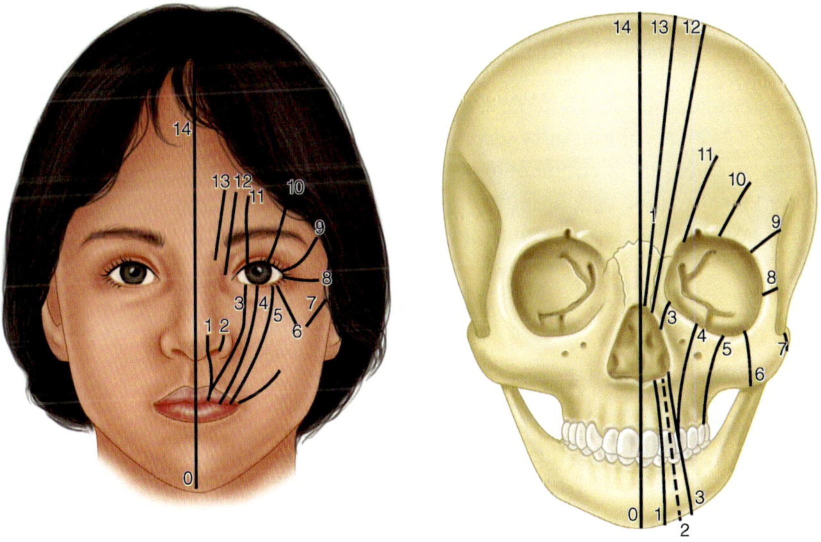

Fig. 17.2 Tessier classification of craniofacial clefts. Treacher Collins syndrome is the result of Tessier clefts 6, 7, and 8. *Left*: soft tissue clefts. *Right*: skeletal clefts

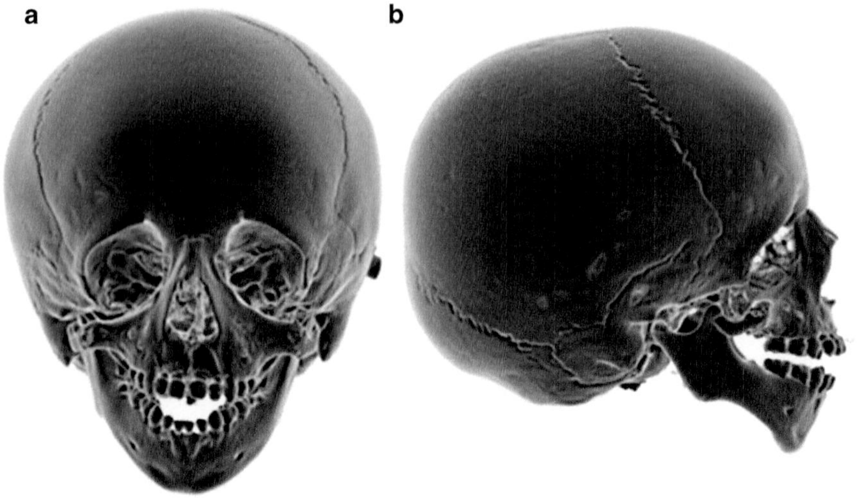

Fig. 17.3 Three-dimensional computed tomography (CT) scan representation of the orbital-zygomatic manifestations of two patients with Treacher Collins syndrome. Note the absent lateral orbital wall, elliptical shape of the orbit with inferolateral rotation (**a**), and the zygomatic deficiency producing a shallow orbit (**b**) (Reprinted with permission from Katowitz and Katowitz [19])

depth in affected patients is deficient, as manifested by decreased lateral orbital wall length, greater exophthalmos, and relative increased medial orbital wall protrusion. Orbital volume and shape are also affected [7]. Significant central orbital and lateral orbital depth deficiency are present, whereas medial orbital depth is unchanged. The lateral orbital depth deficiency correlates with the clinical findings of inferolateral orbital-zygomatic hypoplasia. The central orbital deficiency and normal medial orbit depth can be considered distinctive of the syndrome. Moreover, orbital volumes are decreased in Treacher Collins patients compared to unaffected patients. However, orbital volume in syndromic patients typically normalizes with age, suggesting a catch-up phenomenon may occur with the orbit in these patients [7]. While there is limited data regarding the evolution of the deformity over time, a small case series also demonstrated relative stability with facial growth over time [8].

Ophthalmic Features

A review of the literature demonstrates a paucity of data regarding the ophthalmologic manifestations of Treacher Collins syndrome. The main findings will be discussed, although a comprehensive overview is beyond the scope of this text. Hertle and colleagues presented a case series of 24 patients with Treacher Collins syndrome [9]. All patients had an ophthalmologic abnormality that included refractive errors (58%), vision loss (37%), strabismus (esotropia, exotropia, cranial nerve palsy; 37%), and amblyopia (33%), all of which commonly require treatment. They found that vision loss was likely due to amblyopia. While vision improved with treatment, normal visual acuity was not obtained at follow-up and remained unequal (anisometropia) between the eyes in the majority of patients. Amblyopia may have multiple etiologies, including refractive error, keratopathy from poor ocular surface protection due to eyelid anomalies, and deprivation amblyopia from congenital cataracts and upper eyelid ptosis to name a few. Oblique astigmatism is common in affected patients due to the downward-slanting palpebral fissure, as the slanting of the fissure affects corneal curvature [10, 11].

Congenital cataracts, uveal colobomas, microphthalmos, and anophthalmos have also been documented in Treacher Collins syndrome [9]. Other case reports have reported rare findings including microcornea, retinal detachment, corneal scleralization, and uveal, lens, and retinal dysmorphology [12, 13]. Corneal scarring, exposure keratopathy, ulceration, and ultimately blindness may occur as a result of inadequate globe protection from the lower eyelid colobomata [14]. Assessment for an intact Bell's phenomenon is also important for the integrity of the corneal surface.

Eyelid and Adnexal Features

Initial case reports of Treacher Collins syndrome focused on the ocular and periorbital findings. Indeed, one of the early descriptions of Treacher Collins syndrome was in 1889 by Scottish ophthalmologist Dr. George Andreas Berry, who discussed the congenital lower eyelid colobomas [15]. The periorbital findings were later expanded in Edward Treacher Collins' 1900 case report of two patients [16]. In fact, three of the four necessary features for a diagnosis Treacher Collins syndrome, as asserted by Axelsson in 1963, relate to periorbital findings: antimongoloid palpebral fissures, lower eyelid abnormality (coloboma, deficient lashes), malar hypoplasia, and mandibular hypoplasia [17]. Many still consider the complex soft tissue periorbital features to be characteristic of the syndrome (Fig. 17.4).

The number 6 soft tissue cleft produces the lower eyelid coloboma beginning at the junction of the middle and lateral third of the eyelid; it also contributes to the antimongoloid slant [1, 2]. Studies demonstrate that clefting early in embryogenesis produces larger colobomas and results in greater abnormalities of the developing eye and ocular surface. On the other hand, colobomas occurring later tend to be smaller and are associated with less functional malformations of the underlying globe [18]. Eyelid true colobomas describe congenital, full-thickness defects, and pseudocolobomas refer to hypoplastic subcutaneous tissue and muscle with loss of the posterior lamella. Pseudocolobomas may be the more commonly encountered deformity in Treacher Collins syndrome (Fig. 17.5) [19]. Multiple large series demonstrate that lower eyelid colobomas are found in greater than 50% of cases [20, 21]. The hypoplastic soft tissues associated with pseudocolobomas may result in thin lower eyelid skin and deficient orbicularis oculi muscle, the latter which exacerbates eyelid laxity and predisposes to ectropion [14].

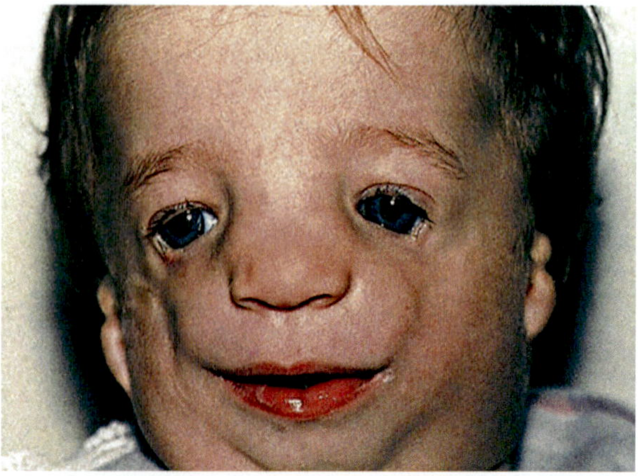

Fig. 17.4 The periorbital features of Treacher Collins syndrome are characteristic of the condition. Noted in this patient are the antimongoloid slant, lateral lower eyelid pseudocoloboma, absence of the medial lower eyelashes, and the orbital-zygomatic hypoplasia (Reprinted with permission from Katowitz and Katowitz [19])

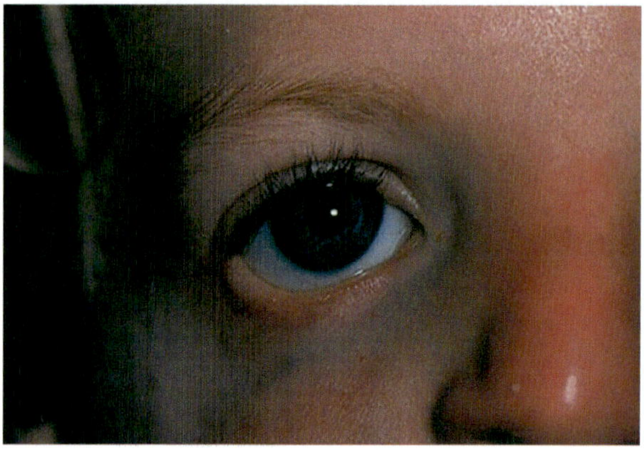

Fig. 17.5 Lateral lower eyelid pseudocolobomas, rather than true colobomas, are more commonly seen in Treacher Collins syndrome. They are characterized by hypoplastic skin and orbicularis with varying involvement of the posterior lamella (Reprinted with permission from Katowitz and Katowitz [19])

The overlying soft tissues in the area of the number 8 cleft at the lateral orbital rim and zygoma are respectively dysmorphic. The orbicularis oculi continuity is disrupted in this region with loss of lateral canthal fixation, lateral canthal dystopia, and eyelid laxity and retraction. In combination with the inferolateral extension of the number 6 cleft, the phenotype presents as a downward-slanting palpebral fissure, producing the distinctive antimongoloid slant. The palpebral fissure morphology has been shown to be the most consistent finding in patients with Treacher Collins syndrome [9, 18, 20]. Lateral canthal dysmorphology and its effects were further elucidated by Bachelor and Kaplan, who noted absent lateral canthal tendon in two patients [22]. It produced lower eyelid retraction with rounding and medialization of the lateral canthus that was more pronounced with forced eyelid closure. Other findings include a shorter horizontal palpebral fissure length at rest with a decrease on closure (termed the "fissure narrowing sign") [10]. The lower eyelid may also be vertically deficient due to tethering of the orbital septum to the inferior orbital rim.

Other soft tissue findings associated with Treacher Collins syndrome include dacryostenosis, blepharoptosis, ectropion and entropion, ciliary abnormalities, and epibulbar dermoids [9, 10, 23]. Lacrimal system dysfunction produces epiphora. Lacrimal anatomy is demonstrated in Fig. 17.6. Bartley identified a high prevalence of inferior punctal and inferior canalicular atresia (Fig. 17.7) in a case series with 70% of patients experiencing epiphora [24]. Complete absence of the inferior lacrimal puncta has also been documented [10]. Congenital blepharoptosis is occasionally seen, and severity ranges from mild to severe, depending on the deficiency of levator palpebrae muscle function. This phenotype may be the result of a variant of Treacher Collins syndrome [10, 25]. Ptosis may also result in amblyopia from visual axis distortion. Ectropion is associated with abnormalities of the eyelid support structures (tarsus and lateral canthal tendon) and anterior lamellar vertical deficiency (Fig. 17.8). Varying degrees of scleral show are observed and can produce

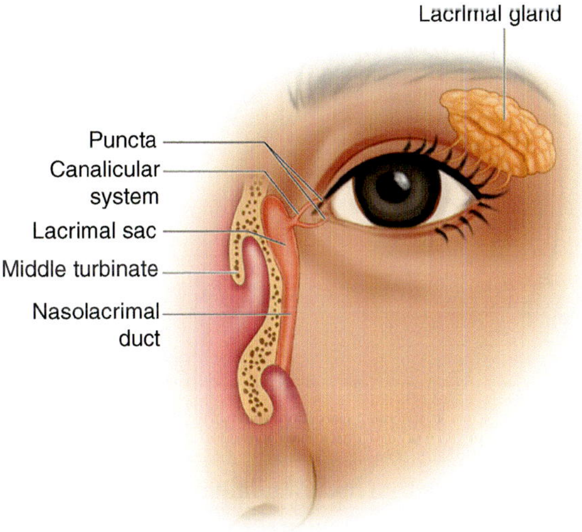

Fig. 17.6 Lacrimal system anatomy. The proximal apparatus is generally affected in Treacher Collins syndrome

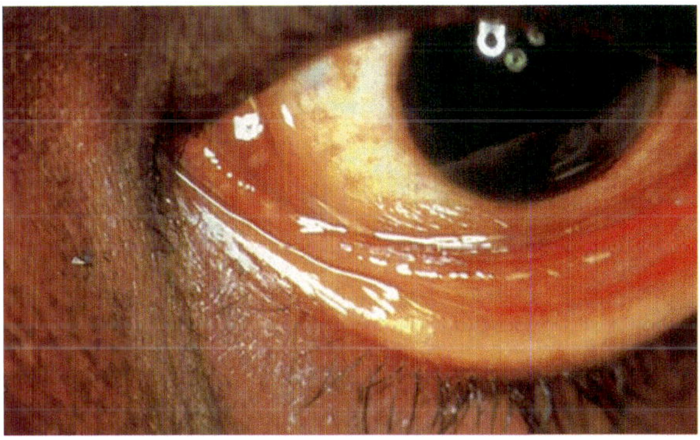

Fig. 17.7 Punctal atresia resulting in epiphora (Reprinted with permission from Katowitz and Katowitz [19])

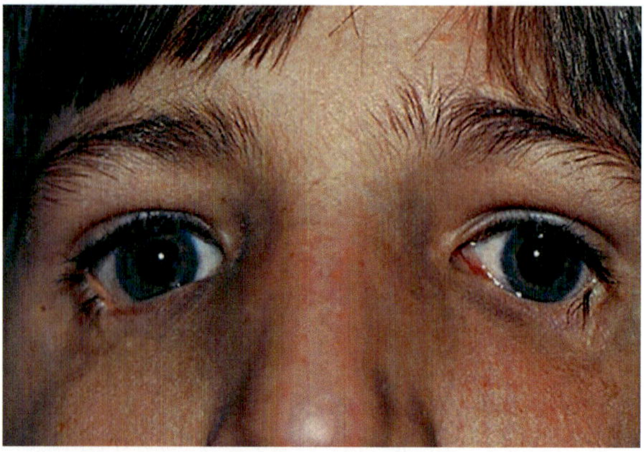

Fig. 17.8 Lower eyelid ectropion and malposition causing epiphora in a patient with Treacher Collins syndrome. Note the true colobomas in this patient (Reprinted with permission from Katowitz and Katowitz [19])

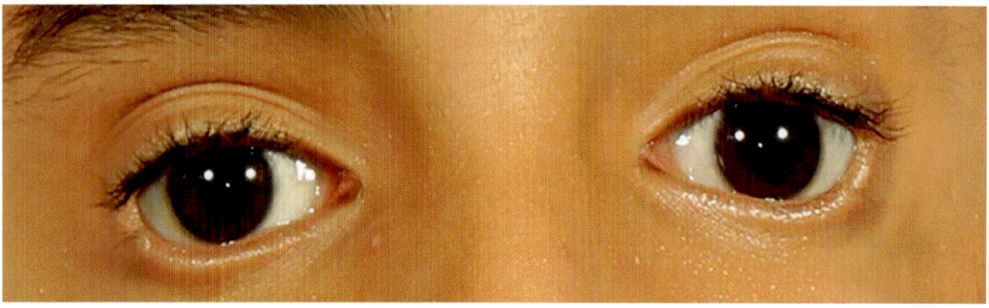

Fig. 17.9 Pathognomonic absence of medial lower eyelid lashes in patients with Treacher Collins syndrome

corneal and conjunctival irritation as well as epiphora due to poor protection of the ocular surface. Entropion is thought to be the result of congenital aberrancy in the attachment of the lower eyelid retractors or posterior lamellar hypoplasia causing corneal irritation from inward turning of the lashes (trichiasis). Other ciliary abnormalities are noted commonly. The hallmark ciliary finding in Treacher Collins syndrome is the deficiency or absence of lashes on the medial third of lower eyelid and is considered to be pathognomonic of the condition (Fig. 17.9). Distichiasis (accessory lashes at the posterior tarsal meibomian orifices) and trichiasis have been also presented in the literature.

Epibulbar dermoids refer to benign masses on the surface of the eye and contain keratinized epithelium, hair follicles, sebaceous glands, and sweat glands. Lipodermoids contain adipose as well but are covered by normal conjunctiva. They are usually located at the superotemporal recess and may extend posteriorly into the orbit to involve extraocular muscles, lacrimal gland, or other orbital structures (Fig. 17.10a). Limbal dermoids are found at the scleral-corneal junction or on the cornea (Fig. 17.10b). The mass encompasses the entire wall thickness. Their size may obstruct vision entirely if excessively large, but more commonly, they may result in a degree of corneal distortion and exposure keratopathy and corneal scarring with moderate-sized masses. As a consequence, astigmatic amblyopia can occur, with deprivational amblyopia occurring for significant lesions.

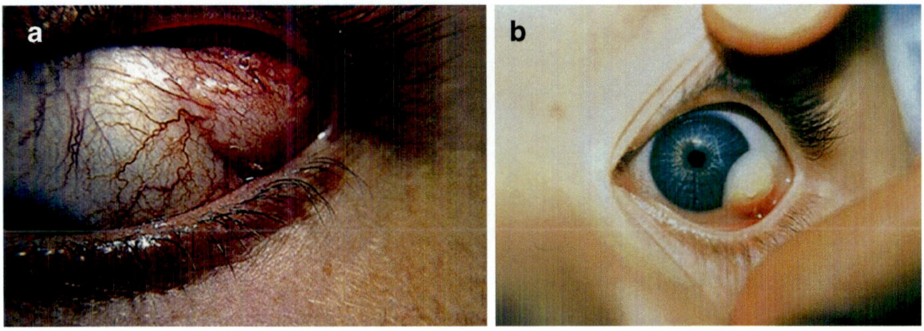

Fig. 17.10 Typical presentation of epibulbar dermoids. (**a**). Lipodermoid. (**b**). Limbal dermoid (Adapted with permission from Katowitz and Katowitz [19])

Treatment

Management Overview

Patients and their families are evaluated in multidisciplinary clinics including craniomaxillofacial surgeons, plastic surgeons, ophthalmologists, oculoplastic surgeons, otolaryngologists, anesthesiologists, dentists, orthodontists, pediatricians, speech therapists, and geneticists. Guidelines have been described to provide a protocol-driven approach to Treacher Collins syndrome. Comprehensive treatment protocols have been established by multiple institutions [26]. The ophthalmologic and periorbital soft tissue treatments will be discussed; a treatment protocol is shown in Fig. 17.11. These patients are often referred to plastic surgeons, craniofacial surgeons, ophthalmologists, or oculoplastic surgeons for treatment.

General treatment goals strive to produce excellent aesthetic and functional results that are long-lasting while minimizing operations and revisions. Treatment for these patients often begins in the neonatal period due to the urgent concern of ocular surface protection and amblyopia risk. Upper face and periorbital reconstruction is the focus through the childhood years (2 through 12) [27]. Ophthalmic treatment begins as early as possible with the goal being to obtain and preserve binocular vision. Periorbital soft tissue management, namely, eyelid reconstruction, can occur early in infancy (first year of life) or deferred until later in childhood (5–7 years), depending on the severity [28, 29]. The treatment of the other adnexal abnormalities outlined above are often dictated by parental concerns or as symptoms arise.

Overall, periorbital soft tissue and ophthalmologic treatment in Treacher Collins syndrome produces variable results. The multiple strategies and surgical techniques for soft tissue management achieve the functional goal of ocular surface protection and vision. Unfortunately, the cosmetic results are one of the main shortcomings in treating affected patients. Residual deformities persist, and multiple revisionary procedures are the rule rather than the exception [29]. Despite being least satisfied with the reconstructed eyelid appearance, most patients are satisfied with their vision [30]. Careful patient and family counseling in this regard is crucial to establishing reasonable expectations.

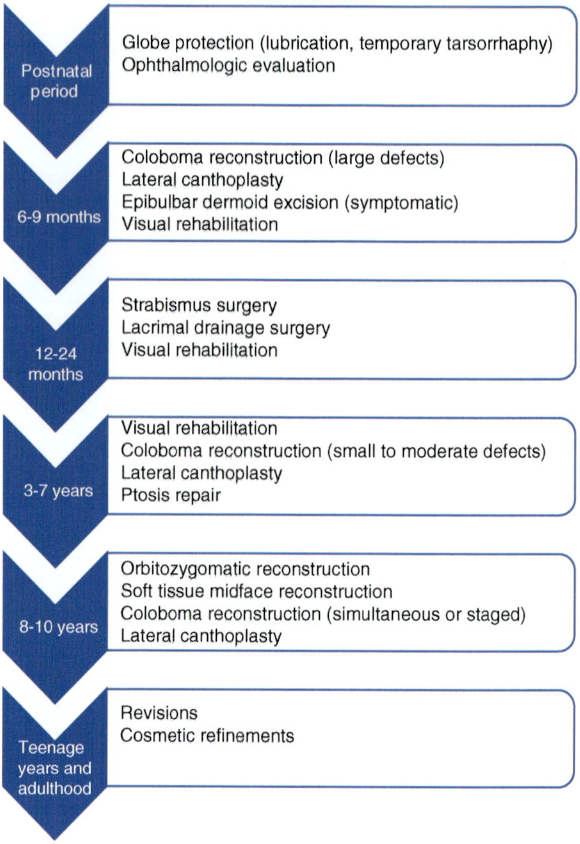

Fig. 17.11 Proposed ophthalmologic and periorbital soft tissue treatment protocol for Treacher Collins syndrome

Ophthalmologic Rehabilitation

Preservation of vision is a primary concern in affected patients, as amblyopia is a common cause of vision loss. Assessment by a pediatric ophthalmologist is prudent. To prevent corneal scarring, ulceration, and vision loss, the initial management in the neonatal period involves lubrication and occasionally moisture chambers if necessary. Should exposure keratitis occur, treatment with topical antibiotics and lubricants can provide rapid improvement. Temporary suture tarsorrhaphy can be performed if conservative measures fail. It is important to be cognizant of iatrogenic causes of deprivational amblyopia that may occur from frequent lubricant application, dressings, tarsorrhaphies, or reconstructive procedures.

Early thorough optometric and ophthalmologic examination in infancy is imperative and will allow prompt, aggressive treatment of refractive errors, amblyopia, and strabismus in an effort to prevent vision loss. Additionally, with the exception of rare cases, the impact on vision observed in Treacher Collins syndrome is predominantly the result of anterior segment, rather than retinal, abnormalities. Manifestly, a good prognosis for vision loss is possible if corrected early [31].

Early surgical treatment is considered if the ocular surface is compromised, risking corneal ulceration or scarring, or deprivation amblyopia as manifested by congenital cataracts or severe ptosis. Treatment may include temporary tarsorrhaphy, ptosis repair, or cataract surgery. Nonsurgical treatment for amblyopia and strabismus is initiated early and includes eyeglasses, prisms, cycloplegic agents (e.g., atropine drops), and occlusion therapy. Strabismus surgery is undertaken early at 12–24 months and after amblyopia and refractive error correction. During strabismus surgery, a fornix rather than limbal incision is preferred by many as it facilitates assessment of all extraocular muscles. A higher index of suspicion for anomalous muscle anatomy (aberrant insertions, hypoplastic muscles, or missing muscles) must be maintained during the procedure.

Ophthalmic outcome is dependent on timely recognition and treatment, as well as patient compliance. In this regard, a few other considerations are worth mentioning. Hertle's group noted that, of the patients that did not achieve equal visual acuity, all had documented poor treatment compliance [9]. They also commented that, for parents, facial profile/cosmetic, airway, and auricular concerns may supersede visual dysfunction, which can consequently limit compliance to vision treatment. Another practical issue that may interfere with treatment includes difficulty with eyewear due to auricular malformations and hearing aids. Finally, given that most patients with Treacher Collins syndrome suffer from conductive hearing loss in addition to amblyopia, there is a risk of cognitive deprivation [32]. As a result, it is clear that patients should be provided with prompt diagnosis and treatment, frequent counseling and follow-up, and support and resources under the guidance of a multidisciplinary care team.

Eyelid Reconstruction

Eyelid reconstruction and protection of the ocular surface is the primary focus of periorbital soft tissue rehabilitation in patients with Treacher Collins syndrome. One of the main components of the reconstructive efforts is lower eyelid coloboma repair. General principles for eyelid reconstruction are maintained for coloboma and pseudocoloboma repair. It is critical to ensure that the bilamellar structure of the lower eyelid is reconstituted, addressing important structures of the anterior lamella (skin and orbicularis oculi muscle) and posterior lamella (tarsus and conjunctiva), as shown in Fig. 17.1b. Skin can be provided from flaps or skin grafts. Local advancement or rotation flaps are utilized from the periorbital area owing to their similar tissue characteristics and quality. They can be limited by their tendency to "pin cushion" at the scar margins and create contour abnormalities, which exacerbates the operated appearance [29]. Skin grafts are full-thickness grafts to minimize secondary contracture and may be harvested from upper eyelid, preauricular, postauricular, and clavicular areas. They are generally reserved as a salvage option following multiple revisions or as an aspect of complication management (e.g., ectropion) due to their patchy appearance [29]. Posterior lamellar eyelid support can be provided from upper tarsus, septal or auricular cartilage, or acellular dermal matrices. Lining can be replaced by buccal or nasal mucosa or amniotic membrane allograft. Additionally, septal composite chondromucosal grafts, hard palate mucosal grafts, and upper eyelid tarsoconjunctival grafts can be utilized to reconstruct the posterior lamella. Care must be taken to preserve the integrity eyelid muscle function including the orbicularis oculi, levator aponeurosis, Mueller's muscle, and lower eyelid retractors.

Timing of eyelid reconstruction is largely dictated by the defect size, extent of globe exposure, and effect on visual function. Small and moderate-sized defects without corneal complications can be observed until school age when more eyelid tissue is available for reconstruction. Early intervention focuses on eyelid reconstruction when the patient is of appropriate age for general anesthesia and can be combined with other procedures such as cleft palate repair. The result may need to be revised at a later age when the orbital framework is reconstructed. Delayed reconstruction permits correction of the hard and soft tissues concurrently. It allows the orbital skeleton and periorbital soft tissues to reach their mature, adult size, which occurs at 8–10 years of age [33]. A staged approach can be employed wherein coloboma repair is performed after zygomatic skeletal and/or soft tissue reconstruction [34]. Eyelid reconstruction and correction of canthal malposition is more accurate following reconstruction of the lateral orbital wall and malar hypoplasia to support the soft tissue repair [14]. More predictable and durable results are presumably achievable with this approach, though a need for revision is not infrequent. Still, many prefer early eyelid reconstruction to provide globe protection and mitigate the stigmata associated with the syndrome.

In the presence of a lateral lower eyelid coloboma, defect size is characterized as small, moderate, or large and directs the reconstructive approach. The size may be overestimated due to the opposing pull of the orbicularis at the edges of the coloboma. Additionally, lateral canthal malposition distorts the eyelid architecture and should be repositioned prior to repairing the defect. In all cases, there may be tethering of the soft tissues to the underlying skeletal framework, necessitating release of the skin, orbicularis oculi, and occasionally the orbital septum to relax the eyelid. Small defects (less than one third of the eyelid) are amenable to primary closure after excision of the coloboma margins. The vertical scar that results can be prone to cicatricial ectropion. Z-plasty techniques minimize this risk by reorienting the central limb along relaxed skin tension lines [35].

Moderate defects (one third to one half of the lower eyelid margin) can be repaired with local flaps but require inclusion of a lateral canthotomy to release the eyelid margin. The Tenzel semicircular flap is commonly utilized for this purpose (Fig. 17.12). It is designed in the lateral orbital area and dissected deep to the orbicularis oculi in this region. After lateral canthotomy and inferior cantholysis, the tissue is advanced and repaired in a full-thickness fashion. It is crucial to secure flap to the lateral rim periosteum to avoid eyelid retraction. Another viable option for moderate to large colobomas are musculocutaneous Tripier transposition flaps (Fig. 17.13). These may be uni- or bipedicled and utilize Z-plasty principles to also reestablish lower eyelid vertical height. Tarsoconjunctival reconstruction is required.

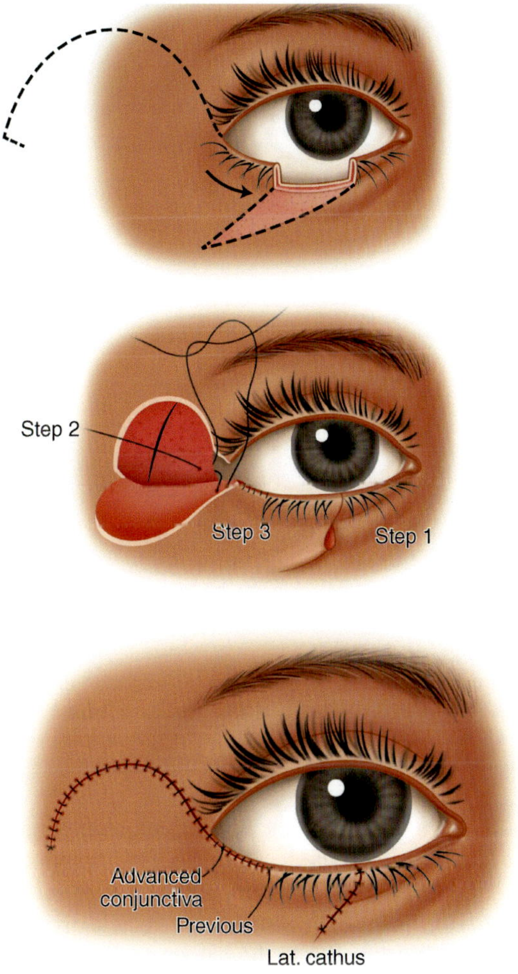

Fig. 17.12 Tenzel semicircular musculocutaneous flap for moderate lower eyelid defects. It is crucial to secure the flap to the lateral orbital rim periosteum after advancement to prevent lower eyelid retraction

The flap is inset into a subciliary incision. With respect to flap design, 20 millimeters of upper eyelid skin should remain to avoid inferior traction on the brow. A composite transposition flap has been described by Ian Jackson based on the upper eyelid that includes a tarsoconjunctival island. The island is small enough to facilitate primary closure of the posterior lamellar defect and does not violate the attachment of the eyelid elevators to the superior tarsal margin [36]. Advancement flaps can be utilized as well for moderate lower eyelid defects; a lateral canthotomy is often necessary to provide mobilization of the lateral flap (Fig. 17.14).

Large defects (greater than half of the lower eyelid margin), though uncommon, may necessitate eyelid-sharing procedures. The Hughes tarsoconjunctival flap is a versatile option for posterior lamellar reconstruction in these cases (Fig. 17.15). The flap is designed from the upper eyelid tarsus and conjunctiva, maintaining 3–4

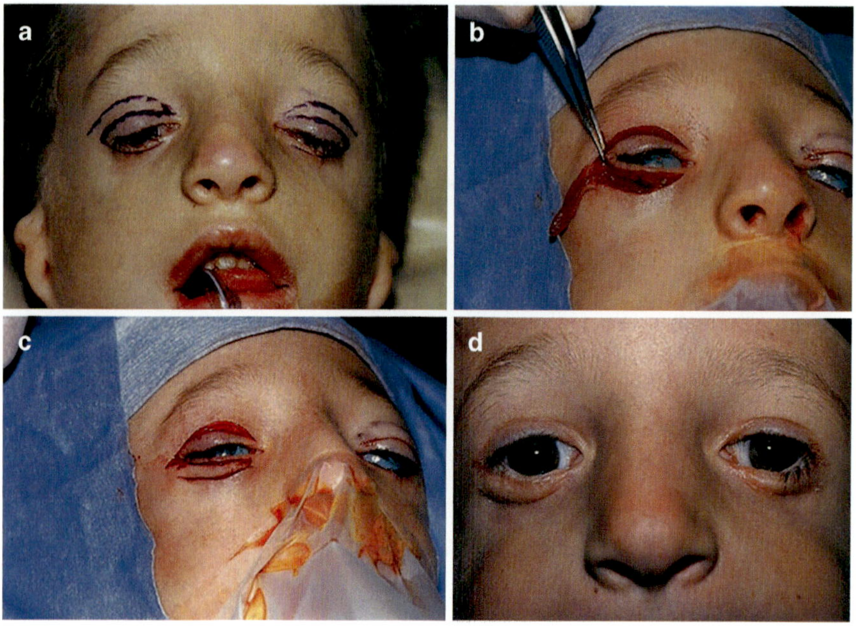

Fig. 17.13 Pseudocoloboma reconstruction using a Tripier transposition flap. (**a**) Flap marking from the upper eyelid. (**b**) Subciliary incision for flap inset and lateral canthal repositioning. (**c**) Flap transposition. (**d**) Post-operative appearance after 1 year. Note the "pin-cushioning" that commonly occurs with local flaps that can compromise the final aesthetic result. (Reprinted with permission from Katowitz and Katowitz [19])

millimeters of tarsus at the eyelid margin for tarsal integrity. The flap is elevated in the plane between the levator palpebrae superioris and the Mueller's muscle and inset into the defect. Anterior lamellar reconstruction can be with a musculocutaneous flap or full-thickness skin graft. Pedicle division is performed after 1 month. As mentioned earlier, due to the risk of deprivational amblyopia eyelid-sharing procedures are avoided in young children unless significant corneal threat is present. In such cases, eyelid-sharing reconstruction can be performed with earlier pedicle division and subsequent intensive amblyopia therapy. The Mustarde cheek rotation-advancement flap is utilized in complex lower eyelid cases where periorbital soft tissues are severely deficient, often in the context of associated anomalies such as cryptophthalmos (Fig. 17.16) [18]. Posterior lamellar reconstruction is required. Tissue expansion with Z-plasties and Y-V advancement flaps can also be considered if tissue recruitment is necessary, such as with combined osseous grafting or for revision cases with significant scar burden to be excised [37].

After correcting the eyelid defect, eyelid cheek junction contour deformities may persist as a result of the malar hypoplasia. Soft tissue and bony reconstruction of the zygoma is discussed further elsewhere, but a few techniques bear mentioning. Dermal or dermis-fat grafts provide better definition to the eyelid, refine the eyelid-cheek junction contour, and improve the overlying skin quality but are limited by

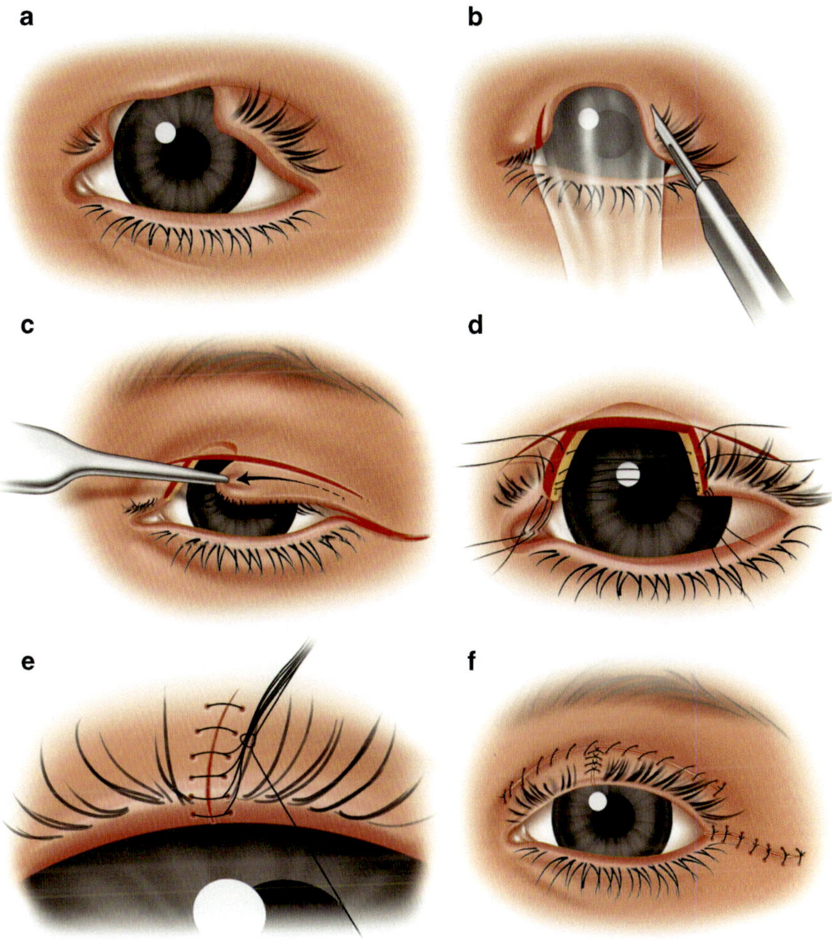

Fig. 17.14 Bilateral advancement flaps are described for the repair of moderate eyelid colobomas (**a**). This technique allows for bilamellar eyelid reconstruction. The eyelid defect skin margins are excised (**b**). The superior flap is created with a skin incision along the natural eyelid crease, and is undermined medially and laterally superficial to the levator muscle to allow the flaps to mobilize. (**c**). Partial thickness sutures are placed through anterior tarsus to close the tarsal defect (**d**) followed by skin closure (**e**). A lateral canthotomy is typically required to allow medial advancement of the lateral flap (**f**)

graft resorption and need for multiple revisions [38]. Autologous fat grafting has gained popularity for soft tissue augmentation and has replaced free tissue transfer in many cases. Additionally, subperiosteal midface lifts can be employed to accentuate the malar region, with fat grafting to remaining areas of deficiency and to smooth areas of transition [39]. These soft tissue procedures are advantageous in that they can be performed at an early age, obviating concerns about completion of orbital skeletal maturity.

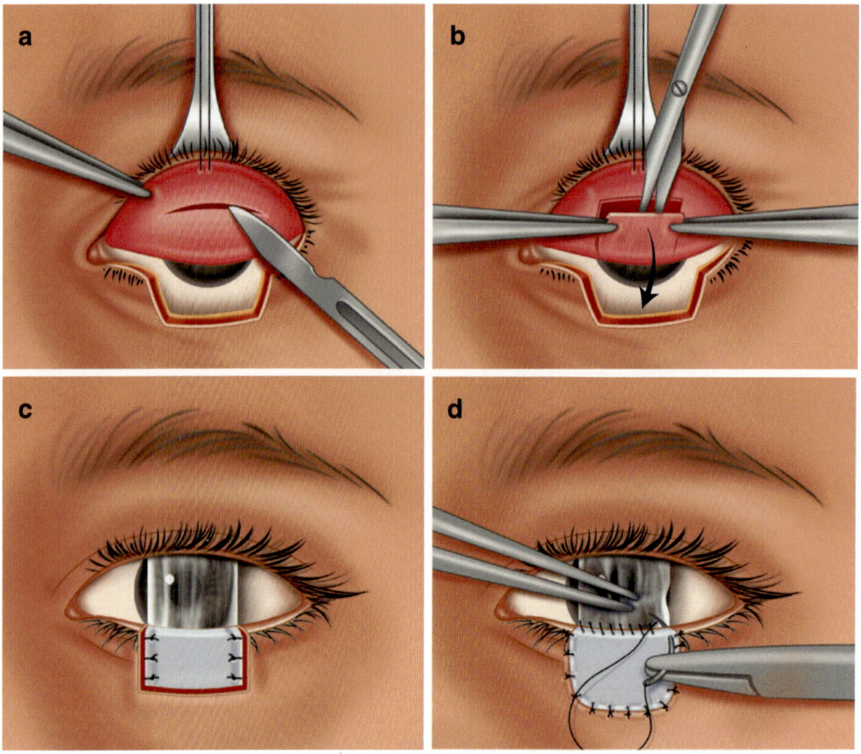

Fig. 17.15 Hughes tarsoconjunctival flap for large lower eyelid defects. The skin edges of the lower eyelid defect are excised. The upper eyelid is everted and a transconjunctival full thickness tarsal horizontal incision is made approximately 4 millimeters above the lash line (**a**). The tarsoconjunctival flap is raised to the superior tarsus leaving attachments to conjunctiva intact for vascular supply (**b**). The flap is secured into place with partial thickness tarsal sutures (**c**). This flap is utilized for posterior lamellar reconstruction. The anterior lamella can be reconstructed with a flap or full-thickness skin graft (shown) (**d**). The pedicle is divided after 1 month

Lateral Canthal Repositioning

Repair of the eyelid defect is one component of correcting the periorbital soft tissue deformity associated with Treacher Collins syndrome. The downward-slanting palpebral fissure, a result of the lateral orbital wall and zygomatic hypoplasia as well as lateral canthal dysmorphology, must be reconstructed with lateral canthoplasty techniques to restore a more aesthetic appearance. Lateral canthal reconstruction can be performed at the same time as coloboma repair or later during orbito-zygomatic reconstruction.

In some cases, the lateral canthus can be simply repositioned. The lateral canthal tendon can be elevated with a cuff of periosteum from the lateral orbital wall [40]. A more common procedure is the tarsal strip canthoplasty (Fig. 17.17). Lateral canthotomy and inferior cantholysis is performed, and the desired eyelid position is determined. In general, lower eyelid position should be 1–2 millimeters above the inferior limbus. A portion of eyelid margin including lashes, conjunctiva, and skin

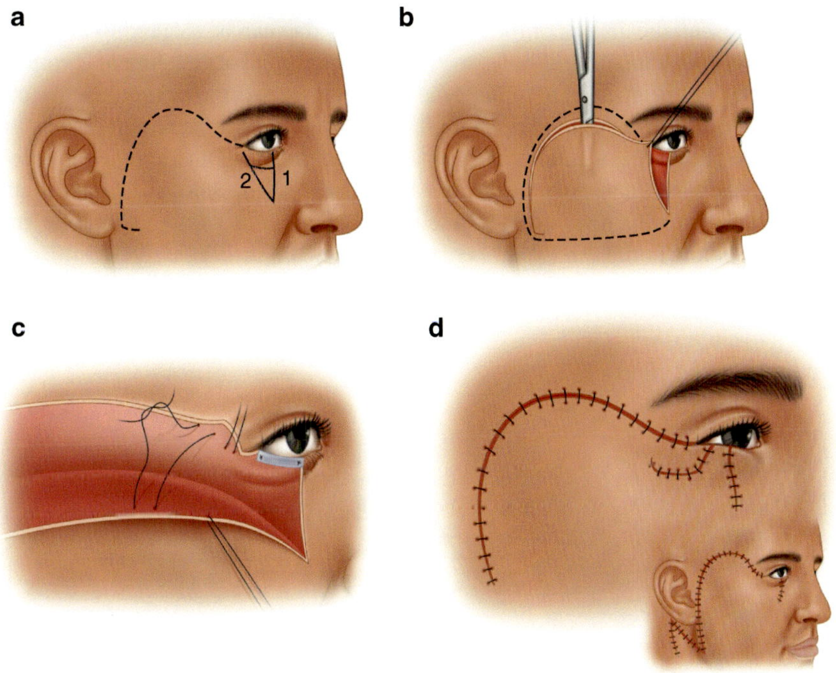

Fig. 17.16 Mustarde cheek rotation-advancement flap for complex lower eyelid and cheek soft tissue deficiency. Posterior lamellar reconstruction is required, which could be achieved with a tarsal graft. The eyelid defect is converted to a triangular defect for the planned Mustarde cheek flap. The flap is designed to course superior to the lateral canthus to prevent inferiorly-directed tension on the lower eyelid (**a**). An incision is made along the skin markings between the lateral canthus and preauricular skin and a skin flap is raised in the subcutaneous plane (**b**). The flap is advanced and rotated medially. The flap should be secured at the lateral orbital rim to prevent lower eyelid retraction (**c**). The transposed flap is then sutured (**d**). If additional mobilization is necessary, the incision can extend posterior to the ear lobule to recruit additional tissue (*inset*)

are removed to "strip" the tarsal segment used for fixation. If eyelid laxity is present, the portion of tarsus can be excised to tighten the eyelid. The fixation point on the inner lateral orbital rim should be at the superior aspect of the pupil with permanent suture to the periosteum or drill holes. The lateral canthal angle should be carefully reestablished between upper and lower eyelid gray lines, and symmetry with the contralateral side should be confirmed. Caution is necessary with this procedure: despite improving eyelid laxity, it may result in excessive shortening in a lower eyelid that is already horizontally deficient. Vertical lengthening with lateral canthal fixation can also be achieved with midface suspension or sub-orbicularis oculi lift to assist in support and proper positioning of the lateral canthal angle.

Other soft tissue techniques for lower eyelid repositioning such as inferior retinacular canthoplasty or dermal-orbicular pennant canthoplasty obviate the eyelid shortening that may occur with the tarsal strip procedure. Still, in maintaining the integrity of the lateral canthal tendon and elevating the lower eyelid, they do not address the underlying lateral canthal deformity. In cases where the lateral canthal tendon is absent, the dermis of the native eyelid or flap can be secured to the lateral orbital rim periosteum or drill holes to create a lateral canthal attachment. Temporal fascia grafts can be utilized to replace the missing tissue. If the lateral orbital rim is severely deficient from the Tessier 8 cleft, the deep temporal fascia can also be utilized for fixation. When canthoplasty is combined with zygomatic osseous reconstruction, the new canthal position will be altered and dependent on final malar positioning. Canthal suspension in these situations requires fixation to a bone graft or alloplastic material and can be performed with drill-hole fixation, suture suspension to miniplates, or Mitek anchor [34]. However, canthoplasty may need to

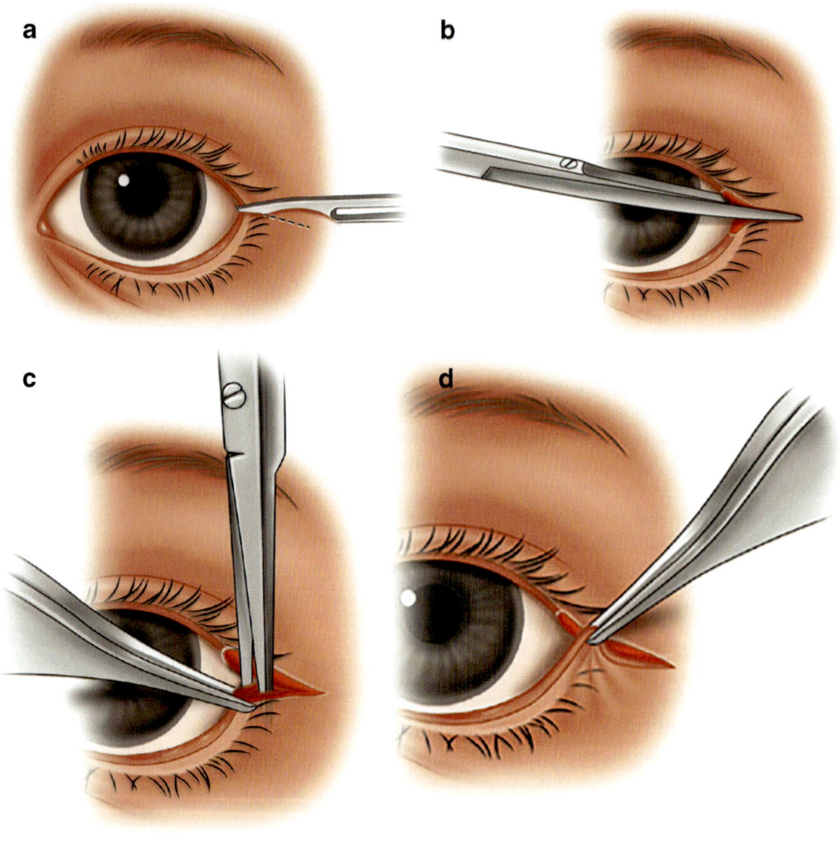

Fig. 17.17 Lateral canthal repositioning with tarsal strip procedure. (**a**) Lateral canthal skin incision. (**b**) Lateral canthotomy is completed with scissors. (**c**) Inferior cantholysis is performed to completely release the lower eyelid from its periorbital attachments. (**d**) Evaluation of desired lateral canthal position. (**e**) Resuspension of the lower eyelid (*inset:* creation of the tarsal strip margin with excision of a portion of anterior lamellar tissues, ciliary margin, and conjunctiva from the tarsus) to the lateral orbital wall periosteum. Drill hole suspension or suspension to the lateral orbital rim periosteum or deep temporal fascia can alternatively be utilized. (**f**) Recreation of the lateral canthal angle at the gray line

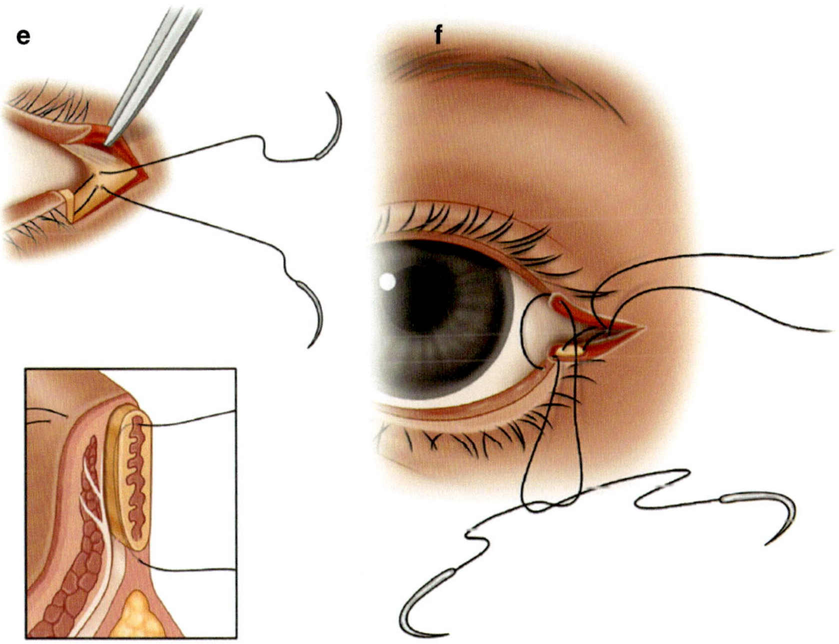

Fig. 17.17 (continued)

be revised after facial growth has completed (i.e., teenage years), especially if it was initially performed early and prior to skeletal reconstruction.

Ptosis and Other Periorbital Treatments

The management of blepharoptosis is dependent on the extent of levator function from downward to upward gaze while stabilizing the brow. Timing is dependent on the severity and the resultant risk of deprivational amblyopia as well as the ability to obtain reliable exam findings. Early correction is favored when significant visual obstruction is identified, whereas asymptomatic patients may be deferred until school age [41]. Patients with mild ptosis and good levator function can be treated with the Fasanella-Servat procedure (tarsoconjunctival mullerectomy). Levator resection and advancement is indicated for moderate ptosis with fair levator excursion. The levator should be advanced 4 millimeters for every millimeter of ptosis and should be centered over the mid-pupil. Severe ptosis with poor or absent levator function requires frontalis suspension with autologous fascia (fascia lata or deep temporal donors) or synthetic materials (Gore-Tex, Prolene suture, silicone). This procedure synchronizes upper eyelid elevation to the frontalis muscle via the brow. It provides static (related to the degree of material tightening) and dynamic (integration with brow elevation) components to the procedure. Multiple techniques have been described for this purpose; the Crawford double triangle is shown in Fig. 17.18.

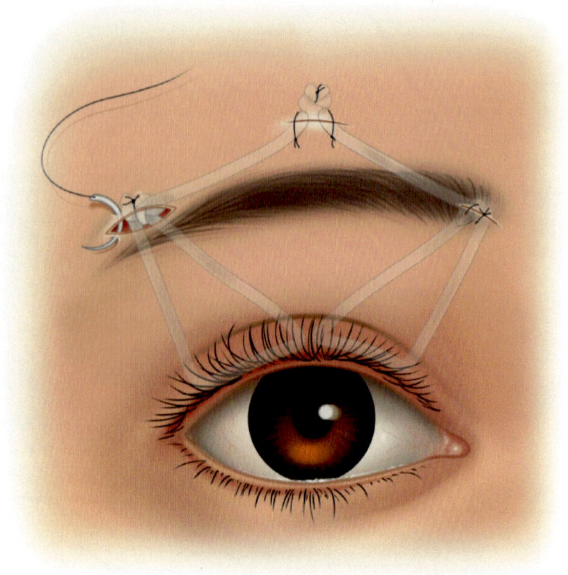

Fig. 17.18 Crawford double triangle technique for frontalis sling for severe ptosis. The static aspect relies on tightening of the material while the dynamic relies on brow elevation

Congenital ectropion and entropion are treated in a fashion similar to acquired cases. Initial management is conservative with lubrication. Hyaluronic acid filler, injected below the anterior lamella, expands the soft tissues of the lower eyelid and can also be considered as a temporizing measure [42]. Surgical intervention is indicated for corneal scarring, exposure keratitis, infection, or for cosmesis. With respect to ectropion, lateral tarsal strip canthoplasty provides tarsoligamentous tightening, and the anterior lamellar soft tissue deficiency can be addressed with skin grafts, flaps, or midface suspension techniques. Some cases may require scar or adhesion release. On the other hand, entropion does not improve over time and requires surgery. It can be treated with excision of excess pretarsal skin and orbicularis which also relieves the associated trichiasis. Another option consists of reattachment of the lower eyelid retractors to the tarsus through a subciliary incision. Lower eyelid lamellar scarring in either case may result in ectropion. If posterior lamellar deficiency is observed, spacer grafts—most commonly hard palate mucosa, allografts, or upper free tarsal grafts—are options to restore the vertical dimensions of the lower eyelid.

Ciliary treatment is required when conjunctival or corneal irritation occurs. If confined to the conjunctiva, primary management consists of lubricating ointment or drops; surgical treatment is recommended for persistent conjunctival irritation. Due to the risk of vision loss, corneal irritation is managed more aggressively with a lower threshold for surgery. Less-invasive treatments for trichiasis and distichiasis include cryotherapy and electroepilation of lash follicles at the posterior tarsal margin. These procedures are prone to recurrence and may also cause pigmentary changes and eyelid distortion [19]. Though there are other surgical options for distichiasis, a more successful treatment consists of excision of the affected strip of eyelid margin (Fig. 17.19). Since the pathology involves the meibomian gland

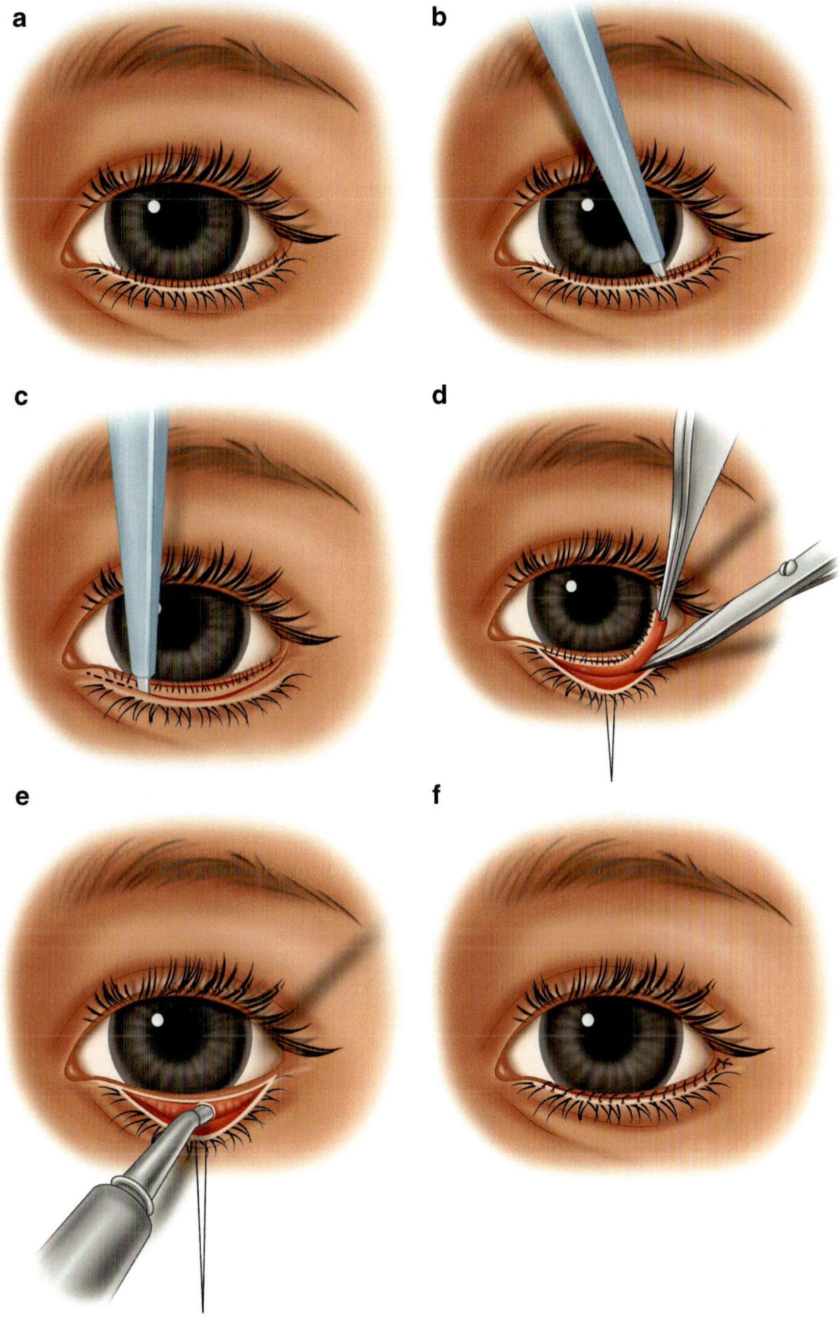

Fig. 17.19 Eyelid excision for treatment of distichiasis. (**a**) Accessory eyelashes originating from Meibomian gland orifices and causing irritation. (**b**) Incision posterior to accessory lashes on lid margin. (**c**) Incision anterior to accessory lashes. (**d**) Full-thickness excision of involved lid margin including a portion of tarsal plate. (**e**) Cryotherapy to destroy residual lash follicles. (**f**) Postoperative appearance after closure

orifices, cryotherapy of the underlying tarsus is recommended to destroy any residual lash follicles.

Epiphora in patients with Treacher Collins syndrome can result from lacrimal system abnormalities proximally in the lower eyelid (punctal or canalicular atresia) or distally (nasolacrimal duct stenosis or atresia). Traditionally, conservative management with massage and topical antibiotics to prevent dacryocystitis are attempted first and have a high rate of success up to 12 months of age. If epiphora persists and the nasolacrimal collecting system is present, then probing and irrigation with stenting can be performed under general anesthesia. Stents are removed in an ambulatory setting or with general anesthesia after 3–6 months depending on the complexity of the obstruction. Dacryocystorhinostomy may be performed if stenting fails to resolve the epiphora.

For proximal lower lacrimal drainage lesions, epiphora may not be seen. Such an observation is the result of demand compensation of a typically normal superior lacrimal puncta and canalicular system, despite the inferior canaliculus being the major outflow source in unaffected patients. As a consequence, many patients do not require treatment for proximal inferior punctal and canalicular atresia. If epiphora is present despite a patent superior outflow system, one treatment option is the creation of a pseudo-punctum on the lower eyelid margin that connects to any patent component of the inferior canaliculus via an open approach to the lacrimal sac. Another procedure is the creation of a new canalicular system from the eyelid margin to the lacrimal sac directly with a hypodermic needle. Following silicone stenting of this new passage, a neopunctum is created in the sac. More severe cases or extensive atresia of the canaliculus, nasolacrimal duct, or of the entire nasolacrimal system may require conjunctivodacryocystorhinostomy or canaliculodacryocystorhinostomy with Jones tube insertion.

Epibulbar dermoids are addressed when causing distorting adjacent structures, astigmatism, cosmetic concern, or visual disturbance. Lipodermoid excision, except for large masses, is largely a cosmetic undertaking. Timing for most tumors is around 6 months of age when anesthetic risk is diminished, though early surgery is needed if vision is affected or if mass effect is noted. Given that the lesion usually extends posteriorly into the orbit and complete resection can damage critical structures in the area (lacrimal gland, lateral rectus muscle, lateral horn of the levator muscle), debulking is often the procedure of choice. The conjunctival surface is preserved, and the visible portion of the lipodermoid up to the level of the fornix is conservatively excised. Since complete excision is not possible in most cases, lipodermoid regrowth may occur as the child ages. Limbal dermoid excision can be more challenging. Superficial keratectomy can be attempted for small, superficial tumors but can result in scarring, corneal vascularization, and pseudopterygium formation [43]. For thicker limbal dermoids, anterior lamellar keratoplasty is required wherein corneal defect is reconstructed with a corneoscleral allograft or amniotic membrane grafts [44, 45]. Most lesions are full thickness, and complete resection is unlikely. While appearance is often improved and vision remains stable, residual corneal stigmata persist.

Conclusion

In conclusion, periorbital soft tissue anomalies associated with Treacher Collins syndrome play a critical role in the classification of this craniofacial disorder. Though ophthalmic manifestations and treatment studies are few, early evaluation of ocular surface and visual function are essential in providing the best functional visual outcome. Coordination with multidisciplinary teams to create an individualized plan for each patient can help assist in reconstructive staging, minimize additional surgeries, and optimize the aesthetic and functional outcome.

References

1. Tessier P. Anatomical classification of facial, cranio-facial, and latero-facial cleft. J Maxillofac Surg. 1976;4(2):69–92.
2. Kawamoto HK. The kaleidoscopic world of rare craniofacial clefts: order out of chaos (Tessier classification). Clin Plast Surg. 1976;3(4):529–72.
3. Franceschetti A, Klein D. The mandibulofacial dysostosis: a new hereditary syndrome. Acta Ophthalmol. 1949;27(2):144–9.
4. Rogers BO. Berry-Treacher-Collin's syndrome: a review of 200 cases. Br J Plast Surg. 1964;17:109–37.
5. Farkas LG, Posnick JC. Detailed morphometry of the nose in patients with Treacher Collins syndrome. Ann Plast Surg. 1989;22(3):211–9.
6. Posnick JC, Al-Qattan MM, Moffat SM, Armstrong D. Cranio-orbito-zygomatic measurements from standard CT scans in unoperated Treacher Collins syndrome patients: comparison with normal controls. Cleft Palate Craniofac J. 1995;32(1):20–4.
7. Levasseur J, Nysjo J, Sandy R, et al. Orbital volume and shape in Treacher Collins syndrome. J Craniomaxillofac Surg. 2018;46(2):305–11.
8. Garner LD. Cephalometric analysis of Berry-TCS. Oral Surg Oral Med Oral Pathol. 1967;23(3):320–7.
9. Hertle RW, Ziylan S, Katowitz JA. Ophthalmic features and visual prognosis in the Treacher-Collins syndrome. Br J Ophthalmol. 1993;77(10):642–5.
10. Wang FM, Millman AL, Sidoti PA, Goldberg RB. Ocular findings in Treacher Collins syndrome. Am J Ophthalmol. 1990;110(3):280–6.
11. Read SA, Collins MJ, Carney LG. A review of astigmatism and its possible genesis. Clin Exp Optom. 2007;90(1):5–19.
12. Holla A, Gonsalves SR, Lobo GJ. Treacher Collins syndrome with microcornea and retinal detachment. BMJ Case Rep. 2013. https://doi.org/10.1136/bcr-2013-202425.
13. Prenner JL, Binenbaum G, Carpentieri DF, et al. Treacher Collins syndrome with novel ophthalmic findings and visceral anomalies. Br J Ophthalmol. 2002;86(4):472–3.
14. Chang CC, Steinbacher DM. Treacher Collins syndrome. Semin Plast Surg. 2012;26(2):83–90.
15. Berry GA. Note on a congenital defect (coloboma?) of the lower lid. R Lond Ophthalmol Hosp Rep. 1889;12:255.
16. Collins ET. Cases with symmetrical congenital notches in the outer part of each lid and defective development of the malar bones. Trans Ophthalmol Soc U K. 1900;20:190–2.
17. Axelsson A, Brolin I, Engstrom H, Liden G. Dysostosis mandibulo-facialis. J Laryngol Otol. 1963;77:575–92.
18. Smith HB, Verity DH, Collin JRO. The incidence, embryology, and oculofacial abnormalities associated with eyelid colobomas. Eye (Lond). 2015;29(4):492–8.

19. Revere KE, Foster JA, Katowitz WR, Katowitz JA. Developmental eyelid disorders. In: Katowitz JA, Katowitz WR, editors. Pediatric oculoplastic surgery. 2nd ed. Cham: Springer; 2018. p. 311–58.
20. Vincent M, Genevieve D, Ostertag A, et al. Treacher Collins syndrome: a clinical and molecular study based on a large series of patients. Genet Med. 2016;18(1):49–56.
21. Teber OA, Gillessen-Kaesbach G, Fischer S, et al. Genotyping in 46 patients with tentative diagnosis of Treacher Collins syndrome revealed unexpected phenotypic variation. Eur J Hum Genet. 2004;12(11):879–90.
22. Bachelor EP, Kaplan EN. Absence of the lateral canthal tendon in Treacher-Collins syndrome. Br J Plast Surg. 1981;34(2):162–4.
23. Aljerian A, Gilardino MS. Treacher Collins syndrome. Clin Plastic Surg. 2019;46:197–205.
24. Bartley GB. Lacrimal drainage anomalies in mandibulofacial dysostosis. Am J Ophthalmol. 1990;109(5):571–4.
25. Hedera P, Toriello H, Petty E. Novel autosomal dominant mandibulofacial dysostosis with ptosis: clinical description and exclusion of TCOF1. J Med Genet. 2002;39(7):484–8.
26. Forrest CR, Hopper RA. Craniofacial syndromes and surgery. Plast Reconstr Surg. 2013;131(1):86e–109e.
27. Thompson JT, Anderson PJ, David DJ. Treacher Collins syndrome: protocol management from birth to maturity. J Craniofac Surg. 2009;20(6):2028–35.
28. Cobb ARM, Green B, Gill D, et al. The surgical management of Treacher Collins syndrome. Br J Oral Maxillofac Surg. 2014;52(7):581–9.
29. Posnick JC, Tiwana PS, Costello BJ. Treacher Collins syndrome: a comprehensive evaluation and treatment. Oral Maxillofac Surg Clin North Am. 2004;16(4):503–23.
30. Plomp RG, Versnel SL, van Lieshout MJ, Poublon RM, Mathijssen IM. Long-term assessment of facial features and functions needing more attention in treatment of Treacher Collins syndrome. J Plast Reconstr Aesthet Sur. 2013;66(8):e217–26.
31. Sharma R, Sharma B, Babber M, Singh S, Jain G. Treacher Collins syndrome: a case report and review of ophthalmic features. Taiwan J Ophthalmol. 2016;6(4):206–9.
32. Black J, Crompton J. Craniofacial abnormalities. In: Lambert SR, Lyons CJ, editors. Taylor and Hoyt's pediatric ophthalmology and strabismus. 5th ed. Edinburgh: Elsevier; 2017. p. 250–66.
33. Waitzman AA, Posnick JC, Armstrong DC, Pron GE. Craniofacial skeletal measurements based on computed tomography: part 1. Accuracy and reproducibility. Cleft Palate Craniofac J. 1992;29(2):112–7.
34. Mitsukawa N, Saiga A, Satoh K. Changing the facial features of patients with Treacher Collins syndrome: protocol for 3-stage treatment of hard and soft tissue hypoplasia in the upper half of the face. Ann Plast Surg. 2014;73(1):39–42.
35. Tessier P. Surgery of the orbit and eyelids. New York: Masson; 1981. p. 169–70.
36. Jackson IT. Reconstruction of the lower eyelid defect in Treacher Collins syndrome. Plast Reconstr Surg. 1981;67(3):365–7.
37. Ueda K, Nuri T, Shigemura Y. Malar reconstruction using Y-V advancement flaps after tissue expansion in Treacher Collins syndrome. Plast Reconstr Surg Glob Open. 2016;4(5):e715–8.
38. Kobus K, Wojcicki P. Surgical treatment of Treacher Collins syndrome. Ann Plast Surg. 2006;56(5):549–54.
39. Franchi G, Kadlub N, Diner PA, Bandini M, Vazquez MP, Picard A. Orbital soft tissue surgery for patients with Treacher-Collins or Nager syndrome. A new surgical approach with early correction of soft tissue: prospective study. Br J Oral Maxillofac Surg. 2015;53(5):421–5.
40. Marsh JL, Edgerton MT. Periosteal pennant lateral canthoplasty. Plast Reconstr Surg. 1979;64(1):24–9.
41. Mehta M, Bauer BS. Congenital and acquired deformities of the eyelids. In: Bentz ML, Bauer BS, Zuker RM, editors. Principles and practice of pediatric plastic surgery. 2nd ed. Boca Raton: CRC Press; 2017. p. 999–1049.

42. Fezza J. Nonsurgical treatment of cicatricial ectropion with hyaluronic acid filler. Plast Reconstr Surg. 2008;121(3):1009–14.
43. Panton RW, Sugar J. Excision of limbal dermoids. Ophthalmic Surg. 1991;22(2):85–9.
44. Spierer O, Gologorsky D, Adler E, Forster RK. Lamellar keratoplasty with corneosceral graft for limbal dermoids. Int J Ophthalmol. 2018;11(3):512–5.
45. Pirouzian A, Holz H, Merrill K, Sudesh R, Karlen K. Surgical management of pediatric limbal dermoids with sutureless amniotic membrane transplantation and augmentation. J Pediatr Ophthalmol Strabismus. 2012;49(2):114–9.

Chapter 18
Correction of Orbital Zygomatic Deformities in the Treacher Collins Patient

Douglas P. Sinn and Danielle Gill

Introduction

Treacher Collins syndrome (TCS) is a relatively rare congenital disorder, but once manifested, it may stigmatize affected individuals with multiple craniofacial features, most notably in the midface region. Zygomatic hypoplasia or, in some cases, zygomatic aplasia and deficiency of the lateral aspect of the orbit are some of the key anomalies. In most cases, these anomalies present bilaterally but not always symmetrically [1]. Surgical reconstruction is deemed necessary in order to achieve the desired cosmetic outcome.

There have been many attempts to come up with both safe and efficient surgical solutions for these individuals, but because of the phenotypic variation of TCS, no gold standard has been established. All surgical techniques provide adequate reestablishment of midfacial and orbital contours but come with varying limitations. Precise anatomical evaluation, timing of surgery, and anticipating the need for future surgeries must be efficiently assessed in order to secure a successful outcome.

This chapter aims to outline the anatomical deformities associated with TCS, classifications associated with these abnormalities, timing associated with intervention, as well as, identifying potential treatment options.

D. P. Sinn (✉)
University of Texas Southwestern Medical Center/Parkland Hospital, Mansfield, TX, USA

D. Gill
Division of Oral and Maxillofacial Surgery, Charlotte, NC, USA

D. M. Yates, M. R. Markiewicz (eds.), *Craniofacial Microsomia and Treacher Collins Syndrome*, https://doi.org/10.1007/978-3-030-84733-3_18

Anatomy

The most significant factors having an impact on the severity of the disease and patients' appearance are associated with the underlying skeletal deformities. To understand how to correct these deformities, it is important to recognize what the distinctive anatomy is for a TCS patient.

The hallmark characteristics of the TCS patient show a degree of hypoplasia of the zygomatic bones, retrusion of the malar region, shortening of the lateral and inferior orbital walls, and narrowing of the facial skeleton in the upper one-third. Flattening or even indentations below the orbits are also very common traits [1–3]. Patients with documented TCS also present with an abnormal shape of the anterior cranial vault due to diminished intercoronal (bitemporal) distance as well as decreased cephalic length [4–6] (Fig. 18.1).

The inferior lateral angle of the orbit is deficient, and the superolateral part of the orbit is displaced caudally. These characteristics give the TCS patient the classic egg-shaped appearance [7]. Other orbital anomalies include moderate protrusion of the eyeballs, orbital hypoplasia, lipodermoids, and limbal dermoids. Colobomata of the lower eyelids and iris, ectropion, absence of eyelashes in the medial aspect of the lid, lacrimal system dysfunction or frank aplasia with resultant epiphora, strabismus, amblyopia, congenital cataracts, refractive errors, and/or vision loss have also been reported [3, 5, 7–9].

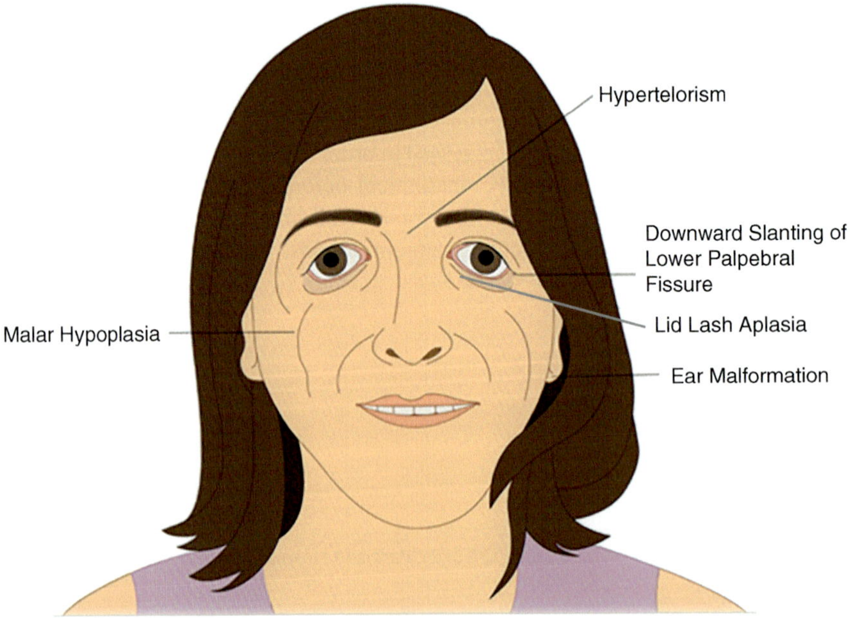

Fig. 18.1 Female Treacher Collins syndrome patient (facial view)

The lid and adnexal abnormalities (canthal dystopia, dacryostenosis, blepharoptosis, lateral lower lid true coloboma, and pseudocolobomas) are found in 96% of TCS patients. Downward slanting of the palpebral fissures have been noted in 89% of cases of TCS, notching of the lower eyelids in 69% of cases, and absence of lid lashes medial to the defect in 69% of cases [7].

Classifications of the Orbitozygomatic Regions

The orbitozygomatic region in a TCS patient can vary in morphology. This can make reconstruction of this region extremely complex. Grouping these patients by their morphological similarities gives the surgeon a comprehensive idea of the underlying anatomy and helps to better determine possible treatment options that may have been successful for these patients [1, 10].

Chang et al. previously published data discussing a classification system based on the orbitozygomatic complex. The type I deformity is represented by a small zygomatic body with all articulations with the exception of the arch [1] (Fig. 18.2a).

The type II deformity has a diminished malar structure and a notable defect along the lateral orbital wall (zygomaticosphenoid suture). The inferolateral orbital rim is preserved, but the arch is incomplete and shows no evidence of the temporal aspect of the zygomatic process (Fig. 18.2b) [1].

Lastly, the type III deformity shows minimal volume with only remnants of the malar apparatus at the zygomaticofrontal or maxillary region. The absence of all

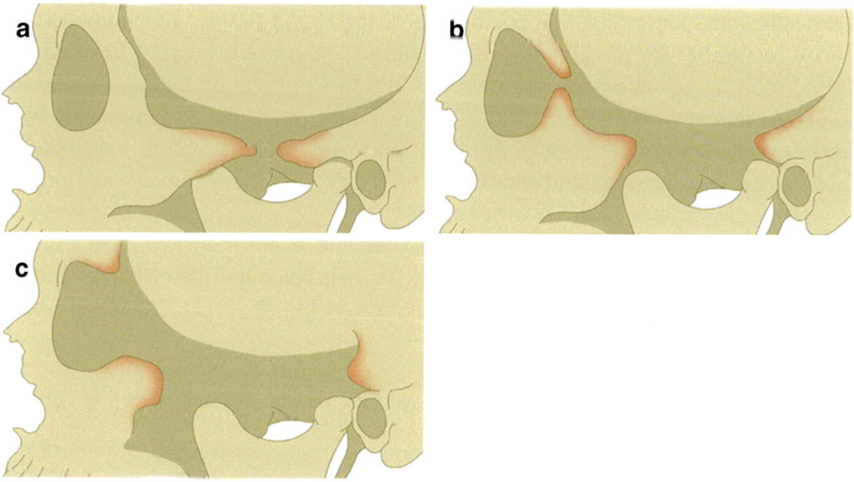

Fig. 18.2 Treacher Collins syndrome classification. (**a**) Small zygomatic body with all articulations except for the arch. (**b**) Diminished malar structure and absence along the lateral orbital wall. Inferolateral orbital rim intact, arch is incomplete. (**c**) Remnants of malar structure at the zygomaticofrontal or maxillary region

ZMC articulations, and the near aplasia of the zygoma, accounts for the classic malar flattening and lid and lateral canthal malposition that is seen in a typical TCS patient. The type III zygoma is the most frequent deformity in the TCS patient (Fig. 18.2c) [1].

Nikkhah and colleagues [10] based their classification system on 3D CT images (Table 18.1). Type 1 defects are mild and are characterized by a hypoplastic or dysplastic orbitozygomatic complex. Most TCS patients that fall within this category can be treated by fat transfer only [10].

Type 2 defects usually have a bony discontinuity of the zygomatic arch with a dysplastic or absent lateral orbital wall. These types of defects require surgery to address the hard tissue defect. These types of defects may warrant a malar osteotomy, alloplast onlay, autograft onlay techniques, or simultaneous osteotomy with an onlay technique [10].

Types 3 and 4 are the most severe defects, and both types require bony or alloplastic augmentation [10]. Type 3 defects have a hypoplastic zygomatic body and a dysplastic orbital wall. The zygomatic temporal process is completely absent in these patients. Type 4 presents with a complete absence of the entire orbitozygomatic complex [10].

Timing of Reconstruction

Once a patient has been diagnosed with TCS, determining when to surgically intervene is important to the overall success of the reconstruction. By 7 years of age, hypoplasia of the lateral wall of the orbit is associated with dislocation of the external canthus and antimongolian positioning of the eyelid fissure. This may be corrected preferably on or after the patient turns 7 years old, bearing in mind the cranio-orbitozygomatic bony maturation is close to completion by the age of 7 [4, 6, 11]. At this age, adult-sized cheekbones may be constructed and implanted with little concern about how growth will alter the result. Other surgeons have recommended various methods and timing for the correction of zygomatic and orbital deformities associated with TCS [6, 12, 13].

Surgical correction before the age of 5 years old is not indicated unless severe corneal exposure problems have occurred [6, 14]. Neonatal tarsorrhaphy can be performed to prevent corneal scarring, ulceration, or blindness [1]. Other periorbital

Table 18.1 Classification system of the orbitozygomatic skeletal deformities seen in Treacher Collins syndrome [10]

Classification	Defect	Surgical procedure
Type 1	Mild	Fat transfer
Type 2	Moderate	Zygomatic osteotomy +/− onlay technique
Type 3/4	Severe	Alloplastic vs. autologous augmentation

corrections should be delayed. This is because the extent of the lower lid skin deficit can be better assessed after skeletal correction.

Given the cosmetic anomalies that TCS can cause, surgeons must also think about the psychosocial concerns of the patients when considering intervention. Weighing the potential for scarring and revision surgery with earlier intervention versus evaluating the mental stability of a patient must be taken seriously. This can often be very a difficult decision when planning for surgical intervention [15].

Treatment Options

Correcting the orbitozygomatic region in a TCS patient can be achieved via an array of surgical interventions. Minimally invasive to invasive techniques have been described to correct or camouflage deficiencies brought about from TCS. Fat grafting and injectables have been used to augment soft tissue. Hard tissue onlays with either autologous bone grafts or alloplastic materials have been used to augment the underlining bony structure of the orbitozygomatic complex [4, 15].

Some authors advocate for the use of vascularized bone graft transpositions from the cranial vault, citing more predictability of the reconstructed area, while other employ the zygomatic osteotomy and protrusion of the orbital margins with simultaneous support of the osteotomized fragments with bone grafts or hydroxyapatite [4].

As a secondary procedure, McCarthy and Hopper [16] have proposed distraction of the zygomatic bone with an onlay graft procedure for reconstruction of these defects [4, 17].

Once the bony augmentation is complete, in order to achieve normal protrusion of the cheeks, temporal region, and lower eyelids, soft-tissue grafts are sometimes transferred under the skin [4].

Each procedure can be used alone, or in conjunction with one another in order to reconstruct these defects and achieve the desired cosmetic outcome. Surgical intervention for these patients is still debated in the literature, and all will be discussed in detail below.

Fat Grafting

Patients that have mild deformities associated with TCS can take advantage of fat transfer. The technique has the benefit of being repeatable as well as the ability to be implemented before skeletal maturity as it does not interfere with bony growth. This is particularly advantageous in the growing child who has psychosocial concerns [1, 18].

Fat transfer also plays a role in more severe defects but must be used in combination with hard tissue augmentation. Protocol for the reconstruction of the orbitozygomatic area in these complex patients must include the following steps in this order: fat grafting, bone reconstruction, and final revisions [18].

Fat grafting, per Konofaos et al. [18], is performed two to three consecutive times every 6 months, after the age of 6 months. Bone reconstruction, using calvarial bone grafts, is then performed 6 months after the last fat transfer procedure. At the revision stage, fat grafting can also be used to augment the orbitozygomatic area [18].

The fat transfer procedure is completed under general anesthesia and typically harvested from the abdomen or the flank. Fat can also be harvested from the thigh or breast regions [19]. The aspirated fat is centrifuged for 3 minutes at 3000 rpm. After the supernatant is removed, fat is transferred into 1 mL syringes and injected immediately into the orbitozygomatic region [18, 20]. The adipose tissue should be evenly distributed subcutaneously in a fan-shaped manner [19]. In the lower eyelids, 1–4 mL is placed, and in the malar area, 5–7 mL of fat is infused [18].

Fat transfer is increasing in popularity due to minimal donor site morbidity as well as its minimally invasive nature. In regard to future orbitozygomatic reconstruction, the idea of fat transplantation, possibly with the use of stem cells, may play an increasingly important role. This may reduce the need for larger reconstructive surgical procedures, significantly reducing associated overall morbidity [19].

Autologous Bone Grafts

The most common recommendation for zygomatic reconstruction in the TCS patient is the traditional autologous bone graft. Autologous bone grafting is a well-known and reliable procedure associated with less than a 1% complication rate in the literature [21]. Resorption is the main limitation of the bone graft, especially in TCS patients requiring large bone volume.

Its noted that, quite often, this procedure has to be repeated due to the significant resorption of the nonvascularized bone [5]. Because the bone graft is not subjected to any functional load as it would be in most mandibular or maxillary osteotomies, the grafted zygomatic region is thought to be less resistant to resorption. While the literature shows a decreased rate of resorption when split or full-thickness calvarial bone grafts are used in reconstruction versus the previously reported use of costochondral grafts, resorption is still a concern [1, 3]. Fan and colleagues [22] have also found a correlation between the age of the patient at time of grafting and degree of resorption. They note that as age increases, the likelihood of bony resorption decreases. There seems to be a correlation with a lower rate of resorption when it is performed after age 12 or at the end of craniofacial growth [22–25].

In an effort to combat excessive resorption, some surgeons recommend prior or early age fat transfer before orbitozygomatic reconstruction to improve the bone graft revascularization [18, 22].

The Posnick and colleagues technique for reconstruction utilizes full-thickness calvarial bone grafts that have been contoured three-dimensionally to form a new zygomatic complex [6]. These are then inset and stabilized with microplate and

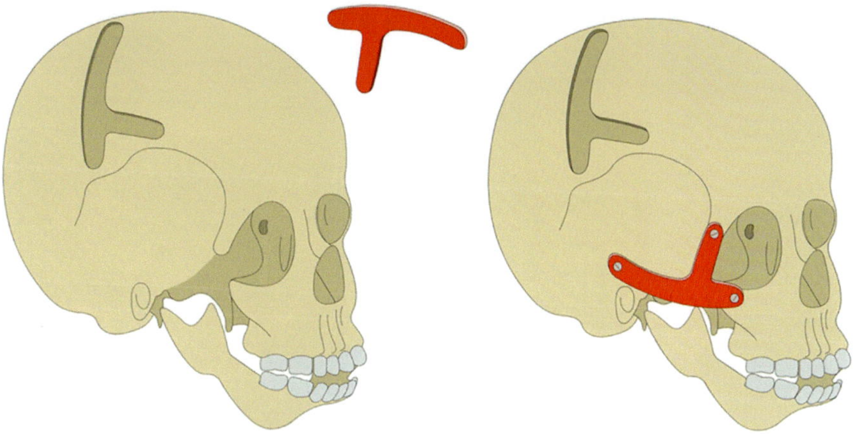

Fig. 18.3 Schematic of a cranial autologous harvest and inset

screw fixation (Fig. 18.3) [6, 14, 26]. Exposure for the reconstruction is provided by a coronal (scalp) incision without periorbital incisions. Orbital floor defects are then reconstructed, and cranial vault graft donor sites are repaired with fixed split-thickness autogenous cranial bone or bone substitutes (i.e., calcium phosphate cements). Lateral canthopexies are completed through the coronal (scalp) incision and secured to each new lateral orbital rim [6].

Preoperative and postoperative CT scanning should be obtained to evaluate the increases in lateral orbital wall length, lateral orbital (rim) distance (width), interzygomatic arch distance (width), and zygomatic arch length for patients [6, 14].

Computer-assisted surgery (CAS) results in better skeletal volumetric analysis that may improve the autologous graft procedure [25].

A presurgical simulation can be performed with a 3D computed tomography (CT) scan. Using this data can allow for the surgeon to obtain optimal shape and volume of the needed bone, cutting guides for the harvest of the bicortical calvaria avoiding critical neurovascular structures, as well as drilling guides and the customized plates for the frontozygomatic fixation [14, 27].

CAS allows for the calvarial harvest and orbitozygomatic reconstruction to be perfectly adapted to each patient's morphology. This provides for the manufacture of custom positioning and cutting guides, avoiding dangerous areas and limiting imprecise graft/bone interface contact, palpable edges, persistent asymmetry, and the need for repeat bone grafting [14].

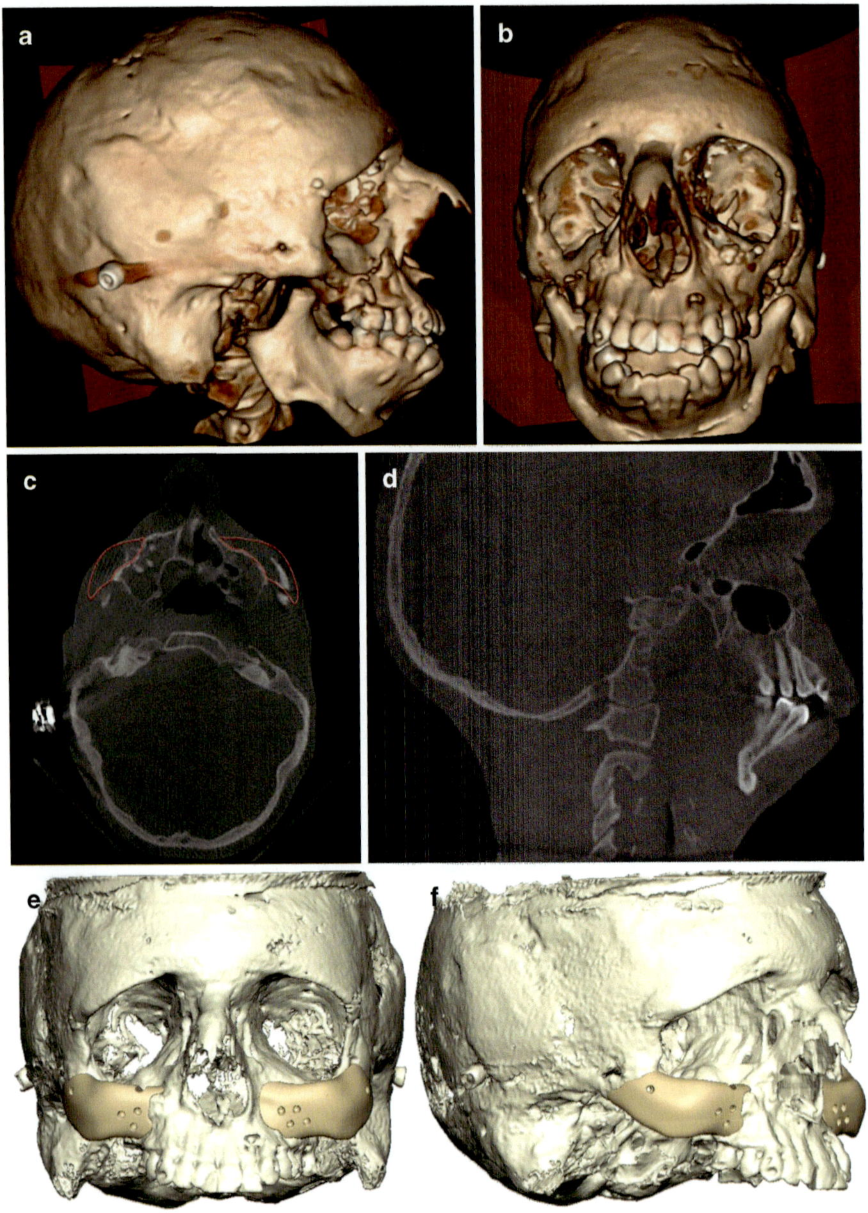

Fig. 18.4 (**a-i**) Alloplastic Implant. (**a**) Preop profile to malar implant reconstruction. (**b**) Preop frontal to malar implant reconstruction. (**c**) Axial view – red outline represents new implant position. (**d**) Sagittal view – red outline represents new implant position. (**e**) Frontal view – proposed implant. (**f**) Right 3/4 view – proposed implant. (**g**) Right profile view – proposed implant. (**h**) Worms view – proposed implant. (**i**) Implant close-up notch made to accommodate infraorbital nerve

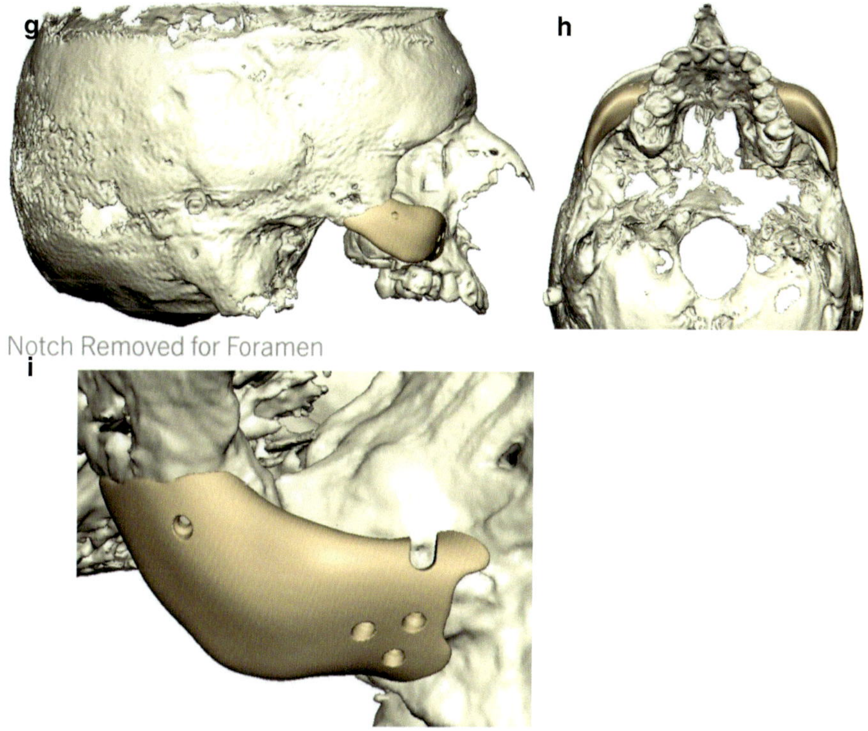

Fig. 18.4 (continued)

Alloplastic Custom Implants

The alloplastic custom implant is an attractive option permitting anatomical reconstruction. Medpore, silicone, or polyether ether ketone (PEEK) can be used (Fig. 18.4) [10, 28]. It is a simple surgery without autologous harvest that would involve donor-site comorbidity [24]. In addition, an implant allows reconstruction that conforms to the mechanical properties of the implantation site and does not suffer from resorption. The downside is that this procedure could produce complications such as chronic inflammation, infection, displacement, or extrusion of the implant [1, 3, 24, 28]. This could require additional surgical procedures in the future, including removal of the implant.

The surgical procedure involves intraoperative access via an upper buccal sulcus incision followed by subperiosteal malar tissue dissection to the periorbita. Further dissection is performed to the lateral orbital rim, with the masseter freed from its anomalous lateral periorbital attachment. The implant is then inserted into the dissected pocket. The position of the implant is then verified clinically and secured with plates and screws. During placement, one must continually assess pupillary diameter and globe hardness [29]. The surgeon should be aware that there is an increased risk of globe compression with implant placement with orbitozygomatic defects. This is especially true in cases where there is a complete absence of the zygoma, and the periorbital soft-tissue boundaries are unaccounted for during the procedure [28].

Zygomatic Osteotomy

The malar osteotomy is another surgical intervention that has been utilized to reconstruct the orbitozygomatic region. It is a simple technique with low patient morbidity and very effective at treating midfacial width. The technique has some limitations in its ability to increase anterior projection of the zygoma [31]. In addition, the vertical height of the zygoma is usually reduced in TCS because of a decrease of bone stock. For those reasons, most surgeons prefer to perform the zygomatic osteotomy in combination with an onlay technique for reconstruction of the orbitozygomatic complex in the TCS patient [10].

The Mommaerts zygomatic osteotomy is a favorite given it does not change orbital volume or widen the orbit [10, 30]. It involves accessing the zygoma by either a LeFort I-type osteotomy approach or by way of a horizontal incision of 1.5 cm length in the upper buccal sulcus [30]. The medial anterior surface of the zygoma is dissected subperiosteally up to the infraorbital rim. The dissection stops cephalad to the semi-horizontal groove palpable below the orbital rim. Laterally, the periosteum is tunneled up to the junction between the frontal and temporal processes. The posterior aspect of the zygomatic crest is also degloved for approximately 2 cm. A vertical osteotomy, through both the anterior and posterior walls of the maxillary sinus. The osteotomy cut stops about 4 mm below the infraorbital rim. An oblique horizontal bone cut is made under raspatory protection, proceeding antero-medially from the junction of the zygomatic arch and body, transecting the sinus walls beneath the orbital floor, and joining the vertical osteotomy at its superior end. The bone cuts are completed with small chisels. A greenstick fracture occurs at the temporo-zygomatic suture. A hydroxyapatite (HA) block or bone grafting material is then carved to a trapezoid of desired width and wedged into the vertical osteotomy space. As a result of this outward rotation, more anterior fullness is created [30, 31].

Vascularized Flaps

To many surgeons, the microvascular soft-tissue approach is effectively considered a salvage effort for persistent suboptimal outcomes instead of a primary reconstructive procedure, but vascularized flaps can provide a long-lasting or even permanent outcome as a primary procedure. Pedicled flaps may be of a little use in facial contouring due to pedicle length and restriction in flap size, but vascularized free flaps, depending on their donor sites, can provide an appropriate bulk that the patient desires without the restriction of the pedicle.

Parascapular Flaps

The parascapular flap is a thin, fasciocutaneous flap with the vascular supply based on the circumflex scapular vessels [32]. The versatility of the parascapular flap allows for detailed contouring of the tissue to address the specific deficiencies in each patient [2]. Good esthetic results can be achieved with minimal complications and minor revisions.

Saadeh and colleagues state that a two-team approach is best but not required to complete the procedure. Procedure begins with simultaneous ipsilateral parascapular flap harvest and facial pocket dissection [2, 33, 34]. A preauricular facelift incision is used for access, allowing for both adequate exposure and a discreet scar, regardless of the soft-tissue requirements. Facial dissection is then carried out in the subcutaneous facelift plane, continuing 1 cm beyond preoperative markings [2].

Once the parascapular flap is harvested, the microvascular anastomoses are completed [2]. Absorbable buried sutures were used to secure the flap to the periosteum near the anastomoses. Absorbable sutures are then used to suspend the flap from the infraorbital rim, lateral orbital rim, and zygoma. The flap should then be secured with tie-over bolster sutures of preplaced 4–0 nylon. The final flap contour and insetting should be confirmed with the patient being upright [2].

Groin Flaps

The use of groin flaps has also been described in the orbital reconstruction of TCS patients. They are advantageous because they require less preoperative planning and have a relatively short operation time [29]. Other hallmarks of the procedure include acceptable donor site morbidity, ability to conceal scars, and primary closure of the donor site, and functional impairment is less likely except for limitation of ambulation during immediate postoperative periods [29, 35, 36].

Heo and colleagues [29] describe the procedure as the following: On each side of the groin, a flap with approximately 13 × 6 cm-sized skin paddle is designed. Flaps are elevated with superficial circumflex iliac artery and vein. Bilateral preauricular incisions were made, and dissection was done above the superficial musculo-aponeurotic system (SMAS) plane. Recipient vascular pedicles used were the superficial temporal artery and vein. De-epithelialization of both flaps is then completed. Donor vascular pedicles are then disconnected on each flap. Microanastomosis is then completed, one flap at a time. This is completed in an end-to-end fashion. Lastly, the de-epithelialized flaps are slid into each defect zone, and the wound is closed in a layered fashion. Negative-pressure closed-suction drain in each side should be placed and sutured before complete closure [29].

Distraction Osteogenesis

Distraction osteogenesis is typically used in secondary cases where there is suboptimal malar projection of a previously reconstructed zygomatic complex. When compared with serial bone grafting, distraction osteogenesis has the benefits of slowly stretching the associated soft-tissue envelope and avoiding the need for repeat bone graft harvest [16].

The disadvantages of this technique are that the vector of distraction may be compromised by the placement of the previous bone grafts. This may lead to a non-union of the zygomatic arch. Additionally, all steps are taken to maintain the periosteal blood supply to the distracted segment, but there is also the risk of devascularization of the bone-grafted segment during the procedure [16].

Tissue Engineering

Tissue engineering of the zygomatic maxillary complex segment may be an additional option to reconstruct the craniofacial skeleton [1, 4, 37, 38]. This could be a critical breakthrough for TCS patients with severe defects of the orbitozygomatic region. Lengthy operations, multiple revision surgeries, and additional donor site morbidity could all be potentially eliminated with advancements in tissue engineering. The ability to provide an exact replica of a missing bone, with normal growth potential, and be resistant to infection is an exciting possibility for TCS patients [38].

Orbital Soft-Tissue Reconstruction

There are several surgical techniques dedicated to the improvement of the soft-tissue deficiencies associated with the eyelid and adnexal regions. Most surgeons prefer staging the surgical correction of the coloboma after zygoma and orbital reconstruction. This is to better assess the extent of lid skin deficit after the skeletal correction [1, 3, 6, 7].

The surgical technique and timing of intervention depend upon the size of the defect and the presence of corneal exposure. Defects are graded as small (less than 25% of the length of lid margin), moderate (25 to 50% defect), and severe (more than 50%) [39].

Depending on the deformity, orbicularis transposition, skin grafting, Z-plasty, and/or canthopexy can be performed [1, 3, 40] (Fig. 18.5). Not all of these procedures have produced the most esthetically pleasing soft-tissue eyelid results [4, 17]. The transposition of pedicled upper eyelid skin muscle flaps to deficient regions of the lower eyelid typically causes adnexal scarring [3, 6]. The scarring can then be severe and may detract from any positive advantages of the procedure [6, 39].

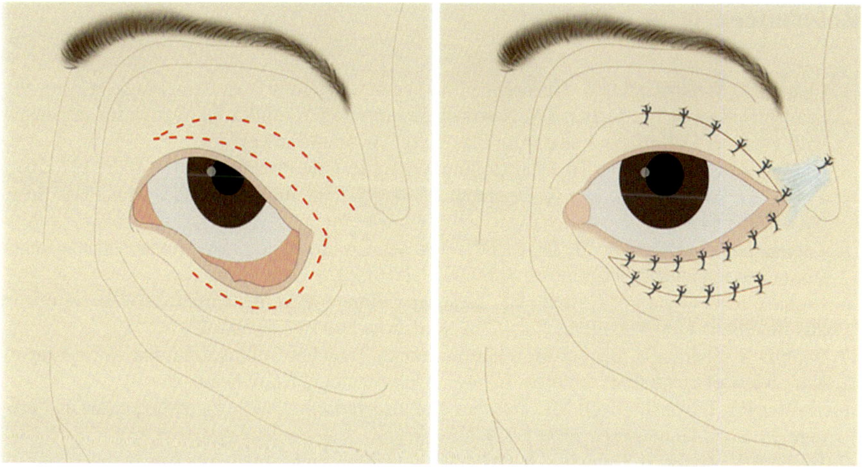

Fig. 18.5 Coloboma correction surgery. Upper eyelid rotational flap followed by results of the flap rotation with lateral canthopexy

Mustarde's cheek rotation flap is particularly useful for reconstruction involving larger, vertical defects of the lower lid. Lower eyelid defects involving the entire lower eyelid may be reconstructed using a Mustarde's cheek rotation flap. A large skin muscle flap is rotated from the cheek to repair large lower eyelid defects while the posterior lamella can undergo reconstruction with tarsoconjunctival, nasal cartilage, or mucous membrane grafts [39].

Full-thickness skin grafts to reconstruct the lower eyelids are another frequently mentioned procedure. This procedure can leave a "patchy" look and should be reserved only for patients with unresolved corneal exposure [6].

With meticulous planning and execution, the transfer of soft-tissue flaps (groin flap) from other body regions, with microvascular reanastomosis, offers an alternative for augmentation of the adnexal, temporal, and cheek soft tissues [33, 34, 41].

Conclusion

Treacher Collins syndrome is a congenital disorder known for significant deficiencies in the midfacial region. Surgical reconstruction is planned based on the morphology and severity of the defects. There are many surgical options available to TCS patients for the correction of midfacial and orbital anomalies. Surgical intervention should not occur before the age of 7; however, psychosocial concerns may warrant earlier intervention. Although there is no gold standard for the reconstruction of these patients, all surgical techniques may provide adequate reestablishment of midfacial and orbital contours. To determine which surgical intervention is best, precise anatomical evaluation, timing of surgery, psychological state, and potential for future surgeries must be adequately assessed.

References

1. Chang CC, Steinbacher DM. Treacher Collins syndrome. Semin Plast Surg. 2012;26(2):83–90.
2. Saadeh P, Reavey PL, Siebert JW. A soft-tissue approach to midfacial hypoplasia associated with Treacher Collins syndrome. Ann Plast Surg. 2006;56(5):522–5.
3. Aljerian A, Gilardino MS. Treacher Collins syndrome. Clin Plast Surg. 2019;46(2):197–205.
4. Kobus K, Wojcicki P. Surgical treatment of Treacher Collins syndrome. Ann Plast Surg. 2006;56(5):549–54.
5. Thompson JT, Anderson PJ, David DJ. Treacher Collins syndrome: protocol management from birth to maturity. J Craniofac Surg. 2009;20(6):2028–35.
6. Posnick JC, Tiwana PS, Costello BJ. Treacher Collins syndrome: comprehensive evaluation and treatment. Oral Maxillofac Surg Clin North Am. 2004;16(4):503–23.
7. Sharma R, Sharma B, Babber M, Singh S, Jain G. Treacher Collins syndrome: a case report and review of ophthalmic features. Taiwan J Ophthalmol. 2016;6(4):206–9.
8. Trainor PA, Dixon J, Dixon MJ. Treacher Collins syndrome: etiology, pathogenesis and prevention. Eur J Hum Genet. 2009;17(3):275–83.
9. Hertle RW, Ziylan S, Katowitz JA. Ophthalmic features and visual prognosis in the Treacher-Collins syndrome. Br J Ophthalmol. 1993;77(10):642–5.
10. Nikkhah D, Ponniah A, Ruff C, Dunaway D. A classification system to guide orbitozygomatic reconstruction in Treacher-Collins syndrome. J Plast Reconstr Aesthet Surg. 2013;66(7):1003–5.
11. Waitzman AA, Posnick JC, Armstrong DC, Pron GE. Craniofacial skeletal measurements based on computed tomography: part II. Normal values and growth trends. Cleft Palate Craniofac J. 1992;29(2):118–28.
12. Zanini S, Viterbo F, Parro F, Tershakowec M. Bone graft of the zygoma in a patient with Treacher-Collins syndrome. J Craniofac Surg. 1994;5(4):270.
13. Freihofer HP. Variations in the correction of Treacher Collins syndrome. Plast Reconstr Surg. 1997;99(3):647–57.
14. Posnick JC, Goldstein JA, Waitzman AA. Surgical correction of the Treacher Collins malar deficiency: quantitative CT scan analysis of long-term results. Plast Reconstr Surg. 1993;92(1):12–22.
15. Cobb AR, Green B, Gill D, et al. The surgical management of Treacher Collins syndrome. Br J Oral Maxillofac Surg. 2014;52(7):581–9.
16. McCarthy JG, Hopper RA. Distraction osteogenesis of zygomatic bone grafts in a patient with Treacher Collins syndrome: a case report. J Craniofac Surg. 2002;13(2):279–83; discussion, 84–6.
17. Ueda K, Nuri T, Shigemura Y. Malar reconstruction using Y-V advancement flaps after tissue expansion in Treacher Collins syndrome. Plast Reconstr Surg Glob Open. 2016;4(5):e715.
18. Konofaos P, Arnaud E. Early fat grafting for augmentation of orbitozygomatic region in Treacher Collins syndrome. J Craniofac Surg. 2015;26(4):1258–60.
19. Hammer-Hansen N, Akram J, Damsgaard TE. The versatility of autologous fat transplantation in correction of facial deformities: a single-center experience. Plast Surg Int. 2015;2015:703535.
20. Coleman SR. Facial recontouring with lipostructure. Clin Plast Surg. 1997;24(2):347–67.
21. Tessier P, Kawamoto H, Matthews D, et al. Autogenous bone grafts and bone substitutes--tools and techniques: I. A 20,000-case experience in maxillofacial and craniofacial surgery. Plast Reconstr Surg. 2005;116(5 Suppl):6S–24S; discussion 92S–94S.
22. Fan KL, Federico C, Kawamoto HK, Bradley JP. Optimizing the timing and technique of Treacher Collins orbital malar reconstruction. J Craniofac Surg. 2012;23(7 Suppl 1):2033–7.
23. Plomp RG, van Lieshout MJ, Joosten KF, et al. Treacher Collins syndrome: a systematic review of evidence-based treatment and recommendations. Plast Reconstr Surg. 2016;137(1):191–204.

24. Herlin C, Doucet JC, Bigorre M, Khelifa HC, Captier G. Computer-assisted midface reconstruction in Treacher Collins syndrome part 1: skeletal reconstruction. J Craniomaxillofac Surg. 2013;41(7):670–5.
25. Pare A, Joly A, Queiros C, Goga D, Laure B. Computer-assisted bilateral Orbitozygomatic reconstruction in a patient with Treacher Collins syndrome using bicortical calvarial graft. JAMA Facial Plast Surg. 2018;20(6):523–5.
26. Tessier P. Complications associated with the harvesting of cranial bone grafts [discussion]. Plast Reconstr Surg. 1995;95:14.
27. Guo Y, Lopez J, Yang R, Macmillan A, Dorafshar AH. The use of virtual surgical planning in total facial skeletal reconstruction of Treacher Collins syndrome: a case report. Craniomaxillofac Trauma Reconstr. 2018;11(3):230–7.
28. Sainsbury DC, George A, Forrest CR, Phillips JH. Bilateral malar reconstruction using patient-specific polyether ether ketone implants in Treacher-Collins syndrome patients with absent zygomas. J Craniofac Surg. 2017;28(2):515–7.
29. Heo JW, Jin US. Contouring of zygomatic soft tissue using bilateral free groin flaps in a Treacher Collins syndrome patient. Arch Craniofac Surg. 2018;19(2):131–4.
30. Mommaerts MY, Abeloos JV, De Clercq CA, Neyt LF. The 'sandwich' zygomatic osteotomy: technique, indications and clinical results. J Craniomaxillofac Surg. 1995;23(1):12–9.
31. Layoun W, Guyot L, Richard O, Gola R. Augmentation of cheek bone contour using malar osteotomy. Aesthet Plast Surg. 2003;27(4):269–74.
32. Chandrasekhar B, Lorant JA, Terz JJ. Parascapular free flaps for head and neck reconstruction. Am J Surg. 1990;160(4):450–3.
33. Siebert JW, Anson G, Longaker MT. Microsurgical correction of facial asymmetry in 60 consecutive cases. Plast Reconstr Surg. 1996;97(2):354–63.
34. Longaker MT, Siebert JW. Microsurgical correction of facial contour in congenital craniofacial malformations: the marriage of hard and soft tissue. Plast Reconstr Surg. 1996;98(6):942–50.
35. Harashina T, Fujino T. Reconstruction in Romberg's disease with free groin flap. Ann Plast Surg. 1981;7(4):289–94.
36. McGregor IA, Jackson IT. The groin flap. Br J Plast Surg. 1972;25(1):3–16.
37. Abukawa H, Shin M, Williams WB, et al. Reconstruction of mandibular defects with autologous tissue-engineered bone. J Oral Maxillofac Surg. 2004;62(5):601–6.
38. Taylor JA. Bilateral orbitozygomatic reconstruction with tissue-engineered bone. J Craniofac Surg. 2010;21(5):1612–4.
39. Kanukollu VM, Ahmad SS. Eyelid Coloboma. Treasure Island: StatPearls; 2020.
40. Goodrich JTHC. Craniofacial anomalies: growth and development from a surgical perspective. New York: Thieme: Medical Publishers; 1995.
41. Longaker MT, Flynn A, Siebert JW. Microsurgical correction of bilateral facial contour deformities. Plast Reconstr Surg. 1996;98(6):951–7.

Chapter 19
Management of the Mandibular Deformity in Growing Patients with Treacher Collins Syndrome

Srinivas M. Susarla, Mark A. Egbert, Hitesh Kapadia, and Richard A. Hopper

Background

Maxillomandibular differences in patients with Treacher Collins syndrome remain challenging for patients and surgeons alike. While mandibular deficiency is a hallmark of the condition ("mandibulofacial dysostosis"), there is a spectrum of presenting phenotypes that are managed by a similarly broad range of interventions, from minimal medical management of mildly hypoplastic skeletal structures to complex, staged interventions for management of severe dysplasias. The phenotypic hallmark of severe maxillomandibular discrepancy is characterized by

S. M. Susarla (✉) · M. A. Egbert
Department of Surgery, Division of Plastic Surgery, University of Washington School of Medicine, Seattle, WA, USA

Department of Oral and Maxillofacial Surgery, University of Washington School of Dentistry, Seattle, WA, USA

Craniofacial Center, Seattle Children's Hospital, Seattle, WA, USA
e-mail: SRINIVAS.SUSARLA@SEATTLECHILDRENS.ORG; MARK.EGBERT@SEATTLECHILDRENS.ORG

H. Kapadia
Craniofacial Center, Division of Craniofacial Orthodontics, Seattle Children's Hospital, Seattle, WA, USA

University of Washington School of Dentistry, Seattle, WA, USA
e-mail: HITESH.KAPADIA@SEATTLECHILDRENS.ORG

R. A. Hopper
Department of Surgery, Division of Plastic Surgery, University of Washington School of Medicine, Seattle, WA, USA

Craniofacial Center, Seattle Children's Hospital, Seattle, WA, USA
e-mail: RICHARD.HOPPER@SEATTLECHILDRENS.ORG

D. M. Yates, M. R. Markiewicz (eds.), *Craniofacial Microsomia and Treacher Collins Syndrome*, https://doi.org/10.1007/978-3-030-84733-3_19

clockwise rotation of a hypoplastic maxillomandibular complex, with concomitant orbitozygomatic hypoplasia (Figs. 19.1a-d) [1–11]. This rotational deformity presents as a long anterior face height, short posterior face height, prominent nasal dorsum, anterior open bite, and a retruded mandible with steep mandibular plane angle with associated microgenia. Hypoplasia (or aplasia) of the zygomatic bones, often with associated soft tissue clefting, contributes to mandibular dysmorphology due to a developmentally deficient glenoid fossa. The primary skeletal differences are frequently accompanied by hypoplasia of the associated lateral facial soft tissues, including the muscles of mastication and facial expression. Dental anomalies are not infrequent within the population of patients with TCS [11].

The anatomic differences associated with maxillomandibular skeletal dysmorphology are frequently translated to pathologic airway obstruction [12–15]. Airway obstruction in patients with TCS is a complex phenomenon but is primarily related

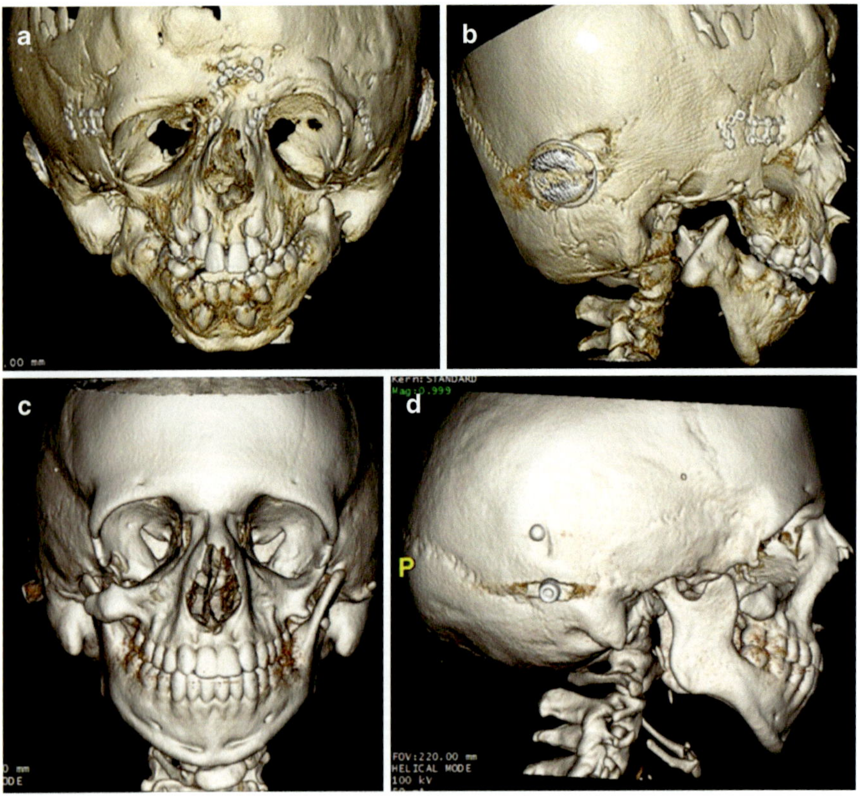

Fig. 19.1 Characteristic facial skeletal dysplasia in a patient with Treacher Collins syndrome. The hallmark of the phenotypic presentation is clockwise rotation of the maxillomandibular complex, resulting in a long anterior face height, short posterior face height, anterior open bite, and steep mandibular and palatal planes. The degree of mandibular dysmorphology drives the clockwise rotational deformity, with more severely foreshortened rami (**a, b**) resulting in a more profound rotational deformity relative to patients with minimal ramus-condyle unit hypoplasia (**c, d**)

to occlusion of the oropharyngeal airway by a hypoplastic skeletal framework, although abnormalities of the entire upper airway can exist [14–15]. Management in infancy is predicated on establishing appropriate upper airway physiology, feeding, hearing, preservation of vision through corneal protection, and management of facial/palatal clefts (if present). The complexity of management of these various components necessitates multidisciplinary care to establish a treatment plan and continually follow progress over time, as surgical interventions can be numerous and extend over the course of many years [2].

Maxillomandibular disharmony plays a critical role in the pathophysiology of TCS. Unlike other congenital craniofacial differences, however, TCS is not generally progressive [11]. The magnitude of the skeletal discrepancy at birth is relatively stable over time. This feature distinguishes TCS from other congenital and developmental conditions involving the maxillomandibular complex, such as craniofacial microsomia, Goldenhar syndrome, and oculo-auriculo-vertebral syndrome. Airway challenges are multifactorial and may include nasal obstruction related to choanal atresia/stenosis, glossoptosis related to micrognathia, and lower airway anomalies such as tracheomalacia. Infants with mild degrees of facial dysplasia may only require noninvasive maneuvers such as special positioning and monitoring of oxygen saturation. In patients with severe presenting phenotypes, airway embarrassment is not infrequent, and tracheostomy placement at birth or infancy is well-described. Interventions in the growing child vary from center to center but share the common goal of establishing an advanced jaw position to facilitate airway expansion.

One critical component of management of the skeletal difference in TCS is recognition of the condition as non-progressive. Roberts and colleagues, in 1975, characterized the morphologic features of TCS using lateral cephalometry [10]. They reported small sella-nasion-B point angles (consistent with marked retrognathia) but relatively normal sella-nasion-A point angles (suggestive of relatively normal maxillary angular position). Facial heights were correspondingly suggestive of a lower facial deficiency with upper facial heights notably normal and total facial heights longer than normal. Sella-nasion to mandibular plane and sella-nasion to palatal plane angles were obtuse, consistent with clockwise rotation of the maxillomandibular complex. These cephalometric parameters were clinically evident as a convex facial profile defined by decreased horizontal length and increased anterior vertical length with associated mandibular deficiency characterized by a truncated ramus height and shortened body length. Remarkably, this constellation of facial differences was age-independent; the characteristic deficiency was relatively unchanged from infancy through skeletal maturity. These preliminary observations were confirmed by a number of other investigators, who documented stability of the mandibular position over time, suggestive of constant growth without "catch-up" potential [7–9, 11]

The clinical observations regarding the lack of accelerated growth normalizing mandibular morphology led many surgeons to consider early mandibular advancement, most recently through the use of distraction osteogenesis. While there is some evidence that early distraction osteogenesis improves airway dynamics to the extent that decannulation is possible in tracheostomy-dependent children, early distraction has also been reported to have potentially detrimental effects on jaw growth, may be prone to relapse, and damage the temporomandibular joints. In this context, some surgeons advocate delaying skeletal reconstruction until maturity, if feasible [3–5, 11].

The magnitude of the mandibular deficiency in TCS has been well-described. The Pruzansky classification of the mandibular deformity in craniofacial microsomia, subsequently modified by Kaban, has been applied to the mandibular difference in TCS [16–17]. Under this paradigm, the severity of the mandibular dysostosis is related to two components: the glenoid fossa and the ramus-condyle unit. In the most mild cases (Type I, Fig. 19.1d), the degree of hypoplasia is minimal – all of the skeletal components are present but may be hypoplastic. These patients may have normal TMJ function. Moderate cases (Type II) have more significant hypoplasia of the individual components and are subdivided according to the stability of the TMJs. In Type IIA differences, the condylar apparatus (glenoid fossa + condylar head) may be dysplastic but has stable joint function. In contrast, Type IIB cases have severe condylar hypoplasia, resulting in unstable TMJ function without a reliable centric relation; this pattern of dysmorphology is relatively infrequent in TCS. The most severe mandibular deficiency (Type III, Fig. 19.1b) results in a ramus-condyle unit and glenoid morphology that is hypoplastic to the extent that no articulation between the mandible and skull base is possible. The adjunctive tissues of the temporomandibular joints – the articular disc, capsule, and glenoid fossa – are not present. The ramus-condyle unit is vertically short, and the sagittal position of the mandible is significantly retruded, with associated clockwise rotation. This degree of dysmorphology is frequently associated with complex airway challenges, frequently necessitating tracheostomy placement at birth or in early infancy.

Paradigms for Skeletal Reconstruction

Timing of skeletal reconstruction of the maxillomandibular deficiency in TCS is largely predicated on the degree of dysmorphology. In patients with mild deficiency, surgical intervention may not be required or may be limited to orthognathic interventions at skeletal maturity. Patients with severe deficiency may benefit from early interventions but frequently require multiple operations to achieve appropriate skeletal positioning. Surgical intervention in growing children is largely predicated on management of severe facial dysplasia and the associated airway compromise.

In this regard, the goals of craniofacial reconstruction in the growing child with TCS are threefold: improve airway physiology by expansion of the skeletal scaffold for the oropharynx and hypopharynx, establish appropriate maxillomandibular relationships and occlusion, and create balanced facial aesthetics. Bimaxillary orthognathic surgery in skeletally mature children with stable temporomandibular joints undergoing smaller rotational movements has been effective in some reports but may not be applicable to many patients with TCS. In contrast, isolated mandibular surgery in growing children with severe deformities, via distraction osteogenesis or skeletal reconstruction with autologous bone grafting and rigid fixation, had initially showed promise, but recent data have demonstrated significant relapse rates as well as incomplete or inadequate resolution of airway obstruction, necessitating multiple interventions with limited potential for success [18–24]. These specific challenges are heightened in the context of data demonstrating a paucity of improvement in the frequency and severity of airway obstruction in TCS with growth, consistent with the non-progressive nature of the deformity and lack of identifiable catch-up growth.

Contextually, early treatment for the tracheostomy-dependent child remains challenging. Interventions should construct appropriate skeletal morphology and improve airway dynamics, while also establishing an appropriate facial balance. Isolated mandibular interventions (e.g., distraction lengthening, genioglossus advancement) have limited utility in this regard, as they do not effectively address the clockwise rotation deformity that is uniformly present in patients with severe disease. Counterclockwise rotational movements of the maxillomandibular complex remain controversial in orthognathic surgery, precisely because of concerns regarding stability over time [25–30]. Prevailing explanations for the instability are related to the muscle pull from the suprahyoid system, as well as proximal segment changes. Confounding the picture is the available evidence suggesting that stability of the rotational movement is predicated on TMJ stability, which many patients with TCS lack a priori [27–29].

Analysis of airway volumes in patients with TCS has clearly demonstrated that the degree of clockwise maxillomandibular rotation and associated hypoplasia contribute to obstruction [14–15]. As such, counterclockwise movements are needed to counteract this primary deficiency. The apex example of conventional surgery for counterclockwise rotation was Tessier and Tulasne's "procedure integral," which incorporated a LeFort II osteotomy with mandibular advancement for composite subcranial rotation [31]. While a valid theoretical approach, this technique failed to gain widespread acceptance, due to high rates of relapse of the maxillary and mandibular plane rotations, the need for extensive bone grafting, and high degree of soft tissue resistance from the deficient lateral facial soft tissues and suprahyoid musculature.

Management of Severe Clockwise Rotation in the Growing Child

A more recent modification of this technique has sought to overcome these specific challenges, utilizing distraction osteogenesis to perform subcranial advancement with associated counterclockwise rotation [32]. Counterclockwise craniofacial distraction osteogenesis (C3DO) is an emerging technique that holds promise for management of tracheostomy dependent children with TCS (Fig. 19.2). The C3DO procedure involves concomitant maxillomandibular rotation via distraction, utilizing a LeFort II osteotomy with bilateral inverted-L mandibular osteotomies. Following completion of the osteotomies, the maxillomandibular complex is rotated in a counterclockwise direction, affording expansion of the oropharynx and hypopharynx, establishing appropriate palatal and mandibular planes, and creating balanced facial proportions.

Preliminary results from this technique have demonstrated successful decannulation in the majority of patients undergoing this procedure, including those with prior failed mandibular distraction. The success attributed to this intervention is believed to be related to the large degree of movement possible with coordinated maxillomandibular distraction. Among the preliminary cohort undergoing this procedure,

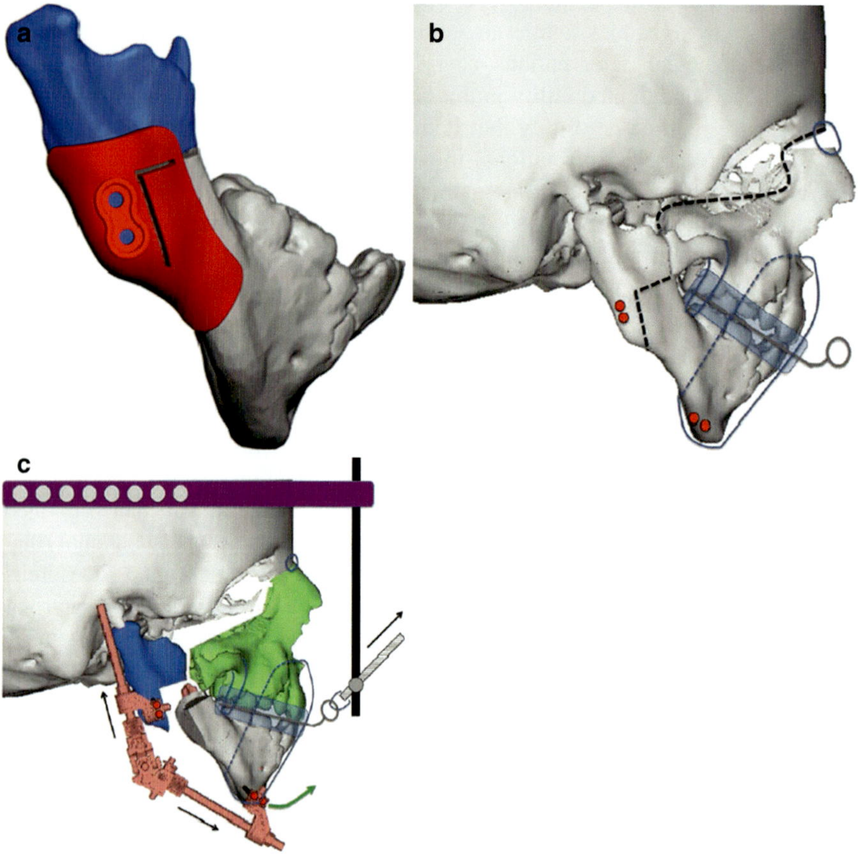

Fig. 19.2 Correction of severe clockwise craniofacial rotation deformities in TCS can be accomplished via synchronous maxillomandibular distraction osteogenesis. Virtual surgical planning is a helpful adjunct for developing cutting guides to plan the mandibular osteotomies and transfacial pin placement (**a**). A LeFort II osteotomy and bilateral mandibular inverted-L osteotomies are completed (**b**), and the maxillomandibular complex is distracted with a counterclockwise rotational movement (**c**). (Reprinted, with permission, from Ref. [33])

the average palatal plane rotation was 17 degrees, and the average facial plane rotation was 14 degrees [32]. Stability of the maxillomandibular position has been demonstrated, with preservation of the anterior facial height and ANB angle changes over time.

In this regard, our treatment protocol for the growing child with TCS characterized by severe Pruzansky-Kaban type III maxillomandibular deficiency (Figs. 19.3a-f) and tracheostomy-dependent airway is as follows [32–33]. In the first stage, appropriate ramus-condyle morphology is established, using autologous rib grafts. Once adequate healing has occurred and stable joint anatomy is established, as evidenced by a reproducible range of mandibular movement and a stable occlusion, counterclockwise craniofacial distraction osteogenesis is performed. After the appropriate maxillomandibular position is established, as evidenced by correction of the palatal and mandibular plane discrepancies, improvement of the anterior and posterior facial height ratios, improved occlusion, and, most importantly, optimized upper airway anatomy, orbitozygomatic reconstruction with calvarial autograft is completed. While effective for management of severe airway obstruction, the end-distraction morphology is prone to 20–30% skeletal relapse, manifested as recurrent anterior open bite (Figs. 19.3e-f). This relapse does not appear to affect airway dynamics but will likely necessitate definitive orthognathic surgery at skeletal maturity for management of the end-stage facial and occlusal dysmorphology [32].

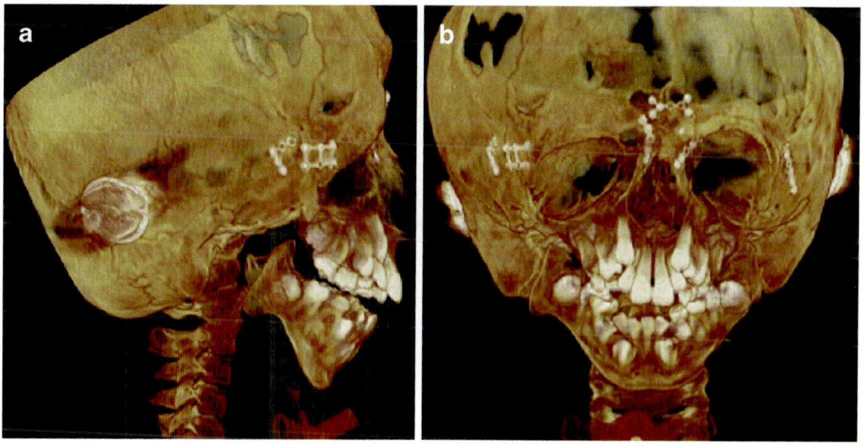

Fig. 19.3 Sequential treatment of a patient with severe maxillomandibular deficiency related to Treacher Collins syndrome. The morphologic presentation is notable for severe ramus-condyle unit dysplasia with no articulating surface (**a-b**), resulting in clockwise rotation of the maxillomandibular complex characterized by a long anterior face height, short posterior face height, anterior open bite, and accentuated palatal and mandibular plane angles. Initial reconstruction with autologous rib grafts establishes appropriate ramus condyle unit height (**c-d**). Following establishment of a stable joint anatomy, synchronous maxillomandibular counterclockwise rotation is performed via distraction osteogenesis. This results in correction of the clockwise rotational deformity and its associated sequelae. Definitive reconstruction of the orbitozygomatic complexes is accomplished at device removal with calvarial bone autograft (**e-f**)

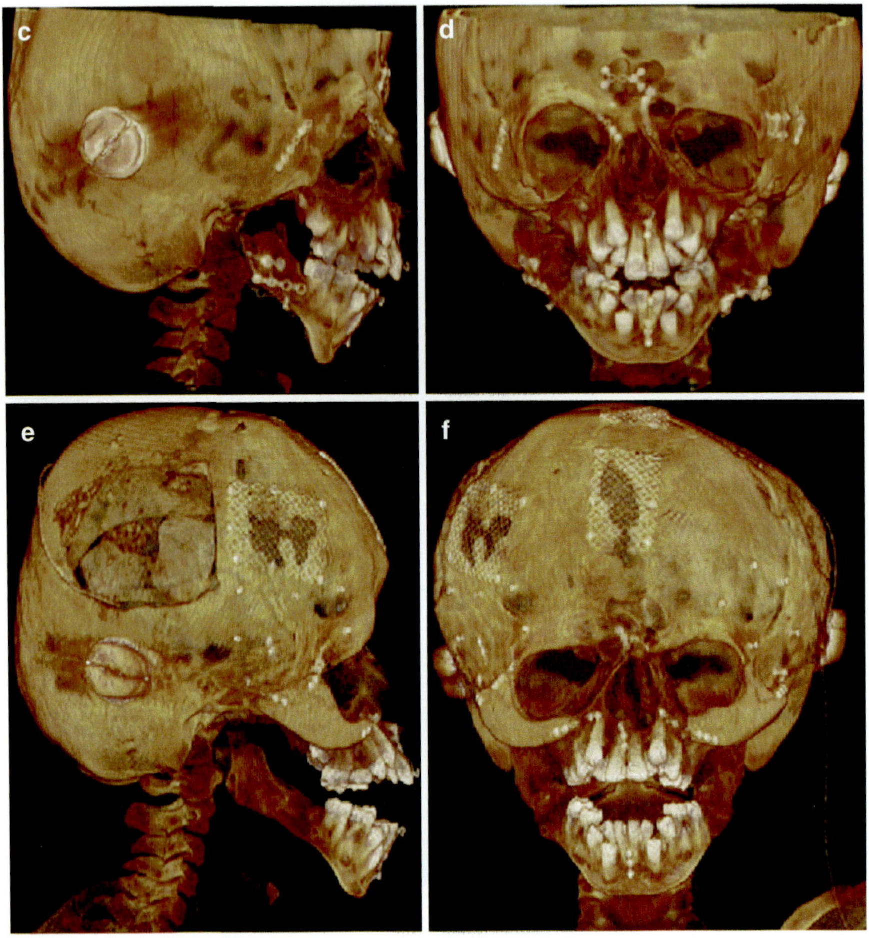

Fig. 19.3 (continued)

Additional modifications to this treatment paradigm are sometimes needed in patients who have sequelae from prior procedures, such as bony ankylosis from mandibular distraction. The complexity of this sequence of interventions necessitates multidisciplinary care and appropriate counseling to the patient and family, establishing the goals of treatment and expectations for recovery.

Management of Mild to Moderate Dysplasia in the Growing and Skeletally Mature Child

In patients with mild to moderate dysmorphology (e.g., minimal clockwise rotation) who do not have severe airway disease, reconstruction of mandibular rami and the orbitozygomatic complex can be completed in the mixed dentition (Figs. 19.4a-b). Definitive correction at skeletal maturity can be reliably accomplished with conventional orthognathic surgery in the form of mandibular ramus osteotomies with autologous bone grafting, midface advancement at the LeFort I level, and advancement genioplasty (Figs. 19.4c-f and 19.5a-h).

Conclusion

Management of the growing child with Treacher Collins syndrome remains challenging. The characteristic facial deficiency is related to clockwise rotation of the maxillomandibular complex, with variable degrees of severity based upon the mandibular ramus-condyle unit morphology. The non-progressive nature of the deformity necessitates careful planning for reconstruction, starting in infancy. Successful treatment is predicated upon establishing a physiologic upper airway, improving facial proportions and occlusion, and balancing facial aesthetics. In growing children with mild to moderate mandibular dysplasia, orbitozygomatic reconstruction and ramus-condyle unit reconstruction in the mixed dentition may be considered, followed by bimaxillary orthognathic surgery at skeletal maturity. For patients with severe, tracheostomy-dependent disease related to excessive clockwise facial rotation, subcranial counterclockwise rotation via synchronous maxillomandibular distraction has emerged as a promising technique.

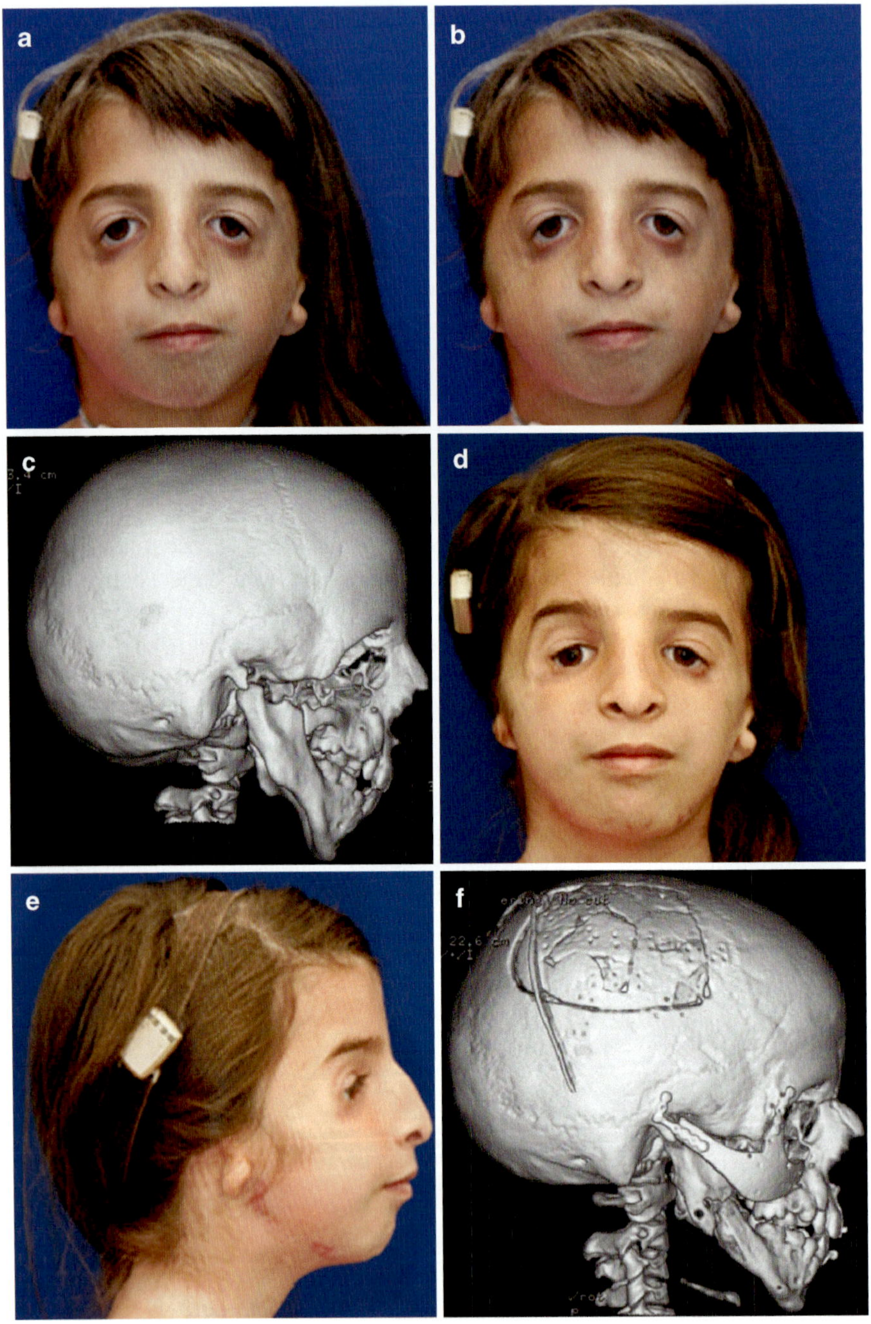

Fig. 19.4 Preoperative clinical (**a**, **b**) and three-dimensional computed tomography (**c**) images demonstrate the typical skeletal deficiency in Treacher Collins syndrome, characterized by clockwise rotation of the maxillomandibular complex. Results following staged reconstruction are shown in panels (**d**–**f**). In the first stage, the maxillomandibular dysplasia is addressed with synchronous counterclockwise distraction via LeFort II osteotomy and bilateral mandibular inverted-L osteotomies. Following consolidation, the zygomas are constructed using calvarial bone autograft as a second stage procedure (Reprinted, with permission, from Ref. [33])

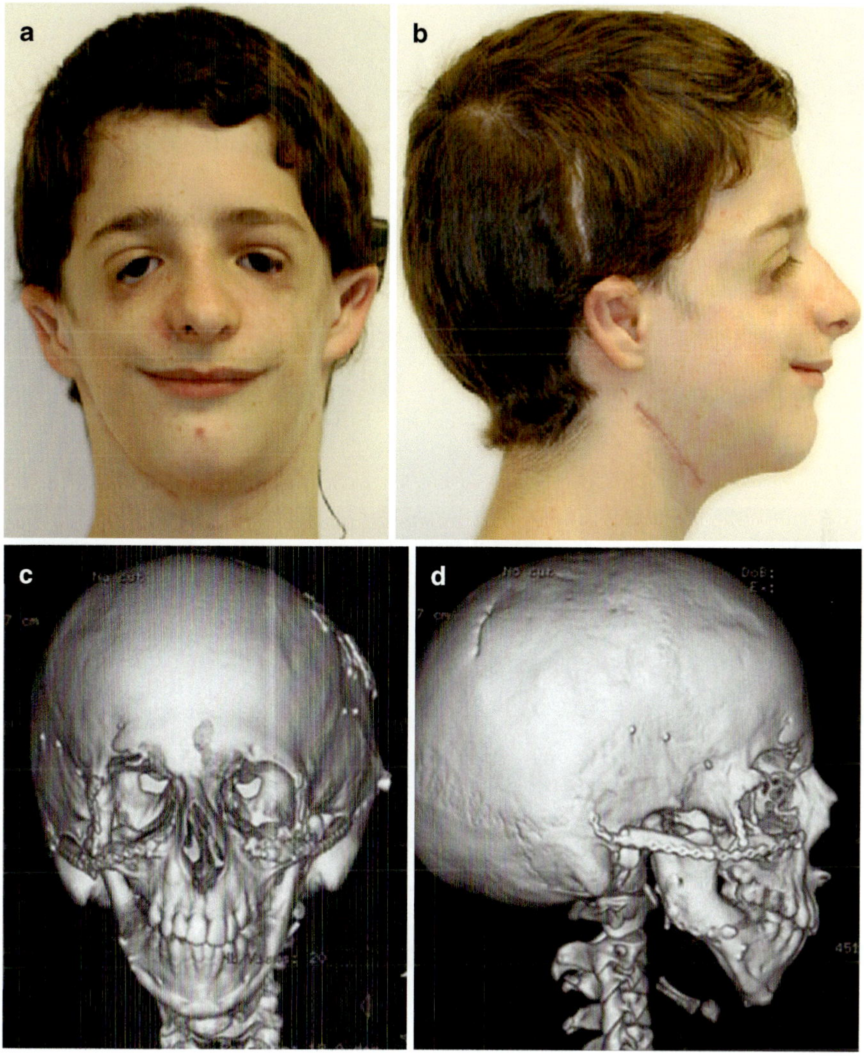

Fig. 19.5 For patients with mild to moderate disease without severe airway obstruction, sequential reconstruction can be pursued with creation of the orbitozygomatic framework and mandibular ramus height (if needed) in the mixed dentition. As the deformity is non-progressive, the end-stage skeletal discrepancy is phenotypically similar to that in the primary and mixed dentition (**a**-**d**). Definitive correction of the clockwise rotational deformity is accomplished via LeFort I osteotomy, bilateral mandibular ramus osteotomies with bone grafting, and genioplasty (**e**-**h**). The maxillomandibular complex is rotated in a counterclockwise fashion, with leveling of the palatal, maxillary, and mandibular planes. Concomitant sagittal advancement of the maxilla, mandible, and chin expands the upper airway

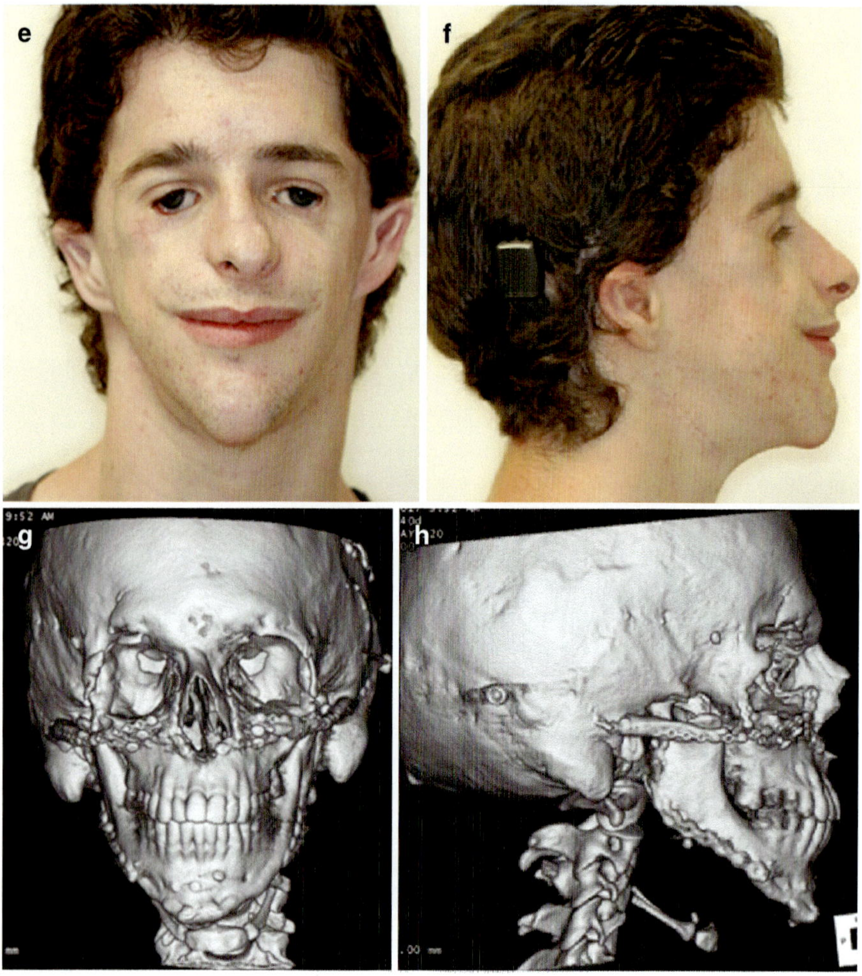

Fig. 19.5 (continued)

References

1. Marszalek B, Wojcicki P, Kobus K, Trzeciak WH. Clinical features, treatment and genetic background of Treacher Collins syndrome. J Appl Genet. 2002;43:223–33.
2. Plomp RG, van Lieshout MJ, Joosten KF, et al. Treacher Collins syndrome: a systematic review of evidence-based treatment and recommendations. Plast Reconstr Surg. 2016;137:191–204.
3. Posnick JC. Treacher Collins syndrome: perspectives in evaluation and treatment. J Oral Maxillofac Surg. 1997;55:1120–33.
4. Posnick JC, Ruiz RL. Treacher Collins syndrome: Current evaluation, treatment, and future directions. Cleft Palate Craniofac J. 2000;37:434. Bibliographic Links [Context Link].
5. Posnick JC, Tiwana PS, Costello BJ. Treacher Collins syndrome: comprehensive evaluation and treatment. Oral Maxillofac Surg Clin North Am. 2004;16:503–23.

6. Thompson JT, Anderson PJ, David DJ. Treacher Collins syndrome: protocol management from birth to maturity. J Craniofac Surg. 2009;20:2028–35.
7. Chong DK, Murray DJ, Britto JA, Tompson B, Forrest CR, Phillips JHA. Cephalometric analysis of maxillary and mandibular parameters in Treacher Collins syndrome. Plast Reconstr Surg. 2008;121:77e–84e.
8. Arvystas M, Shprintzen RJ. Craniofacial morphology in Treacher Collins syndrome. Cleft Palate Craniofac J. 1991;28:226–30.
9. Peterson-Falzone SJ, Figueroa AA. Longitudinal changes in cranial base angulation in mandibulofacial dysostosis. Cleft Palate J. 1989;26:31–5.
10. Roberts FG, Pruzansky S, Aduss H. An x-radiocephalometric study of mandibulofacial dysostosis in man. Arch Oral Biol. 1975;20:265–81.
11. Posnick JC. Treacher Collins syndrome: evaluation and treatment. In: Posnick JC, editor. Orthognathic surgery: principles and practice. London: Elsevier; 2014. p. 1059–194.
12. Akre H, Overland B, Asten P, Skogedal N, Heimdal K. Obstructive sleep apnea in Treacher Collins syndrome. Eur Arch Otorhinolaryngol. 2012;269:331–7.
13. Plomp RG, Bredero-Boelhouwer HH, Joosten KF, et al. Obstructive sleep apnoea in Treacher Collins syndrome: prevalence, severity and cause. Int J Oral Maxillofac Surg. 2012;41:696–701.
14. Ma X, Forte AJ, Persing JA, Alonso N, Berlin NL, Steinbacher DM. Reduced three-dimensional airway volume is a function of skeletal dysmorphology in Treacher Collins syndrome. Plast Reconstr Surg. 2015;135:382e–92e.
15. Ma X, Forte AJ, Berlin NL, Alonso N, Persing JA, Steinbacher DM. Reduced three-dimensional nasal airway volume in Treacher Collins syndrome and its association with craniofacial morphology. Plast Reconstr Surg. 2015;135:885e–94e.
16. Kaban LB, Mulliken JB, Murray JE. Three-dimensional approach to analysis and treatment of hemifacial microsomia. Cleft Palate J. 1981;18(2):90–9.
17. Figueroa AA, Pruzansky S. The external ear, mandible and other components of hemifacial microsomia. J Maxillofac Surg. 1982;10(4):200–11.
18. Sorin A, McCarthy JG, Bernstein JM. Predicting decannulation outcomes after distraction osteogenesis for syndromic micrognathia. Laryngoscope. 2004;114:1815–21.
19. Steinbacher DM, Kaban LB, Troulis MJ. Mandibular advancement by distraction osteogenesis for tracheostomy-dependent children with severe micrognathia. J Oral Maxillofac Surg. 2005;63(8):1072–9.
20. Kaban LB, Seldin EB, Kikinis R, Yeshwant K, Padwa BL, Troulis MJ. Clinical application of curvilinear distraction osteogenesis for correction of mandibular deformities. J Oral Maxillofac Surg. 2009;67(5):996–1008.
21. Miloro M. Mandibular distraction osteogenesis for pediatric airway management. J Oral Maxillofac Surg. 2010;68:1512–23.
22. Heller JB, Gabbay JS, Kwan D, et al. Genioplasty distraction osteogenesis and hyoid advancement for correction of upper airway obstruction in patients with Treacher Collins and Nager syndromes. Plast Reconstr Surg. 2006;117:2389–98.
23. Tessier P. Tulasne JFStability in correction of hypertelorbitism and Treacher Collins syndromes. Clin Plast Surg. 1989;16:195–204.
24. Shetye PR, Warren SM, Brown D, Garfinkle JS, Grayson BH, McCarthy JG. Documentation of the incidents associated with mandibular distraction: introduction of a new stratification system. Plast Reconstr Surg. 2009;123:627–34.
25. Proffit WR, Turvey TA, Phillips C. Orthognathic surgery: a hierarchy of stability. Int J Adult Orthodon Orthognath Surg. 1996;11:191–204.
26. Proffit WR, Turvey TA, Phillips C. The hierarchy of stability and predictability in orthognathic surgery with rigid fixation: an update and extension. Head Face Med. 2007;3:21.
27. Al-Moraissi EA, Wolford LM. Is counterclockwise rotation of the maxillomandibular complex stable compared with clockwise rotation in the correction of dentofacial deformities? A systematic review and meta-analysis. J Oral Maxillofac Surg. 2016;74:2066.e1–2066.e12.

28. Al-Moraissi EA, Wolford LM. Does temporomandibular joint pathology with or without surgical management affect the stability of counterclockwise rotation of the maxillomandibular complex in orthognathic surgery? A systematic review and meta-analysis. J Oral Maxillofac Surg. 2017;75:805–21.
29. Goncalves JR, Cassano DS, Wolford LM, Santos-Pinto A, Marquez IM. Postsurgical stability of counterclockwise maxillomandibular advancement surgery: affect of articular disc repositioning. J Oral Maxillofac Surg. 2008;66:724–38.
30. Nguyen PD, Caro MC, Smith DM, Tompson B, Forrest CR, Phillips JH. Long-term orthognathic surgical outcomes in Treacher Collins patients. J Plast Reconstr Aesthet Surg. 2016;69:402–8.
31. Tulasne JF, Tessier PL. Results of the Tessier integral procedure for correction of Treacher Collins syndrome. Cleft Palate J. 1986;23(Suppl 1):40–9.
32. Hopper RA, Kapadia H, Susarla S, Bly R, Johnson K. Counterclockwise craniofacial distraction osteogenesis for tracheostomy-dependent children with Treacher Collins Syndrome. Plast Reconstr Surg. 2018;142(2):447–57.
33. Hopper RA, Kapadia H, Susarla SM. Surgical-orthodontic considerations in subcranial and Frontofacial distraction. Oral Maxillofac Surg Clin North Am. 2020;32(2):309–20.

Chapter 20
TMJ Total Joint Prosthesis in Treacher Collins Syndrome and Hemifacial Microsomia

Adam Wandell, Daniel Perez, and Aaron Liddell

Introduction

Total joint replacement utilizing endoprostheses has become the standard of care for diseased diarthrodial joints, providing predictable outcomes with long-term function and stability. In the 1890s, the German surgeon Thermistocles Gluck championed total joint replacement utilizing ivory as a replacement for osseous bone substrate. Through the mid-1900s, Sir John Charnley led the development, implementation, and refinement of operative techniques of total hip arthroplasty. These modifications were spurred by advancements in aseptic technique and material science [1]. Improvement in material biocompatibility and decreased surgical time produced predictable outcomes, improving function and patient satisfaction while, at the same time, reducing the occurrence and severity of complications [2]. Many of the advancements in orthopedic total joint replacement have carried over into craniomaxillofacial (CMF) surgery. Both Dr. Louis G. Mercuri and Dr. Larry Wolford have contributed a tremendous amount of research and clinical work in total joint replacement surgery. Although not without growing pains (including catastrophic failures in material biocompatibility), contemporary alloplastic total joint replacement of the TMJ has borne out to be safe and predictable and provides long-term stability that is difficult to reproduce with autograft or conventional osteotomies. Advancements in CT imaging and the implementation of virtual surgical planning platforms have enhanced the predictability of the most complex cases. These advances make it possible to replace temporomandibular joints (TMJ) in patients who suffer from a myriad of craniofacial deformities, including congenital, developmental, and post-traumatic. The aim of

A. Wandell · D. Perez (✉)
Oral and Maxillofacial Surgery Department, UT Health San Antonio, San Antonio, TX, USA
e-mail: wandell@uthscsa.edu, Perezd5@uthscsa.edu

A. Liddell
Private Practice. Colorado Oral and Maxillofacial Surgery, Denver, CO, USA

D. M. Yates, M. R. Markiewicz (eds.), *Craniofacial Microsomia and Treacher Collins Syndrome*, https://doi.org/10.1007/978-3-030-84733-3_20

this chapter is to describe a combined or staged approach utilizing orthognathic surgery and TMJ TJR in patients with TCS and CFM.

Background

Treacher Collins syndrome (TCS) is a condition that, with variable expressivity, results in a variety of growth aberrancies of the craniofacial skeleton. Notably, patients with TCS have symmetrical abnormalities within the first and second branchial arches. In addition to a myriad of soft tissue abnormalities, facial skeletal growth abnormalities often affect the cranio-orbital-zygomatic complex (including hypoplastic growth with/without clefting) and can be as proximal as the glenoid fossa of the temporal bone (Fig. 20.1a, b). Often, hypoplastic growth tendencies of the maxilla and mandible result in "clockwise" rotation of the maxillomandibular complex [3]. These changes are frequently exaggerated by dysmorphologic or aplastic growth patterns of the mandibular condyles, resulting in apertognathia and significant deprojection of the skeletal chin point [4]. The aforementioned findings result in significant masticatory impairment, cosmetic deformities, malocclusion, and in some cases severe breathing disorders.

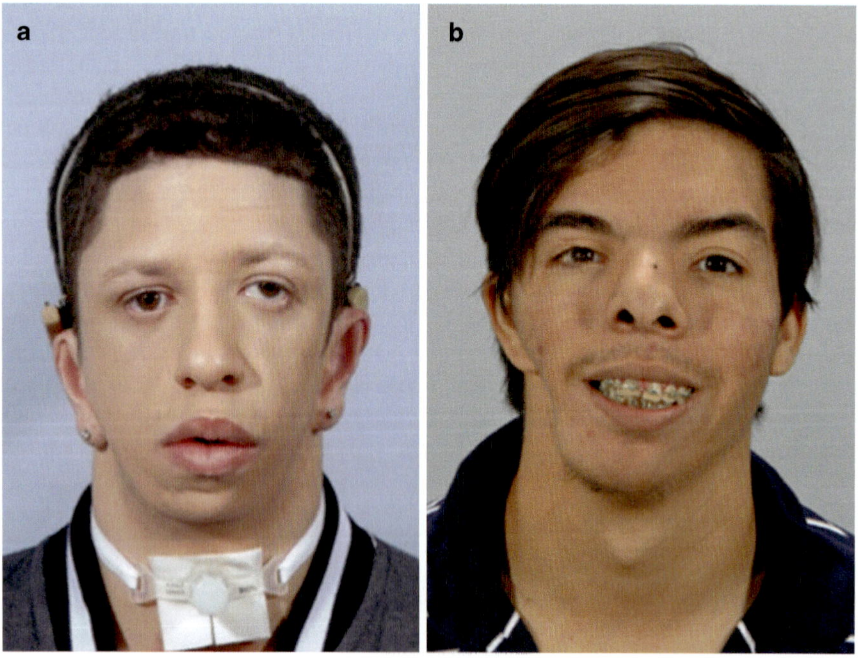

Fig. 20.1 (**a**) 16-year-old patient with TCS. (**b**) 17-year-old patient with HFM

Craniofacial microsomia (CFM) is part of the oculoauriculovertebral spectrum (OAVS) and like TCS involves growth disruption of the first and second branchial arches. Like patients with TCS, growth and developmental abnormalities can involve the craniozygomatic region in addition to the maxillomandibular complex and auricular soft tissues. In this population, there is significant variability in phenotypic expressivity. Consequently, cases can be very minor, with minimal facial asymmetry, or severe, involving complex clefting patterns of the lateral facial skeleton. Because of the typically unilateral expression, significant facial asymmetries are frequently noted, which progress until facial skeletal maturity is attained [4]. A full description of the multitude of classification systems and associated deformities in CFM are beyond the scope of this chapter; suffice it to say most involve varying degrees of hypoplasia of the ramus-condyle unit and glenoid fossa. This atypical formation of the ramus-condyle and glenoid fossa results in significant unilateral hypoplasia and in marked asymmetrical growth tendencies into both the maxilla and mandible.

In both TCS and HFM, the reconstruction of the ramus-condyle unit and the correction of the significant facial asymmetry and malocclusion present the biggest challenge. It is difficult to be predictable and consistent with your surgical results, and the timing of reconstruction is a subject of controversy among clinicians [5, 6].

Reconstruction Considerations

A variety of surgical approaches have historically been used to reconstruct the craniofacial abnormalities associated with TCS and CFM. Additionally, the timing and techniques for addressing these patients continue to evolve. Improvements in rigid internal fixation techniques and material science evolution have, in many instances, changed classical paradigms. Surgical treatments should be tailored to the severity of the skeletal deformity. There is no doubt that conventional mandibular orthognathic surgery osteotomies (inverted L and sagittal split ramus osteotomies) can frequently be employed to achieve functional, stable, and esthetic outcomes when defects are mild. However, with increased mandibular/skull base dysmorphology, or when the demands of mandibular movement exceed the parameters of stability that conventional osteotomies afford, practitioners have historically been left with distraction osteogenesis, microvascular surgery, or autografts. Although excellent outcomes can and have been achieved with each of these modalities, the interventions are exceedingly technique sensitive and often require multiple procedures to address relapse or persistent asymmetry.

As three-dimensional imaging capabilities have improved and virtual planning software has evolved, the ability to manage the maxillomandibular growth aberrancies in TCS and HFM patients has been dramatically enhanced. Specifically, the ability to utilize patient-fitted customized TMJ prostheses enables surgeons to reconstruct an aplastic or dysmorphological glenoid fossae as well as malformed or hypoplastic abnormalities associated with the ramus-condyle unit of the mandible (Fig. 20.2) [7–12]. Virtual surgical planning, in this context, enables these

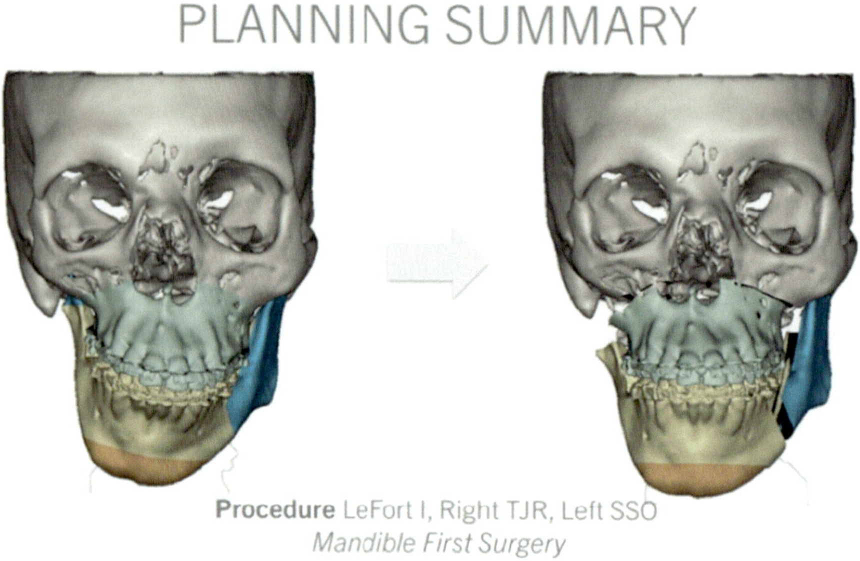

Fig. 20.2 Example of virtual surgical planning of a patient with HFM who will receive a right TJR, left BSSO, and LeFort 1

procedures to be completed in a single stage procedure with stable and predictable long-term outcomes, minimizing the morbidity associated with staged surgical treatment modalities.

In the most complex cases, especially when function is severely limited, consideration should be given to a staged approach, usually reconstructing the articulation first, followed immediately by aggressive physical therapy. Malocclusions can be addressed with conventional orthognathic surgery osteotomies after improved function has been achieved.

Timing of the Surgery

When utilizing total joint replacement combined with orthognathic surgery techniques, interventions should be completed at the cessation of anticipated skeletofacial growth. This is not always possible, particularly when the quality of life for the patient supersedes conventional reconstruction paradigms. In some severe cases, TMJ TJR may be performed in very young patients with the understanding that a revision or replacement is likely to be required in the future [13]. In TCS and CFM, the degree of malformation present at birth is presumed to be relatively stable and not progressive, outside of changes that are noted secondary to hypoplastic growth tendencies. Based on these observations, early intervention (outside of intervention based on airway concerns), including conventional osteotomies and distraction osteogenesis, will frequently require secondary revision. Accordingly, whenever possible, definitive interventions should be completed when facial growth is presumed to be complete [5, 14, 15]. In females, this entails waiting on surgical intervention until the age of 15–16 years, whereas in males, definitive surgical interventions would be held until 17–18 years (Fig. 20.1) [4, 5, 15].

Orthodontic Considerations and Virtual Surgical Planning

Early orthodontic intervention (so-called "phase 1" therapy) in patients with CFM and TCS should be avoided whenever it is feasible, outside of correcting transverse deficiencies in the maxilla. Transverse issues can be corrected prior to skeletal maturation using conventional expansion mechanics. Subsequently, traditional decompensation techniques should be started as patients are nearing skeletal maturity and are completed in the standard fashion of presurgical orthodontics, with aims of leveling, aligning, and uprighting the teeth over the basal skeletal bone. When orthodontic decompensation has been completed, virtual surgical planning can be initiated.

Over the last decade, virtual surgical planning has widely replaced conventional model surgery and can be used to plan both standard orthognathic surgery and orthognathic surgery combined with TMJ replacement [8, 16, 17]. Virtual 3D model renderings are used to design the TMJ prostheses in addition to intermediate and final positioning splints.

Virtual surgical planning begins with a non-contrast CT scan of the patient's craniofacial skeleton, utilizing 1 mm or smaller cuts and zero gantry tilt. The DICOM files from the CT scan along with dental models (or intraoral scans of the patient's dentition) are rendered using software tools that allow the surgeon to visualize the impact of adjustments to the patient's vertical and anterior/posterior maxillomandibular positions. The software makes it possible to simulate translational adjustments of yaw, pitch, and cant in order to achieve optimal skeletal positioning. As in conventional model surgery, decisions regarding the surgical movements of the maxilla and mandible should be made based on clinical evaluation, dental models (or scans), and patient goals. Soft tissue surgeries should be delayed after the final bony reconstruction has healed, allowing for a more predictable cosmetic result.

After the desired positions of the maxilla and mandible have been optimized utilizing computer simulation software, a digital file is created that enables fabrication of a stereolithographic model that is used to fabricate the custom TMJ prostheses (Fig. 20.3). Once the joint(s) have been designed, the data is then used to facilitate production of intermediate and final splints, based on the newly designed rotation point of the neo-condyle and fossa. It is important to keep the occlusion in a holding pattern with no changes in the bite once the fabrication of the device has been initiated. Two to three weeks prior to the planned surgery, a new set of models or scanned occlusion should be uploaded and compared with the original plan to assure that the splints will fit. It is at this time that the splints should be printed.

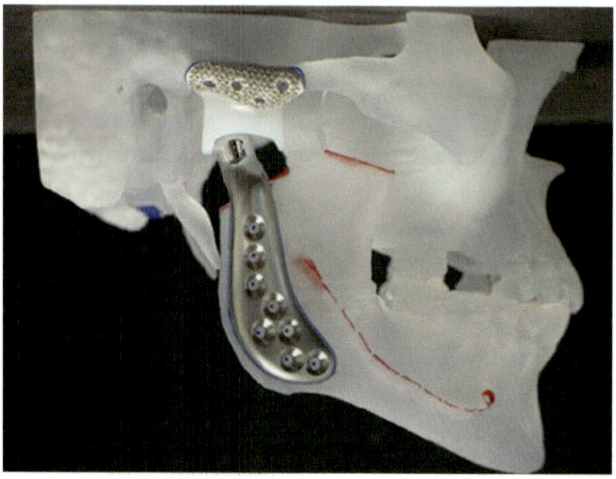

Fig. 20.3 Stereolithic model with joint prosthesis

Surgical Protocol

This section describes the steps used in our surgical protocol.

Preparation

The surgery for completing TMJ TJR with concomitant orthognathic surgery begins with standard naso-endotracheal intubation, using a nasal RAE tube. In many instances, patients with CFM and TCS have reduced mandibular range of motion and, consequently, require nasal fiberoptic intubation. Airway management, in these cases, can be difficult; therefore, careful selection of an anesthesia provider that is comfortable/competent in nasal fiberoptic technique is critical. On occasion, where airway anatomy is significantly abnormal or where multiple attempts at nasal intubation have been made without success, a standard tracheostomy can be used to safely procure a stable airway. Following nasal intubation, the endotracheal tube is sutured to the nasal septum above the columella with a 2-0 or 3-0 silk suture. The patient's head is placed in a supine position, with the neck in a neutral to slightly flexed position (Fig. 20.4a). The patient's head is wrapped using a standard surgical towel, and the endotracheal tube is secured to the head wrap with standard 2″ silk tape. It is important to assure that there are no pressure spots where the tube is secured. Local anesthetic is then infiltrated into the preauricular region and via auriculotemporal nerve block. Subsequently, the face, neck, mouth, ears, and nose are scrubbed with a betadine solution, and the face is isolated and draped with sterile towels (Fig. 20.4b). To assure that the ear canals have been adequately prepared, a cotton-tip applicator is used to clean the external auditory area with betadine solution. A cotton ear plug is then fashioned and soaked in mineral oil or betadine solution and gently packed into the external auditory canal. The mouth and nose are covered using an Ioban wrap to prohibit contamination of the TMJ surgical field with oral/nasal microbial flora.

Surgical Approaches for the TMJ Prosthesis

Multiple approaches to the temporomandibular joint have been described, a full elaboration of which is beyond the scope of this paper [18–20]. Our standard approach utilizes an endaural incision, which we have found enables rapid, predictable access to the TMJ capsule minimizing the risk of damaging cranial nerve VII, the superficial temporal artery, and the cartilaginous external auditory canal (Fig. 20.5a). That being said, one of the challenges in TCS and HFM patients is that frequently the external auricular anatomy is either abnormal or missing entirely. Therefore, standard anatomic landmarks that are conventionally used in the dissection are frequently not present, which may include osseous structures such as the zygomatic process of the temporal bone and the lateral glenoid fossa. Accordingly, intraoperative nerve monitoring may be required during the surgical approach to

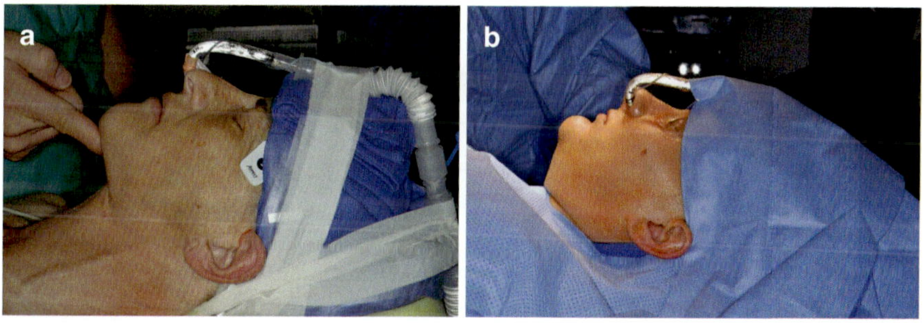

Fig. 20.4 (**a**) Patient's head is in a supine position, with the neck neutral to slightly flexed. (**b**) Patient with proper towel draping

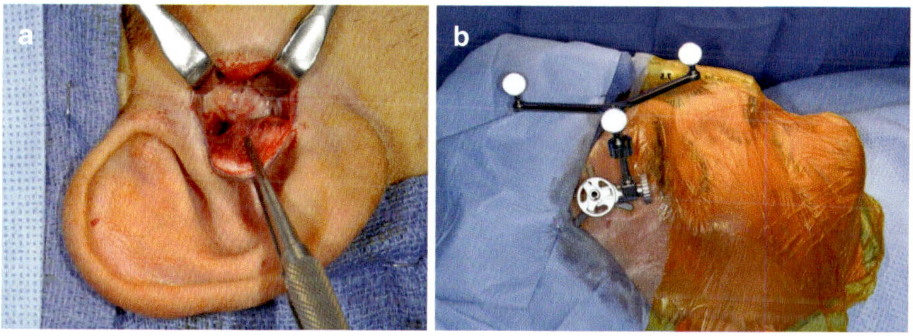

Fig. 20.5 (**a**) Endaural site outlined prior to incision. (**b**) Intraoperative navigation used for a patient with missing external ear anatomy

minimize trauma to cranial nerve VII. Additionally, in cases where the external ear is not present and the temporal bone anatomy is significantly atypical, computer-assisted intraoperative navigation can be considered to assure that site preparation for the glenoid fossa component occurs in the appropriate position along the caudal aspect of the temporal bone [21, 22] (Fig. 20.5b).

We utilize a submandibular incision in order to introduce and fixate the ramus component (Fig. 20.6). This incision provides access to the inferior-lateral area of the ramus. The submandibular incision is placed 2 cm inferior to the lower border of the mandible and is generally 2 cm in length. Dissection is carried to the level of the platysma. The platysma is then sharply divided, monitoring the nerve activity of the marginal mandibular nerve. In the subplatysmal plane, dissection is carried superiorly on the superficial layer of the deep cervical fascia to the inferior border of the mandible. Frequently, the facial artery and vein can be left intact; however, if needed, these vessels can be ligated and separated. At the mandible, the pterygomasseteric sling is divided along the inferior border of the mandible, and dissection is carried in a subperiosteal plane to connect to the superior dissection cavity. Any contouring of the lateral ramus can then be completed, as per the virtual surgical plan to facilitate passive adaptation of the ramus component.

Site Preparation for Prosthesis Insertion

In cases when the mandibular condyle is present, a condylectomy is performed according to the virtual surgical plan. Cutting guides, which can be fabricated during the surgical planning, can be used to assure that the condyle resection mimics the virtual plan. Once the condylectomy has been completed, the joint space is prepared to facilitate placement of the prosthesis. Because of the vertical elongation of the ramus that frequently occurs with prosthesis placement in the TCS and CFM population, adequate space is usually procured for placement of the fossa and ramus

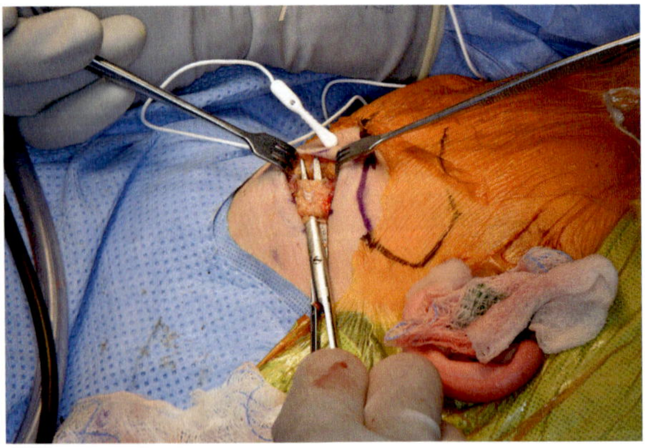

Fig. 20.6 Submandibular incision and approach

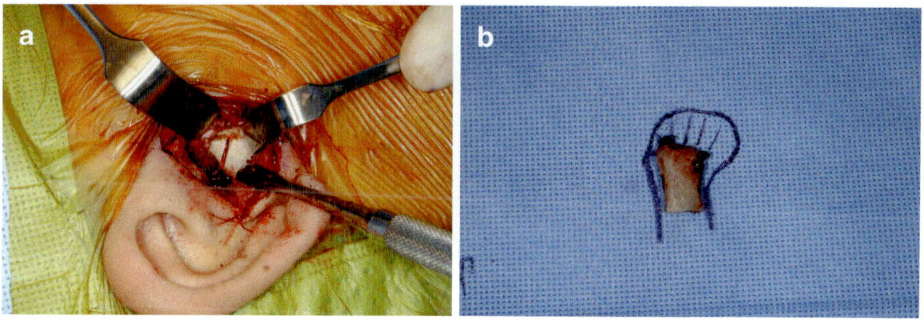

Fig. 20.7 (**a**) Condylectomy osteotomy in order to gain 20 mm of space for the prosthesis (**b**) Resected right condyle

components of the prosthesis. If vertical lengthening of the ramus is not significant, a minimum 20 mm space is needed for passive fit of the prosthetic components, measuring from the superior aspect of the cut ramus to the base of skull (Fig. 20.7). During site preparation at the skull base, careful attention should be given to the superior aspect of the parotid gland during this phase of site preparation. This gland is a reproducible landmark that suggests proximity to the superior branches of the facial nerve [23].

Through the endaural access, a coronoidectomy can be also performed. We have found that by using a piezoelectric saw, the risk of damaging underlying vasculature during the coronoidectomy is minimized. The aims of coronoidectomy are to detach the temporalis muscle which facilitates a larger and more passive advancement of the mandible. Bone from the condylectomy and coronoidectomy may be saved and used to graft bone defects that may be present following fixation of the maxillary osteotomy.

At this point, it should be noted that many TCS and CFM patients require significant counterclockwise rotation of the maxillomandibular complex. When this is the case, significant effort may be required to fully mobilize the mandible to attain passive fit of the intermediate splint. Aggressive intraoperative "stretching" of the mandible can be quite cumbersome and requires patience and persistence. Frequently, the vertical elongation of the mandibular ramus can result in a significant increase in the distance from the foramen ovale to the lingula. Patients must be informed that paresthesia to the inferior alveolar nerve is a significant risk during this procedure due to the nature of the counterclockwise rotation necessary to optimize function and esthetics [24].

Mobilization of the Uninvolved Side Where Indicated

In TCS patients, the above noted protocol is followed for both sides, in anticipation of bilateral TJR. However, in patients with CFM, frequently the uninvolved side has developed normally and is amenable to conventional sagittal ramus osteotomy to enable occlusal plane leveling and counterclockwise rotation of the maxillomandibular complex. This osteotomy, when indicated, can be completed using a

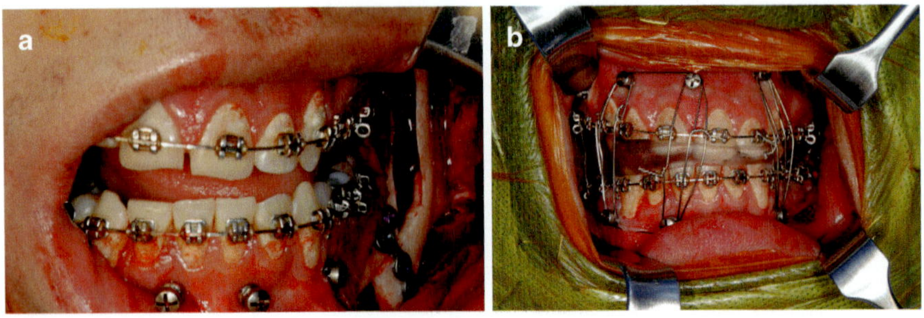

Fig. 20.8 (**a**) Fixated sagittal split osteotomy (**b**) Patient in IMF in intermediate splint

transmucosal intraoral incision, as described by Obwegeser, with modifications as described by DalPont and Hunsuck [25–27] (Fig. 20.8a). It is important that instruments used for the intraoral aspect of the procedure be placed on a separate table and not be mixed with or contaminate instruments that were used to access the TMJ. Prior to entering the oral cavity, the TMJ access site(s) are covered with a large Tegaderm, and the face is draped with new surgical towels, such that only the oral cavity is exposed. The Ioban which was placed over the mouth and nose at the beginning of the procedure is divided in order to gain access to the oral cavity. Subsequently, a unilateral sagittal split osteotomy is performed, the proximal and distal segments are separated, and then the patient is placed into intermaxillary fixation utilizing the intermediate splint (Fig. 20.8b). Once the mandible has been passively rotated into the intermediate splint, the mandible is wired to the maxilla and the proximal segment is seated into centric relation. The segments are fixated, as per the surgeons' preference. Following fixation of the mandible, the surgeons re-scrub and change gowns and gloves, and the mouth and nasal complex are sealed off with Ioban, such that sterility can be maintained for placement of the TMJ prosthesis.

Placing and Fixating the Prostheses

Once the oral and nasal cavities have been covered, the surgeon places the fossa component of the prosthesis into the patient's glenoid fossa, when present, or onto the base of the temporal bone when there is significant glenoid dysmorphology. The component is fixated with four screws whose length is predetermined according to the virtual surgical plan. The condylar component is then placed through the submandibular incision (Fig. 20.9). Careful attention must be paid to assure that the prosthetic condylar head is in the most posterior-superior aspect of the fossa prosthesis. The mandibular component is then secured to the lateral ramus using eight screws of predetermined length. We have found that placement of the first screw with a posterior-superior offset relative to the screw hole facilitates positioning the joint into centric relation.

Preventing Heterotopic Bone Formation

One of the concerns in orthopedic reconstruction relates to the development of heterotopic bone at the site of surgery. This phenomenon has been reported in the context of TMJ TJR and can be difficult to manage [28]. Accordingly, our protocol prefers to obliterate any dead space surrounding the fossa-condyle interface with free fat graft. A variety of techniques and harvest sites have been described [28, 29]. We have found that a simple technique involves either a suprapubic or periumbilical harvest of free fat. The technique is very simple and involves a curvilinear incision adjacent to the umbilicus or a linear incision in the suprapubic region. The incision is carried through the skin into the subcutaneous fat. Sharp dissection is completed with curved mayo scissors in this plane, leaving a layer of fat superficially at the fat-dermis junction. An additional dissection plane is created deep to this plane, in the subcutaneous fat, and approximately 5–10 cc free fat is harvested. Hemostasis is verified, and the wound is irrigated and closed. The fat is then immediately transferred to the periprosthetic region and packed via the preauricular incision around the prosthesis, both medially and laterally (Fig. 20.10). The endaural incision is then closed in layers. Following closure of the endaural incision, the submandibular site

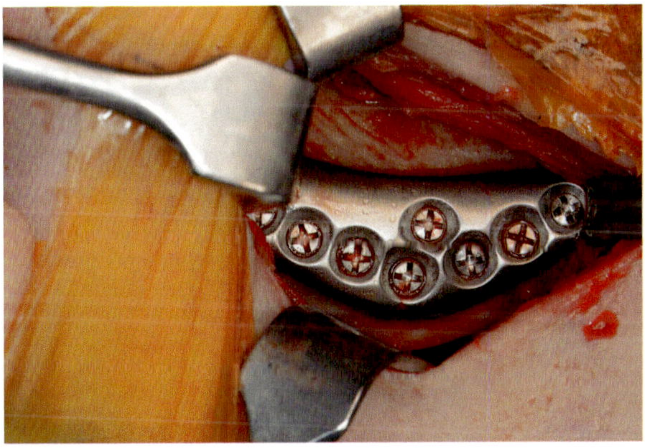

Fig. 20.9 Plating of the prosthesis through the submandibular incision site

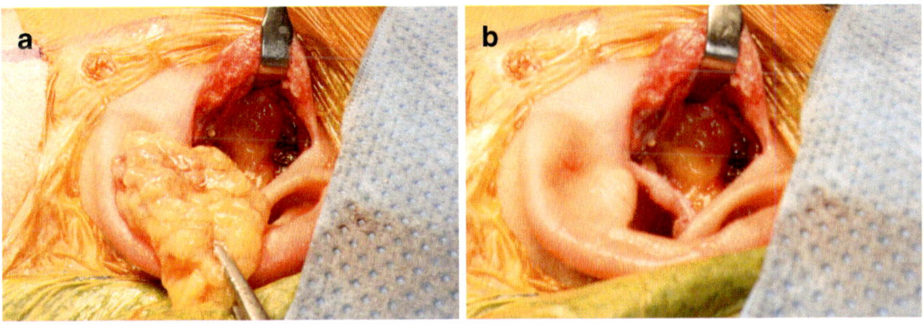

Fig. 20.10 (**a** and **b**) Autologous fat (left) placed into periprosthetic region (right)

is irrigated and closed. Attempts should be made at re-suspending the pterygomasseteric sling over the ramus of the mandible. On occasion, a bicortical hole may be drilled through the caudal aspect of the mandibular ramus, and the masseter may then be sutured to the mandible through this hole using 2-0 Vicryl. Layered closure of the remaining tissue planes can then be completed.

Moving the Maxilla into Final Position

Once the joints have been placed and the extraoral wounds have been closed, the maxilla may then be repositioned. This repositioning is completed based on the final splint that was fabricated during the virtual planning. Once the extraoral wounds have been closed, there is no longer a risk of instrument contamination. The maxilla is typically repositioned at the LeFort 1 level, using conventional orthognathic surgical techniques (Fig. 20.11). A septoplasty may also be performed at this time. Once the maxilla has been adequately mobilized, the maxilla is wired to the mandible using the "final" splint, which may be wired in place if done in the context of segmental maxillary osteotomies, and the mandible is autorotated to position the maxilla relative to the uncut midface. A K-wire, which is placed at the nasofrontal junction, can be used as a fixed vertical reference point for repositioning of the vertical location of the central incisor. Once vertical positioning has been established, the maxilla is fixated in place, and bone grafting to facilitate bone to bone contact is completed. Tissue closure is then initiated with careful attention to complete an alar cinch suture and V-Y advancement of the upper lip [30].

Occasionally, the decision is made to complete the maxillary osteotomy in a delayed fashion. This decision is made based on the ability to rapidly restore passive mandibular range of motion in cases where preoperative range of motion is significantly restricted, and early aggressive physical therapy is required. We have found that heavy fulcruming off a recently osteotomized/fixated maxilla causes maxillary

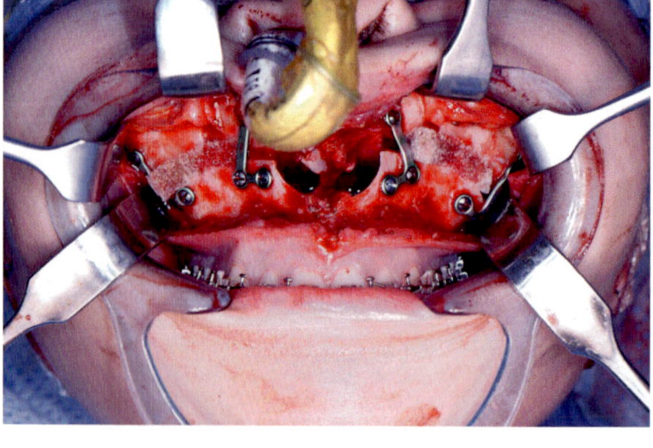

Fig. 20.11 Fixated LeFort 1 osteotomy

movement and increases the risk for long-term malocclusion secondary to movement of the maxilla. Accordingly, in these cases, early aggressive physical therapy is advised, and the maxillary osteotomy is completed in a delayed fashion once adequate mandibular range of motion has been attained. In these select cases, we have found that patients tolerate the intermediate malocclusion well, for the short period required to optimize mandibular function.

Complications

Like conventional orthognathic surgery, there are a variety of known risks associated with total joint replacement. In this section, these risks are discussed, in addition to techniques that we have used to mitigate (or at least minimize) these risks in the preoperative, intraoperative, and postoperative periods.

Nerve Injury

Injuries to cranial nerve V are a well-known risk associated with any orthognathic surgical procedure [31]. In addition to cranial nerve V trauma, patients who undergo TJR surgery are at increased risk of damage to cranial nerve VII, particularly in cases where external anatomic landmarks are not present, as described above. Accordingly, the surgical approaches are designed to avoid encountering and injuring these nerves. Additionally, as described previously, intraoperative nerve monitoring is frequently employed in an attempt to minimize risk. Nonetheless, patients must be aware of the risk of damage to the fronto-temporal branches, which may be encountered during the endaural approach, in addition to injury to the marginal mandibular nerve, which may be encountered during the submandibular approach [32]. In many cases, traction neuropraxia injuries are nearly inevitable. That being said, in most cases, with intraoperative monitoring and careful dissection, many of these injuries are transient and return to full function.

Infection

A comprehensive discussion regarding infections in the context of total joint replacement is beyond the scope of this article. In brief, prosthetic joint infections have plagued orthopedic surgery for decades. These include acute and/or chronic infections. Pertaining to TJR infections involving the TMJ, multiple articles have suggested an infection rate from 2% to 5% [31]. Many hypothesize that these infections are related to biofilms on the prosthesis, which result in infections that become difficult to treat with antibiotics alone. Accordingly, well-defined protocols have been elucidated, including early wash out/debridement in the context of acute infections and removal/replacement of the prosthesis in the case of chronic or nonresponsive infections [33].

Allergic Reactions

Metal allergies associated with TMJ prostheses are well-documented. Accordingly, patients should be asked prior to surgery if they have had any previous metal hypersensitivity. Where there is concern, patients should be sent to an allergy/immunologist prior to the placement of the prosthesis for appropriate testing. The diagnosis and management of allergic reactions may be difficult and should be managed in conjunction with an allergy specialist [34].

Heterotopic Bone Formation

Heterotopic ossification is another well-documented phenomenon in the context of TJR, both in conventional orthopedic replacement and in TMJ reconstruction. The underlying pathophysiology is poorly understood; however bone formation that occurs surrounding the fossa/ramus components can lead to decreased range of motion, pain, and, in some cases, joint ankylosis [35]. Multiple modalities have been described that aim to mitigate risk, including placement of free fat surrounding the joint, as described above, utilizing a piezoelectric saw for resections and osseous contouring and meticulous hemostasis. Additionally, the use of low-dose indomethacin has been proposed in high-risk cases [36]. In instances where patients have developed heterotopic ossification and will be debrided, focused external beam radiation to the site has been utilized with some success, combined with surgical debridement and possible joint replacement.

Secondary Soft Tissue Management

Patients with CFM and TCS often need secondary soft tissue reconstruction to achieve optimal esthetic results. There are a number of approaches to reconstructing depressed/hypoplastic areas in patients with congenital malformations. These include the use of autologous tissue grafts, allogenic tissue grafts, and alloplastic materials.

Autologous tissue grafting can be used to achieve proper contour of the face, improving symmetry with fewer complications and shorter operating times than microvascular free flaps [37]. Surgeons typically use the lower anterior abdominal wall as the donor harvesting fat site. Usually, fat is infiltrated into the recipient tissue until an overcorrection is achieved in areas of under projection (Fig. 20.12). Fat

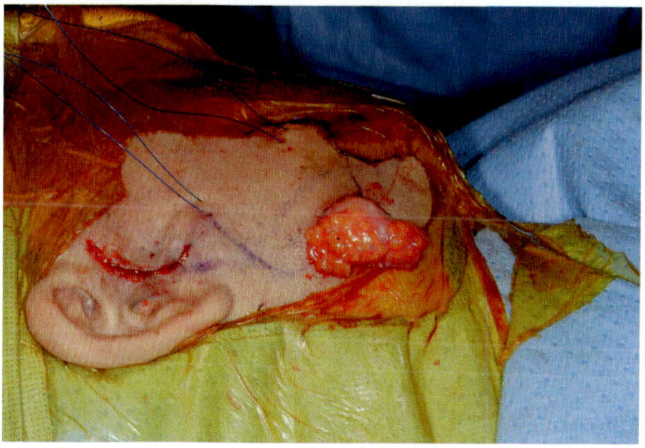

Fig. 20.12 Autologous fat placed in the soft tissue

injections can produce high-quality immediate postoperative results, although long-term success is not guaranteed. Horl et al. (1991) reported greater than 50% volume loss when measured 6 months post injection with magnetic resonance imaging (MRI) [38]. Postoperative physiotherapy prevents soft tissue contraction in some cases, and additional less-invasive fat transfer can take place in the future if it is necessary to make adjustments.

Implants made from alloplastic materials such as silicone, Medpor, and expanded polytetrafluorethylene implants (ePTFE) can improve the soft tissue projections in a deficient area, but each of these materials poses their own unique challenges for congenital facial deformities. Silicone is soft and tends to change shape and shift over time. Medpor implants are stiff and are mainly recommended for bone contour deformities. EPTFE implants can be placed beneath the superficial temporal fascia and over the superficial musculoaponeurotic system in the zygomatic region, mandible, and cheek. EPTFE meshes may prove promising in the future, however, like all alloplastic materials, it poses higher risks for inflammatory cell reactions and bacterial microfilm contamination [39].

Autologous tissue grafting remains the most effective technique to recreate soft tissue contours and can be performed in conjunction with orthognathic and TJR procedures.

Patient Expectations

The surgical treatment of both TCS and HFM patients requires great preparation and surgical skill. Even in the hands of the most skilled surgeons, these cases are difficult to treat. It is imperative to understand the goals and expectations of the patients and their families in order to prepare them for realistic outcomes. Below are some case examples of patients who have undergone surgical treatment of TCS and HFM (Figs. 20.13 and 20.14).

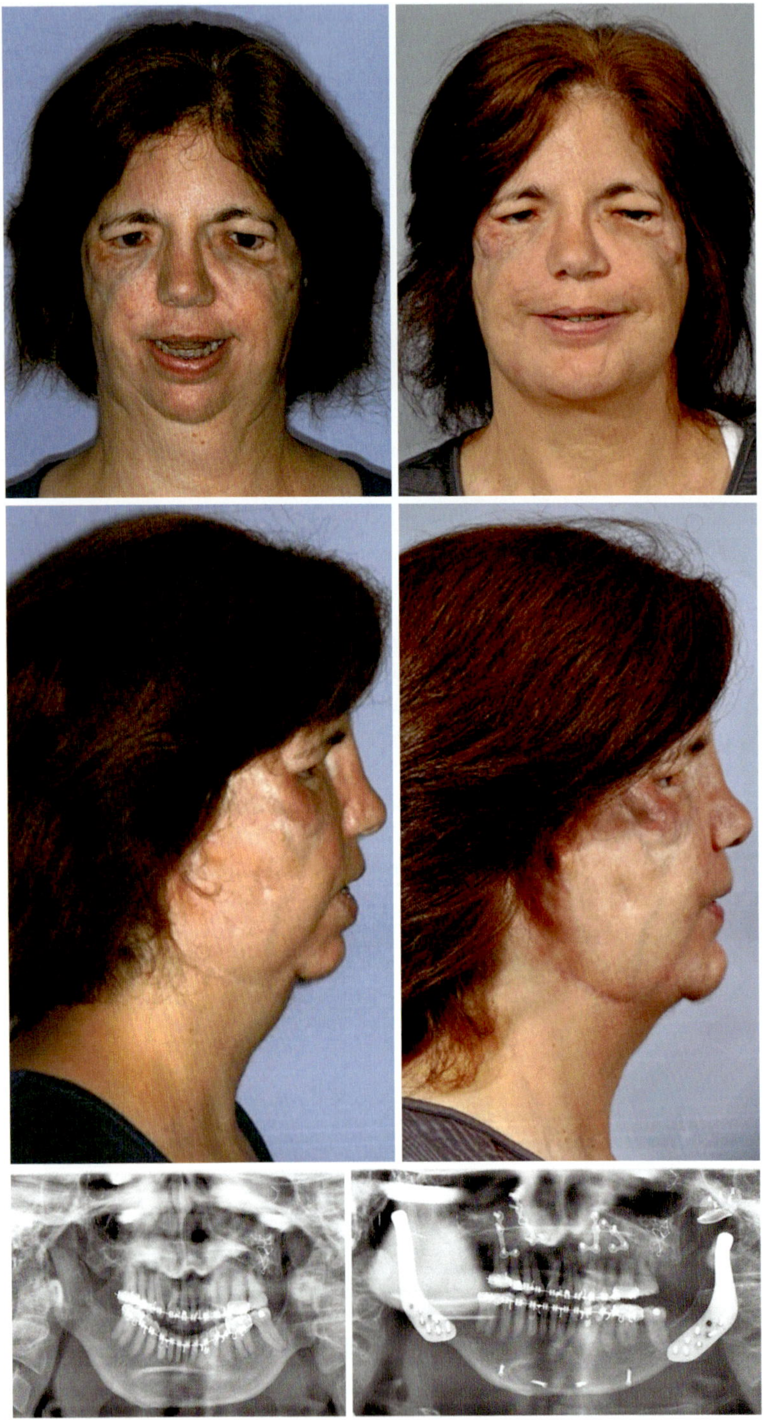

Fig. 20.13 Patient before (left) and 1-year postoperative treatment (right) with bilateral TJR and fat graft placement

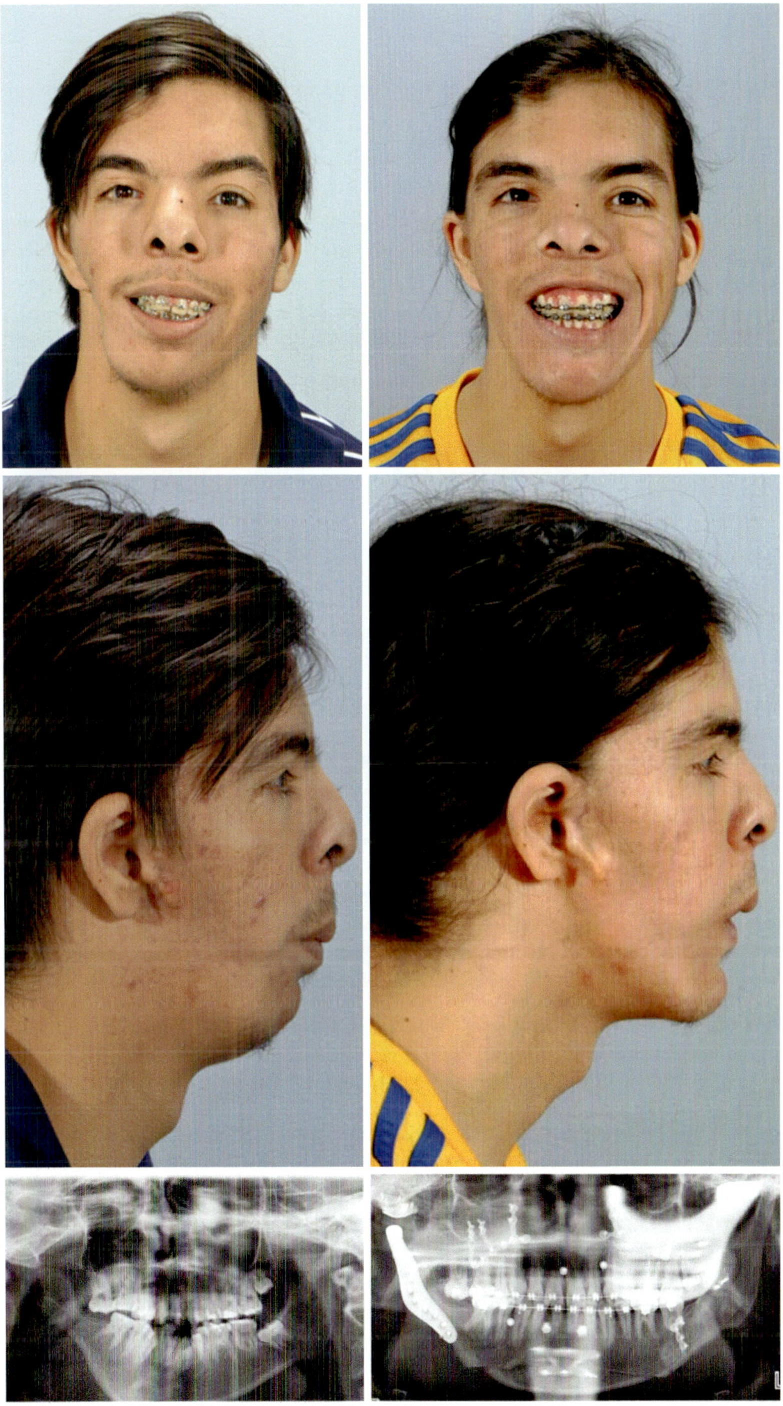

Fig. 20.14 Patient before (left) and 1-year postoperative treatment (right) with unilateral TJR and fat graft placement

Summary

- Total joint replacement (TJR) with concomitant orthognathic surgery has proven to be a stable alternative to conventional distraction or osteotomies and can improve the function/esthetics of patients with moderate to severe Treacher Collins syndrome (TCS) and craniofacial microsomia (CFM).
- Both TJR and orthognathic surgery can be accomplished in a single operation.
- Where feasible, surgery should be delayed until skeletal maturity in patients with TCS and CFM, so as to minimize the need for additional revision surgery.
- Virtual surgical planning (VSP) plays a critical role in creating a custom-fitted prosthesis and planning the concomitant orthognathic surgery.
- We describe and illustrate the surgical approach and protocol for total joint replacement (TJR) with orthognathic surgery and discuss possible complications.

References

1. Charnley J. Low friction arthroplasty of the hip: theory and practice. New York: Springer-Verlag; 1979.
2. Knight SR, Aujla R, Biswas SP. Total hip arthroplasty – over 100 years of operative history. Orthop Rev (Pavia). 2011. https://doi.org/10.4081/or.2011.e16.
3. Wolford LM, Perez DE. Surgical management of congenital deformities with temporomandibular joint malformation. Oral Maxillofac Surg Clin North Am. 2015. https://doi.org/10.1016/j.coms.2014.09.010.
4. Posnick JC. Hemifacial microsomia: evaluation and treatment. Orthognath Surg Princ Pract. 2013. https://doi.org/10.1016/B978-1-4557-2698-1.00028-9.
5. Wolford LM, Karras SC, Mehra P. Considerations for orthognathic surgery during growth, part 1: mandibular deformities. Am J Orthod Dentofac Orthop. 2001. https://doi.org/10.1067/mod.2001.111401.
6. Wolford LM, Karras SC, Mehra P. Considerations for orthognathic surgery during growth, part 2: maxillary deformities. Am J Orthod Dentofac Orthop. 2001. https://doi.org/10.1067/mod.2001.111400.
7. Movahed R, Teschke M, Wolford LM. Protocol for concomitant temporomandibular joint custom-fitted total joint reconstruction and orthognathic surgery utilizing computer-assisted surgical simulation. J Oral Maxillofac Surg. 2013. https://doi.org/10.1016/j.joms.2013.07.024.
8. Stokbro K, Aagaard E, Torkov P, Bell RB, Thygesen T. Virtual planning in orthognathic surgery. Int J Oral Maxillofac Surg. 2014. https://doi.org/10.1016/j.ijom.2014.03.011.
9. Schendel SA. Computer simulation in the daily practice of orthognathic surgery. Int J Oral Maxillofac Surg. 2015. https://doi.org/10.1016/j.ijom.2015.05.022.
10. Swennen GRJ, Mollemans W, Schutyser F. Three-dimensional treatment planning of orthognathic surgery in the era of virtual imaging. J Oral Maxillofac Surg. 2009. https://doi.org/10.1016/j.joms.2009.06.007.
11. Hodzic Z, Törnwall J, Leikola J, Heliövaara A, Suojanen J. Alloplastic temporomandibular Joint reconstruction in Congenital Craniofacial deformities. Journal of Craniofacial Surgery, 2021;32(6). https://doi.org/10.1097/scs.0000000000007533.

12. Zanakis NS, Gavakos K, Faippea M, Karamanos A, Zotalis N. Application of custom-made tmj prosthesis in hemifacial microsomia. J Oral Maxillofac Surg. 2009;38(9):988–92. https://doi.org/10.1016/j.ijom.2009.04.012.
13. Mercuri LG, Swift JQ. Considerations for the use of alloplastic temporomandibular joint replacement in the growing patient. J Oral Maxillofac Surg. 2009. https://doi.org/10.1016/j.joms.2009.05.430.
14. Posnick JC. Treacher Collins syndrome: evaluation and treatment. Orthognath Surg Princ Pract. 2013. https://doi.org/10.1016/B978-1-4557-2698-1.00027-7.
15. Posnick JC, Tiwana PS, Costello BJ. Treacher Collins syndrome: comprehensive evaluation and treatment. Oral Maxillofac Surg Clin North Am. 2004. https://doi.org/10.1016/j.coms.2004.08.002.
16. Farrell BB, Franco PB, Tucker MR. Virtual surgical planning in orthognathic surgery. Oral Maxillofac Surg Clin North Am. 2014. https://doi.org/10.1016/j.coms.2014.08.011.
17. Chandran R, Keeler GD, Christensen AM, Weimer KA, Caloss R. Application of virtual surgical planning for total joint reconstruction with a stock alloplast system. J Oral Maxillofac Surg. 2011. https://doi.org/10.1016/j.joms.2010.03.010.
18. Kreutziger KL. Surgery of the temporomandibular joint. I. Surgical anatomy and surgical incisions. Oral Surgery, Oral Med Oral Pathol. 1984. https://doi.org/10.1016/0030-4220(84)90027-6.
19. Morizono T. Endaural approaches. Oper Tech Otolaryngol Head Neck Surg. 1996. https://doi.org/10.1016/S1043-1810(96)80065-0.
20. Bhalla RK, Lesser THJ. Simple, painless, cosmetic closure of endaural incisions. J Laryngol Otol. 2003. https://doi.org/10.1258/002221503321046685.
21. Sun Y, Du W, Xu C, Lin Y, Liu X, Luo E. Applications of computer-aided design/manufacturing technology in treatment of hemifacial microsomia. J Craniofac Surg. 2020. https://doi.org/10.1097/scs.0000000000006335.
22. Nijmeh AD, Goodger NM, Hawkes D, Edwards PJ, McGurk M. Image-guided navigation in oral and maxillofacial surgery. Br J Oral Maxillofac Surg. 2005. https://doi.org/10.1016/j.bjoms.2004.11.018.
23. Terence M Myckatyn, Susan E Mackinnon. A review of facial nerve anatomy. Semin Plast Surg. 2004. https://doi.org/10.1055/s-2004-823118
24. Movahed R, Wolford LM. Protocol for concomitant temporomandibular joint custom-fitted total joint reconstruction and orthognathic surgery using computer-assisted surgical simulation. Oral Maxillofac Surg Clin North Am. 2015. https://doi.org/10.1016/j.coms.2014.09.004.
25. Trauner R, Obwegeser H. The surgical correction of mandibular prognathism and retrognathia with consideration of genioplasty. Part I. Surgical procedures to correct mandibular prognathism and reshaping of the chin. Oral Surgery, Oral Med Oral Pathol. 1957. https://doi.org/10.1016/S0030-4220(57)80063-2.
26. DAL PONT G. Retromolar osteotomy for the correction of prognathism. J Oral Surg Anesth Hosp Dent Serv. 1961;19:42–7.
27. Hunsuck EE. A modified intraoral sagittal splitting technic for correction of mandibular prognathism. J Oral Surg. 1968;26(4):250–3.
28. Wolford LM, Cassano DS. Autologous fat grafts placed around Temporomandibular Joint (TMJ) total joint prostheses to prevent heterotopic bone. Autologous Fat Transf Art Sci Clin Pract. 2010. https://doi.org/10.1007/978-3-642-00473-5_48.
29. Wolford LM, Morales-Ryan CA, Morales PG, Cassano DS. Autologous fat grafts placed around temporomandibular joint total joint prostheses to prevent heterotopic bone formation. Baylor Univ Med Cent Proc. 2008. https://doi.org/10.1080/08998280.2008.11928404.
30. Hackney FL, Timmis DP, Van Sickels JE. Esthetic evaluation of frontal labial morphology after double V-Y closure following le fort I osteotomy. J Oral Maxillofac Surg. 1989. https://doi.org/10.1016/0278-2391(89)90723-4.
31. Bouloux GF. Complications of temporomandibular joint surgery. Complicat Temporomandibular Jt Surg. 2017. https://doi.org/10.1007/978-3-319-51241-9.

32. Hoffman D, Puig L. Complications of TMJ surgery. Oral Maxillofac Surg Clin North Am. 2015. https://doi.org/10.1016/j.coms.2014.09.008.
33. Wolford LM, Rodrigues DB, McPhillips A. Management of the infected temporomandibular joint total joint prosthesis. J Oral Maxillofac Surg. 2010. https://doi.org/10.1016/j.joms.2010.05.089.
34. Hassan S, Mercuri LG, Miloro M. Does metal hypersensitivity have relevance in patients undergoing TMJ prosthetic replacement?. J Oral Maxillofac Surg. 2020. https://doi.org/10.1016/j.joms.2020.01.020.
35. Mercuri LG, Caicedo MS. Material hypersensitivity and alloplastic temporomandibular joint replacement. J Oral Maxillofac Surg. 2019. https://doi.org/10.1016/j.joms.2019.01.042.
36. Amstutz HC, Fowble VA, Schmalzried TP, Dorey FJ. Short-course indomethacin prevents heterotopic ossification in a high- risk population following total hip arthroplasty. J Arthroplast. 1997. https://doi.org/10.1016/S0883-5403(97)90058-9.
37. Lim AA, Fan K, Allam KA, Wan D, Tabit C, Liao E, Kawamoto HK, Bradley JP. Autologous fat transplantation in the craniofacial patient: the UCLA experience. J Craniofac Surg. 2012. https://doi.org/10.1097/SCS.0b013e31824e695b.
38. Horl HW, Feller AM, Biemer E. Technique for liposuction fat reimplantation and long-term volume evaluation by magnetic resonance imaging. Ann Plast Surg. 1991. https://doi.org/10.1097/00000637-199103000-00007.
39. Liu X, Zhang Y, Wang S, Lei Z, Li X, Fan D. The use of expanded polytetrafluoroethylene in depressed deformities of the face. Exp Ther Med. 2016. https://doi.org/10.3892/etm.2016.3771.

Chapter 21
Definitive Correction of Associated Maxillomandibular Deformities in Treacher Collins Syndrome

E. Weston Santee and Vernon Burke

Treacher Collins syndrome is a distinct genetic disorder characterized by abnormalities in the structures of the first and second branchial arches. It is eponymously named after Edward Treacher Collins, a renowned English ophthalmologist, who was the first to cohesively describe the essential findings of the condition in 1900. The condition is also known as mandibulofacial dysostosis, which is the term that was used by Adolphe Franceschetti and David Klein when they characterized the same condition in 1949 [1]. The clinical findings include downward sloping palpebral fissures, inferiorly positioned lateral canthi, a prominent nose, a severely convex facial profile, and long sideburns or tongues of hair extending onto the face. See Fig. 21.1 of an individual with characteristic findings.

The extent of the abnormalities can vary, but there are characteristic maxillomandibular findings that include malar and midface hypoplasia, a hypoplastic and irregularly shaped mandible, and hypoplasia of the structures of the temporomandibular joint. Affected individuals often have severe skeletal and dental malocclusions with large anterior open bites. The constellation and severity of the abnormalities in the facial skeleton create a maxillomandibular complex that has unique features and requires an orthognathic surgical plan that is tailor-made for the individual patient.

E. W. Santee (✉)
High Desert Oral and Facial Surgery and El Paso Children's Hospital 2019-2020, El Paso, TX, USA

V. Burke
High Desert Oral and Facial Surgery, El Paso Children's Hospital, El Paso, TX, USA
e-mail: burke@hdofs.com

D. M. Yates, M. R. Markiewicz (eds.), *Craniofacial Microsomia and Treacher Collins Syndrome*, https://doi.org/10.1007/978-3-030-84733-3_21

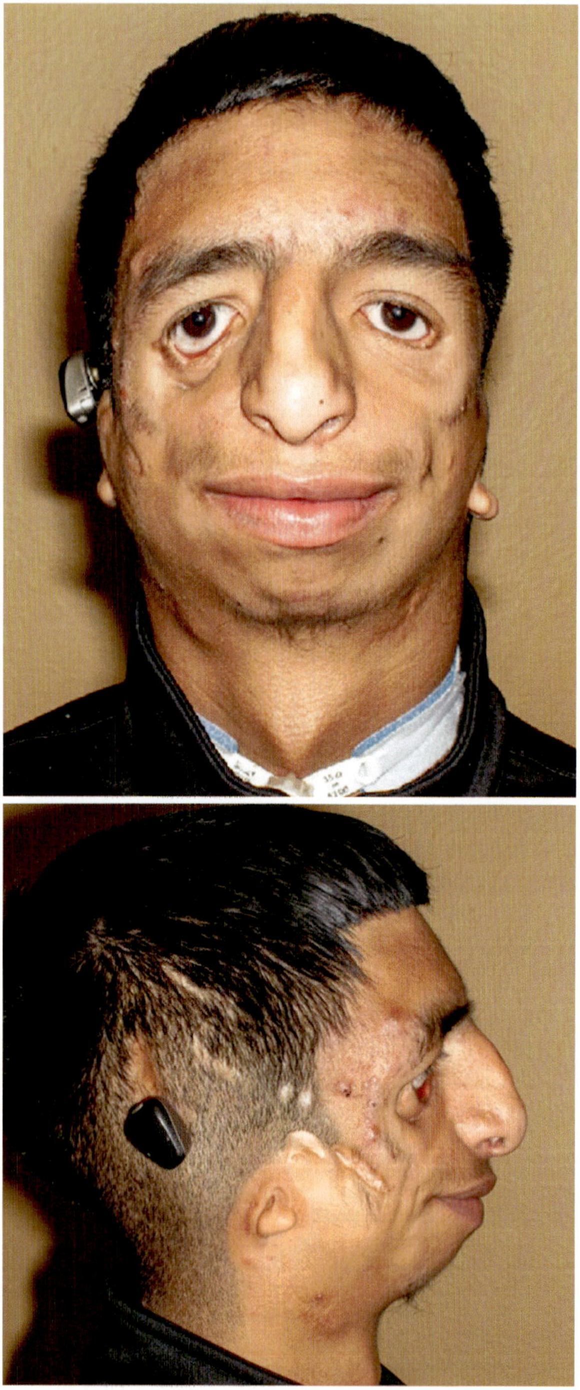

Fig. 21.1 Patient with characteristic findings of Treacher Collins syndrome

Cephalometric Findings

Individuals with Treacher Collins syndrome have characteristic cephalometric findings. For an affected individual, the length of both the maxilla and mandible is short. The mandible is inescapably rotated downward and backward. There is premature occlusion of the posterior dentition due to the short ramus height and severely enlarged mandibular plane angle. Consequently, anterior open bites are frequently present. The nasopharyngeal and oropharyngeal spaces are diminished due to the short posterior facial height in conjunction with the aforementioned findings [2]. Basilar kyphosis has also been demonstrated as a frequent finding, which likely has adverse effects on the upper airway spaces [3, 4]. It is important to utilize lateral cephalograms and computer software to objectively quantify skeletal abnormalities. The extent of hypoplasia and skeletal abnormalities can be more easily appreciated. See Fig. 21.2a and b for an example of a traced lateral cephalogram and the accompanying cephalometric analysis data.

It appears that females tend to have more severe mandibular abnormalities and present with more significant mandibular retrusion in relation to the relative position of the maxilla and skull base. Typically, the maxilla is quite retruded in female subjects, as well. The changes in the growth and shape of the mandible are severe in all dimensions. See Fig. 21.3 for a sample 3D reconstruction from a CT scan. The vertical ramus height, length of the horizontal ramus, volume of bone in the horizontal ramus, and position of the chin prominence were all shown to be significantly affected in a study by Chong et al. from The Hospital for Sick Children in Toronto, Canada. Indeed, the shortened posterior facial height is one of the most notable differences when compared to controls [7].

A comprehensive assessment of cephalometric findings in 20 patients with Treacher Collins syndrome was published in 2013 by Dr. Kapadia from Seattle Children's Hospital and Dr. Shetye, Dr. Grayson, and Dr. McCarthy at New York University. They were able to present their findings on 20 unoperated patients, from age 5 to 16 years, for whom diagnostic quality lateral cephalograms were available. A summary of their findings can be found in Table 21.1

Several important observations included the abnormal position of the tongue superiorly and posteriorly secondary to severe mandibular retrognathism and a much smaller mandibular ramus height. The mandibular length is also greatly reduced [8]. The hypoplastic maxilla has deleterious effects on the nasal airway and possibly causes choanal stenosis or atresia. The hypoplastic maxilla combined with the hypoplastic mandible creates an unfavorable airway that is highly susceptible to obstructive sleep apnea [10]. Please see Chap. 15 regarding management of the pediatric airway for patients with Treacher Collins syndrome.

A whole host of pernicious effects of obstructive sleep apnea can plague individuals with Treacher Collins syndrome throughout childhood and adulthood. Obstructive sleep apnea in children can manifest as behavioral and cognitive problems leading to poor performance in school. Long-term effects can cause hypertension, type 2 diabetes, coronary heart disease, cerebrovascular disease, arrhythmias,

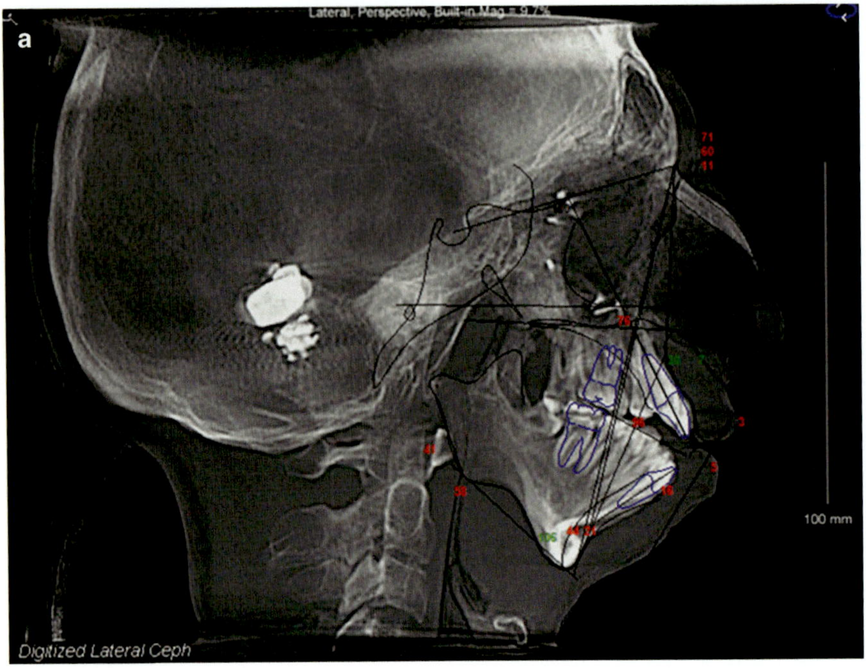

b

Group/Measurement	Value	Norm	Std Dev	Dev Norm
SNA (°)	70.8	82.0	3.0	-3.7 ***
SNB (°)	60.0	80.0	3.0	-6.7 ******
ANB (°)	10.8	1.6	1.5	6.1 ******
Facial Angle (FH-NPo) (°)	76.3	89.4	3.0	-4.4 ****
FMA (MP-FH) (°)	40.9	26.0	5.0	3.0 ***
Mand Plane to SN (°)	57.9	31.5	4.7	5.6 *****
U1 - SN (°)	100.5	103.0	5.5	-0.5
U1 - NA (mm)	7.2	4.3	2.7	1.1 *
U1 - NA (°)	29.6	22.8	5.7	1.2 *
L1 - NB (mm)	21.0	4.0	1.8	9.5 ******
L1 - NB (°)	43.7	25.2	4.0	4.6 ****
L1 Protrusion (L1-APo) (mm)	16.2	0.0	2.0	8.1 ******
U-Incisor Protrusion (U1-APo) (mm)	15.3	6.0	2.2	4.2 ****
IMPA (L1-MP) (°)	105.8	95.0	7.0	1.5 *
Interincisal Angle (U1-L1) (°)	95.9	130.0	5.0	-6.8 ******
Lower Lip to E-Plane (mm)	5.0	-2.0	2.0	3.5 ***
Upper Lip to E-Plane (mm)	2.6	-7.4	2.0	5.0 *****

Fig. 21.2 (**a**). Lateral ceph with tracing. (**b**). Cephalometric measurements

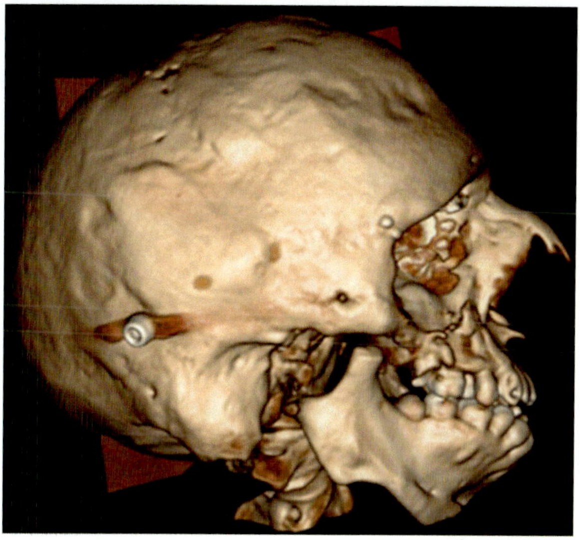

Fig. 21.3 3D recon of CT scan

and heart failure [11]. Certainly, if our goal is to minimize long-term morbidity for these patients, a key component of their surgical care will involve surgically correcting the maxillomandibular complex to treat obstructive sleep apnea.

Stability of Orthognathic Surgery

Many surgeons who have had the privilege to care for individuals with Treacher Collins syndrome will undoubtedly relate their personal experiences with frustrating long-term stability issues. Indeed, separate and respective studies published by Dufresne and Stelnicki confirm that even with early surgical intervention the Treacher Collins mandible has a profound tendency to relapse [5, 6]. There seems to be something influencing the stability of orthognathic surgery in patients with Treacher Collins syndrome, but at this time the cause is not fully elucidated.

The surgical movements typically needed to advance the maxillomandibular complex for an individual with TCS include maxillary advancement, mandibular advancement, and a counterclockwise rotation of the complex, which does include inferior movement of the posterior maxilla. A genioplasty with or without the inclusion of the genioglossus muscles is also typically performed. This is a similar treatment for individuals with a class II malocclusion with mandibular retrognathia and an open bite. Individuals with Treacher Collins syndrome have characteristic malocclusions. See Chap. 22 for more information regarding orthodontic treatment.

Data from the 2007 publication by Proffit, Turvey, and Phillips indicated that with rigid fixation mandibular advancement is a very stable and predictable surgical movement. Maxillary advancement is also considered stable, but moving the

Table 21.1 Treacher Collins syndrome cephalometric findings [8]

Cranial base	
Anterior cranial base (S-Na)	Decreased by 8.44 mm
Total cranial base (Na-Ba)	Decreased by 13.36 mm
Length of posterior cranial base (S-Ba)	Decreased by 1.29 mm
Cranial base (Na-S-Ba) angle	Decreased by 9.09 degrees
Maxilla	
Maxillary length (ANS-PNS)	Decreased by 6.98 mm
S-ANS	Decreased by 10.39 mm
Ba-ANS	Decreased by 16.42 mm
SNA	Decreased by 1.99 degrees
Anterior face height (Na-ANS)	Decreased by 3.53 mm
Posterior face height (SE-PNS)	Decreased by 9.89 mm
Maxillary plane (SN/ANS-PNS)	Tipped upward anteriorly by 10.45 degrees
Functional occlusal plane (SN-FOP)	Tipped upward anteriorly by 14.98 degrees
Mandible	
Ramus length (co to go)	Decreased by 13.08 mm
Ramus length (Cr to go)	Decreased by 13.03 mm
Mandibular body length (go-Pog)	Decreased by 17.78 mm
Total mandibular length (co-Pog)	Decreased by 22.73 mm
Anteroposterior ramus width	Decreased by 7.53 mm
SNB	Decreased by 8.95 degrees
Ba-Pg (mandible related to skull base)	Decreased by 31.62 mm
Lower face height (ANS-ME)	Decreased by 3.19 mm
Mand. Plane angle to SN plane (MP-SN)	Increased by 21.49 degrees
Mand. Plane to max. Plane (MP-ANS/PNS)	Increased by 10.70 degrees
Gonial angle (Ar-go-me)	Increased by 18.28 degrees

S sella, *Na* nasion, *Ba* basion, *ANS* anterior nasal spine, *PNS* posterior nasal spine, *SNA* sella, nasion, A point, *SNB* sella, nasion, B point, *SE* Sella entrance, *SN* sella - nasion, *FOP* functional occlusal plane, *Co* condylion, *Cr* coronoid, *Go* gonion, *Pog* pogonion, *ME* menton, *Ar* articulare, *MP* mandibular plane [8]

maxilla inferiorly is considered problematic [12]. While this assignment of hierarchical stability may still apply to the Treacher Collins patient in general, there seem to exist multiple factors that contribute to more profound relapse than in the subjects in that study.

Nguyen et al. published their findings on the long-term stability of bimaxillary orthognathic surgery in Treacher Collins patients in 2015. They performed a retrospective review for patients treated by a single surgeon from 1993 to 2007. There was a female predominance in the group that underwent surgery, which was not surprising given that females with TCS tend to have more severe skeletal abnormalities than males. Significant relapse was noted at SNA, palatal plane angle, and

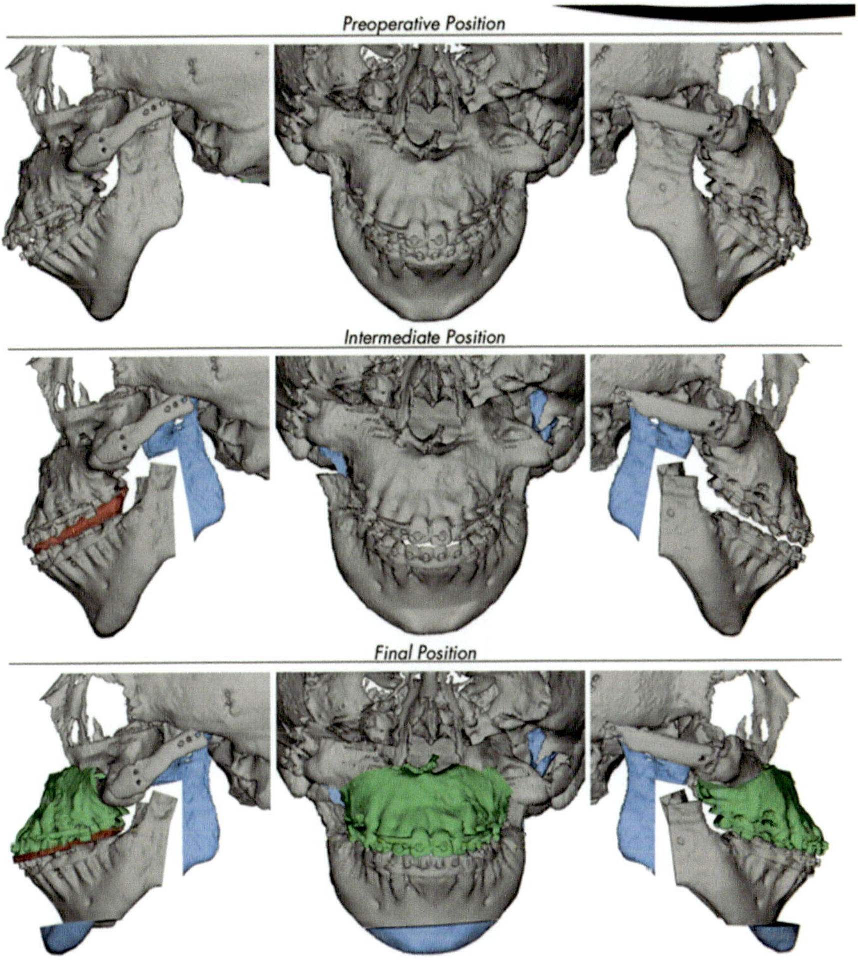

Fig. 21.4 Typical workflow summary for orthognathic surgery. In this individual with TCS, inverted L osteotomies bilaterally were planned

midface length. The decreases that were not statistically significant were the gonial angle and mandibular length. [9].

The soft tissue envelope should not be underestimated as a challenge to large advancements and is a formidable foe of long-term stability. Many times individuals with TCS have undergone prior surgeries by the time of definitive maxillomandibular orthognathic surgery, and each iteration of surgical scarring adds to the limitation of the soft tissue to accommodate a large advancement in the maxillofacial skeleton.

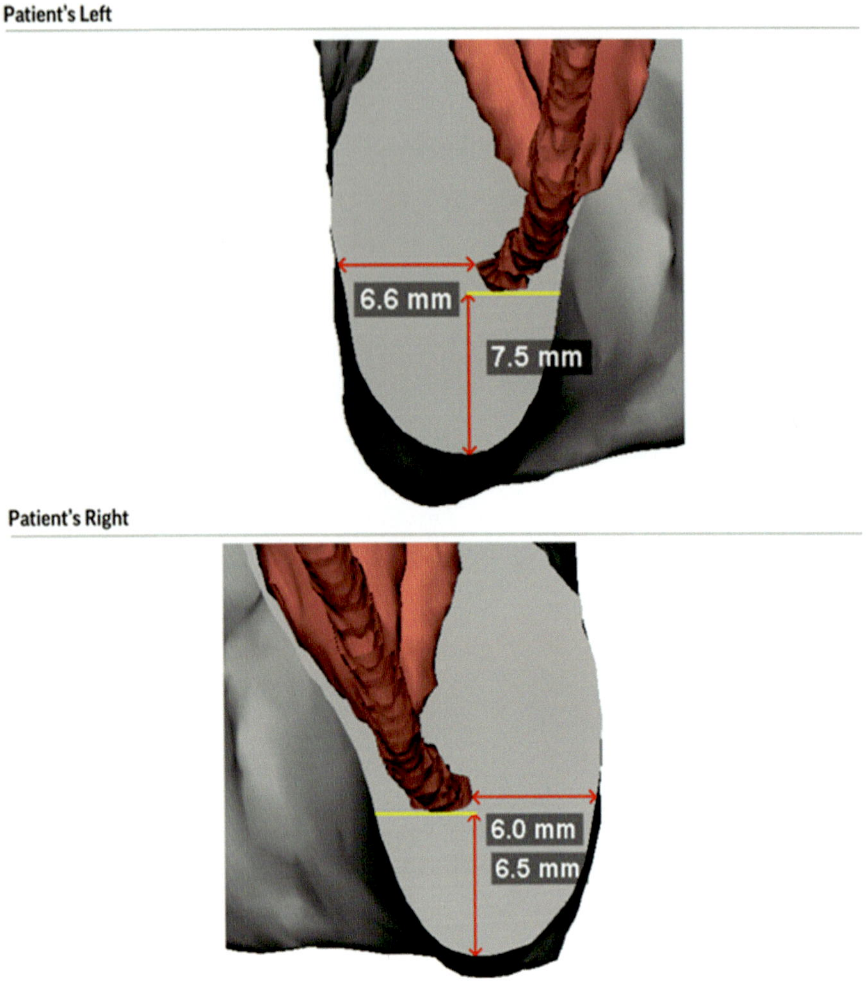

Fig. 21.5 Example of computer-aided planning helping visualize vital structures, in this case the inferior alveolar nerve

Surgery Protocol

At our institution, we strongly believe that each patient with Treacher Collins syndrome should be treated as a unique individual. The degree of psychosocial impact of having Treacher Collins syndrome will vary among affected individuals, and these children should ideally have access to the appropriate specialists. We recommend and invite all patients with Treacher Collins syndrome to be seen and evaluated by our ACPA-approved cleft and craniofacial team. Individuals with Treacher Collins syndrome are candidates for specialized surgical and nonsurgical intervention from numerous specialists and are likely to benefit from being seen in a multidisciplinary team setting.

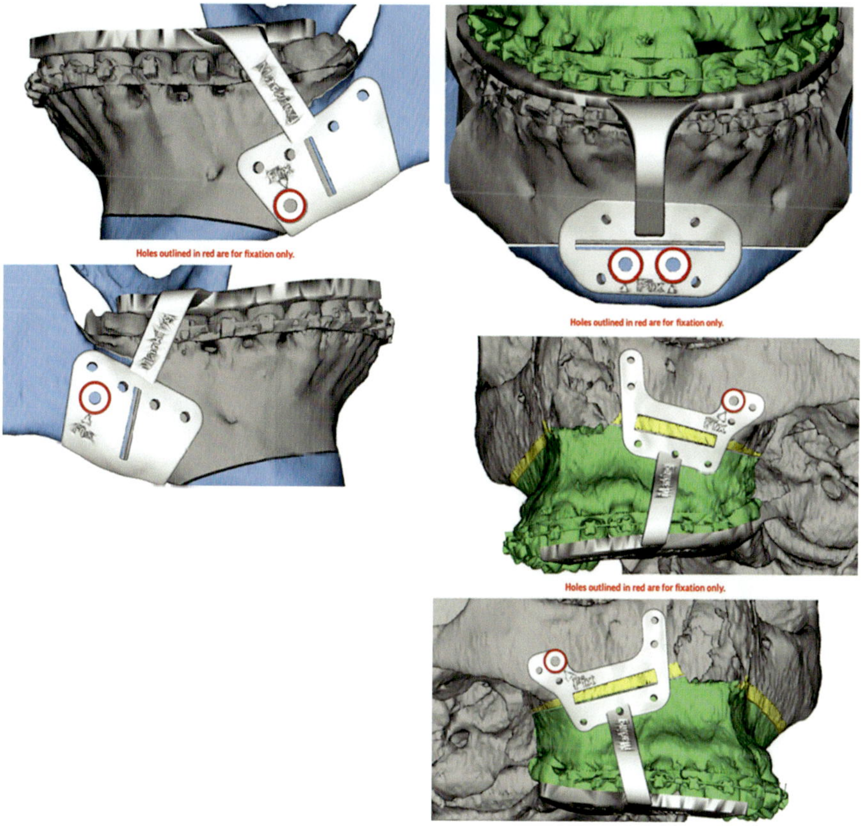

Fig. 21.6 Custom surgical cutting guides

In general, we adhere to the principle of postponing maxillomandibular orthognathic surgery until skeletal maturity. However, children with significant obstructive sleep apnea are considered candidates for orthognathic surgery, knowing full well that growth may be unpredictable and a second or even third operation may be indicated in the future. We refer children in whom we suspect obstructive sleep apnea to a sleep medicine specialist who can help determine the severity of OSA and offer to the child and family nonsurgical options that can be considered as stop gaps until either growth of the mandible occurs or skeletal maturity is reached.

We recommend every patient with Treacher Collins syndrome to start seeing a pediatric or general dentist when the primary dentition begins to erupt. Routine, thorough evaluations should continue through early childhood, and at the appropriate age, these patients should be evaluated by an orthodontist who routinely performs surgical orthodontic treatment. Severe open bites with a reverse curve of Spee are routinely encountered, and nearly all of these individuals will be candidates for surgical orthodontics and bimaxillary orthognathic surgery. Fig. 21.11 shows a typical open bite malocclusion seen in a TCS individual. Please see Chap. 22 regarding orthodontic treatment for an individual with Treacher Collins.

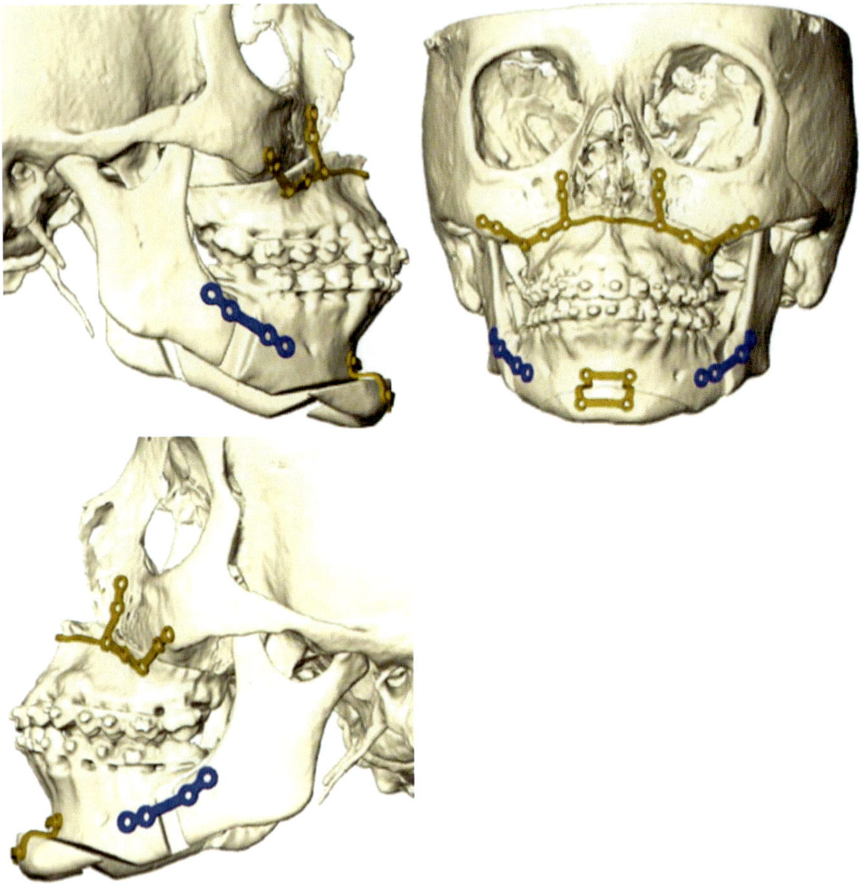

Fig. 21.7 Custom-designed fixation plates

Once it has been determined that a patient is a candidate for orthognathic surgery, the decision is then made to pursue a surgery-first approach or the traditional three-stage approach with presurgical orthodontics, surgery, and post-surgery orthodontics. At our institution, in the majority of cases, we treat patients with the traditional three-stage approach.

Some form of maxillomandibular orthognathic surgery will be indicated for these individuals. Mandibular osteotomies such as the bilateral sagittal split osteotomy and the inverted L osteotomy are two options. See Figs. 21.8, 21.9, and 21.10 for lateral and profile photos, as well as 3D recons for an individual treated with bilateral inverted L osteotomies, LeFort I osteotomy, and genioplasty. Bicortical fixation screws with bilateral sagittal split osteotomies may not lend themselves well for large mandibular advancements. For patients who are having severe airway obstruction, we will consider performing neonatal mandibular distraction. For more on the pediatric airway, see Chap. 15 and mandibular distraction see Chap. 19.

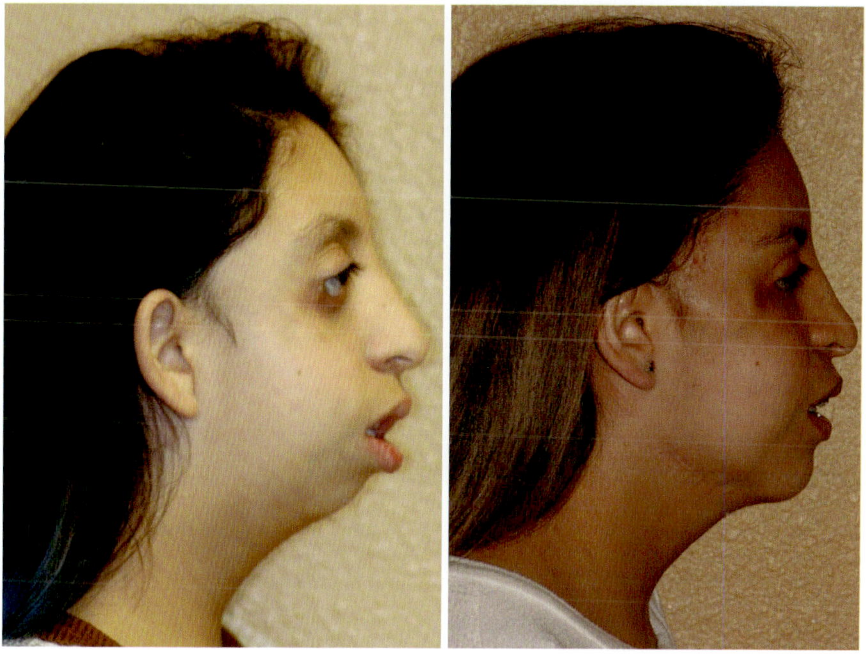

Fig. 21.8 Profile view before and after bilateral inverted L osteotomies and genioplasty for patient X. She had also undergone a Kufner osteotomy and calvarial bone harvest and grafting to the zygomatic arches

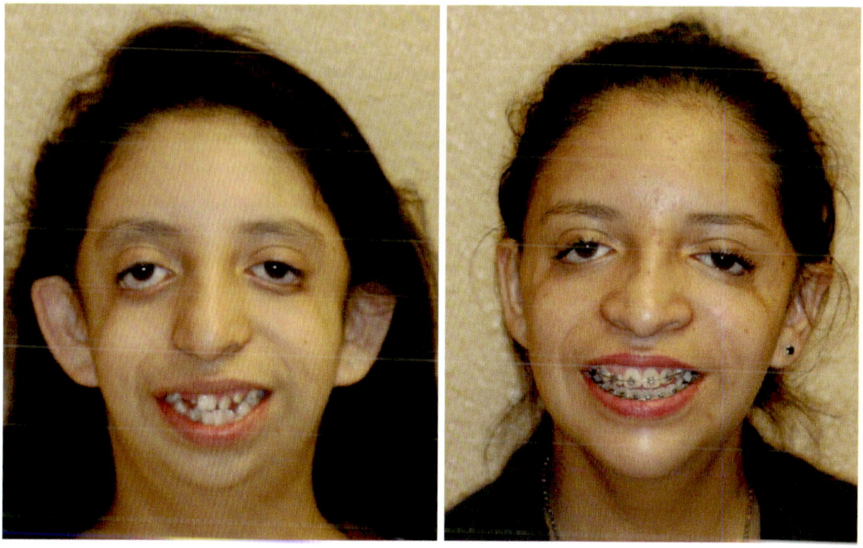

Fig. 21.9 Frontal views of the same patient

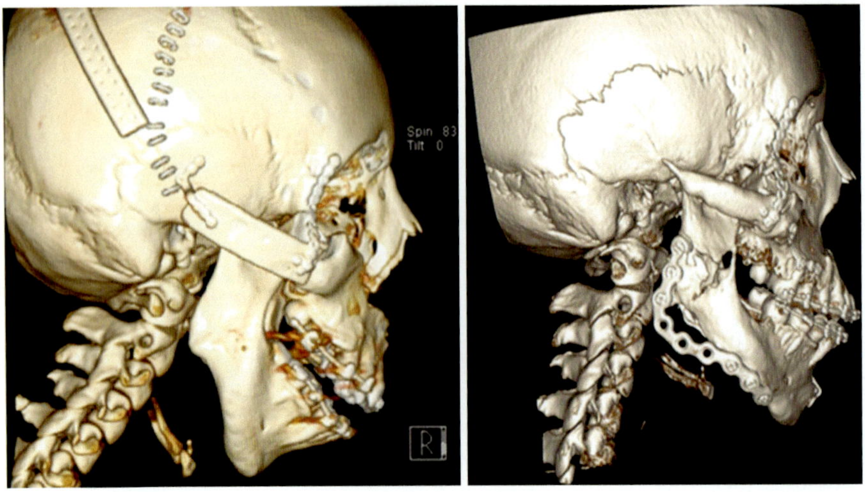

Fig. 21.10 Before and after 3D reconstructions of the same patient. Notice the amount of counterclockwise rotation and the occlusal plane change. Note the recon plate appears maladapted to the mandibular angle; there was significant resorption of the bone graft at the site

Table 21.2 TCS severity and osteotomy options

Severity	Surgical treatment
Mild	BSSO, LeFort, +/− genioplasty
Moderate	Bilateral inverted L, LeFort, genioplasty
Severe	TMJ TJR, LeFort, genioplasty

In order to appropriately treat each patient, it is crucial to identify the severity of the skeletal deformity and understand the limitations of the various treatment modalities available to the patient. See Table 21.2 for a summary of our osteotomy options. For mild deformities, we strongly consider use of more traditional bimaxillary surgery, which includes bilateral sagittal split osteotomies, LeFort I osteotomy, and +/− genioplasty.

In individuals with a moderate degree of deformity, we opt for use of bilateral inverted L osteotomies, in order to maximize the advancement and counterclockwise rotation. See Fig. 21.4 for a typical virtual workflow including LeFort I, inverted L osteotomies, and a genioplasty. Sufficient ramus height is necessary, and the stability of the TMJ is also important to consider. If the TMJ is a Kaban type I or type IIa, then this is our preferred approach. This is done in conjunction with a LeFort I osteotomy and a genioplasty.

Individuals with severe hypoplasia and deformity of the temporomandibular joint complex, such as in Kaban type IIb and III joints, will benefit from total joint replacement in conjunction with a LeFort osteotomy. We have significant concern for further remodeling of the TMJ and for significant relapse if a large advancement is performed without addressing the joint with a prosthetic reconstruction in these

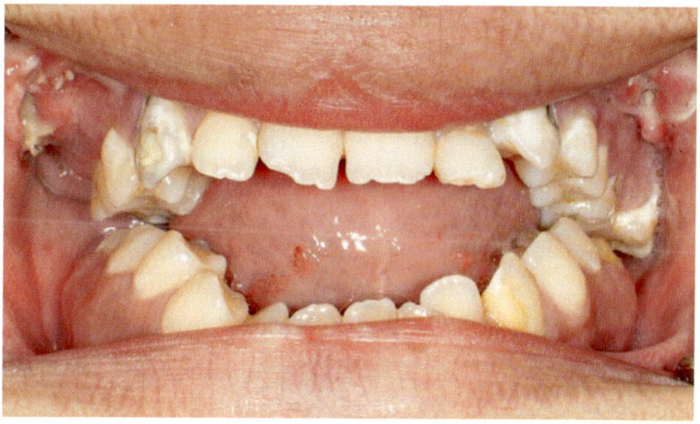

Fig. 21.11 Typical open bite for TCS

individuals. For further details regarding temporomandibular joint total joint replacement for the patient with Treacher Collins syndrome, please see Chap. 20.

Our clinical workflow in preparation for surgery includes the following:

1. Obtain full medical history.
2. Clinical measurements.
3. CBCT.
4. Intraoral scanning.
5. Clinical photos.
6. Cephalometric evaluation.
7. Computer-aided surgical planning.
8. Fabrication of computer-designed occlusal splints, cutting guides, and patient-specific plates (for large advancements with inverted L osteotomy) or custom TMJ total joint prosthesis with TMJ concepts (Ventura, CA).

In order to optimize stability for large advancements and improve bone growth in the large gaps at the osteotomy sites, we utilize several strategies. First, appropriately rigid plates are utilized. These can either be stock recon plates that are pre-bent off 3D printed models or can be custom-made plates. Next, allogeneic or autogenous bone grafting is performed at the osteotomy gap. Recombinant human bone morphogenetic protein-2 (rhBMP-2) on a collagen sponge is also mixed with the bone graft. We also use a similar technique in large maxillary advancements with cortical blocks of bone wedged and often fixated with screws and then covered with sheets of rhBMP-2 in a collagen sponge.

Summary

The morphologic characteristics of the maxillomandibular complex, the degree of hypoplasia, the challenging malocclusions, and the restrictive soft tissue envelope create a constellation of surgical challenges for the Treacher Collins patient. The growth potential of the TCS mandible is diminished, and the mandible tends to remain diminutive despite the pubertal growth spurt that tends to help with mandibular growth in other craniofacial syndromes [13]. It is imperative that these individuals receive treatment based on a team approach with access to the medical and surgical specialists who can address the specific needs of the affected individual. Obstructive sleep apnea that cannot be treated nonsurgically or psychosocial problems may expedite the need to perform surgery prior to skeletal maturity.

The goals of definitive maxillomandibular surgical treatment should include eliminating obstructive sleep apnea, providing a functional occlusion, and creating a facial profile that is within normal limits. Some individuals with more severe deformities will need temporomandibular total joint reconstruction. Others will be appropriately treated with bilateral inverted L osteotomies or bilateral sagittal split osteotomies, with concomitant LeFort I osteotomy and genioplasty. In general, the surgical movements are forward in the maxilla and mandible with a counterclockwise rotation.

Surgical planning should include 3D imaging with CBCT or CT scan, intra-oral scanning, clinical photos, and clinical measurements. Computer-aided planning should be utilized to fully appreciate the skeletal deficiencies, to plan movements accordingly, and to appreciate vital structures (Fig. 21.5). The fabrication of custom cutting guides and plates (Figs. 21.6 and 21.7) is widely available.

In an effort to lower the burden of care for patients and their family, the surgery-first approach in orthognathic surgery is an option. In select patients, the overall treatment time can be drastically reduced. Also, it may be appropriate to consider the surgery-first approach for individuals with severe obstructive sleep apnea who can benefit from an expedited surgical date and realize the benefits of an expanded airway sooner, rather than potentially years of presurgical orthodontics [14]. The conventional approach typically takes 27 to 35 months of orthodontic treatment [15–17]. The surgery-first approach can require on average 10 months of orthodontics [18, 19].

With technological advancements providing for a fully digital workflow with computer-aided planning, patient-specific osteotomy cutting guides and fixation devices, and the use of growth factors, the future is promising that more predictable and more stable maxillomandibular surgical outcomes can be achieved for individuals with Treacher Collins syndrome.

Disclosure The authors have nothing to disclose.

References

1. Franceschetti A, Klein D. Mandibulo-facial dysostosis: new hereditary syndrome. Acta Ophthalmol. 1949;27:143–224.
2. Arvystas M, Shprintzen RJ. Craniofacial morphology in Treacher Collins syndrome. Cleft Palate Craniofac J. 1991;28:226.
3. Peterson-Falzone SJ, Figueroa AA. Longitudinal changes in cranial base angulation in mandibulofacial dysostosis. Cleft Palate J. 1989;26:31.

4. Roberts FG, Pruzansky S, Aduss H. An x-radiocephalometric study of mandibulofacial dysostosis in man. Arch Oral Biol. 1975;20:265.
5. Dufresne C, Richtsmeier JT. Interaction of craniofacial dysmorphology, growth, and prediction of surgical outcome. J Craniofac Surg. 1995;6:270.
6. Stelnicki EJ, Lin WY, Lee C, Grayson BH, McCarthy JG. Long-term outcome study of bilateral mandibular distraction: a comparison of Treacher Collins and Nager syndromes to other types of micrognathia. Plast Reconstr Surg. 2002;109:1819.
7. Chong DK, Murray DJ, Phillips JH, et al. A cephalometric analysis of maxillary and mandibular parameters in treacher collins syndrome. Plast Reconstr Surg. 2008;121:77e.
8. Kapadia H, Shetye PR, Grayson BH, McCarthy JG. Cephalometric assessment of craniofacial morphology in patients with Treacher Collins syndrome. J Craniofac Surg. 2013;24:1141–5.
9. Nguyen PD, Caro MC, Smith DM, Tompson B, Forrest CR, Phillips JH. Long-term orthognathic surgical outcomes in Treacher Collins patients. J Plast Reconstr Aesthet Surg. 2016;69:402–8.
10. Posnick JC, Tiwana PS, Costello BJ. Treacher Collins syndrome: comprehensive evaluation and treatment. Oral and Maxillofac Surg Clin North Am. 2004;16:503–23.
11. Gottlieb DJ, Punjabi NM. Diagnosis and management of obstructive sleep apnea, a review. J Am Med Associat. 2020:323(14).
12. Proffit WR, Turvey RA, Phillips C. The hierarchy of stability and predictability in orthognathic surgery with rigid fixation: an update and extension. Head Face Med. 2007;3:2.
13. Rogers GF, Lim AA, Mulliken JB, Padwa BL. Effect of a syndromic diagnosis on mandibular size and sagittal position in Robin sequence. J Oral Maxillofac Surg Off J Am Assoc Oral Maxillofac Surg. 2009;67:2323–31.
14. Uribe FA, Farrell B. Surgery-first approach in the Orthognathic patient. Oral and Maxillofacial Surg Clin N Am. 2020;32:89–103.
15. Diaz PM, Garcia RG, Gias LN, et al. Time used for orthodontic surgical treatment of dentofacial deformities in white patients. J Oral Maxillofac Surg. 2010;68(1):88–92.
16. O'Brien K, Wright J, Conboy F, et al. Prospective, multi-center study of the effectiveness of orthodontic/orthognathic surgery care in the United Kingdom. Am J Orthod Dentofac Orthop. 2009;135(6):709–14.
17. Slavnic S, Marcusson A. Duration of orthodontic treatment in conjunction with orthognathic surgery. Swed Dent J. 2010;34(3):159–66.
18. Hernandez-Alfaro F, Guijarro-Martínez R, Peiro-Guijarro MA. Surgery first in orthognathic surgery: what have we learned? A comprehensive workflow based on 45 consecutive cases. J Oral Maxillofac Surg. 2014;72(2):376–90.
19. Uribe F, Adabi S, Janakiraman N, et al. Treatment duration and factors associated with the surgery first approach: a two center study. Prog Orthod. 2015;16:29.

Chapter 22
Principles of Orthodontic Management of Treacher Collins Syndrome

Veerasathpurush Allareddy, James Maclaine, and Mohammed H. Elnagar

Introduction

Treacher Collins syndrome (TCS), frequently referred to as mandibulofacial dysostosis, is a disorder of craniofacial development attributed to mutations in the "treacle" gene (TCOF1) on chromosome 5q32 (TCS-1), POLR1D gene on chromosome 13q12 (TCS-22), POLR1C gene on chromosome 6p21 (TCS-3), or POLR1B gene on chromosome 2q14 (TCS-4) [1–4]. A vast majority of cases of TCS are due to mutations in TCOF1, and the incidence of TCS is about 1 in 50,000 live births [Caluseriu 2013] [5]. TCS-1 and TCS-4 are inherited as an autosomal dominant disorder, TCS-3 is inherited as an autosomal recessive disorder, while TCS-2 can be inherited either as autosomal dominant or autosomal recessive [1–4]. There is variable involvement of craniofacial structures derived from the first and second branchial arches [6, 7]. The involvement of craniofacial structures is usually symmetric. TCS has a high penetrance and variable expressivity [8–10]. Those with TCS require care from a multidisciplinary team comprised of orthodontists, pedodontists, craniofacial surgeons, oral and maxillofacial surgeons, etc. [11]. The earliest clinical interventions could start as early as infancy, and the continuum of care could last

V. Allareddy (✉)
Department of Orthodontics, Department of Orthodontics, College of Dentistry, University of Illinois at Chicago, Chicago, IL, USA
e-mail: sath@uic.edu

J. Maclaine
Clinical Instructor, Department of Developmental Biology, Boston Children's Hospital and Harvard School of Dental Medicine, Boston, MA, USA
e-mail: James.Maclaine@childrens.harvard.edu

M. H. Elnagar
Department of Orthodontics, College of Dentistry - University of Illinois at Chicago, Chicago, IL, USA
e-mail: melnagar@uic.edu

D. M. Yates, M. R. Markiewicz (eds.), *Craniofacial Microsomia and Treacher Collins Syndrome*, https://doi.org/10.1007/978-3-030-84733-3_22

into adulthood with comprehensive phase or orthodontic treatment and orthognathic surgeries performed in the late teenage years or in the early 20s. The below sections provide an overview of the common orofacial features and the principles of orthodontic management of TCS.

Orofacial Features

The phenotypic expression of TCS is highly variable [12–17]. Frequently, those with TCS present as Class II skeletal malocclusions, marked convexity of face (due to a prominent nasal dorsum and retrognathic mandible), and an anterior open bite. Some of the common facial features (Fig. 22.1) include downward-slanting palpebral fissures, euryblepharon, absence of lower medial third of eyelashes, coloboma, hypoplasia of the zygomatic arches, maxillary hypoplasia, external ear malformations, accessory skin tags, and external ear malformations [12–17]. Tessier type 6–8 clefts can also be seen in those with severe manifestations of TCS. The typical oral features (Fig. 22.2) include anterior open bite, crowding of maxillary and mandibular arches, Class II molar relationship, ectopic eruption of maxillary first molars, congenitally missing teeth, high-arched palate, shortened soft palate, and cleft palate (estimated to occur in 35% of patients) [12, 16–18]. About 30 to 40% of those with TCS have velopharyngeal incompetence, and 25% have obstructive sleep apnea [12]. The classic lateral cephalometric features include (Fig. 22.3) reduced cranial base angle, steep mandibular plane angle, antegonial notching, clockwise rotation of occlusal plane, short ramus, obtuse gonial angle, increased lower anterior facial height, reduced posterior facial height, and increased ANB angle [10, 19].

Principles of Orthodontic Management

Those with TCS present with occlusal/skeletal disharmony in all three dimensions, transverse, sagittal, and vertical, and are very challenging to treat orthodontically. Depending on the variability and complexity of malocclusions, orthodontic

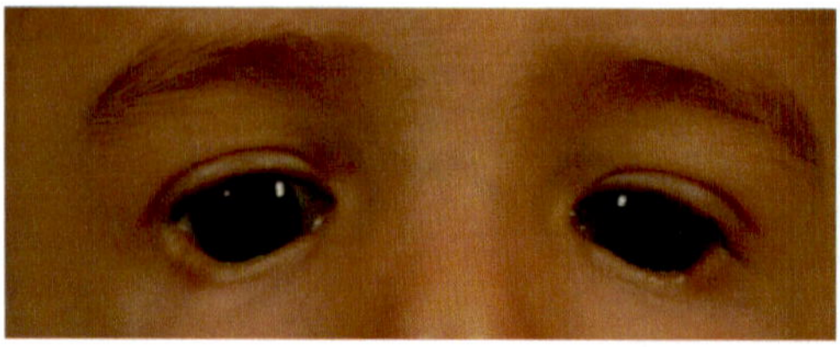

Downward slanting palpebral fissures and absence of lower medial third of eyelashes

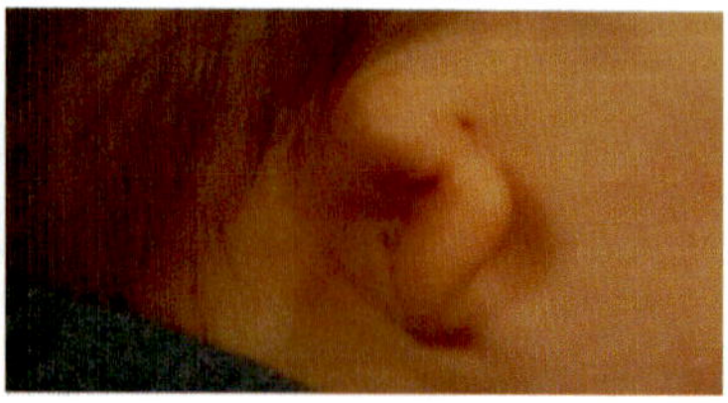

External ear malformations

Fig. 22.1 Facial Features

treatment is frequently required in conjunction with orthognathic surgery. A brief overview of timeline of various orthodontic interventions is provided below:

Time point	Care	Objectives
Birth to 1 year	Examination of patient by the orthodontist along with craniofacial team (orthodontists play a pivotal role in the continuum of care and hence should be a part of the craniofacial team	Know the patient and parents
	Distraction osteogenesis if appropriate skull base condylar stop is present	To address airway issues
	Establishment of a dental home by 1 year of age	Follow up on development of dentition
1 year to early mixed dentition	Periodic examinations annually	Follow up on growth and development, eruption of teeth, and oral hygiene
Mixed dentition	Maxillary expansion	To correct posterior cross bites and establish compatible arch forms
	Limited phase of orthodontic treatment	To facilitate eruption of permanent teeth into the arch, correct traumatic occlusions, and functional shifts
Permanent dentition	Comprehensive phase of orthodontic treatment with or without orthognathic surgery	Restoration of facial balance obtaining balanced and functional occlusion
	Final restorative treatment (e.g., implants and implant supported crowns, etc.)	For addressing missing teeth and restorative needs

Maxillary Expansion

Frequently, those with TCS tend to have a high-arched palate and about 30% have a cleft palate [12, 16–18]. Consequently, the maxillary arch is constricted which manifests as posterior crossbites. Depending on severity of constriction, there is crowding. Some of the objectives of orthodontic treatment are to establish the maxillary arch form, make maxillary and mandibular arch forms compatible, correct crossbites, and resolve crowding. These objectives can be realized by expansion of maxilla. The type of expansion that needs to be done is dependent on the arch form and area of constriction (anterior versus posterior). Those with a cleft palate and alveolus tend to have collapsed arch segments in the anterior region. In such situations, differential expansion (more expansion in the anterior region versus posterior region) is required. On the other hand, a symmetrical expansion will be required if there is constriction in both anterior and posterior regions. Fan-shaped expanders are used to obtain differential expansion (Fig. 22.4). Symmetrical expansion can be achieved by a wide variety of expansion appliances such as hyrax expanders, Haas expanders, etc. (Fig. 22.5). Below is a step-by-step process recommended for accomplishing maxillary expansion:

- **Clinical examination**: The importance of a good clinical examination cannot be overemphasized. The severity of crossbite can range from a single tooth to

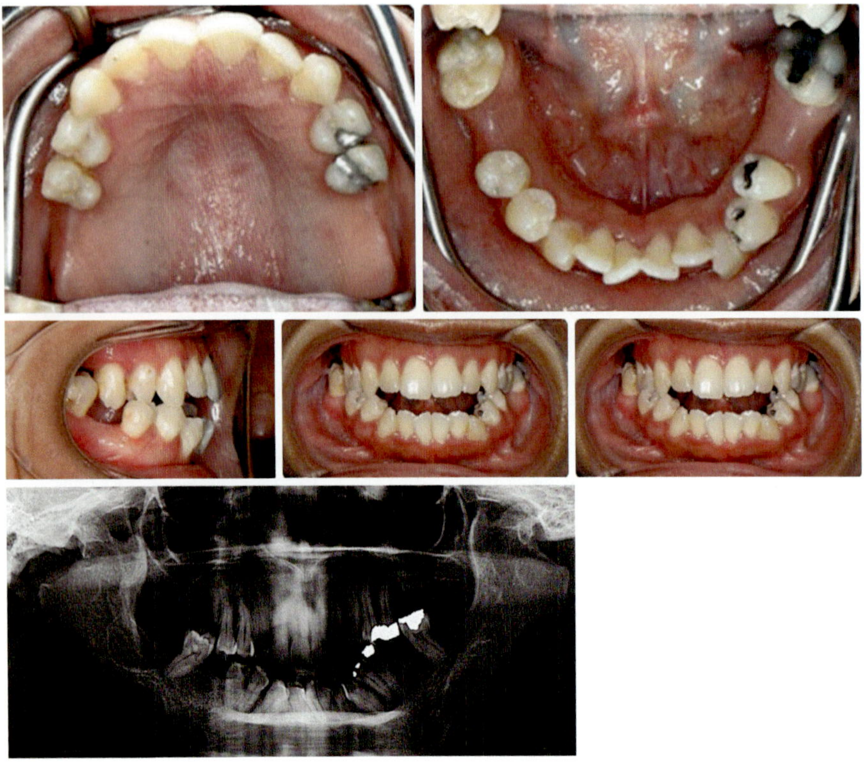

Fig. 22.2 Common Oral Features

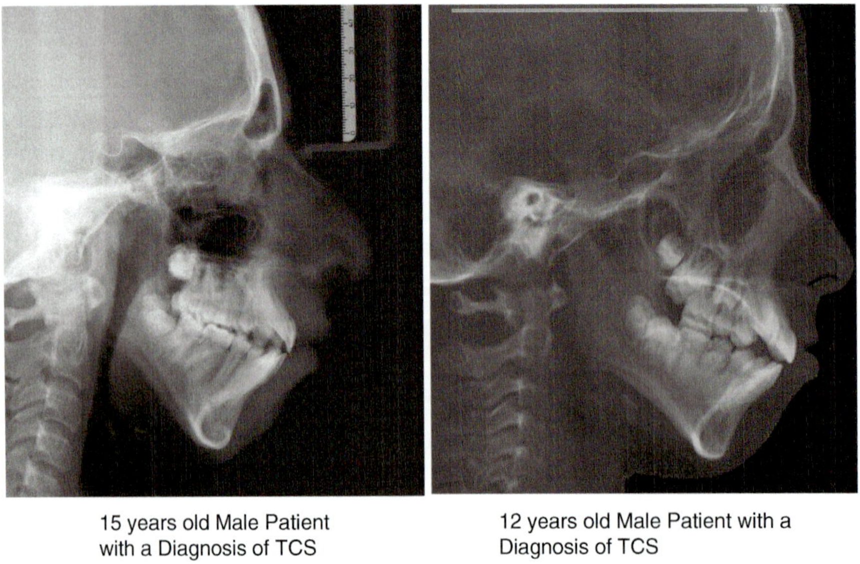

Fig. 22.3 Lateral Cephalometric Images of TCS

Fig. 22.4 Fan Shaped Expander

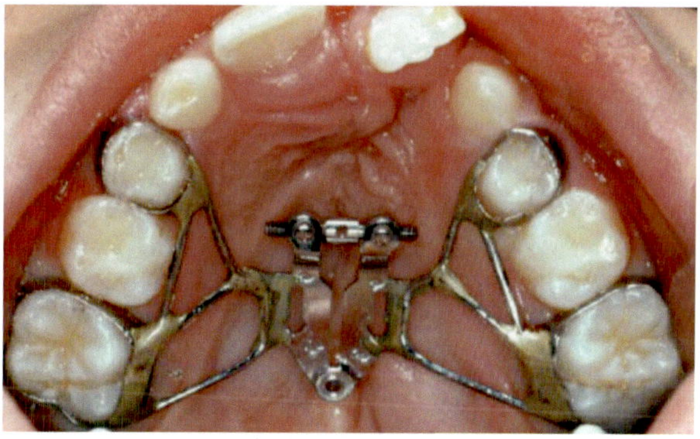

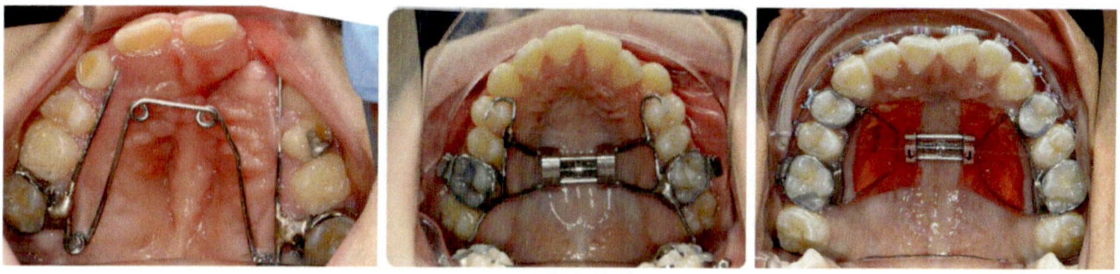

Fig. 22.5 Different Types of Expansion Appliances

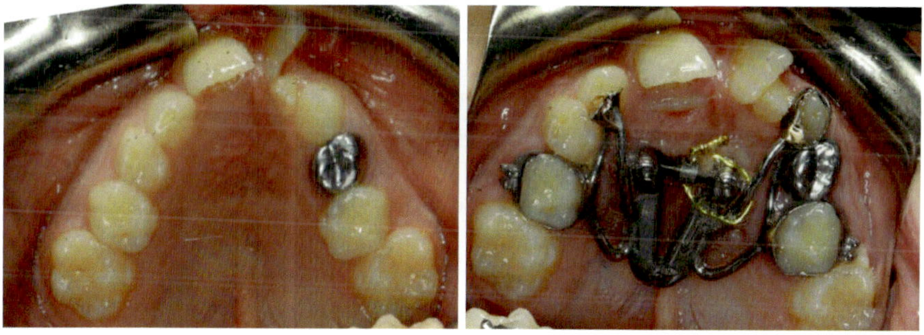

Fig. 22.6 Differential Expansion with Fan Shaped Expander

involving an entire segment. A crossbite that involves only a single tooth or a couple of teeth typically are dental crossbites and can be effectively addressed with orthodontic aligning/leveling and use of cross elastics. On the other hand, if multiple teeth or an entire segment is involved, then maxillary skeletal expansion will be required. It is vital to assess the maxillary arch form and its compatibility with the mandibular arch. The type of expander that needs to be used is dependent on these factors. As mentioned earlier, those with TCS have Class II skeletal and dental manifestations. Consequently, on clinical examination in maximum intercuspation, there may not be an apparent posterior crossbite since the maxillary arch articulates with a narrower segment of the mandibular arch. It is recommended that the patient positions the mandible anteriorly (into a Canine Class I relationship) and then the transverse relationship be examined. When the mandible is positioned anteriorly to as close as possible to the future desired position, the maxilla articulates with a wider segment of the mandible and the true relative maxillary/mandibular transverse discrepancy can be appreciated.

- **Diagnostic aids**: The amount and type of maxillary expansion that need to be obtained are dependent on a multitude of factors such as severity of constriction of maxillary arch, amount of arch length teeth size discrepancy (crowding), type of maxillary arch form and its compatibility with mandibular arch, and compensations of posterior teeth (usually maxillary molars are buccally tipped while the mandibular molars are lingually tipped). We recommend that diagnostic models be obtained and assessed for the above factors. As mentioned in the clinical examination step, the models should be articulated (mandible moved anteriorly into the future desired position) in a Class I canine relationship, and then the amount of posterior crossbite should be quantified. The degree of compensations of the maxillary and mandibular molar teeth and amount of crowding should also be accurately assessed, and the planned amount of expansion should be established accordingly. One other key diagnostic aid is a postero-anterior cephalometric radiograph. This enables us to assess the amount of relative skeletal maxillary/mandibular transverse discrepancy.
- **Maxillary expansion appliance designs**: A wide variety of maxillary expansion appliances are in use, and the specific design should be based on the type and timing of expansion. Expansion can be done during the mixed dentition stages using a simple quad-helix or W-shaped expander. Typically hyrax and Haas-type expanders are done before the age of 15 years. Beyond this age, the median palatine suture tends to interlock, and it is difficult to obtain pure skeletal expansion. In such scenarios, temporary anchorage device-assisted expansion appliances can be used. As explained earlier, fan-shaped expansion appliances can be used to obtain differential expansion (more expansion in the canine region compared to in the molar region) (Fig. 22.6). The positioning of the fulcrum of the expansion screw in relation to the distal abutments determines the amount of anterior versus posterior expansion. As the fulcrum is placed more anteriorly in relation to the distal abutment, more anterior expansion relative to the posterior expansion can be achieved. We have conducted extensive lab experiments in an attempt to compute the relative anterior and posterior expansions obtained by varying the position of the fulcrum [20]. When the fulcrum of the expansion screw is placed 10 mm behind a line drawn from and to the central pits of the distal abutment teeth (usually the maxillary first permanent molars), an anterior to posterior expansion ratio of 1.95 to 1.9 is obtained. If the fulcrum is placed 5 mm behind the distal abutment, the anterior to posterior expansion ratio is 5.20:1, and if the fulcrum is placed 3 mm behind the distal abutment, the anterior to posterior

expansion is 27.33:1.9. Regardless of the type of expansion appliance used (hyrax, Haas type, or fan-shaped), we recommend using four abutment teeth to support the expansion appliance. We use the maxillary first molars as the distal abutment and the maxillary first premolars (or maxillary first primary molars) as the mesial abutments for hyrax and Haas-type expanders. For fan-shaped expanders (usually used only in those with a cleft palate), we use the maxillary first molars as distal abutments and the primary canines as the mesial abutments.

- **Activation protocol**: For most patients, a rapid maxillary expansion is done. The recommended activation protocol is one turn activation of the expansion screw each day. We have obtained consistently good clinical outcomes with this approach. Occasionally, we have used two activations of expansion screw each day. The total number of activations will be dependent on the amount of expansion required. Typically, each activation will yield about 0.25 mm of expansion. It is critical that the total amount of expansion need to correct the transverse discrepancy be computed prior to cementing the expansion appliance. The length of the expansion screw is dependent on this and should be taken into consideration while designing the appliance. In those with cleft palate, where there is an increased likelihood of opening palatal fistulas with rapid expansion, we tend to do slow expansion. We activate the expansion by one turn every 3 or 4 days to minimize opening of large fistulas. Our rationale is that the slow expansion protocol enables the palatal tissues to adapt to the stresses placed by the expansion appliance.
- **Retention**: Maxillary expansion is one of the least stable orthodontic movements, and there is significant amount of relapse. It is our practice to over-expand by about 25% to account for possible relapse. Following completion of maxillary expansion, we use brass wires or composite to seal the expansion screw and have the appliance in place for about 3 months. After this, we remove the maxillary expansion appliance and cement a fixed trans-palatal arch with mesial extension arms (up to the maxillary canines). The trans-palatal arch is made of rigid stainless steel wire. This is in place until the commencement of comprehensive phase of orthodontic treatment when fixed orthodontic appliances are banded/bonded.

Limited Orthodontic Treatment

A limited phase of orthodontic treatment (usually only in the maxillary arch) while not an absolute essential is usually recommended if there are any anterior crossbites leading to functional shifts and traumatic occlusion and to facilitate eruption of permanent teeth. Frequently, those with TCS have hypoplastic maxilla and mandible, and there is relative arch length/teeth size discrepancies. The severe crowding may lead to ectopic eruption of teeth and/or blocked/impacted teeth. In such situations, a limited phase of orthodontic treatment is usually done to facilitate eruption of teeth into their appropriate positions in the arch. The case illustrated in Figs. 22.7a–c is a female patient aged 12 years. It is evident that there is severe crowding in the maxillary arch, constriction of the maxillary arch, posterior crossbite, premature loss of maxillary right second primary molar which resulted in the first permanent molar drifting anteriorly, palatal eruption of maxillary second

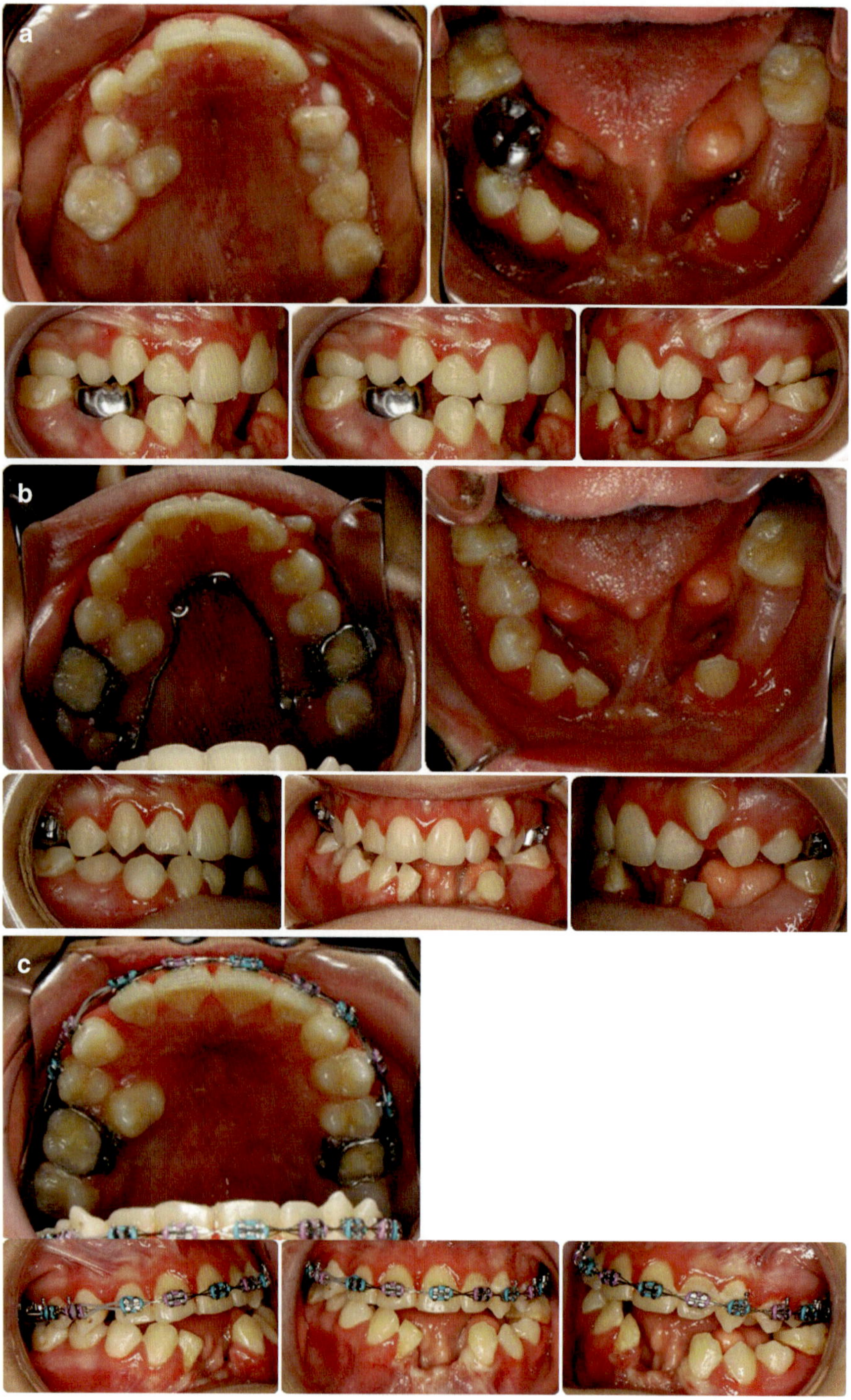

Fig. 22.7 (**a**) Initial Presentation. (**b**) Progress (Maxillary Expansion). (**c**) Limited Orthodontic Treatment

premolar, and labial eruption of maxillary left canine. The goals of the limited phase of orthodontic treatment were to expand the maxillary arch to make it compatible with the mandibular arch, align and level the maxillary arch, and create space for the maxillary left permanent canine to erupt into the arch. Limited orthodontic treatment was commenced by expanding the maxillary arch with a quad helix appliance. This is usually done by banding the first molars. Following expansion, brackets were bonded on the maxillary arch teeth, and light nitinol wires are used to align the teeth, and stainless steel wires are used to level the arches. Open coil springs and power chains were used to create/consolidate spaces and help facilitate the eruption of maxillary left canine into the arch. During the limited orthodontic treatment phase, the definitive anterio-posterior correction (correction of Class II skeletal/occlusal relationship) and vertical correction (anterior open bites) are seldom corrected. These are usually best treated during the comprehensive phase of orthodontic treatment.

Occasionally, mandibular distraction osteogenesis can be performed in childhood. This is usually indicated in patients with obstructive sleep apnea. This procedure could obviate the need for a future orthognathic surgery. Illustrated in Figs. 22.8, 22.9, 22.10, 22.11, 22.12, and 22.13 is a case of TCS that was treated with mandibular distraction osteogenesis in the mixed dentition stage. The patient presented initially at age 9 years. This patient also had a submucous cleft palate with subsequent velopharyngeal insufficiency (VPI). At age 10 years, in order to improve the VPI, a pharyngeal flap was planned. However, the patient also developed snoring, and this created concern that he would develop obstructive sleep apnea due to the pharyngeal flap. Therefore, in an attempt to open up the posterior airway space, bilateral mandibular osteotomies were done to advance the mandible with the use of curvilinear distraction devices, in order to achieve both advancement and

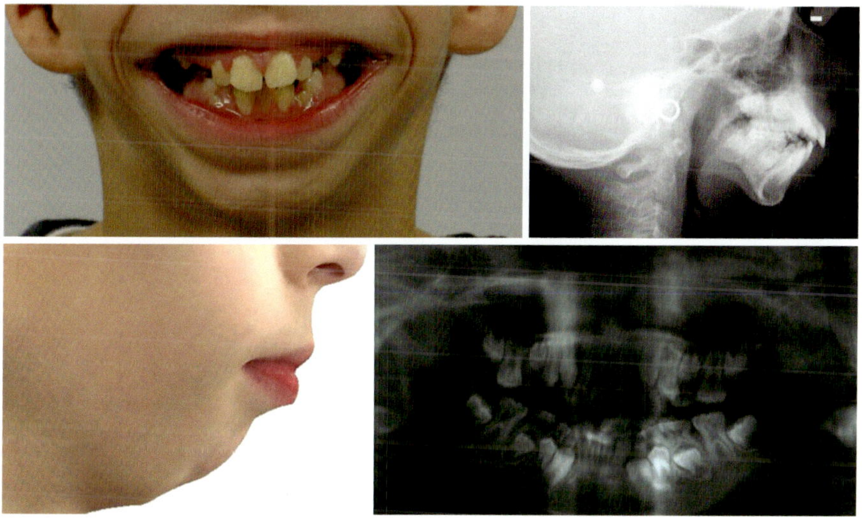

Fig. 22.8 Initial Presentation of 9 Year Old Patient with TCS and SubmucousCleft

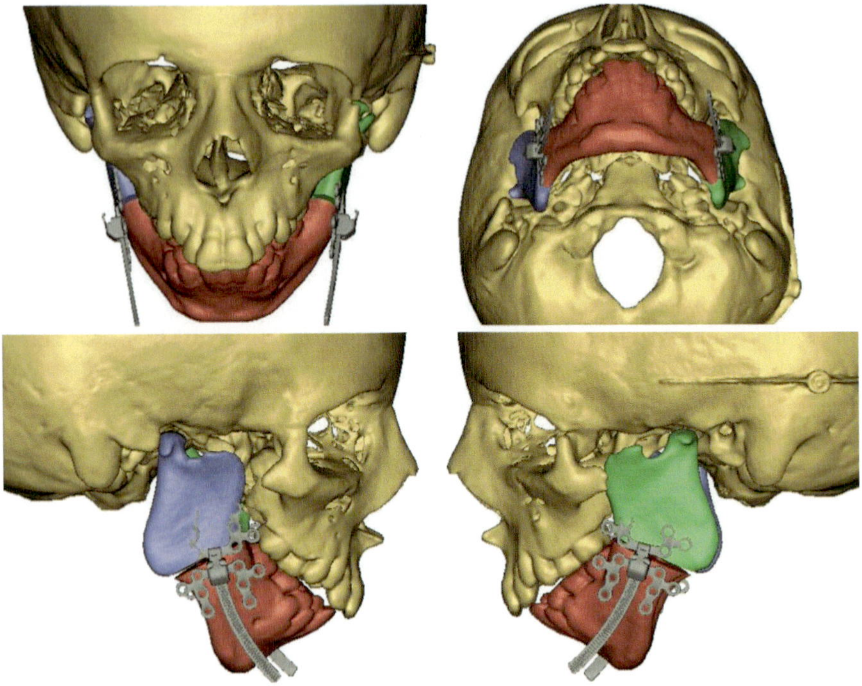

Fig. 22.9 Pre-Operative Distraction Planning

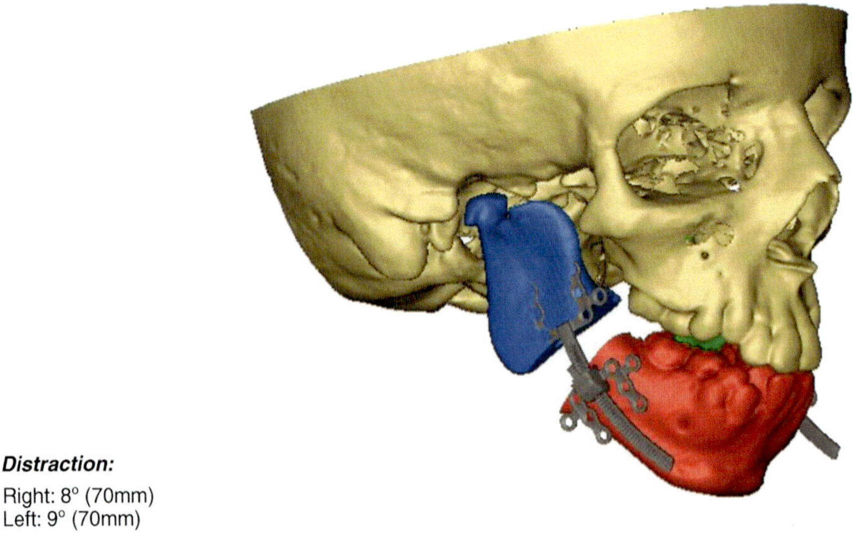

Fig. 22.10 Planned Distraction

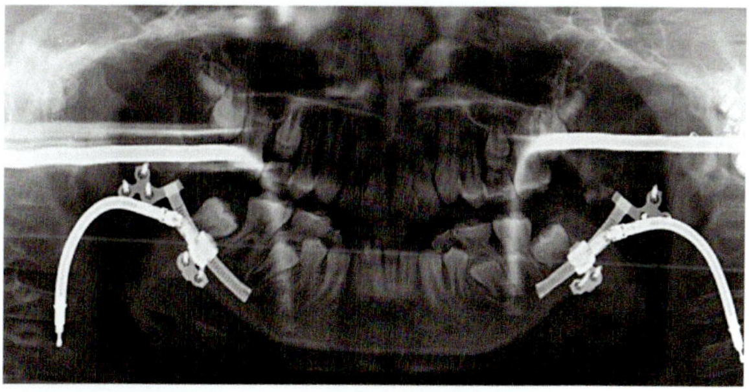

Fig. 22.11 Mid Distraction

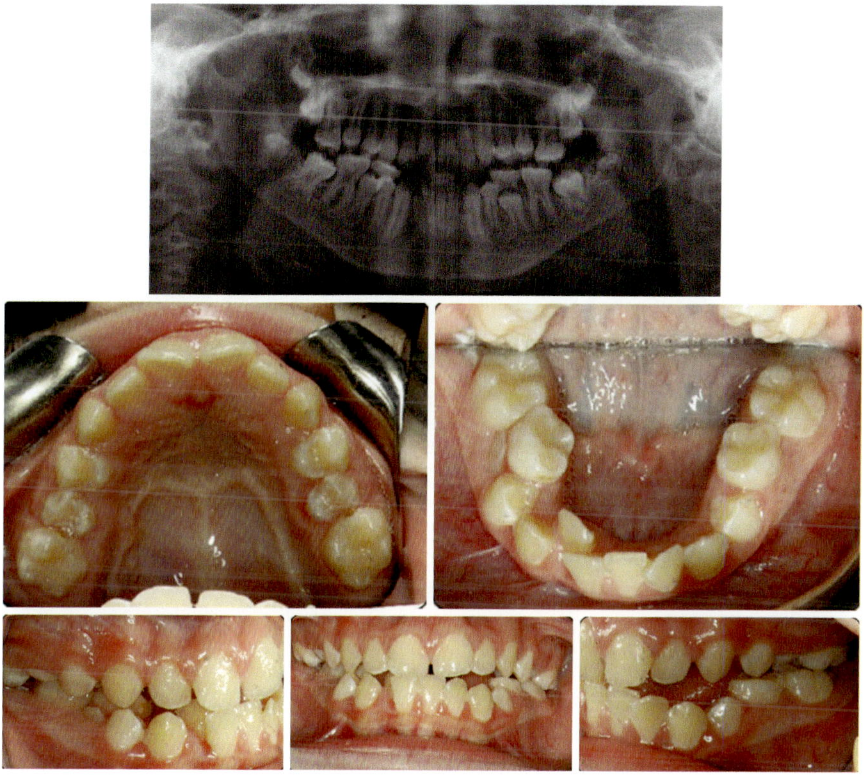

Fig. 22.12 Follow-up Post-Distraction at Age 12 Years

counterclockwise rotation. The bilateral devices were inserted under a general anesthetic, and then activated by 1 mm per day for 20 days, until a negative overjet was achieved. The arms of the distractor were removed shortly following cessation of activation, while the device footpads remained secured to the mandible for a 6-month period of consolidation. The patient was periodically followed up and eventually had a comprehensive phase of orthodontic treatment (without

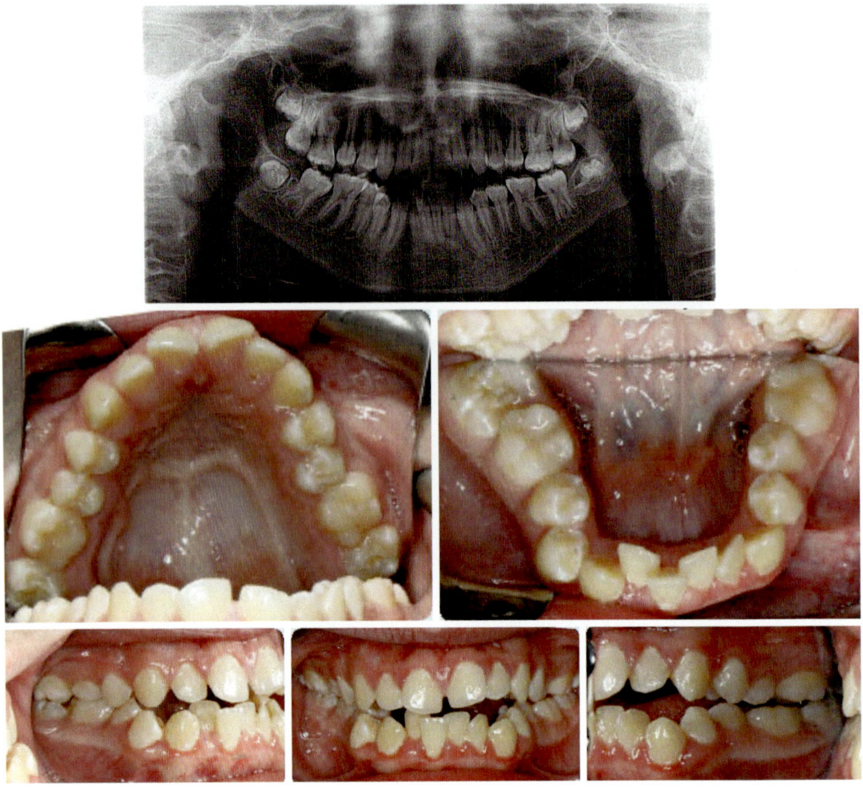

Fig. 22.13 Follow-up at Age 15 Years

orthognathic surgery) initiated at 15 years of age. Crowding in the mandibular arch was resolved by extraction of first premolars.

Comprehensive Orthodontic Treatment

The degree of malformation of different structures impacted in TCS is thought to be stable and does not worsen with age [21]. However, growth cannot be predicted with certainty. Consequently, it is best to initiate the comprehensive phase of orthodontic treatment (with fixed appliances in both maxillary and mandibular arches) at close to completion of growth. The primary objectives of the comprehensive phase of orthodontic treatment are to help restore facial imbalance and correct malocclusions. More often than not, those with TCS require orthodontic treatment in conjunction with an orthognathic surgery to address the skeletal imbalances. Those with TCS present with a wide range of malocclusions, and reviewing every type of orthodontic correction will be beyond the scope of this chapter. A brief overview of orthodontic preparation for orthognathic surgeries is provided below.

Maxillary Expansion Using Temporary Anchorage Devices As mentioned earlier, it is best to correct the transverse discrepancies earlier during the mixed dentition stage when the median palatine suture is still patent and not significantly interlocked. Usually, the comprehensive phase of orthodontic treatment is initiated at close to cessation of growth. As a result, the maxillary expansion appliances which use teeth as anchorage are not very effective at obtaining skeletal expansion of the maxillary arch. What is typically obtained is dentoalveolar bending and tipping of teeth. To overcome the dentoalveolar undesirable side effects and maximize skeletal expansion potential, a nonsurgical miniscrew-assisted rapid palatal expansion (MARPE) technique was introduced [22]. The role of the miniscrews to provide expansion with less tipping, reducing the excessive pressure on the buccal plates of the anchor teeth, MARPE is tooth-and-bone-borne expander. The MARPE design is a combination of hyrax expansion appliance with four extension arms made of 0.9 mm round rigid stainless steel soldered under the body of the jackscrew for the accommodation of four miniscrews adjacent to the median palatine suture, two mesial and two distal to the expanding screw (Figs. 22.14 and 22.15) [22]. The bicortical insertion of the miniscrews is recommended to obtain anchorage in internal cortical plates of the palate and nasal fossa. The fixation in both cortical plates is fundamental to aid the anchorage during expansion and to surpass the resistance of maxillary bones to separation [23]. Correct selection of miniscrew location and length by analyzing the bone thickness and height of median palatine suture is pivotal for the success of MARPE. Below is the recommended protocol for this procedure:

- An impression or scan with the bands on the first premolars and first molars should be obtained.
- Using CBCT, the location of the four miniscrews is selected to provide good skeletal anchorage and stability; measurements of the bone thickness and soft tissue thickness are essential for choosing appropriate miniscrew length. Usually 1.6 to 2 mm diameter is appropriate.

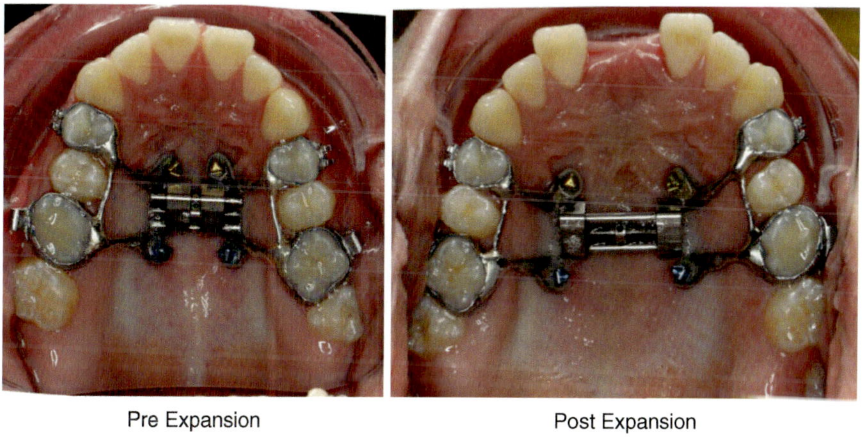

Fig. 22.14 MARPE (TAD Assisted)

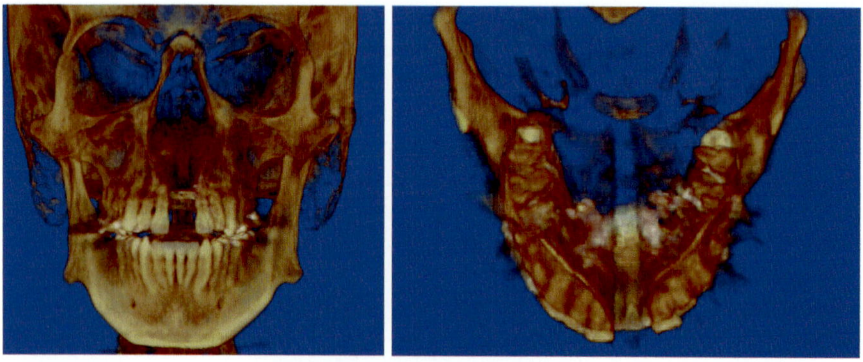

Notice split of median palatine suture
and maxillary midline diastema

Fig. 22.15 Effects of MARPE (TAD Assisted)

- The locations of miniscrews are transferred to the cast over which a conventional hyrax expander is fabricated. Four rigid connectors made of stainless steel wire with helical hooks are soldered on the base of the hyrax screw body. Two anterior hooks are positioned on the rugae region, and the two posterior hooks are placed on the parasagittal area. The hooks should be adjusted for passive contact with the underlying tissues.
- The MARPE appliance is cemented on the first premolars and first molars. Orthodontic miniscrews are placed in the center of the helical hooks under local infiltration anesthesia.
- The activation rate of hyrax expansion screw is once a day to provide about 0.25 mm of expansion per day.
- After active expansion, the MARPE can be maintained for 3 months to allow bone formation in the separated sutural areas.
- Since MARPE is performed during the comprehensive orthodontic phase, the fixed orthodontic appliances with continuous main arch wire can prevent relapse.

Orthognathic Surgery Those with a TCS typically present with a skeletal Class II malocclusion with anterior open bites. Depending on the severity of skeletal discrepancies, a single jaw or a bimaxillary surgery is required in conjunction with orthodontic treatment. The LeFort I osteotomy can correct the transverse, anteroposterior, and posterior vertical discrepancies [10, 21]. Counterclockwise rotation of the occlusal plane helps to improve the tooth-lip relationship while increasing the height of the posterior maxilla which is usually short in those with TCS. The frequently performed mandibular surgery is a bilateral sagittal split osteotomy that advances the mandible and rotates the mandible in a counterclockwise direction to close the anterior openbite [21]. Bilateral extraoral inverted "L" ramus osteotomies with bone grafts have also been used successfully to treat the skeletal discrepancies in those with TCS [24].

Presurgical Orthodontics The goal of presurgical orthodontics is to prepare the patient for the surgical procedure by placing the teeth in a good position relative to their supporting bone and to arrange the teeth so they will not interfere with setting of the jaws. This requires aligning the arches to make them compatible and establishing the anteroposterior and vertical position of the incisors [25]. Leveling of arches is fundamental. Extrusion generally is done more easily postsurgically, whereas intrusion must be accomplished presurgically. For those with TCS, there is an abnormal clockwise rotation of mandible and a very steep mandibular plane. Consequently, in those with TCS, the leveling of arches must be accomplished presurgically. Leveling of the mandibular arch should be accomplished by intrusion of incisors. The posterior teeth should not be extruded. In those with an open bite who will have vertical repositioning of the maxilla and multiple segment surgery, presurgical leveling of the upper arch should be done only within each segment, and then the segments are leveled at surgery. Extrusion of anterior teeth prior to surgery must be avoided [26, 27].

The anteroposterior position of the incisors determines where the mandible will be placed relative to the maxilla during surgery. For mandibular advancements, retraction of protruding lower incisors before surgery is required to provide adequate overjet for advancing the mandible. In some cases, lower first or second premolar extractions will be required. When several surgical segments are planned for the maxilla, the axial inclination of the upper incisors and canines should be established presurgically so that major rotation of the anterior segment at operation can be avoided [25–27].

After presurgical orthodontic preparation, minor adjustments can be made to avoid interferences. Stabilizing wires are full-dimension edgewise wires (i.e., 17 × 25 steel in the 18-slot appliance and 21 × 25 steel in the 22-slot appliance). Hooks as attachments are crimped to the archwires as needed [27].

For the final surgical planning, surgical guide CBCT is used to simulate surgical movements and evaluate the resulting soft tissue profile. When the satisfactory functional and esthetic balance has been achieved, the surgical movements are applied in the virtual or actual model surgery, and the surgical splint is fabricated according to the dental relationships it establishes [28].

Postsurgical Orthodontics After the initial healing, the finishing stage is initiated. Light vertical elastics are needed initially to allow the teeth to settle into better interdigitation. Elastics should not be discontinued until a solid occlusion has been established. Elastics can be discontinued during any further detailing of the occlusion. A TMA wire can be used for final detailing [27].

Orthodontics Retention Anterior open bite malocclusions which are typical manifestations of TCS tend to be very challenging to retain with traditional retainers such as Hawley appliances. We recommend bonded fixed lingual retainers (canine to canine in mandibular arch and lateral incisor to lateral incisor in maxillary arch) along with clear retainers. The clear retainers prevent extrusion of posterior teeth and are ideal for retaining open bites. We recommend retainer wear (24 hours) for the first year, and thereafter the clear retainers can be worn at night times only.

Stability Both traditional orthognathic surgeries and distraction osteogenesis can be successfully used to correct the skeletal discrepancies of the maxilla and mandible. There is a paucity of studies that have prospectively evaluated the stability of surgical corrections in those with TCS. Most of the published literature are either case reports/series or retrospective evaluations [29–31]. Nguyen and colleagues conducted a retrospective analysis of 22 patients with TCS who underwent orthognathic surgery between 1993 and 2007 [31]. Patients were followed up for 1 to 3 years. They found that superior repositioning of the maxilla is most stable followed by mandibular advancement. Mandibular counterclockwise rotations tended to be stable over time, and there was no significant relapse of the mandibular length. Significant relapse of the palatal plane was found. They concluded that the overall relapse rates following bimaxillary orthognathic surgery correction of TCS were comparable to typical Class II corrections [31]. Gursoy and colleagues examined the long-term stability of mandibular distraction osteogenesis on the dentofacial structure of syndromic children and concluded that while excellent short-term results can be achieved the results are not stable during growth in syndromic children [30]. They recommended mandibular distraction osteogenesis for addressing airway issues as opposed to for improving facial esthetics.

References

1. OMIM (# 154500). TREACHER COLLINS SYNDROME 1; TCS1. WWW link is https://omim.org/entry/154500. Date of access is 08/30/2020.
2. OMIM (# 613717). TREACHER COLLINS SYNDROME 2; TCS2. WWW link is https://omim.org/entry/613717. Date of access is 08/30/2020.
3. OMIM (# 248390). TREACHER COLLINS SYNDROME 3; TCS3. WWW link is https://omim.org/entry/248390. Date of access is 08/30/2020.
4. OMIM (# 618939). TREACHER COLLINS SYNDROME 4; TCS4. WWW link is https://omim.org/entry/618390. Date of access is 08/30/2020.
5. Caluseriu O, Lowry BR, McLeod R, Lamont R, Parboosingh JS, Bernier FP, Innes AM. The Hutterite variant of Treacher Collins syndrome: a 28-year-old story solved. Am J Med Genet A. 2013;161A(11):2855–9. https://doi.org/10.1002/ajmg.a.36172.
6. Horiuchi K, Ariga T, Fujioka H, Kawashima K, Yamamoto Y, Igawa H, et al. Mutational analysis of the TCOF1 gene in 11 Japanese patients with Treacher Collins syndrome and mechanism of mutagenesis. Am J Med Genet A. 2005;134:363–7.
7. Dahl E, Kreiborg S, Björk A. A morphologic description of a dry skull with mandibulofacial dysostosis. Scand J Dent Res. 1975;83(5):257–66. https://doi.org/10.1111/j.1600-0722.1975.tb00435.x.
8. Arvystas M, Shprintzen RJ. Craniofacial morphology in Treacher Collins syndrome. Cleft Palate Craniofac J. 1991;28(2):226–31. https://doi.org/10.1597/1545-1569_1991_028_0226_cmitcs_2.3.co_2.
9. Behrents RG, McNamara JA, Avery JK. Prenatal mandibulofacial dysostosis (Treacher Collins syndrome). Cleft Palate J. 1977;14(1):13–34.

10. Posnick JC, Tiwana PS, Costello BJ. Treacher Collins syndrome: comprehensive evaluation and treatment. Oral Maxillofac Surg Clin North Am. 2004;16(4):503–23. https://doi.org/10.1016/j.coms.2004.08.002.
11. Hylton JB, Leon-Salazar V, Anderson GC, De Felippe NL. Multidisciplinary treatment approach in Treacher Collins syndrome. J Dent Child (Chic). 2012;79(1):15–21.
12. Martelli-Junior H, Coletta RD, Miranda RT, Barros LM, Swerts MS, Bonan PR. Orofacial features of Treacher Collins syndrome. Med Oral Patol Oral Cir Bucal. 2009;14(7):E344-8. Published 2009 Jul 1.
13. Marszałek B, Wójcicki P, Kobus K, Trzeciak WH. Clinical features, treatment and genetic background of Treacher Collins syndrome. J Appl Genet. 2002;43(2):223–33.
14. Bartzela TN, Carels C, Maltha JC. Update on 13 Syndromes Affecting Craniofacial and Dental Structures. Front Physiol. 2017;8:1038. Published 2017. https://doi.org/10.3389/fphys.2017.01038.
15. Teber OA, Gillessen-Kaesbach G, Fischer S, et al. Genotyping in 46 patients with tentative diagnosis of Treacher Collins syndrome revealed unexpected phenotypic variation. Eur J Hum Genet. 2004;12(11):879–90. https://doi.org/10.1038/sj.ejhg.5201260.
16. Magalhães MH, da Silveira CB, Moreira CR, Cavalcanti MG. Clinical and imaging correlations of Treacher Collins syndrome: report of two cases. Oral Surg Oral Med Oral Pathol Oral Radiol Endod. 2007;103(6):836–42. https://doi.org/10.1016/j.tripleo.2006.04.011.
17. Arvystas M, Shprintzen RJ. Craniofacial morphology in Treacher Collins syndrome. Cleft Palate Craniofac J. 1991;28(2):226–31. https://doi.org/10.1597/1545-1569_1991_028_0226_cmitcs_2.3.co_2.
18. Shete P, Tupkari J, Benjamin T, Singh A. Treacher Collins syndrome. J Oral Maxillofac Pathol. 2011;15(3):348–51. https://doi.org/10.4103/0973-029X.86722.
19. Esenlik E, Plana NM, Grayson BH, Flores RL. Cephalometric predictors of clinical severity in Treacher Collins syndrome. Plast Reconstr Surg. 2017;140(6):1240–9. https://doi.org/10.1097/PRS.0000000000003853.
20. Allareddy V, Bruun R, MacLaine J, Markiewicz MR, Ruiz R, Miller MA. Orthodontic preparation for secondary alveolar bone grafting in patients with complete cleft lip and palate. Oral Maxillofac Surg Clin North Am. 2020;32(2):205–17. https://doi.org/10.1016/j.coms.2020.01.003.
21. Cobb AR, Green B, Gill D, et al. The surgical management of Treacher Collins syndrome. Br J Oral Maxillofac Surg. 2014;52(7):581–9. https://doi.org/10.1016/j.bjoms.2014.02.007.
22. Lee KJ, Park YC, Park JY, Hwang WS. Miniscrew-assisted nonsurgical palatal expansion before orthognathic surgery for a patient with severe mandibular prognathism. Am J Orthod Dentofac Orthop. 2010;137(6):830–9. https://doi.org/10.1016/j.ajodo.2007.10.065.
23. Lee RJ, Moon W, Hong C. Effects of monocortical and bicortical mini-implant anchorage on bone-borne palatal expansion using finite element analysis. Am J Orthod Dentofac Orthop. 2017;151(5):887–97. https://doi.org/10.1016/j.ajodo.2016.10.025.
24. Chung JY, Cangialosi TJ, Eisig SB. Treacher Collins syndrome: a case study. Am J Orthod Dentofac Orthop. 2014;146(5):665–72. https://doi.org/10.1016/j.ajodo.2014.06.019.
25. Proffit WR, Phillips C, Turvey TA. Stability after mandibular setback: mandible-only versus 2-jaw surgery. J Oral Maxillofac Surg. 2012;70:e408–14.
26. Hernandez-Alfaro F, Guijarro-Martinez R, Piero-Guijarro MA. Surgery first in orthognathic surgery: what have we learned? A comprehensive workflow based on 45 consecutive cases. J Oral Maxillofac Surg. 2014;72:376–90.
27. Proffit WR, White RP Jr. Contemporary treatment of Dentofacial deformity. St. Louis: Mosby; 2003.
28. Elnagar MH, Aronovich S, Kusnoto B. Digital workflow for combined orthodontics and Orthognathic surgery. Oral Maxillofac Surg Clin North Am. 2020;32(1):1–14. https://doi.org/10.1016/j.coms.2019.08.004.
29. Tessier P, Tulasne JF. Stability in correction of hypertelorbitism and Treacher Collins syndromes. Clin Plast Surg. 1989;16(1):195–204.

30. Gürsoy S, Hukki J, Hurmerinta K. Five year follow-up of mandibular distraction osteogenesis on the dentofacial structures of syndromic children. Orthod Craniofac Res. 2008;11(1):57–64. https://doi.org/10.1111/j.1601-6343.2008.00415.x.
31. Nguyen PD, Caro MC, Smith DM, Tompson B, Forrest CR, Phillips JH. Long-term orthognathic surgical outcomes in Treacher Collins patients. J Plast Reconstr Aesthet Surg. 2016;69(3):402–8. https://doi.org/10.1016/j.bjps.2015.10.036.

Chapter 23
Hearing Loss and Aural Rehabilitation in Patients with Treacher Collins Syndrome

Kevin Chow, Randi Tepper, Jaymee Franknecht, Lauren Kaplan, and Maura Cosetti

Introduction

Hearing loss is a ubiquitous manifestation of first and second pharyngeal arch dysgenesis in Treacher Collins syndrome (TCS). Malformations of the cartilaginous auricle and temporal bone are both common and highly variable in this population. Patients with TCS usually present with varying degrees of symmetric and bilateral malformations of the external and middle ears, most commonly resulting in mild to profound conductive hearing loss [1]. Early identification and diagnosis of both the type and degree of hearing loss is crucial to facilitating speech and language development in these children. While the intellectual abilities of TCS patients are unaffected, language and speech development become impaired in the absence of timely screening and treatment of hearing loss. It has been well-documented that

The original version of the chapter has been revised. A correction to this chapter can be found at https://doi.org/10.1007/978-3-030-84733-3_27.

K. Chow
McGovern Medical School, University of Texas Health Science Center at Houston, Houston, TX, USA
e-mail: Kevin.Chow@uth.tmc.edu

R. Tepper · L. Kaplan
Ear Institute, New York Eye and Ear of Mount Sinai, New York, NY, USA
e-mail: rtepper@nyee.edu; lkaplan@NYEE.EDU

J. Franknecht
Department of Otolaryngology-Head and Neck Surgery, Columbia University Medical Center, New York, NY, USA
e-mail: jmf2264@cumc.columbia.edu

M. Cosetti (✉)
Ear Institute, New York Eye and Ear of Mount Sinai, New York, NY, USA

Department of Otolaryngology-Head and Neck Surgery and Neurosurgery, Icahn School of Medicine at Mount Sinai, New York, NY, USA
e-mail: maura.cosetti@mountsinai.org

D. M. Yates, M. R. Markiewicz (eds.), *Craniofacial Microsomia and Treacher Collins Syndrome*, https://doi.org/10.1007/978-3-030-84733-3_23

intervention in auditory impairment before 3–6 months of age is vital to improve expressive and receptive language outcomes in children [2].

A multitude of unique amplification options are available which address conductive hearing loss in these patients. These should be initiated as soon as hearing loss is identified in early childhood. Surgical correction of auricular deformities and aural atresia is also possible in many children and typically occurs in later childhood depending on patient-specific anatomic and hearing loss considerations. Individualized surgical interventions may include any combination of atresiaplasty, ossicular chain reconstruction, or placement of bone-anchored hearing implants. Overall, optimal management of hearing loss in this patient population requires a multidisciplinary team of specialists in neurotology, audiology, and speech language pathology.

This chapter discusses otologic manifestations of TCS, diagnostic testing, and available treatment options for hearing loss, with an emphasis on evidence-based audiologic and surgical options to improve language and speech development through childhood.

Otologic Manifestations of Treacher Collins Syndrome

Outer Ear/Auricle

Both external auditory canals (EAC) and auricles are commonly dysmorphic and malpositioned in cases of TCS (85 to 100% of cases), with a high degree of variance existing in presentation of microtia (small or malformed) or anotia (absence) of the auricle [3, 4]. Although microtia is typically a unilateral malformation, in TCS microtia is often bilateral and symmetric, occurring in up to 85% of TCS patients [3–5]. Ears may present with malformed, typically low-lying and rotated pinna, fistulas, preauricular tags, and missing landmarks. The Marx microtia classification is the most commonly used assessment of the auricular remnant (Fig. 23.1) and uses

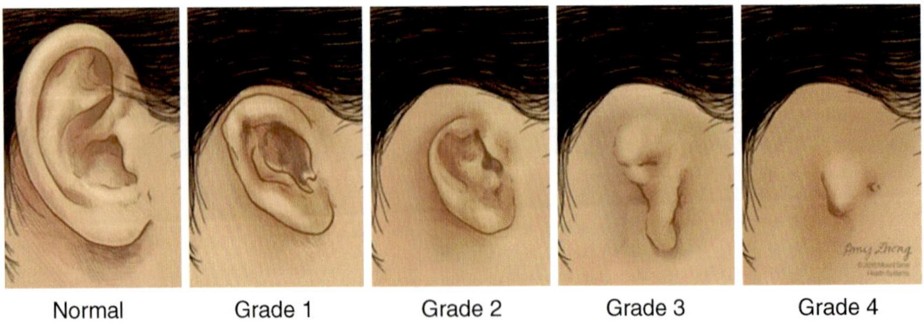

Fig. 23.1 Marx grading system for microtia. The most common auricular manifestation of Treacher Collins syndrome is Grade 3. (Printed with permission from ©Mount Sinai Health System)

a 4-point scale. A small peanut-shaped ear remnant (Grade 3) is the most common presentation of microtia in TCS [5].

Congenital aural atresia, or the complete absence of the ear canal, is present in 54–78% of cases and is often bilateral (Fig. 23.2). Less frequently, stenosis or narrowing of the ear canal may occur in 22–31% of cases with bilaterally deformed tympanic membranes [3–6].

Middle Ear

By the nature of their anatomy, patients with aural atresia have no tympanic membrane and typically have bilateral, often symmetric hypoplasia of the middle ear cavity (Fig. 23.2). The bones of the middle ear, including the malleus, incus, and stapes, are typically fused, malformed, or absent (22–67%) [4, 6]. Specific deformities reported in the ossicular chain include monopodal stapes, stapes ankylosis (33–82%), underdeveloped ossicles, and fusion of the malleus and incus [6]. The presence and condition of the ossicular chain are important factors in the evaluation of TCS patients for surgical correction of the ear canal (e.g., atresiaplasty) (described in more detail below). Aural atresia is often associated with aberrant paths of the

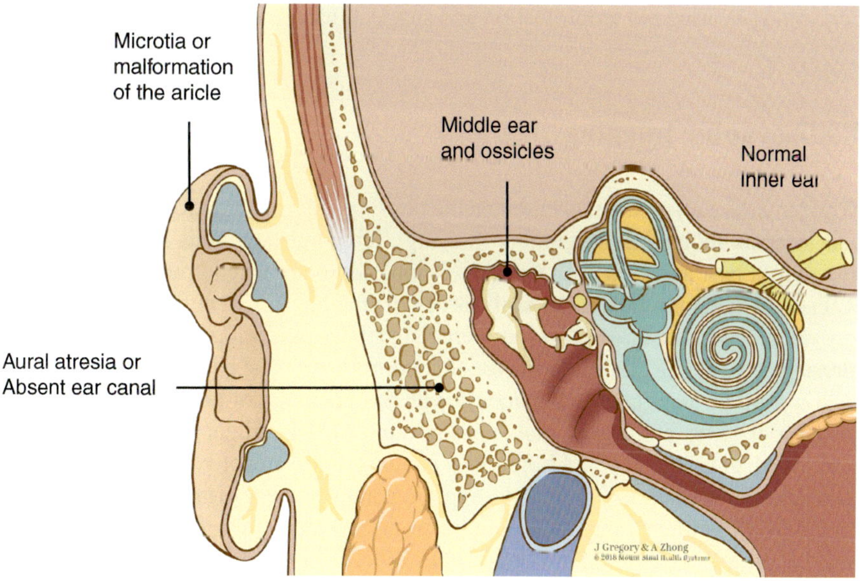

Fig. 23.2 Diagram of external auditory canal atresia demonstrating the most common abnormalities of the external ear in Treacher Collins syndrome (TCS), specifically microtia or malformation of the auricle and atresia or absence of the external auditory canal. A contracted middle ear and normal inner ear are also typical of TCS. (Printed with permission from ©Mount Sinai Health System)

facial nerve in both the middle ear (tympanic segment) and mastoid (descending portion) [3, 7]. An understanding of the facial nerve location is crucial, as this knowledge will influence or impede surgical decision-making in atresiaplasty.

Inner Ear

Because of their different embryologic origins, the morphology and function of the inner ear, specifically the cochlea and semicircular canals, is largely preserved in TCS patients. In general, the type and degree of hearing loss is guided by the anatomic malformations. Patients with TCS typically present with *conductive* hearing loss (CHL) due to aural atresia and normal inner ear structures. Even in TCS patients with normal or stenotic ear canals, CHL may result from eustachian tube dysfunction, middle ear fluid, or abnormalities of the ossicular chain [8]. About 96% of individuals with TCS have unilateral or bilateral conductive hearing loss, usually moderate or maximal up to 60 dB [3–6]. Because the inner ear is typically unaffected, *sensorineural hearing loss* (SNHL) is rare but has been seen in up to 7% of children with TCS. In all cases, the SNHL was present with an anatomic abnormality of the outer ear, resulting in a mixed (meaning combined conductive and sensorineural) hearing loss [6]. The understanding of anatomy and hearing loss has important implications for the type and timing of treatment, influencing decisions concerning hearing aid amplification and surgical intervention.

Radiographic Imaging

While microtia assessment is based on the physical exam, evaluation of aural atresia and stenosis requires radiographic imaging. Temporal bone and skull base bony anatomy is best assessed with fine cut (1 mm) non-contrast computed tomography (CT) of the temporal bone. The analysis of CT imaging and identification of various key middle ear structures serves as a crucial step in deciding patient candidacy for atresiaplasty [7] (Fig. 23.3). However, this information must be used in conjunction with a hearing assessment, as patients with SNHL may not benefit from surgical creation of an external ear canal. Because atresiaplasty surgery is not commonly performed until age 6–7, radiographic imaging for conductive hearing loss and aural atresia is often deferred until approximately 5 years of age [9]. Due to the complexity of craniofacial abnormalities in TCS, many children may obtain imaging that evaluates the temporal bone at an earlier age. Scoring systems such as the well-known Jahrsdoerfer scale aid in surgical candidacy assessments by predicting the likelihood of hearing improvement following atresiaplasty (Table 23.1) [5]. The presence of a normal stapes and middle ear space demonstrates improved hearing outcomes in comparison to their lower-scoring counterparts following atresiaplasty [10]. Ultimately, the presence of an aerated middle ear is considered the most

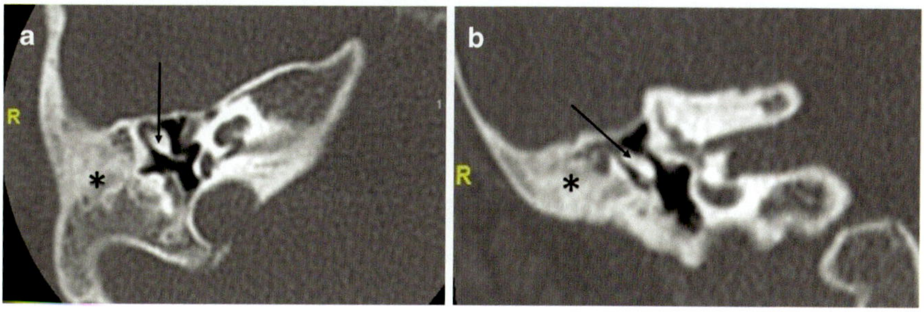

Fig. 23.3 Axial (**a**) and coronal (**b**) non-contrast computed tomography images of the temporal bone demonstrating a right side external auditory canal atresia. Asterisk (*) identifies the atretic ear canal and the black arrow identifies the malformed ossicular mass in the middle ear

Table 23.1 Jahrsdoerfer scoring criteria

Radiographic finding	**Points**
Presence of stapes	2
Open oval window	1
Middle ear space	1
Normal facial nerve	1
Malleus-incus complex present	1
Pneumatized mastoid	1
Incus connected to stapes	1
Normal round window	1
Appearance of external ear	1
Total points	**Surgical candidacy status**
10	Excellent
9	Very good
8	Good
7	Fair
6	Marginal
≤5	Poor

important factor in a successful atresiaplasty. [9, 11] Nevertheless, the majority of TCS patients are poor candidates for atresiaplasty based on imaging [7]. Calvarial thickness can also be assessed with CT and has important implications for placement of bone anchored hearing implants (discussed in detail, below).

Imaging may also identify the presence of a cholesteatoma, a collection of squamous epithelium that can become trapped during atypical embryologic development and maybe associated with congenital aural stenosis in up to 20% of patients with diameter < 2 mm [12]. External ear cholesteatoma is rare, and, while benign, it may lead to bone erosion, ongoing infection, and various complications inside and outside the temporal bone [13]. CT imaging may be suggestive of cholesteatoma in TCS with characteristic findings of smooth margins of erosion. Magnetic resonance imaging (MRI) is less commonly employed to delineate temporal bone anatomic malformations but may be used to assess for presence or abnormalities of the cochlear nerve when sensorineural hearing loss is diagnosed. Additionally, specific MRI sequences, including non-echo planar diffusion weighting imaging, may be employed to detect the presence of cholesteatoma when suggested by CT findings [14].

Hearing Loss in Treacher Collins Syndrome

While the rate of being deaf or hard of hearing increases from 1.2/1000 in newborns to 3/1000 in early school age, the incidence of hearing loss among those with Treacher Collins syndrome (TCS) is greater. An estimated 1 in 55,000 newborns is born with TCS with up to 97% presenting with some degree of hearing loss [6]. Access to sound is a requisite for successful development of speech and language in young children, and this relationship underlies the motivation for establishing universal newborn hearing screening. The universal newborn hearing screening (UNHS) is a state-mandated standard test designed to screen newborn hearing status shortly after birth. Ideally, screening of newborns is conducted before leaving the hospital, or before 1 month of age in cases of home births. Early detection, especially for those at risk of hearing loss, is crucial. The Joint Committee on Infant Hearing (JCIH) 2019 stresses the importance of early hearing detection and intervention for all infants, especially those at risk of being deaf or hard of hearing, as well as those with risk factors for delayed onset and progressive hearing loss [8, 15]. In all cases of TCS, ear anomalies dictate that additional audiologic testing beyond the UNHS is required.

Because of the complexity of craniofacial anomalies in TCS, hearing loss is not the only factor affecting speech and language development in young children. Abnormalities of orofacial musculature, voice and breadth, suction, and chewing and swallowing functions may all influence receptive and expressive speech acquisition. Therefore, prompt and accurate audiologic assessment and multidisciplinary intervention, including speech language therapy, are essential to maximize speech and hearing outcomes. For infants with TCS and bilateral conductive hearing loss, a comprehensive evaluation of auditory function is warranted. Behavioral, electrophysiological, and acoustic immittence measures can be utilized in isolation or in combination with one another in the evaluation process. These tests aim to determine the degree, configuration, and type of hearing loss.

Age-Based Audiological Testing

Various audiological tests are available when assessing pediatric patients, the modality of which depend on age, cognitive, and developmental abilities. Often, multiple visits are required to obtain a complete understanding of the child's auditory function.

For infants, the most accurate method to measure auditory function is through electrophysiological testing. This type of noninvasive testing includes auditory brainstem response testing (ABR) and auditory steady-state response (ASSR). This testing requires the patient to be still and quiet, ideally in a deep sleep, but can also be performed with sedation if natural sleep cannot be achieved. Testing is typically conducted with sticker electrodes placed on the child's ears or mastoid bone and forehead. When there is a patent ear canal, the stimulus is presented through an inserted earphone, and the response of the auditory nerve is measured at the site of electrode placement. Because of the many craniofacial abnormalities associated with TCS, including atresia of the ear canal, it is often not possible to test air conduction. As a result, only bone conduction threshold testing is performed in most cases. This testing involves presenting a vibrating stimulus on the child's mastoid bone, which bypasses the outer and middle ear and directly stimulates the cochlea. Based on the combined results of air and bone conduction testing, the type and degree of hearing loss can be determined. These results are necessary to guide treatments pertaining to amplification selection and fitting.

As a child develops, more subjective behavioral testing techniques are preferred over (or in combination with) electrophysiological assessment. When testing younger children, audiologists will utilize visual reinforcement audiometry (VRA) for children 5–24 months old and conditioned play audiometry (CPA) for 2–5 year olds [16]. Of note, age ranges may vary depending on the patient's developmental status. VRA is an operant-conditioned response that capitalizes on a child's natural instinct to respond to auditory stimuli with a head turn [17]. When a child responds with a head turn, reinforcement is provided for that response in the form of lighting and/or activation of a movie/motorized toy by the audiologist [18, 19]. While this technique for eliciting responses to auditory stimuli is used in children aged 5–24 months, this age range may vary depending on the patient's developmental status. Since CPA relies on the use of a play-based motor activity to establish a time-locked conditioned response to an auditory signal, the test assistant may provide the child with a positive social reinforcement to further shape the response behavior [20]. For children aged 5 years or older, standard adult behavioral audiometry is performed, which involves conditioning the child to raise a hand in response to a sound.

Speech audiometry is an essential component of the audiologic test battery performed at approximately 6 months developmental age and older to examine speech awareness, speech discrimination, and speech recognition [21]. Speech audiometry assesses a child's ability to perceive speech or speech-like stimuli, aids in determination of pure-tone threshold reliability, and helps to monitor the child's progress with amplification.

Auditory Rehabilitation Options

Traditional Hearing Aid Amplification

Amplification options depend on the type and degree of hearing loss and the patient's ear anatomy. Hearing technology is complex. To that end, there are several different types of hearing devices that may be appropriate for children with TCS, the first of which is a traditional hearing aid. Simply put, this is a type of hearing aid that fits behind the ear and is connected to a soft, plastic custom earmold that fits inside the ear. This hearing aid design can be worn by children with any type or degree of hearing loss as long as there is an ear canal that can fit and hold the earmold securely. Traditional amplification is appropriate for children with grade 1 or 2 microtia and a patent ear canal. Hearing aid use can begin as soon as hearing loss is diagnosed and characterized, ideally before 3 months of age.

Bone-Anchored Hearing Amplification

In more severe cases where a patient presents with grade 3 or 4 microtia, or in cases where there is an atretic or absent canal, traditional amplification is not an option. In these cases, bone-anchored or bone conduction hearing aids should be recommended. This type of hearing aid is indicated for children with CHL or some forms of mixed hearing loss (combination of sensorineural hearing loss and CHL). Use of a bone conduction hearing device is a necessity for normal speech and language development in children with bilateral aural atresia [9, 22]. When utilized, a bone-anchored hearing aid is worn behind the ear or auricular remnant. Sound is received by the hearing aid and is transmitted through the skull directly to an intact, functioning cochlea, after which it travels along the remaining intact auditory pathway to the cortex. Because bone-anchored implants bypass abnormal outer and middle ear anatomy, they are frequent options for aural rehabilitation in patients with TCS [4].

There is a myriad of surgical and non-surgical options for bone-anchored hearing devices from multiple manufacturers. The options are highlighted below and vary by device strength and size, in addition to surgical and wear options unique to each manufacturer.

Non-surgical devices can be fit on children as young as newborns and involve wearing a hearing aid on a specific type of headband (Fig. 23.4). The "softband" is the most common non-surgical option and uses an adjustable, elastic soft band (Fig. 23.4a). Two alternatives include the hardband SoundArc ™ (Cochlear Americas, Englewood CO) recommended for older school-aged children and the AdHear ™ (MEL-EL, Austria) which adheres to the skin with adhesive (Fig. 23.4b, c).

Surgical options involve placing an implant into the calvarium, which then osseointegrates and transmits sound from a processor to the functioning inner ear (Fig. 23.5). Sound can be transmitted to the osseointegrated implant directly through an abutment or transcutaneously through the skin with a magnet. Currently, viable options include percutaneous osseointegrated bone conduction devices such as the BAHA Connect (Cochlear, NSW, Australia) and Ponto implant (Oticon, Copenhagen, Denmark), as well as the BoneBridge (MED-EL, North Carolina, USA), BAHA Attract, and newer OSIA (Cochlear, NSW, Australia) (Fig. 23.5). FDA indications for recipient age vary by device, but all begin at 5 years of age. Although the exact details regarding surgical candidacy for the aforementioned

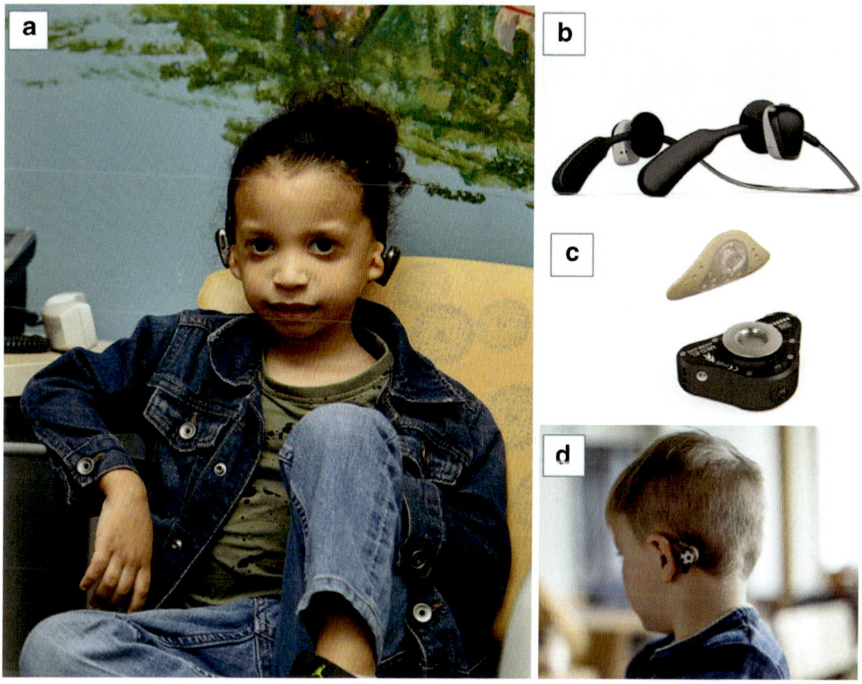

Fig. 23.4 Non-surgical options for bone conduction hearing aids. (**a**) 6-year-old with Treacher Collins syndrome and bilateral microtia and atresia wearing bilateral bone conduction hearing aids (BAHA ™) from Cochlear Americas (Englewood, CO) on a softband. (**b**) An alternative to the softband: the hardband SoundArc ™ (Cochlear Americas, Englewood CO) recommended for older school-aged children. (**c, d**) The AdHear ™ MEL-EL, Austria), a non-surgical alternative which adheres to the skin with adhesive

implants are beyond the scope of this chapter, it should be noted that additional options frequently enter the US marketplace. For patients with TCS, the choice of device often involves additional considerations such as calvarial thickness, mastoid aeration, and hearing loss. Furthermore, global development and the need for other surgeries that may take precedent over implantable hearing devices must be addressed [23]. Overall, the determination to proceed with an osseointegrated device, as well as the specific choice of device, is a highly individualized process. Decision-making should be directed by the patient's family in consultation with a multidisciplinary care team.

Whether surgical or non-surgical, an important feature of all bone conduction devices is the ability connect to hearing-assistive technology (HAT). This is extremely important for children in educational settings because it helps reduce the signal to noise ratio, thus reducing the negative effect of background noise on the child's learning environment. A hearing education specialist (HES) is also needed to ensure the child's device and HAT are paired successfully with additional technology and fully functional.

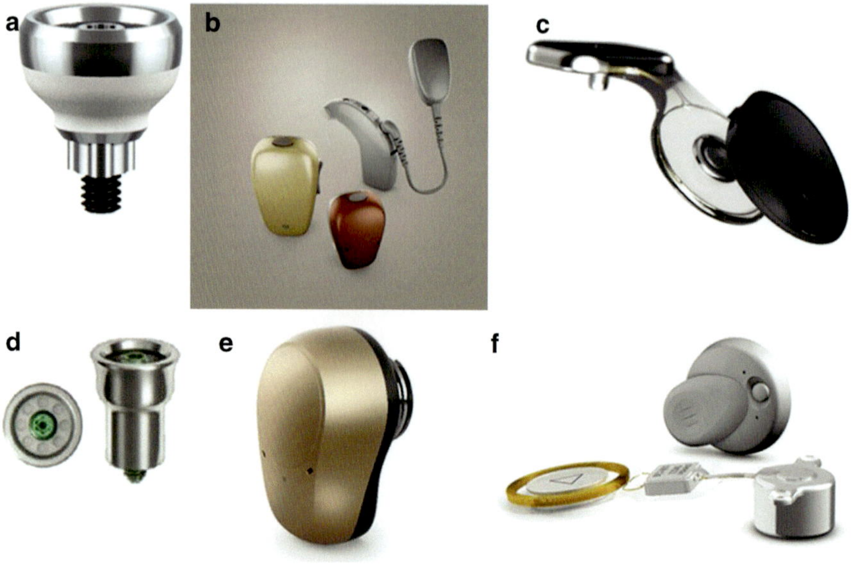

Fig. 23.5 (**a**) BAHA Connect™ percutaneous bone-anchored hearing implant and (**b**) available device processors from Cochlear, NSW, Australia; (**c**) the Osia™, a transcutaneous magnetic implant and processor from Cochlear, NSW, Australia; (**d**) percutaneous bone-anchored hearing implant and (**e**) Ponto™ processors from Oticon, Copenhagen, Denmark; (**f**) the BoneBridge, a transcutaneous magnetic bone conduction implant and processor from MED-EL, North Carolina, USA

Atresiaplasty or Canalplasty

Surgical creation of an external ear canal in congenital aural atresia is guided by the patient's hearing assessment and temporal bone anatomy as determined by radiographic imaging. In cases of ear canal stenosis or narrowing, surgery may be necessary due to concern for cholesteatoma. Surgery in these cases is typically variable and is guided by the degree of stenosis and amount of preserved anatomy. This includes bony or cartilaginous ear canal remnants in addition to ossicular involvement.

For patients with complete atresia to be considered for atresiaplasty, they must have normal inner ear function without significant SNHL. Surgery is not recommended until the child is approximately age 6–7 years old due to the need for compliance during postoperative debridement, resolution of age-related eustachian tube dysfunction, and decrease in bony regrowth [9]. Radiographic imaging, specifically CT, serves as the basis of candidacy for atresia surgery. As described above, imaging should note both middle ear anatomy and facial nerve position. If the facial nerve position traverses the planned location for the new canal or blocks ossicular assessment and reconstruction, atresiaplasty should not be attempted [7, 9]. Recommendations for surgery in non-syndromic atresia from the International

Microtia and Atresia Workgroup (IMAW) supports the use of the Jahrsdoerfer grading scale and recommends surgery for children scoring 7 or higher [22, 24]. No published guidelines exist for patients with TCS. Additionally, and especially in cases of TCS, the timing of atresiaplasty must be balanced with other planned surgical interventions, including possible microtia or external ear reconstruction.

Conclusion

Children with TCS manifest a variety of otologic manifestations, the most common and important of which is bilateral aural atresia resulting in bilateral maximal CHL. Early and accurate audiologic assessment is crucial and should occur as soon as possible in the newborn period to facilitate early amplification. Initiation of amplification is crucial to assist with speech and language development in this complex syndrome. Decisions about surgical intervention are highly individualized and are typically based on radiographic assessments of otologic anatomy. Due to the complexity of craniofacial anomalies, these children are best managed by a multidisciplinary team with experience assessing and treating patients with TCS.

References

1. Cobb ARM, Green B, Gill D, Ayliffe P, Lloyd TW, Bulstrode N, et al. The surgical management of Treacher Collins syndrome. Br J Oral Maxillofac Surg. 2014;52:581–9.
2. Yoshinaga-Itano C, Sedey AL, Coulter DK, Mehl AL. Language of early- and later-identified children with hearing loss. Pediatrics. 1998;102:1161–71.
3. Aljerian A, Gilardino MS. Treacher Collins syndrome. Clin Plast Surg. 2019;46:197–205.
4. Rosa F, Coutinho MB, Ferreira JP, Sousa CA. Ear malformations, hearing loss and hearing rehabilitation in children with Treacher Collins syndrome. Acta Otorrinolaringol Esp. 2016;67:142–7.
5. Jahrsdoerfer RA, Jacobson JT. Treacher Collins syndrome: otologic and auditory management. J Am Acad Audiol. 1995;6:93–102.
6. Plomp RG, van Lieshout MJS, Joosten KFM, Wolvius EB, van der Schroeff MP, Versnel SL, et al. Treacher Collins syndrome. Plast Reconstr Surg. 2016;137:191–204.
7. Takegoshi H, Kaga K, Kikuchi S, Ito K. Facial canal anatomy in patients with microtia: evaluation of the temporal bones with thin-section CT. Radiology. 2002;225(3):852–8.
8. Joint Committee on Infant Hearing. Year 2000 position statement: principles and guidelines for early hearing detection and intervention programs. Pediatrics. 2000;106:798–817.
9. Ruhl DS, Kesser BW. Atresiaplasty in congenital aural atresia: what the facial plastic surgeon needs to know. Facial Plast Surg Clin North Am. 2018;26:87–96.
10. Jahrsdoerfer RA, Yeakley JW, Aguilar EA, Cole RR, Gray LC. Grading system for the selection of patients with congenital aural atresia. Am J Otol. 1992;13:6–12.
11. Oliver ER, Lambert PR, Rumboldt Z, Lee F-S, Agarwal A. Middle ear dimensions in congenital aural atresia and hearing outcomes after atresiaplasty. Otol Neurotol. 2010;31:946–53
12. Casale G, Nicholas BD, Kesser BW. Acquired ear canal cholesteatoma in congenital aural atresia/stenosis. Otol Neurotol. 2014;35:1474–9.

13. Mann W, Al-Nawas B, Wriedt S, Mann S, Koutsimpelas D. Cholesteatoma of the hypotympanum in a patient with Treacher Collins syndrome. Auris Nasus Larynx. 2014;41:101–4.
14. Li PM, Linos E, Gurgel RK, Fischbein NJ, Blevins NH. Evaluating the utility of non-echo-planar diffusion-weighted imaging in the preoperative evaluation of cholesteatoma: a meta-analysis. Laryngoscope. 2013;123:1247–50.
15. Smith J, Wolfe J. Highlights in 2019 pediatric audiology literature. The Hearing J. 2020;73:14.
16. Sabo DL. The audiologic assessment of the young pediatric patient: the clinic. Trends Amplif. 1999;4:51–60.
17. Widen JE, O'Grady GM. Using visual reinforcement audiometry in the assessment of hearing in infants. The Hearing J. 2002;55:28–36.
18. Moore JM, Thompson G, Thompson M. Auditory localization of infants as a function of reinforcement conditions. J Speech Hear Disord. 1975;40:29–34.
19. Moore JM, Wilson WR, Thompson G. Visual reinforcement of head-turn responses in infants under 12 months of age. J Speech Hear Disord. 1977;42:328–34.
20. Bonino AY, Leibold LJ. Behavioral assessment of hearing in 2 to 4 year-old children: a two-interval, observer-based procedure using conditioned play-based responses. J Vis Exp. 2017;119:54788.
21. Mendel LL. Current considerations in pediatric speech audiometry. Int J Audiol. 2008;47:546–53.
22. Zhang T, Bulstrode N, Chang KW, Cho Y-S, Frenzel H, Jiang D, et al. International consensus recommendations on microtia, aural atresia and functional ear reconstruction. J Int Adv Otol. 2019;15:204–8.
23. Marsella P, Scorpecci A, Pacifico C, Tieri L. Bone-anchored hearing aid (Baha) in patients with Treacher Collins syndrome: tips and pitfalls. Int J Pediatr Otorhinolaryngol. 2011;75:1308–12.
24. Shonka DC Jr, Livingston WJ III, Kesser BW. The Jahrsdoerfer grading scale in surgery to repair congenital aural atresia. Arch Otolaryngol Head Neck Surg. 2008;134:873–7.

Chapter 24
Reconstruction of the Ear Deformities Associated with Treacher Collins Syndrome

Kristan P. Alfonso, Yi-Chun Carol Liu, and Rodrigo C. Silva

Background

Treacher Collins syndrome (TCS) has a high degree of penetrance but variable expressivity. A range of craniofacial manifestations may be observed. This chapter serves to discuss the identification and management of manifestations related to the external ear. These manifestations may include periauricular anomalies like accessory appendages or pits, auricular deformities like cup ear, or malformations like microtia or atresia (Fig. 24.1).

TCS affects the development of first and second branchial arch structures. The external ear arises from the 6 hillocks of His, with the first 3 hillocks arising from the first branchial arch and the second 3 hillocks arising from the second branchial arch. The hillocks lead to development of the tragus, helix, concha cymba, antihelix, and antitragus. Thus, any alteration in the development of the first and second branchial arch will be reflected in the mature external ear anatomy.

After diagnosis of TCS, a comprehensive physical examination should be undertaken (Fig. 24.2). It is important for the patient and family to establish care with a reconstructive surgeon, who is a key part of the multidisciplinary team. Early identification of auricular deformities and malformations is important in providing the

K. P. Alfonso (✉)
Department of Otolaryngology- Head and Neck Surgery, Emory University, Atlanta, GA, USA

Division of Pediatric Otolaryngology, Children's Healthcare of Atlanta, Center for Advanced Pediatrics, Atlanta, GA, USA
e-mail: Kristan.alfonso@emory.edu

Y.-C. C. Liu · R. C. Silva
Department of Otolaryngology-Head and Neck Surgery, Baylor College of Medicine, Houston, TX, USA

Division of Pediatric Otolaryngology, Texas Children's Hospital, Houston, TX, USA
e-mail: yi-chun.liu@bcm.edu; rodrigo.silva@bcm.edu

D. M. Yates, M. R. Markiewicz (eds.), *Craniofacial Microsomia and Treacher Collins Syndrome*, https://doi.org/10.1007/978-3-030-84733-3_24

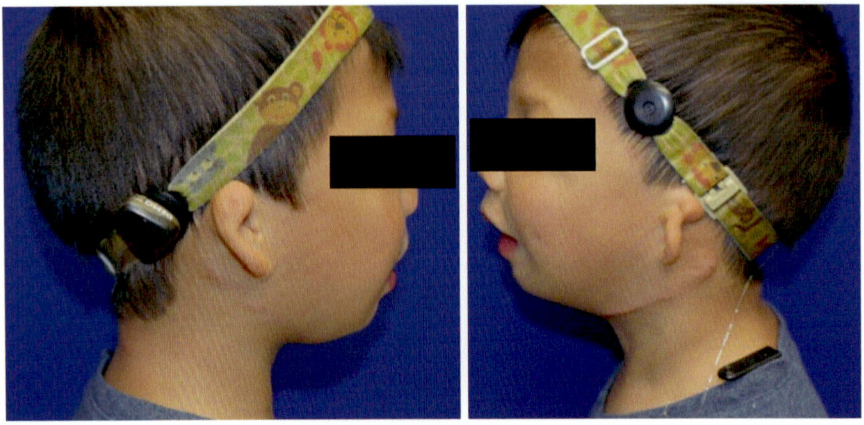

Fig. 24.1 A child with TCS demonstrating bilateral microtia. The patient is wearing bilateral softband bone conduction devices

Fig. 24.2 A patient with TCS exhibiting multiple craniofacial anomalies, including retrognathia and grade 3 microtia

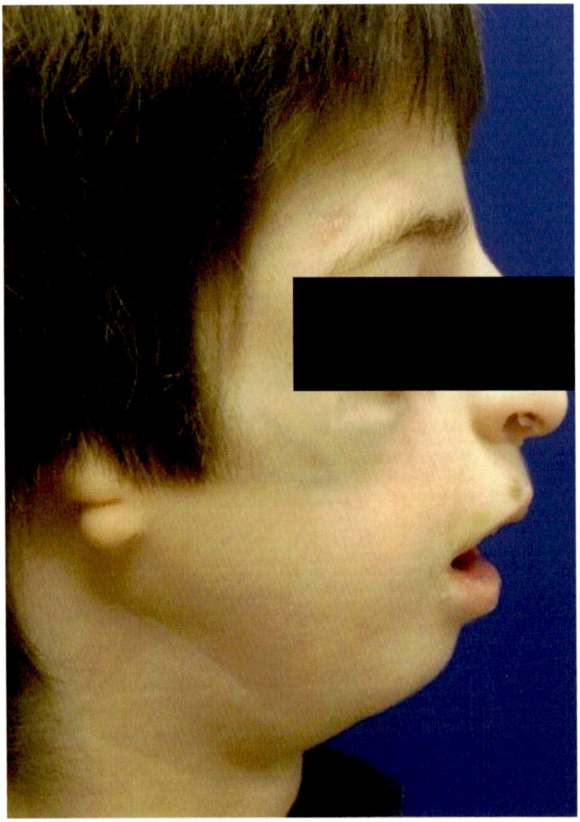

family reassurance and discussion of plans for future management. Auricular malformations may also portend worse hearing, as the more formed the external ear is, the more formed the middle ear [9]. These may be observed on prenatal ultrasound, allowing for earlier diagnosis and counseling [10].

Some deformities may respond to early intervention, like molding, and need to be instituted in the first week of life. Malformations, like microtia, are intervened upon later in life but early discussion with the family will improve decision-making and preparation and help set expectations.

Periauricular Anomalies

Periauricular Accessory Appendages

Periauricular accessory appendages occur in up to 30 to 40% of the TCS population [2]. These anomalies may be referred to by one of several names, including accessory tragus, supernumerary tragus, accessory auricle, or ear tag. They may appear as single or multiple (Figs. 24.3 and 24.4). They may be sessile (flat against the skin) or pedunculated (raised by a stalk). They may be soft (with little to no cartilage) or firm (with cartilage). These appendages often involve cartilage, versus an

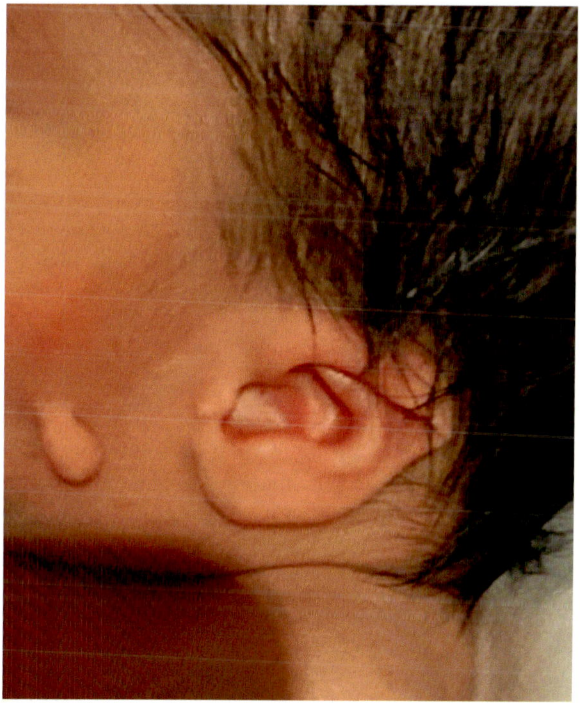

Fig. 24.3 An accessory auricle located anterior to the tragus and another at the angle of the mandible

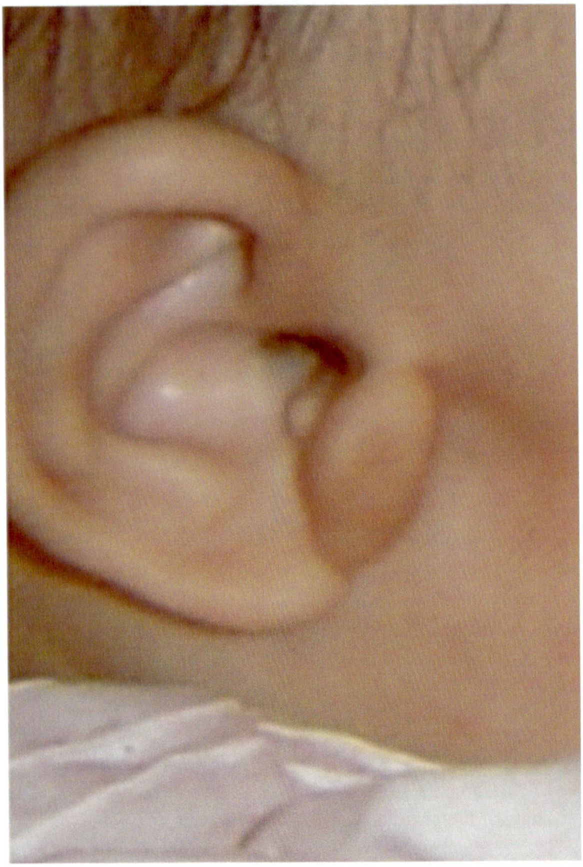

Fig. 24.4 Another example of a preauricular appendage emanating from the natural tragus

acrochordon, also known as a skin tag. In one study of over 1000 accessory auricles, the authors found that 78.4% contained cartilage [8].

These appendages arise from first branchial cleft anomaly and may be located anywhere along a triangle from the ear to the lip, along the mandible. The appendage may be pedunculated via a very thin stalk and fall off naturally as the lesion itself becomes ischemic with growth. Generally, surgical excision under sedation will be performed after the age of 3 due to the elective nature of the operation or in combination with other procedures (i.e., auricular reconstruction). Earlier excision could be considered during the first several months of life under local anesthesia.

Elliptical excision surrounding the base of the appendage, with undermining, allows for approximation of the skin without tension. It is important to avoid deep dissection, particularly in the preauricular area, for risk of injuring the parotid, facial nerve, or superficial temporal artery. This method of excision generally leads to a satisfactory aesthetic result. Use of absorbable sutures with surgical tape or glue use improves cooperation in the postoperative period. It also prevents the need for suture removal, which reduces patient discomfort and possible need for further sedation.

Preauricular Pits

Preauricular pits may also be noticed at or near the root of the helix (Fig. 24.5). The pit may have a blind-ended pouch or continue as a deeper sinus to attach to the auricular cartilage.

Surgical excision may be offered, particularly if the patient has suffered a prior infection of the pit or sinus. This may be done in conjunction with other procedures or as an ambulatory procedure. An elliptical incision can be designed surrounding the pit or sinus, after probing with a lacrimal probe. Dissection must continue along the tract to its base, which typically inserts into cartilage. A small area of cartilage should be removed to prevent recurrence. Primary closure is then performed.

Auricular Deformities

The auricle in the TCS patient may appear anomalous secondary to a deformity (Fig. 24.6). Deformities may include cryptotia, prominauris, lop ear, or cup ear [16]. These anomalies are less commonly seen than microtia in the TCS population, however.

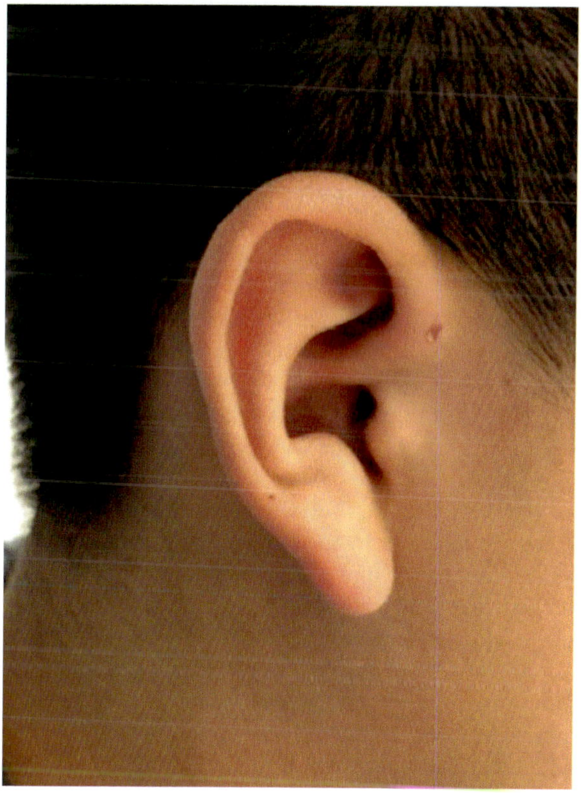

Fig. 24.5 A preauricular pit located at the root of the helix

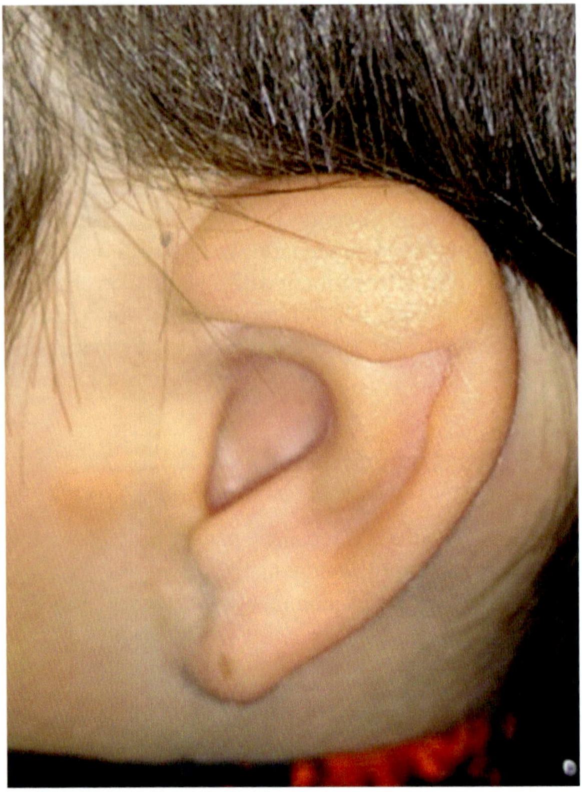

Fig. 24.6 Auricular deformities may be identified like lop ear, shown here. Prominent auricles or cup ear may also be identified in the TCS patient

If identified early enough, auricular molding procedures can be performed. Molding is much more successful if instituted within 1 week of birth. Due to circulating maternal exogenous estrogen, infant cartilage is more pliable. Estrogen levels peak around 3 days after birth and then begin to fall. The manner in which estrogen influences the auricular cartilage is due to the increase in hyaluronic acid within the cartilage [11]. Once estrogen levels decline, the ear then becomes firmer and molding techniques are less likely to succeed.

Various materials may be used to stent the auricle into the desired shape, such as silastic tubing with dental wire, dental wax, or an endotracheal tube stylet (Fig. 24.7). Commercial kits are also available, including EarBuddies (Ear Buddies Ltd., London, UK) and EarWell (Becon Medical, Batavia, Illinois). These may be placed by the physician or by the family. The stent should be changed at least biweekly to allow examination of the underlying skin and ensure no breakdown or infection has occurred. This also allows for assessment of progress. Molding will generally take place for 2 to 6 weeks depending on how early the process was initiated.

Otoplasty may be considered in these patients if they are too old for molding procedures. Otoplasty is generally undertaken around 5–6 years of age, once the auricle has reached around 85–90% of adult size. Various techniques may be used and individually designed to address the deformity.

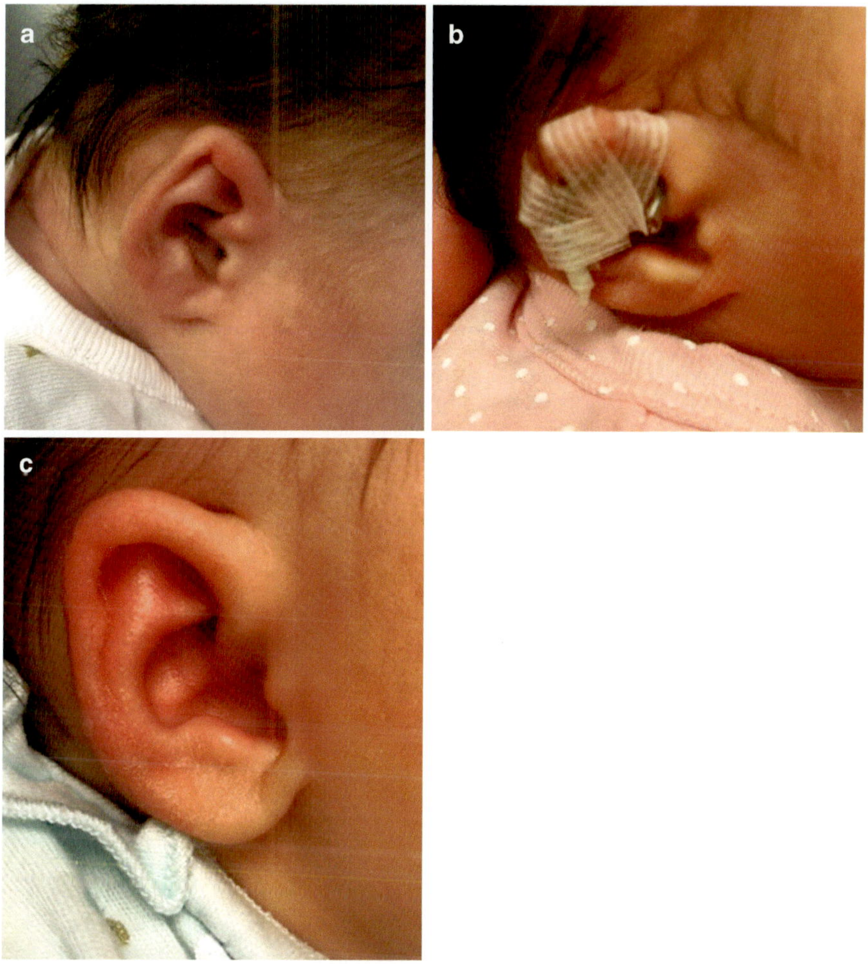

Fig. 24.7 Molding of an auricular deformity in an infant. An auricular deformity was identified anterior to the antihelix (**a**). A custom splint of silastic with dental wire was created and adhered via surgical tape (**b**). The outcome after molding process was completed (**c**)

Microtia

Microtia is the most common auricular malformation and has been reported to occur in up to 85% of TCS patients [3]. In an assessment of Nagata's auricular reconstruction clinic, 9.1% of the syndromic patients with microtia had TCS [17].

One commonly adopted grading system, originally described by Weerda and simplified by Aguilar, classifies the deformity based on the appearance of the vestigial remnants. Grade 1 microtia has a mild reduction of size compared to a normal ear. Grade 2 microtia has a volume loss with reduced cartilage and skin. Landmarks are not as easily identified. Grade 3 microtia is also known as "peanut ear" as only

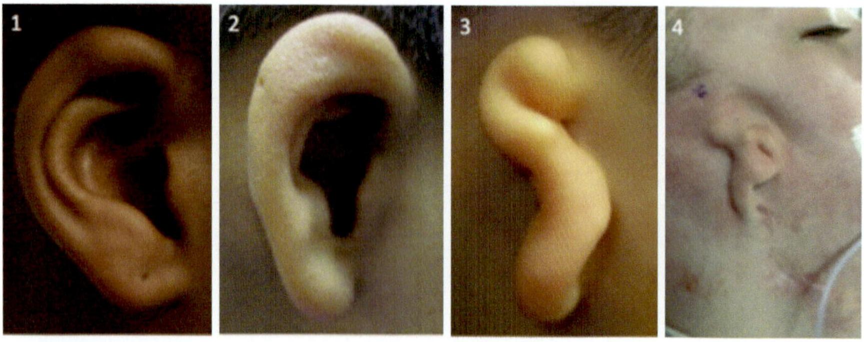

Fig. 24.8 The grading of microtia. Grade 1 microtia with a smaller than normal ear, but landmarks are easily identifiable (1). Grade 2 microtia with further volume loss and landmarks are not as easily identified (2). Grade 3 microtia with a small remnant auricle and lobule (3). Grade 4 microtia or "anotia," with no external auricule (4). (Reprinted from Clinics in Perinatology. 45 (4). Hartzell L, Chinnadurai S. Microtia and Related Facial Anomalies, 679–697, 2018, with permission from Elsevier)

a small remnant remains, with a lobule. Grade 4 microtia is the absence of any external ear, also known as anotia (Fig. 24.8).

The family of a TCS patient should be fully informed of the reconstructive options. These include no intervention, prosthetics, porous polyethylene (MedPor) implantation, or autologous rib reconstruction.

Prosthetics

Prosthetics may allow for an excellent aesthetic result without the requirement for surgical intervention. Interested patients and families may be referred to an anaplastologist, or one may be already incorporated into the reconstructive team. An anaplastologist is a clinical specialist experienced in prosthetic design and creation for the replacement of an absent or malformed body part.

Auricular prostheses are generally constructed from silicone after molds have been created. The template may be the patient's contralateral ear or that of a family member. The prosthetic may be secured in place using adhesive or implantable magnets or abutments. Adhesive may allow for the prosthetic use at an early age, as young as age 3. The adhesive is typically painted onto the prosthetic, allowed to dry partially, and then the prosthetic can be applied. Adhesive-applied prosthetics are the most conservative method of auricular reconstruction [15]. Risks associated with adhesives include a failure of the adhesive to hold, particularly in a humid or hot environment, or skin reactions.

Implantable magnets or osseointegrated (bone-anchored) abutments are placed after age 5 (Fig. 24.9). One such abutment option is the VistaFix system (Cochlear, Sydney, Australia). It is important to consider the bone integrity, particularly in the TCS population. These patients are more likely to have poor bone integrity or irregularity [13]. A "sleeper" screw may be helpful in case of poor osseointegration or

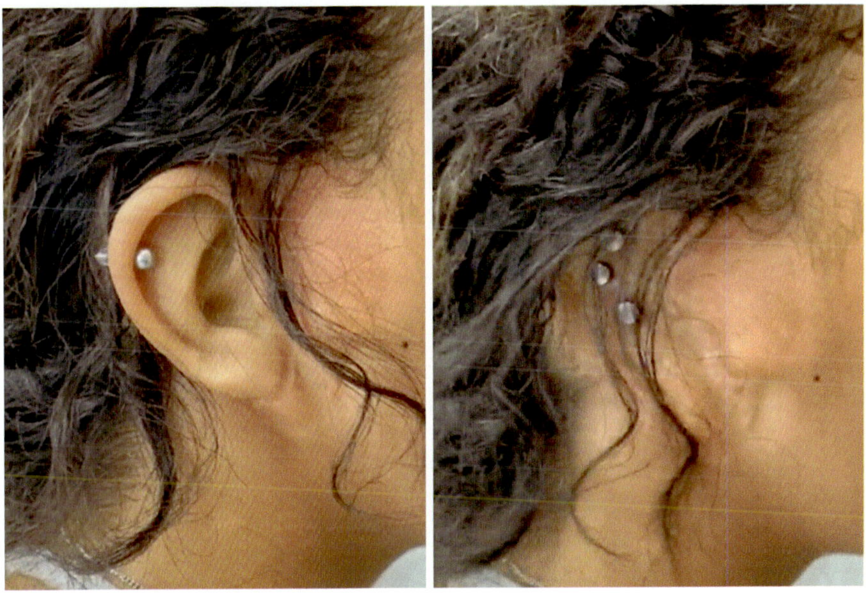

Fig. 24.9 An example of a patient with an auricular prosthesis (left image) that is secured via osseointegrated abutment technology. There are 3 abutments to which the prosthesis can fixate (right image)

potential trauma of the other screw. Additionally, a two-stage procedure is recommended in this population: the first to place the screw and the second to attach the abutment 4 to 6 months later after osseointegration is achieved.

The surgeon must work closely with the anaplastologist in deciding the best placement of the prosthetic and abutments. Auricular remnants may need to be excised or altered depending on the prosthetic design. Sometimes the prosthesis can be designed to incorporate the auricular remnant. A tragus may also need to be constructed. This can be done via cartilage harvest from the contralateral concha cavum.

The prosthetic is also an ideal option in the case of a failed porous polyethylene implant or rib reconstruction, post-traumatic cases, and following excision of malignancies and irradiation. Limitations include daily prosthetic care, daily application and removal of the prosthetic, and the need for prosthetic replacement every 4–5 years due to wear. The prosthetic should be removed during water activities, bathing, and sleeping.

Implantable Reconstruction

Early alloplastic implants used for auricular reconstruction were based in silicone. However, these had a high rate of infection and extrusion. Porous high-density polyethylene (MedPor [Stryker, Kalamazoo, MI]) implantation became available in the 1990s. The material is more resilient to trauma. Disadvantages include using nonnative tissue and there is still a risk for future infection or extrusion compared to autologous tissue.

The surgery can be performed as early as 3–5 years old and is generally performed in a single stage. The implant requires a temporoparietal fascia (TPF) flap for coverage. The course of the superficial temporal artery is identified using Doppler and marked on the patient (Fig. 24.10).

The incisions are made and the skin pocket is developed. The TPF flap is raised carefully from posterior to anterior, making sure to keep a wide base around the vascular pedicle. By keeping a wide base, postoperative edema and risk of vascular compression are reduced. The rudimentary cartilage is then removed from the auricle, and the implant is assembled (Fig. 24.11). The implant comes in two parts, one as the base and one as the helix. These are customized as necessary and then secured together with non-absorbable suture. The implant is inserted with the TPF flap providing anterior coverage (Fig. 24.12). Any area without epithelial coverage may be reconstructed with a split or full-thickness skin graft, which may be harvested from the postauricular region or thigh. A bolster is applied, and the patient is seen back in the office 1 week later for removal.

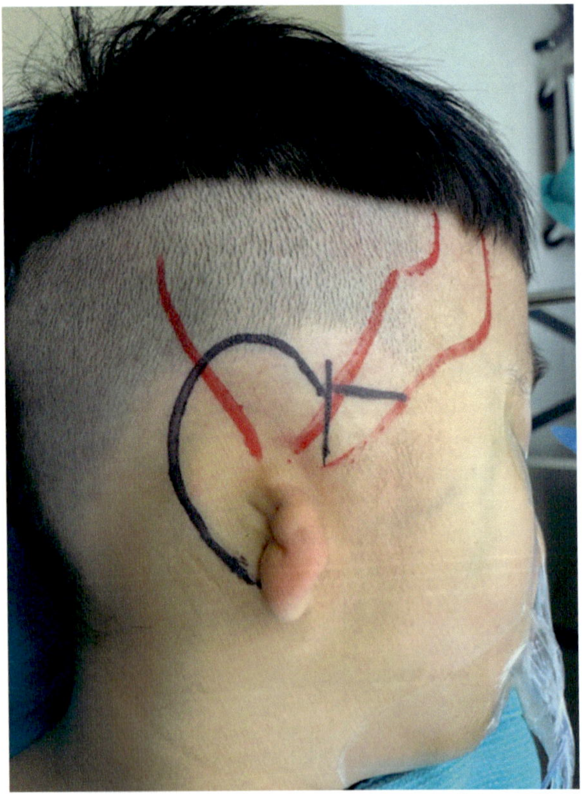

Fig. 24.10 An example of the marking of the course of the superficial temporal artery (seen in red). The incisions are marked as well as the skin pocket for the MedPor implant (seen in black)

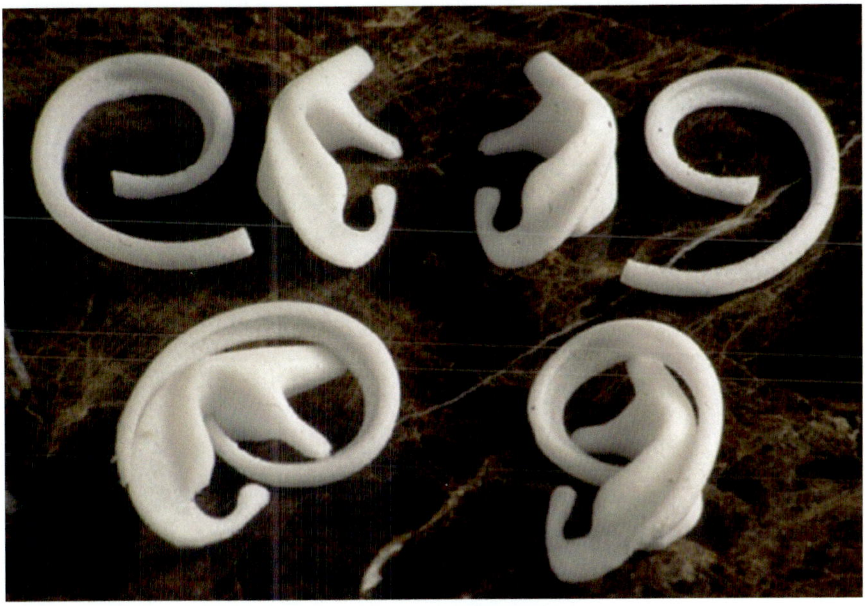

Fig. 24.11 Porous high-density polyethylene auricular implants come with 2 components: the base and the helix. (Reprinted from Facial Plastic Surgery Clinics of North America. 22 (4). Cabin J, Bassiri-Tehrani M, Sclafani A, et al. Microtia Reconstruction Autologous Rib and Alloplast Techniques, 679–697, 2014, with permission from Elsevier)

Autologous Rib Reconstruction

Autologous rib reconstruction techniques have been described by numerous surgeons, including Tanzer, Brent, Nagata and Firmin [4, 7, 14, 18]. The benefit of using autologous tissue includes less risk of extrusion, infection, or failure due to trauma in patients implanted over several decades. Disadvantages include donor site morbidity, more than one procedure, and less predictable aesthetic result.

Surgery generally requires several stages, ranging from two stages in the Nagata and Firmin techniques to four stages in the Brent technique. In our practice, the two-stage Firmin method is followed. The first stage combines framework construction, lobule transposition, and tragal reconstruction. Framework elevation and postauricular skin grafting occurs in the second stage.

The first stage starts with harvest of section of costal cartilage from ribs 6 through 9. A template is designed from the contralateral ear if normal, or a previously selected model ear, such as that of a parent. The template is drawn on radiograph film and soaked in betadine (Fig. 24.13). Harvest may be from the ipsilateral or contralateral chest, but preferably on the same side. The sixth and seventh ribs form a synchondrosis which is harvested for use as the base of the construct (Fig. 24.14). The floating eighth and ninth ribs are harvested for use as the helix, antihelix, tragus and antitragus. A portion may also be used as a projection piece. During harvest, the

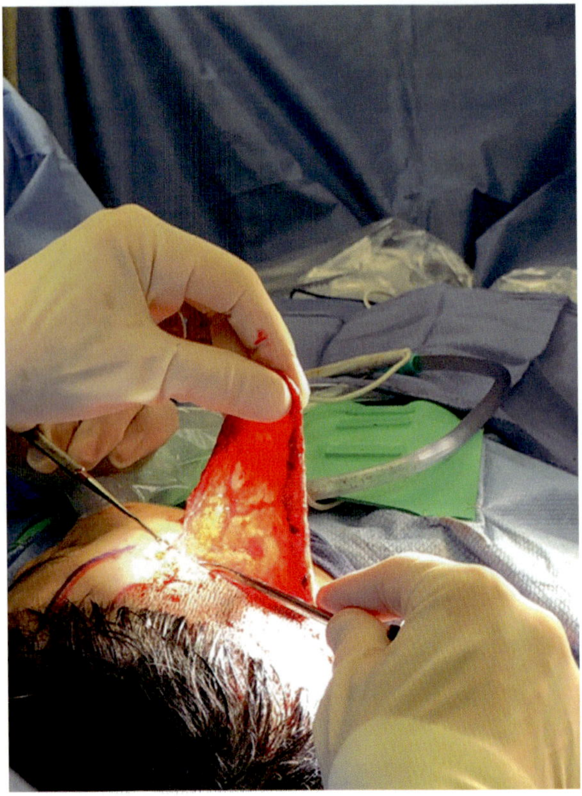

Fig. 24.12 A TPF flap about to be positioned over the implant. The wide base as well as thin, pliable nature of the flap with vasculature is demonstrated here

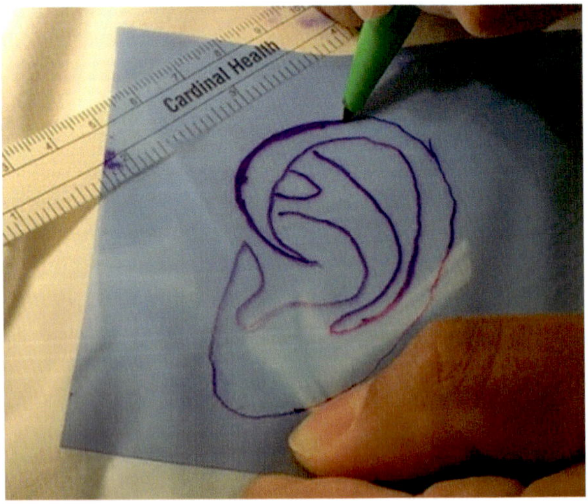

Fig. 24.13 Template designed on a radiograph film. This will be soaked in betadine prior to use as a template for the auricular construct

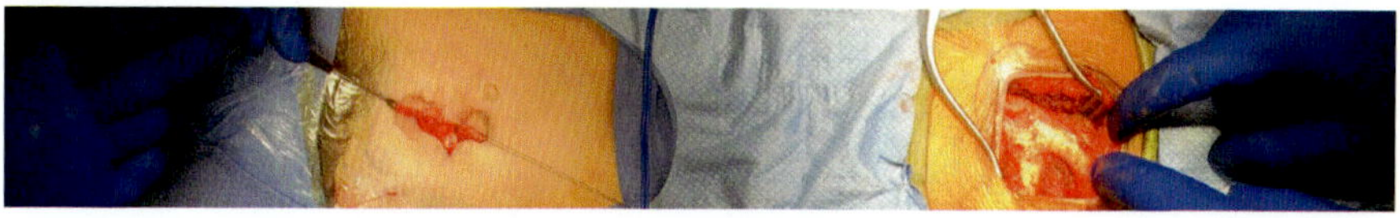

Fig. 24.14 Image depicting the skin envelope being developed and vestigial cartilage removed by one surgeon, while the second surgeon harvests the rib cartilage from the donor site. The sixth and seventh ribs form a synchondrosis which is pictured here

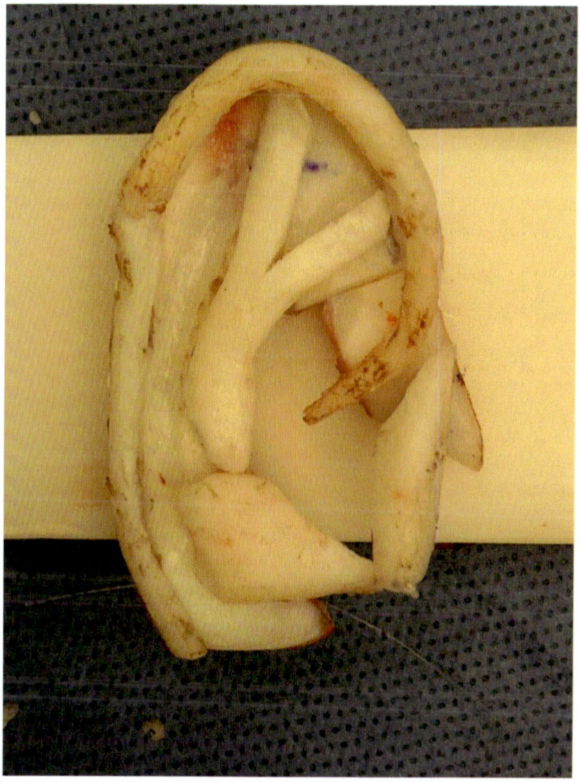

Fig. 24.15 Cartilage construct after completion

perichondrium of the ribs is preserved medially. The donor site is checked for any pleural leaks with irrigation and Valsalva maneuvers prior to closure. Next, the incision is closed in multiple layers with closure of the muscle and aponeurosis, subcutaneous tissue and epidermis.

The auricular construct is then carefully carved on the back Table. A template based on the normal side is used. The base is constructed from the sixth and seventh ribs. The helix is constructed and secured to the base using surgical steel or clear nylon sutures. The antihelix is also constructed as a separate piece and secured. Finally, the tragus and antitragus are constructed on a contiguous cartilage piece and secured (Fig. 24.15). A projection piece may be placed posteriorly at this time if

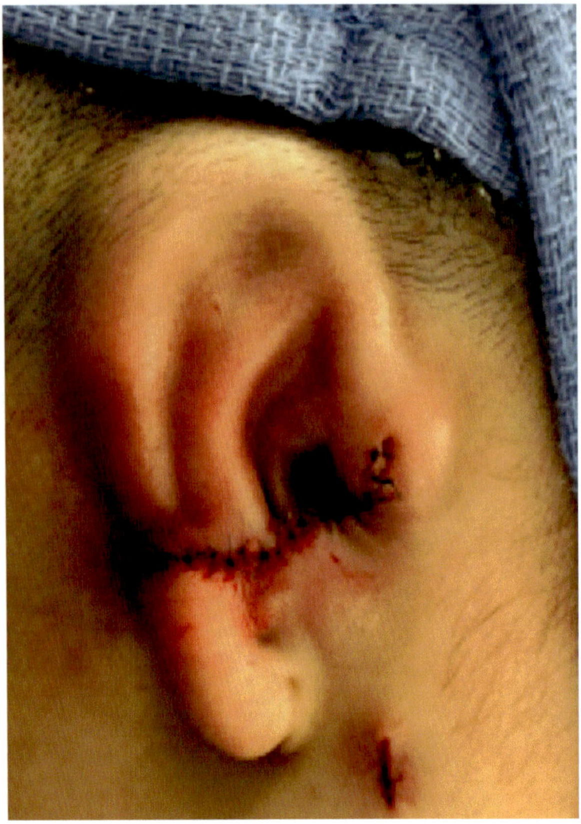

Fig. 24.16 Once the construct is placed under the skin envelope, the drains are placed on suction. In this patient, a preauricular appendage was also excised

there is enough laxity of the skin envelope. The construct is then positioned within the skin envelope. Drains are placed to suction and seal the skin onto the construct (Fig. 24.16).

At the second stage, the framework is elevated and skin grafting performed. This typically occurs at least 6 months after the first stage and can be done as an ambulatory procedure. At the second stage, implantation of an osseointegrated hearing device may also be considered. The hair is shaved surrounding the temporal area. A thin split thickness skin graft (0.015 in) is designed and taken from the posterior scalp. The hair is removed using gentle pressure with a wet sponge. A nonstick dressing is placed over the donor site. Next, an incision is made around the helix of the framework. The soft tissue on the posterior aspect of the construct is left intact and dissection continues anteriorly to raise the helix until the area of conchal bowl. The skin posteriorly is widely undermined and brought anteriorly to the new post-auricular area and is sutured in place. The skin graft is then applied to the posterior auricle and sutured in place. A bolster is placed around the ear of petroleum gauze. The split-thickness skin graft donor site is then covered with a Mepilex Ag foam dressing (Mölnlycke, Norcross, Georgia, USA) and the foam is sutured in place with 3–0 Prolene (Ethicon, Somerville, New Jersey, USA) suture. The patient is seen back in the clinic setting around 1 week later for an ear dressing and Mepilex Ag foam dressing removal.

Considerations on Timing and the Patient Perspective

Patients with TCS typically present with several craniofacial anomalies, not simply related to the external ear. Timing for surgical intervention of the external ear does not need to be different for the patient with TCS than a non-syndromic patient [1]. However, the average TCS patient undergoes five different surgeries during their reconstructive process [12]. A general approach to the overall operative timeline involves airway management, oropharyngeal repair, and then midface and auricular reconstruction [6]. Hearing should be assessed early with necessary amplification provided during the first year of life, which has been discussed elsewhere in this text.

A study by Lodovichi et al. sought to explore the TCS patient perspective on their ear deformity [12]. Twelve patients with TCS were divided into two groups, those with normal ears and those without, and then asked to complete the World Health Organization (WHO) quality-of-life questionnaire. Despite a small sample size, the study demonstrated an intermediate quality of life for both groups without a statistically significant difference.

The benefit of awaiting until the patient is older for auricular reconstruction is increased maturity and cooperation with post-procedural care, increased size of ribs (ideally a chest circumference greater than 60 cm), and patient assent for the procedure. An argument against this is the desire for repair prior to starting school when patients may experience bullying [5]. Overall, it is most important for a patient and family to find a reconstructive surgeon who considers their concerns and desires for reconstruction and is comfortable with his or her skills in auricular reconstruction.

References

1. Aljerian A, Gilardino MS. Treacher Collins syndrome. Clin Plast Surg. 2019;46(2):197–205. https://doi.org/10.1016/j.cps.2018.11.005.
2. Amirhassankhani S, Lloyd MS. Accessory auricles: systematic review of definition, associated conditions, and recommendations for clinical practice. J Craniofac Surg. 2018;29(2):372–5. https://doi.org/10.1097/SCS.0000000000004201.
3. Arvystas M, Shprintzen RJ. Craniofacial morphology in Treacher Collins syndrome. Cleft Palate Craniofac J. 1991;28(2):226–30; ; discussion 230-221. https://doi.org/10.1597/1545-1569_1991_028_0226_cmitcs_2.3.co_2.
4. Brent B. Microtia repair with rib cartilage grafts: a review of personal experience with 1000 cases. Clin Plast Surg. 2002;29(2):257–71, vii. https://doi.org/10.1016/s0094-1298(01)00013-x.
5. Cabin JA, Bassiri-Tehrani M, Sclafani AP, Romo T. Microtia reconstruction: autologous rib and Alloplast techniques. Facial Plast Surg Clin North Am. 2014;22(4):623–38. https://doi.org/10.1016/j.fsc.2014.07.004.

6. Chang CC, Steinbacher DM. Treacher Collins syndrome. Semin Plast Surg. 2012;26(2):83–90. https://doi.org/10.1055/s-0032-1320066.
7. Firmin F. Ear reconstruction in cases of typical microtia. Personal experience based on 352 microtic ear corrections. Scand J Plast Reconstr Surg Hand Surg. 1998;32(1):35–47. https://doi.org/10.1080/02844319850158930.
8. Hwang J, Cho J, Burm JS. Accessory auricle: classification according to location, protrusion pattern and body shape. Arch Plast Surg. 2018;45(5):411–7. https://doi.org/10.5999/aps.2018.00430.
9. Kountakis SE, Helidonis E, Jahrsdoerfer RA. Microtia grade as an indicator of middle ear development in aural atresia. Arch Otolaryngol Head Neck Surg. 1995;121(8):885–6. https://doi.org/10.1001/archotol.1995.01890080053010.
10. Kubo S, Horinouchi T, Kinoshita M, Yoshizato T, Kozuma Y, Shinagawa T, Ushijima K. Visual diagnosis in utero: prenatal diagnosis of Treacher-Collins syndrome using a 3D/4D ultrasonography. Taiwan J Obstet Gynecol. 2019;58(4):566–9. https://doi.org/10.1016/j.tjog.2019.05.024.
11. Lennon C, Chinnadurai S. Nonsurgical management of congenital auricular anomalies. Facial Plast Surg Clin North Am. 2018;26(1):1–8. https://doi.org/10.1016/j.fsc.2017.09.001.
12. Lodovichi FF, Oliveira JP, Denadai R, Raposo-Amaral CA, Ghizoni E, Raposo-Amaral CE. Traz a deformidade de orelha impacto negativo na qualidadede vida em indivíduos com síndrome de Treacher Collins? Cien Saude Colet. 2018;23:4311–8.
13. Marsella P, Scorpecci A, Pacifico C, Tieri L. Bone-anchored hearing aid (Baha) in patients with Treacher Collins syndrome: tips and pitfalls. Int J Pediatr Otorhinolaryngol. 2011;75(10):1308–12. https://doi.org/10.1016/j.ijporl.2011.07.020.
14. Nagata S. Total auricular reconstruction with a three-dimensional costal cartilage framework. Ann Chir Plast Esthet. 1995;40(4):371–99; discussion 400-373
15. Raju M, Shetty M, Prasad DK. Prosthetic rehabilitation of a patient with congenitally deformed ears. J Indian Prosthodont Soc. 2014;14(Suppl 1):264–7. https://doi.org/10.1007/s13191-013-0325-z.
16. Rosa F, Coutinho MB, Ferreira JP, Sousa CA. Ear malformations, hearing loss and hearing rehabilitation in children with Treacher Collins syndrome. Acta Otorrinolaringologica (English Edition). 2016;67(3):142–7. https://doi.org/10.1016/j.otoeng.2016.05.001.
17. Shibazaki-Yorozuya R, Nagata S. Preferential associated malformation in patients with Anotia and Microtia. J Craniofac Surg. 2019;30(1):66–70. https://doi.org/10.1097/SCS.0000000000004915.
18. Tanzer RC. Total reconstruction of the auricle. The evolution of a plan of treatment. Plast Reconstr Surg. 1971;47(6):523–33. https://doi.org/10.1097/00006534-197106000-00001.

Chapter 25
Rhinoplasty in Patients with Treacher Collins Syndrome

Alexander P. Marston and Andrew R. Scott

Introduction

Failure of neuroepithelial proliferation as a result of mutations in the TCOF1 gene leads to incomplete development of the first and second pharyngeal arches in individuals with Treacher Collins syndrome (TCS). Although this has a more direct effect on the mandibular and midfacial anatomy, there are significant secondary consequences on nasal anatomy, function, and aesthetics. The timing and order for surgical correction of the complex TCS deformities are initially based on priorities of airway stabilization, followed by staged procedures based on skeletal growth and psychosocial needs [14]. Airway obstruction is most commonly due to mandibular hypoplasia and secondary posterior positioning of the tongue base; however, choanal atresia is variably present in patients with TCS [1, 11] and may contribute to early respiratory difficulty. If choanal atresia significantly impacts respiratory function, this may require an endonasal surgical intervention early in life. Mild cases of choanal atresia can be surgically treated later in childhood with associated improved outcomes and less risk of revision surgery [10, 19]. In the absence of choanal atresia, surgical nasal intervention, such as septorhinoplasty, is delayed until after skeletal maturity is achieved. As a result of multiple severe anatomic deficiencies that take precedence over the nasal sequelae of TCS, few available studies on rhinoplasty techniques and results are published in the literature.

A. P. Marston (✉) · A. R. Scott
Tufts University School of Medicine, Department of Otolaryngology – Head and Neck Surgery, Division of Pediatric Otolaryngology, Division of Facial Plastic and Reconstructive Surgery, Boston, MA, USA
e-mail: amarston@tuftsmedicalcenter.org; ascott@tuftsmedicalcenter.org

D. M. Yates, M. R. Markiewicz (eds.), *Craniofacial Microsomia and Treacher Collins Syndrome*, https://doi.org/10.1007/978-3-030-84733-3_25

Nasal Anatomy

Although the nose is typically less dysplastic than the surrounding facial and cranial anatomy in patients with TCS, intrinsic and extrinsic nasal structures can be severely affected. There are reports of arhinia [7] and choanal atresia [1, 11], but more commonly there is moderate nasal obstruction that results from midfacial hypoplasia [14] and septal and/or external deviation. A thorough understanding of the adjacent dysplastic facial anatomy is an important component of rhinoplasty assessment, planning, and patient counseling. Regardless of the severity of the facial malformations at birth, these generally remain stable into adulthood [16]. Although the facial deformity is bilateral, there are typically asymmetric features with one side demonstrating more severe involvement. Prominent features that secondarily impact nasal anatomy in patients with TCS result from orbitozygomatic hypoplasia, retrognathia, and microgenia leading to relative prominence of the nasal dorsum and an overall convex facial profile [14]. A reduced cranial base angle further contributes to the convexity of the facial profile and apparent prominence of the nose [8]. Cephalometric analyses demonstrate that the lower anterior facial height is long and the posterior facial height is short due to mandibular dysplasia and chin retrusion [4]. The upper anterior facial height is typically normal. Hypertelorism may be present, and the globes appear protruded as a result of midfacial hypoplasia and dysplastic lateral orbital walls. Soft tissue deficiencies of the eyelids, cheek skin, and temporal fossa are additionally important factors to consider [4].

More careful analysis of the nasal anatomy on frontal view often reveals external deviation of the nose due to underlying asymmetries of the midface and orbitozygomatic complexes. The width of the upper third of the nose is often increased [5] (Fig. 25.1), and this deformity is further accentuated if hypertelorism is present. The nasal tip may appear boxy or bulbous and is classically bifid in appearance (Fig. 25.2) [13]. Furthermore, the alar bases are often narrow and constricted. On profile view, there is a characteristic mid-dorsal hump composed of both bone and cartilage (Fig. 25.3) [5]. The length of the nose from the radix to the tip is often long with ptosis of the nasal tip and deficient projection. Underlying midfacial hypoplasia and incomplete superior rotation of the maxilla lead to a deficient and downward-oriented nasal spine that further contributes to nasal tip ptosis. In cases of severe underprojection, the nasofronal angle is greater than 135 degrees (the generally accepted upper limit of normal) (Fig. 25.4) [15]. Ptosis of the nasal tip can additionally cause an acute nasolabial angle. The nasofacial angle, represented by the intersection of a line from the nasal tip to the nasion and a vertical line from the pogonion to the glabella, has a range of normal between 30 and 40 degrees. As a result of micrognathia, the pogonion is posteriorly positioned, which leads to an obtuse nasofacial angle in most TCS patients. An optimal chin-nose relationship places the pogonion and glabella along the same vertical line that is perpendicular to the Frankfurt horizontal [3]. As a result, the retrodisplaced chin among individuals with TCS contributes significantly to their nasal aesthetics.

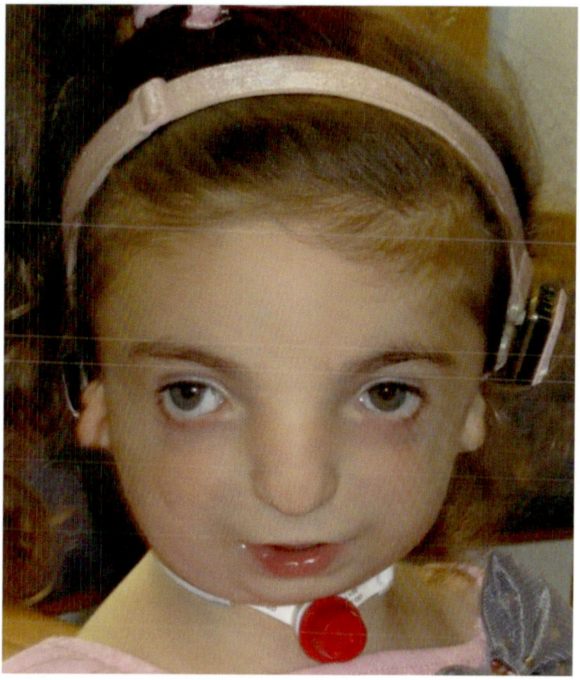

Fig. 25.1 Front view demonstrating a broad nasal dorsum that is further emphasized in the setting of hypertelorism

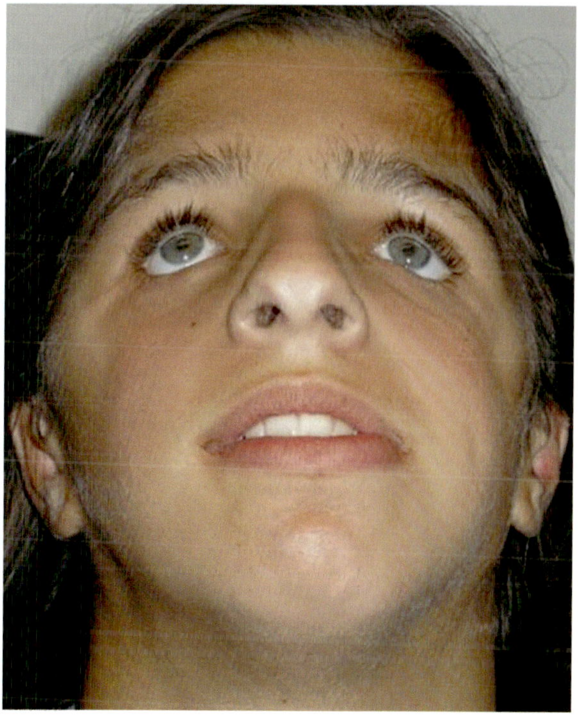

Fig. 25.2 Base view with evidence of the nasal tip bifidity

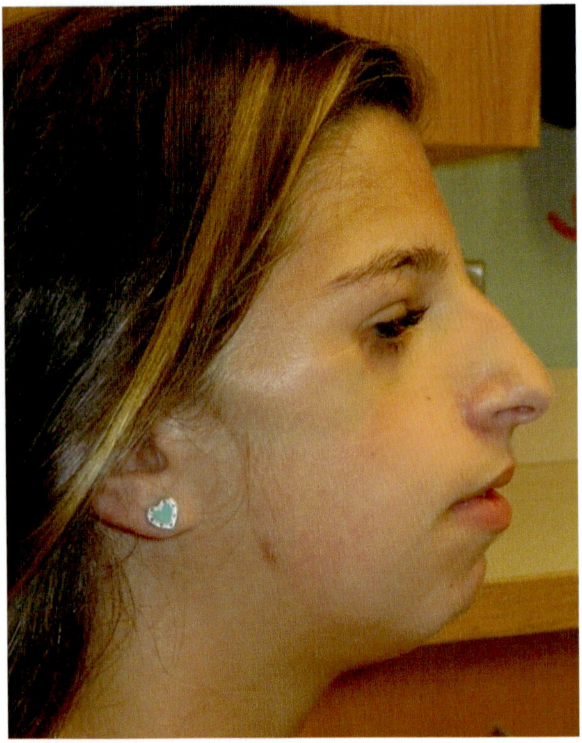

Fig. 25.3 Profile view with evidence of a prominent dorsal hump, convex facial profile, and microgenia

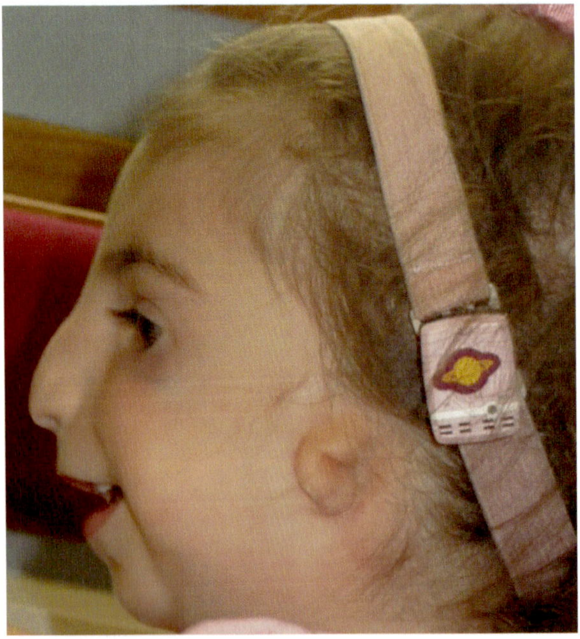

Fig. 25.4 Profile view demonstrating an obtuse nasofrontal angle due to severe underprojection of the nasal tip

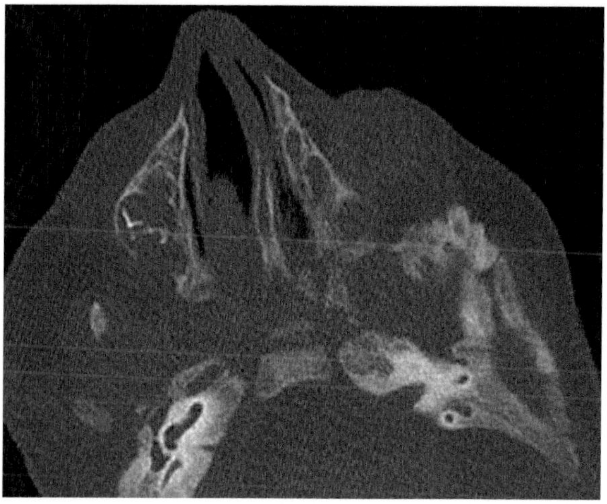

Fig. 25.5 Non-contrast CT image revealing severe deviation of the nasal septum, involving both the quadrangular cartilage and vomer

Few publications are available on the specific nasal characteristics of patients with TCS. One such report from 2015 by Plomp et al. included 11 TCS patients and found that 73% had a dorsal hump, 55% had external nasal deviation, 55% had a bulbous or bifid nasal tip, and 36% had under-rotation of the nasal tip [13]. On profile view, approximately one-third of patients had an under-rotated nasal tip leading to a reported "droopy" appearance. Endonasal examination demonstrated an 82% incidence of septal deviation (Fig. 25.5). This same study also used the Nasal Appearance and Function Evaluation Questionnaire (NAFEQ) to assess the satisfaction of nasal function and appearance among this cohort of 11 TCS patients compared to 151 controls. When compared to controls, TCS patients had significantly lower satisfaction scores for the following metrics: nasal position, nostril size, color of the nose, and total nasal appearance. Nine of 11 (81%) TCS patients indicated they were "satisfied" with their "total nasal appearance." Interestingly, the two individuals who were unsatisfied were the two patients who had undergone prior rhinoplasty procedures.

Rhinoplasty

Similar to standard rhinoplasty workup and preoperative counseling, particular care is taken to understand the patient's priorities and expectations, appreciate the nuances and variability of the nasal anatomy, and create a well-outlined surgical plan. It is important to carefully advise the patient on how a potential rhinoplasty intervention is expected to alter their facial aesthetics. Due to adjacent midfacial and orbitozygomatic anatomic deficiencies, there are obvious limitations in how nasal surgery will impact overall appearance among patients with TCS. Preoperative computer-simulated morphing is a valuable way of gaining a better understanding of the patient's wishes [9], allows for demonstration of the anticipated outcome, and depicts how the procedure might improve their overall facial form. An honest approach to preoperative image morphing is critical in order to create realistic goals [3]. Patients with TCS require a myriad of surgical interventions throughout their childhood and adolescent years; rhinoplasty should be considered only after skeletal maturity has been attained and, if necessary, orthognathic surgery has been completed [14].

Definitive rhinoplasty often requires an open approach in TCS patients to allow for correction of external nasal deviation and severe nasoseptal obstruction. Dorsal hump reduction typically necessitates resection of both cartilage and bone with osteotomies and medialization of the bony vault to close the resulting open roof deformity (Fig. 25.6). Osteotomies additionally achieve a more natural appearing nasal width, which is increased at baseline in individuals with TCS. According to a TCS nasal analysis paper by Farkas et al., the nasal root width should be reduced by up to 7 mm for an ideal aesthetic result [5]. Decreased nasal tip projection and under-rotation are best addressed with a caudal septal extension graft in the authors' experience. Greater projection, rotation, and long-term stability can be accomplished with a caudal extension graft as compared to a floating columellar strut [2].

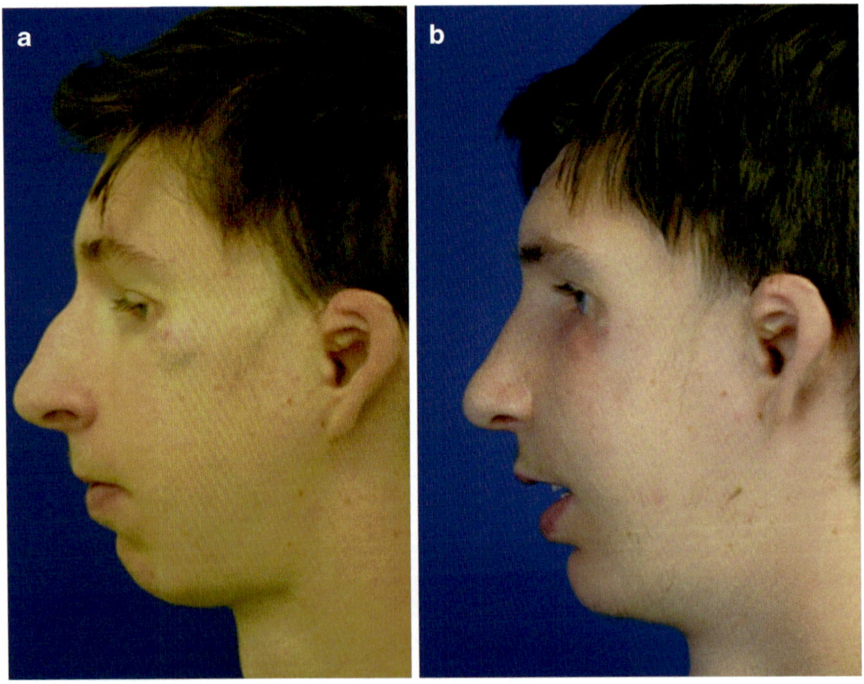

Fig. 25.6 Preoperative (**a**) and postoperative (**b**) septorhinoplasty photographs. The primary interventions included dorsal hump takedown, caudal septal extension graft, extended spreader grafts, chin implant placement, and free fat grafting to the cheeks. (Courtesy of Krishna G. Patel, MD, PhD, at the Medical University of South Carolina in Charleston, SC)

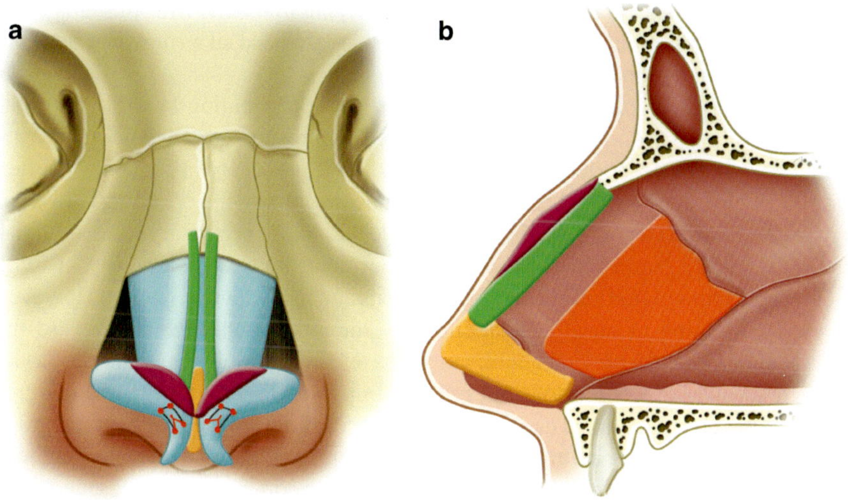

Fig. 25.7 Gunter diagrams depicting example septorhinoplasty interventions. The front view (**a**) shows medial and lateral osteotomies (blue) these are not present need to be drawn on by author, extended spreader grafts (green), caudal septal extension graft (orange), cephalic trim of the lateral crura (magenta), and intradomal sutures for tip definition (red). The sagittal view (**b**) demonstrates dorsal hump takedown (magenta), extended spreader graft (green), caudal septal extension graft (orange), and septal cartilage graft harvest (red-orange)

According the Farkas et al., the tip projection ought to be increased by up to 4 mm in this patient population. Nasal tip definition improves as a result of increasing tip projection and can be further refined through conservative trimming of the cephalic margin of the lower lateral cartilages and dome suturing techniques (Fig. 25.7). Lastly, the surgeon and patient should discuss chin retrodisplacement as a contributing factor of their nasal aesthetic and consider alloplastic chin augmentation or genioplasty in conjunction with septorhinoplasty.

Implications of Nasal Dysfunction

Consequences of the TCS nasal deformity and dysfunction can have wide ranging implications from speech disturbance and obstructive sleep apnea to exacerbation of psychosocial-related outcomes. Abnormalities of speech are common among TCS individuals, primarily due to the high incidence of cleft palate and conductive hearing loss, with a prevalence ranging between 21–33% [17, 18, 23] and 83–92% [18, 23], respectively. If one or both of these features are present, there is a significant risk for speech delay and/or velopharyngeal insufficiency (VPI). For those with a history of cleft palate and VPI, this is typically manifested in the form of hypernasal speech. However, in cases of severe TCS midfacial hypoplasia and/or repaired choanal atresia, secondary constriction of the nasal cavities can actually lead to hyponasality of speech [20]. Although the underlying midfacial hypoplasia is difficult to correct, septorhinoplasty can lead to an increase in nasal airflow and possible improvement in hyponasality.

Nasal obstruction can additionally manifest as a contributing factor of obstructive sleep apnea (OSA). The prevalence of OSA among pediatric and adult patients with TCS has been reported to be 54% and 41%, respectively [12]. There is often multilevel obstruction with the most prominent contributing factors being midfacial hypoplasia, as well as oro- and hypo-pharyngeal collapse secondary to mandibular deformities [12]. Nasal obstruction can further contribute to the severity of OSA secondary to constricted nasal cavity dimensions and nasoseptal deviation. However, surgical correction of nasal obstruction only imparts a minor benefit toward the treatment of OSA. As previous publications have demonstrated, nasal surgery as an isolated surgical treatment does not reliably improve OSA by objective measures [6]. Nevertheless, subjective measures of nasal breathing and snoring often improve following nasal surgery with a possible reduction in pressure titrations for those treated with continuous positive airway pressure support for OSA [6]. Due to the known high prevalence of OSA and the frequent occurrence of nasal obstruction in individuals with TCS, septorhinoplasty interventions should aim to improve not only nasal breathing and aesthetics but also sleep- and OSA-related metrics.

Improvements in speech and OSA severity are important potential outcomes of nasal surgery; however, perhaps the most significant result can be observed in optimization of a patient's psychosocial health. Patients with congenital facial deformities have been found to be significantly less satisfied with their facial appearance [21]. This can then lead to low self-esteem and high fear of negative appearance evaluation by others, both of which are strong determinants of psychological functioning [21]. An emphasis should be made on preoperative counseling to impart realistic surgical expectations, but a definitive goal of the nasal procedure should include an improvement in patient satisfaction so as to optimize their long-term psychosocial well-being [22].

Conclusion

Although TCS nasal deformities are typically less severe than the adjacent mandibulofacial dysostosis, there are significant implications of the altered nasal function and aesthetics. Therefore, septorhinoplasty is an important aspect in the staged surgical management of TCS patients. Narrowing of the nasal dorsal width, dorsal hump takedown, and correction of external nasal and septal obstruction can lead to marked improvement in nasal function and appearance.

Acknowledgments The authors thank the patients who have consented to publication of their photographs in this chapter. The images in Fig. 25.6 are courtesy of Krishna Patel, MD, PhD, from the Medical University of South Carolina in Charleston, SC.

Disclosure Statement None of the authors have any commercial or financial conflicts of interest, and no external funding sources were obtained.

References

1. Andrade EC, Junior VS, Didoni AL, Freitas PZ, Carneiro AF, Yoshimoto FR. Treacher Collins syndrome with choanal atresia: a case report and review of disease features. Braz J Otorhinolaryngol. 2005;71(1):107–10. https://doi.org/10.1016/s1808-8694(15)31296-9.
2. Atighechi S, Sajadinejad BS, Baradaranfar MH, Dadgarnia MH, Shahbazian H. Caudal extension graft versus columellar strut with plumping graft for acute nasolabial angle correction in rhinoplasty surgery. Eur Arch Otorhinolaryngol. 2015;272(7):1673–7. https://doi.org/10.1007/s00405-014-3218-9.
3. Azizzadeh B. Master techniques in rhinoplasty. Philadelphia: Elsevier/Saunders; 2011.
4. Cobb AR, Green B, Gill D, Ayliffe P, Lloyd TW, Bulstrode N, Dunaway DJ. The surgical management of Treacher Collins syndrome. Br J Oral Maxillofac Surg. 2014;52(7):581–9. https://doi.org/10.1016/j.bjoms.2014.02.007.
5. Farkas LG, Posnick JC. Detailed morphometry of the nose in patients with Treacher Collins syndrome. Ann Plast Surg. 1989;22(3):211–9. https://doi.org/10.1097/00000637-198903000-00008.
6. Friedman M, Tanyeri H, Lim JW, Landsberg R, Vaidyanathan K, Caldarelli D. Effect of improved nasal breathing on obstructive sleep apnea. Otolaryngol Head Neck Surg. 2000;122(1):71–4. https://doi.org/10.1016/S0194-5998(00)70147-1.
7. Hansen M, Lucarelli MJ, Whiteman DA, Mulliken JB. Treacher Collins syndrome: phenotypic variability in a family including an infant with arhinia and uveal colobomas. Am J Med Genet. 1996;61(1):71–4. https://doi.org/10.1002/(SICI)1096-8628(19960102)61:1<71::AID-AJMG14>3.0.CO;2-T.
8. Kapadia H, Shetye PR, Grayson BH, McCarthy JG. Cephalometric assessment of craniofacial morphology in patients with treacher Collins syndrome. J Craniofac Surg. 2013;24(4):1141–5. https://doi.org/10.1097/SCS.0b013e3182860541.
9. Lekakis G, Hens G, Claes P, Hellings PW. Three-dimensional morphing and its added value in the rhinoplasty consult. Plast Reconstr Surg Glob Open. 2019;7(1):e2063. https://doi.org/10.1097/GOX.0000000000002063.
10. Marston AP, Patel T, Nguyen SA, White DR. Short-term risk factor profile of pediatric Choanal atresia repair using ACS-NSQIP National Database. Ann Otol Rhinol Laryngol. 2019;128(9):855–61. https://doi.org/10.1177/0003489419848457.
11. Moorman-Voestermans K, Vos A. Bilateral choanal atresia in two members of one family. J Pediatr Surg. 1983;18(2):175–6. https://doi.org/10.1016/s0022-3468(83)80546-6.
12. Plomp RG, Bredero-Boelhouwer HH, Joosten KF, Wolvius EB, Hoeve HL, Poublon RM, Mathijssen IM. Obstructive sleep apnoea in Treacher Collins syndrome: prevalence, severity and cause. Int J Oral Maxillofac Surg. 2012;41(6):696–701. https://doi.org/10.1016/j.ijom.2012.01.018.
13. Plomp RG, Mathijssen IM, Moolenburgh SE, van Montfort KA, van der Meulen JJ, Poublon RM. Nasal sequelae of Treacher Collins syndrome. J Plast Reconstr Aesthet Surg. 2015;68(6):771–81. https://doi.org/10.1016/j.bjps.2015.02.029.
14. Posnick JC, Ruiz RL. Treacher Collins syndrome: current evaluation, treatment, and future directions. Cleft Palate Craniofac J. 2000;37(5):434. https://doi.org/10.1597/1545-1569(2000)037<0434:TCSCET>2.0.CO;2.
15. Powell N, Humphreys B. Proportions of the aesthetic face. The American Academy of facial plastic and reconstructive surgery. New York: Thieme-Stratton; 1984.
16. Roberts FG, Pruzansky S, Aduss H. An x-radiocephalometric study of mandibulofacial dysostosis in man. Arch Oral Biol. 1975;20(4):265–81. https://doi.org/10.1016/0003-9969(75)90124-7.
17. Splendore A, Silva EO, Alonso LG, Richieri-Costa A, Alonso N, Rosa A, Carakushanky G, Cavalcanti DP, Brunoni D, Passos-Bueno MR. High mutation detection rate in TCOF1 among Treacher Collins syndrome patients reveals clustering of mutations and 16 novel pathogenic changes. Hum Mutat. 2000;16(4):315–22. https://doi.org/10.1002/1098-1004(200010)16:4<315::AID-HUMU4>3.0.CO;2-H.

18. Teber OA, Gillessen-Kaesbach G, Fischer S, Bohringer S, Albrecht B, Albert A, Arslan-Kirchner M, Haan E, Hagedorn-Greiwe M, Hammans C, Henn W, Hinkel GK, Konig R, Kunstmann E, Kunze J, Neumann LM, Prott EC, Rauch A, Rott HD, Seidel H, Spranger S, Sprengel M, Zoll B, Lohmann DR, Wieczorek D. Genotyping in 46 patients with tentative diagnosis of Treacher Collins syndrome revealed unexpected phenotypic variation. Eur J Hum Genet. 2004;12(11):879–90. https://doi.org/10.1038/sj.ejhg.5201260.
19. Teissier N, Kaguelidou F, Couloigner V, Francois M, Van Den Abbeele T. Predictive factors for success after transnasal endoscopic treatment of choanal atresia. Arch Otolaryngol Head Neck Surg. 2008;134(1):57–61. https://doi.org/10.1001/archoto.2007.20.
20. Thompson JT, Anderson PJ, David DJ. Treacher Collins syndrome: protocol management from birth to maturity. J Craniofac Surg. 2009;20(6):2028–35. https://doi.org/10.1097/SCS.0b013e3181be8788.
21. Versnel SL, Duivenvoorden HJ, Passchier J, Mathijssen IM. Satisfaction with facial appearance and its determinants in adults with severe congenital facial disfigurement: a case-referent study. J Plast Reconstr Aesthet Surg. 2010;63(10):1642–9. https://doi.org/10.1016/j.bjps.2009.10.018.
22. Versnel SL, Plomp RG, Passchier J, Duivenvoorden HJ, Mathijssen IM. Long-term psychological functioning of adults with severe congenital facial disfigurement. Plast Reconstr Surg. 2012;129(1):110–7. https://doi.org/10.1097/PRS.0b013e3182361f64.
23. Vincent M, Genevieve D, Ostertag A, Marlin S, Lacombe D, Martin-Coignard D, Coubes C, David A, Lyonnet S, Vilain C, Dieux-Coeslier A, Manouvrier S, Isidor B, Jacquemont ML, Julia S, Layet V, Naudion S, Odent S, Pasquier L, Pelras S, Philip N, Pierquin G, Prieur F, Aboussair N, Attie-Bitach T, Baujat G, Blanchet P, Blanchet C, Dollfus H, Doray B, Schaefer E, Edery P, Giuliano F, Goldenberg A, Goizet C, Guichet A, Herlin C, Lambert L, Leheup B, Martinovic J, Mercier S, Mignot C, Moutard ML, Perez MJ, Pinson L, Puechberty J, Willems M, Randrianaivo H, Szakszon K, Toutain A, Verloes A, Vigneron J, Sanchez E, Sarda P, Laplanche JL, Collet C. Treacher Collins syndrome: a clinical and molecular study based on a large series of patients. Genet Med. 2016;18(1):49–56. https://doi.org/10.1038/gim.2015.29.

Chapter 26
An Overview of Treatment Recommendations for the Treacher Collins Syndrome Patient

David M. Yates and Sediqua Bufford

Introduction

Similar to craniofacial microsomia described in Section 1, Treacher Collins syndrome (TCS) is an entity that affects derivatives of the first and second branchial arches. TCS occurs in 1:50,000 live births and has no gender predilection. Sixty percent of cases of TCS arise from de novo mutations and 40% of cases are familial (40%) [1, 2] (Table 26.1).

Etiology and Pathogenesis

TCS most commonly results from a mutation in the treacle ribosome biogenesis factor 1 (TCOF1) gene which leads to a defective treacle protein resulting in mass apoptosis (death) of the neural crest cells. These neural crest progenitor cells are responsible for the creation of the craniofacial bones, tissues, and structures residing within the first and second branchial arches. The first, or mandibular, branchial arch gives rise to the muscles of mastication, stylohyoid, anterior belly of the digastric, tensor tympani, and tensor veli palatini muscles, the malleus, incus, and Meckel's cartilage, as well as the third division of the trigeminal nerve (V3). The

D. M. Yates (✉)
Division of Cranial and Facial Surgery, El Paso Children's Hospital, El Paso, TX, USA

Paul Foster School of Medicine El Paso, El Paso, TX, USA

Oral and Maxillofacial Surgery, University of Texas Health Sciences Center, San Antonio, TX, USA
e-mail: yates@hdofs.com

S. Bufford
Morehouse School of Medicine, Atlanta, GA, USA

D. M. Yates, M. R. Markiewicz (eds.), *Craniofacial Microsomia and Treacher Collins Syndrome*, https://doi.org/10.1007/978-3-030-84733-3_26

Table 26.1 Treacher Collins Associated Deformities

Associated facial deformity	Incidence in Treacher Collins patients
Malar hypoplasia	100%
Ocular manifestations	
Eyelid deformities	
Downslanting palpebral fissures	Common
Colobomas	50–89%
Hypoplastic lower eyelid	96%
Absence of eyelashes on medial portion of lower lid Dacrostenosis	Pathognomonic. Common
Ophthalmic features	
Strabismus	Common
Vision loss	37%
Amblyopia	33%
Anisometropia	17%
Refractive errors	58%
Ear deformity	
Outer ear/auricle	
Microtia	78–85%
Preauricular tag	30–40%
Preauricular tongue of hair	Common
External auditory canal atresia/stenosis.	54–78%
Deformed tympanic membranes.	22–31%
Middle ear	
Ossicular malformations/hypoplasia of the middle ear	22–67%
Inner ear - Generally preserved in TCS	
Conductive hearing loss	96%
Sensorineural hearing loss	7%
Oral complex	
Macrostomia Clefting of secondary palate Dental anomalies Tooth agenesis Enamel deformities Malposition of max first Mol Hypoplastic and retropositioned tongue Micrognathia	15% 36% 60% 60% 20% 13% Common 78–89%
Nasal deformity	
Choanal atresia Dorsal hump External nasal deviation Bulbous or bifid nasal tip Under-rotation of nasal tip Narrow alar base Septal deviation	Variable (28%) 73% 55% 55% 36% Common 82%

Table 26.1 (continued)

Associated facial deformity	Incidence in Treacher Collins patients
Soft tissue deficiencies	
Preauricular region Temporal fossa region Parotid dysgenesis	Variable Variable 48%
Cranial base abnormalities	Basilar kyphosis – reduction in cranial base Abnormal head shape –not associated with cranial synostosis
Cardiac anomalies	12% needed major cardiovascular surgery
Other findings	
Normal to above average intelligence Sleep apnea (generally obstructive)	Majority of TCS patients 46–100%
Anomalies of kidneys, limb, calvarium, brain, cryptorchidism	Rare

[2–22]

second, or hyoid, branchial arch provides the muscles of facial expression, stapedius, stylohyoid, and posterior belly of the digastric muscle, as well as the stapes, styloid cartilage, lesser cornu of the hyoid bone, and Reichert's cartilage, and the facial (VII) nerve. This occurs within the first 5–8 weeks of fetal development. For a thorough discussion on this topic, please refer to Chap. 13 under the Treacher Collins section of this book.

Clinical Features

The clinical features of TCS result from a hypoplasia of the orbits, midface, mandible, ears, skull base, and soft tissues of the face (Figs. 26.1a–c and 26.2a–d). More specifically, orbito-malar/zygomatic arch hypoplasia is present in all patients with TCS. This results in a more inferior position of the lateral canthus and thereby the hallmark downslanting of the palpebral fissures. Coloboma, a structural defect of the eyelid or the eye that appears as a cleft in the lid margin or the iris, while not present in every case, is highly specific for TCS. Lacrimal system anomalies are also common with atresia of the lacrimal puncta and cannaliculi being typical. The mandible is also a prominent feature of the phenotype with characteristic micrognathia that features marked antegonial notching and a steep mandibular plane. The TMJ may also be hypoplastic and/or dysplastic. The ears are typically bilaterally involved with microtia/anotia, atresia of the auditory canal, and anomalous middle ear ossicles leading to a bilateral conductive hearing loss. Also common are preauricular skin tags and preauricular hair displacement. Less common features include cleft palate, maxillary hypoplasia, and an over-projected nasal dorsum. Intelligence is usually normal in affected individuals. For a thorough discussion on this topic, please refer to Chap. 14 from which the above excerpt was taken.

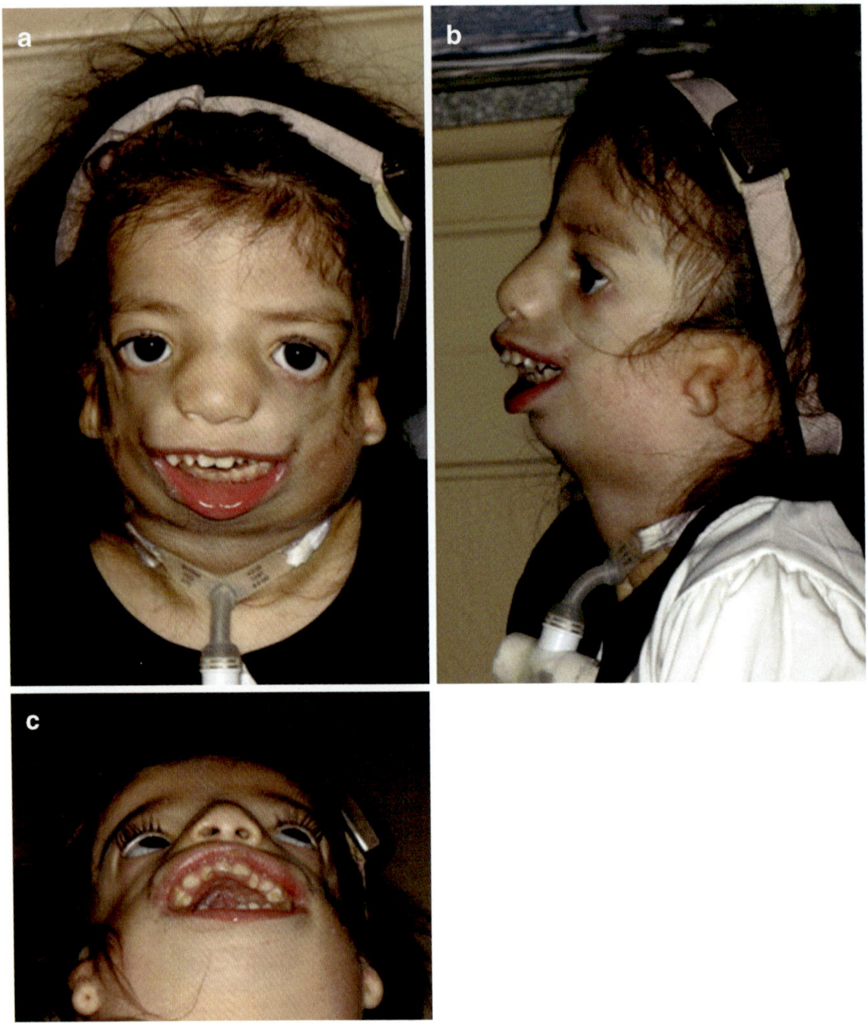

Fig. 26.1 Typical Facies of Severe Treacher Collins Syndrome. Treacher Collins syndrome – (**a**) frontal view, (**b**) profile view, (**c**) worm's-eye view (child with severe Treacher Collins syndrome demonstrating severe mandibular retrognathia (Kaban III), Grade III microtia, zygomatic hypoplasia, macrostomia, cleft palate, downslanting palpebral fissures, coloboma, absence of eyelashes medial third of eyelid, preauricular extending tongue of hair) [22]

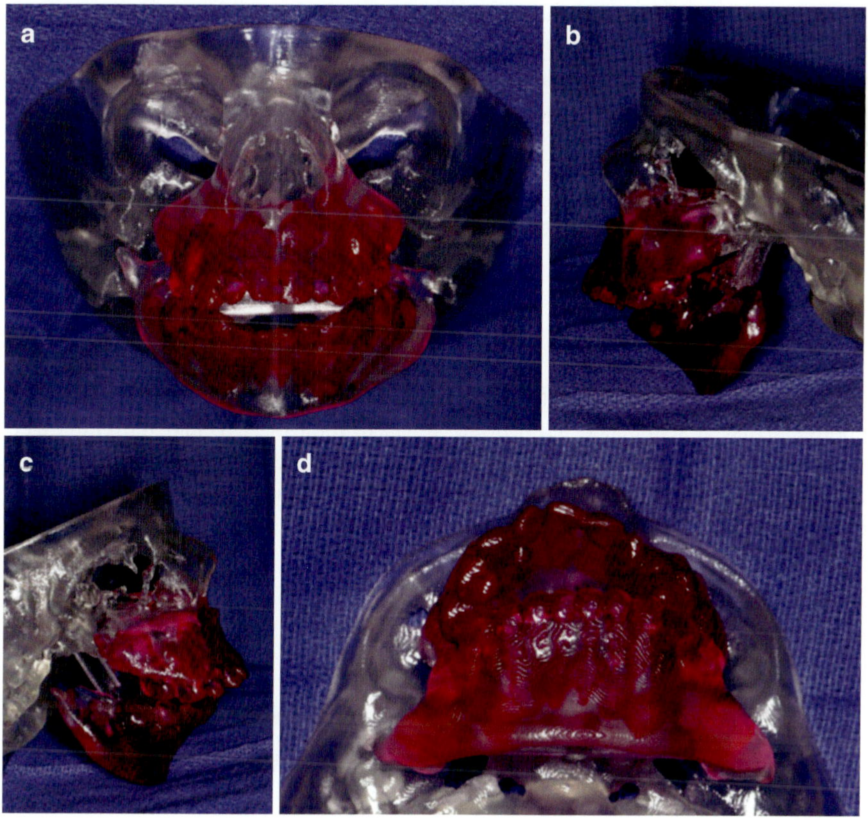

Fig. 26.2 Model Skull Severe Treacher Collins Phenotype. Kaban Type III mandible (**a**) frontal view, (**b**) left profile view, (**c**) right profile view, (**d**) worm's eye view (Demonstrates the skeletal features of TCS including the clockwise rotation of the facial skeleton contributing factors include: mandibular retrognathia, hypoplasia of the bilateral mandibular ramus, condyle, and glenoid fossa, zygomatic arch aplasia with associated orbital and skull base deformities.) [22]

Functional Concerns

These anatomical aberrations lead to a myriad of functional concerns, which must be considered during the initial evaluation of a newborn with suspected TCS. The micrognathia may result in airway obstruction, feeding, and swallowing problems. The orbito-malar hypoplasia combined with colobomas of the eyelids may result in exposure keratopathy and visual disturbances. The auricular and ossicular anomalies typically lead to a bilateral conductive hearing loss which jeopardizes normal speech and language development. As the child grows, these functional concerns will need to be monitored and interventions timed and planned so as to minimize morbidity and treatment burden and maximize benefit. Long-term dependence on tracheostomies and gastrostomies are not infrequent and often the focus of these interventions. Speech and language development must be monitored along with hearing. Jaw function should be observed as well for the impact of malocclusions and limitations in mouth opening. Neuropsychological monitoring is essential to support psychological and mental development and to identify any cognitive delays or deficits [7]. For a thorough discussion on this topic, please refer to Chap. 3 under the Treacher Collins section of this book.

Treatment Guidelines

It is important to understand that treatment of TCS requires a multidisciplinary approach that is sequenced appropriately based upon the age and individualized needs of the patient. The craniofacial team evaluating these patients should include a pediatric otolaryngologist, ophthalmologist, geneticist, audiologist, a speech pathologist, cranio-maxillo-facial surgeon, orthodontist, social worker, neuropsychologist, pediatric dentist, and care coordinator. Airway, nutrition, ocular concerns, speech, and hearing are generally the most critical and recurrent needs in this patient population. At every appointment, these areas should be addressed.

Guiding Principles:

1. *Regular multidisciplinary craniofacial team evaluation.*
2. *In general, reducing the number of surgeries during active growth will result in better functional and cosmetic outcomes (do not burn bridges).*
3. *Ensuring that the patient is supported and able to feed, hear, and speak as soon as physically possible is critical to overall success.*
4. *Providing appropriate social and psychological support systems for the child as they develop emotionally and physically.*

Prenatal Evaluation (Second-Third Trimester)

Diagnosis of at-risk families or suspected fetuses may be accomplished by chorionic villus sampling. It is critical to determine the extent of mandibular retrognathia/micrognathia prior to delivery to prevent poor airway outcomes at birth. 3D-4D sonographic imaging may be used to demonstrate a decreased inferior facial angle (IFA). The IFA is a reliable predictor of retrognathia as measured on ultrasound (US). It is measured by taking the intersection of two lines: (1) a line perpendicular to the vertical part of the forehead, drawn at the level of the nasal and frontal bone suture, and (2) a line from the tip of the menton and the anterior border of the more protrusive lip. An IFA of >2 standard deviations from normal (65.5 degrees) corresponds with an angle of <50 degrees and is a reliable indicator for retrognathia. Of neonates presenting with micrognathia, 54% require immediate airway support from simple positioning to tracheotomy. If concern exists for severe micrognathia based on an IFA, an ex utero intrapartum treatment (EXIT) procedure should be ready to be performed at birth.

Airway

At birth if the inferior facial angle (IFA) < 50 degrees on prenatal US, prepare for an EXIT procedure (Fig. 26.3a, b). If IFA > 50 degrees, EXIT procedure is likely unnecessary, but it is recommended to have an airway specialist present at birth. Immediate helpful interventions may include prone positioning, placement of a nasal trumpet, or an oral airway with use of supplemental oxygen therapy. Should these interventions fail to provide relief, a tongue stitch or intubation may be required. Upon initial examination, if the patient is unable to maintain their airway and a severe mandibular deformity is present (Kaban IIB or III), consider tracheotomy. If the mandible is a Kaban I or IIa and the patient's airway is unable to be maintained, judicious mandibular distraction may be considered. It is noted that

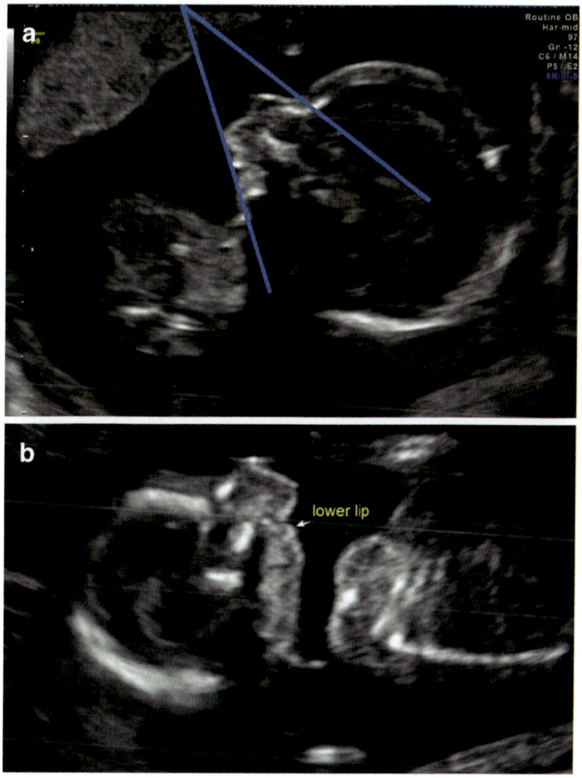

Fig. 26.3 Severe Micrognathia Noted on US in TCS Fetus (**a**) Mid-sagittal view of prenatal ultrasound demonstrating severe micrognathia and inferior facial angle (IFA) of 20 degrees. (**b**) Severe micrognathia – mid-sagittal view – prenatal ultrasound

mandibular distraction in Treacher Collins patients is much less reliable than in the straightforward Pierre Robin sequence population. This is likely secondary to the U-shaped mandible often present and the lack of mandibular stop secondary to a hypoplastic cranial base in the region of the glenoid fossa (Fig. 26.4a, b). TCS patients may also have choanal atresia which may contribute to their airway distress; if present, surgical correction is performed. Useful exams to determine the

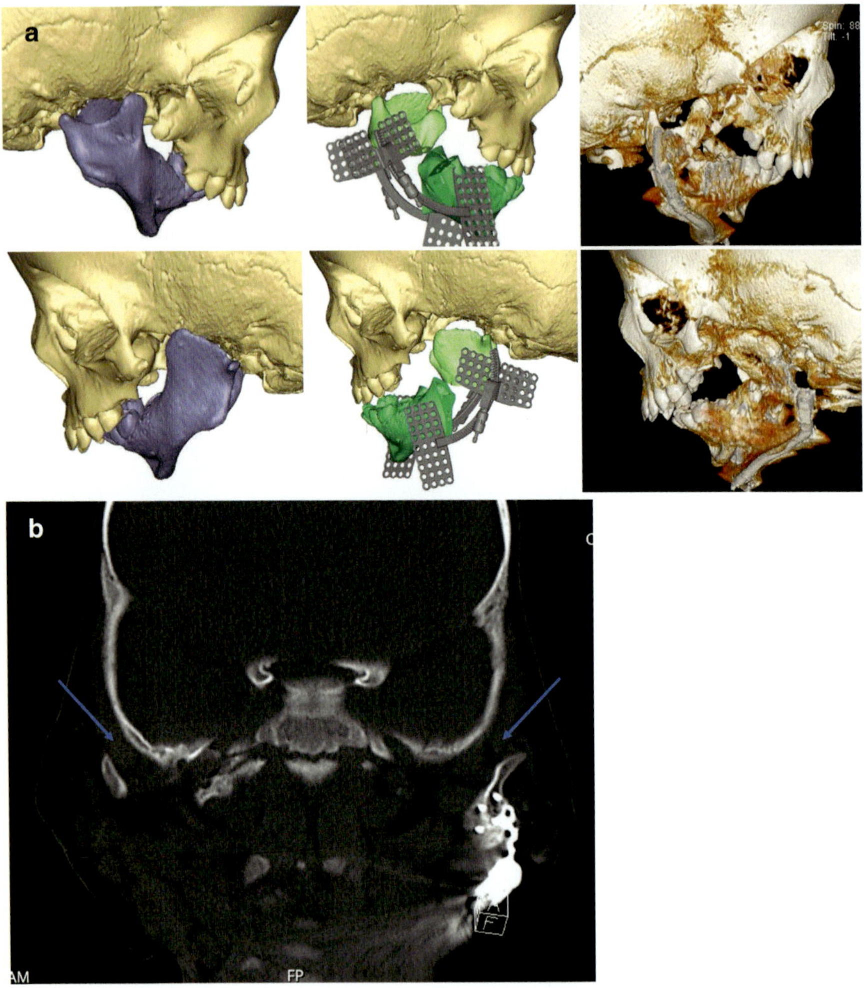

Fig. 26.4 Failed Mandibular Distraction in Kaban III Mandible (**a**) Far left images – preoperative position of the mandible prior to distraction Kaban III mandible (severe malformation of ramus, condyle, and glenoid fossa). Center images – virtual surgical plan (VSP) demonstrates projected mandibular position after 25 mm of curvilinear distraction. Far right images – actual postoperative position after 25 mm of curvilinear distraction differs greatly from projected mandibular position resulting in suboptimal mandibular projection. (**b**) Glenoid fossa atrophic, unable to achieve condylar stop resulting in distraction of proximal segment lateral to the cranial base. This resulted in suboptimal projection of the mandible. Despite 25 mm of curvilinear distraction, only about 2–5 mm of anterior mandibular pogonion projection is obtained

extent of the mandibular and airway deformity include CT maxillofacial, nasendoscopy, and polysomnography. For a thorough discussion on this topic, please refer to Chap. 15 under the Treacher Collins section of this book.

During infancy and early childhood, obstructive sleep apnea signs and symptoms warrant evaluation with polysomnography. The craniofacial team may consider judicious mandibular distraction if necessary. It is important to minimize mandibular surgeries – final cosmetic and functional outcome depends upon this principle. Tracheotomy may be considered if worsening airway concerns are present which are not able to be addressed with mandibular distraction, tonsillectomy, or other effective surgical treatment.

In late childhood if a tracheostomy is present, consider mandibular reconstruction to obtain decannulation if possible. It is emphasized that mandibular reconstruction at this age is avoided when possible. Only airway concerns legitimize mandibular surgery at this time (Fig. 26.5). TMJ and ramus reconstruction can be achieved with costochondral grafting >9–10 years of age. Additionally, early (prior to skeletal maturity) TMJ alloplastic reconstruction may be considered. Judicious mandibular distraction may also be used to augment mandibular growth.

Once skeletal maturity is reached, definitive maxillomandibular surgery is performed which will provide adequate airway support. It is recommended to have a yearly PSG since TCS patients represent an at-risk population.

Speech/Nutrition

During the initial evaluation at birth, it is critical for speech/nutrition to be an active part of the team evaluating these patients. Due to the often-present significant mandibular retrognathia, it is common for patients with TCS to aspirate when feeding, and many will suffer from failure to thrive. Adequate nutrition is key in promoting physical development. In the neonatal period, bedside and videofluoroscopic swallow studies may be performed, and a PEG is placed if the child is unable to maintain appropriate nutrition.

During infancy, cleft palate repair may be considered and should be performed ideally by 18 months of age. However, airway concerns must also be taken into account prior to repair. The use of Sign language is encouraged in this population and careful attention to the child's growth curve during this period are encouraged.

During early childhood, speech is encouraged, and if tracheostomy dependent, the use of a Passy Muir is advised. The child continues speech therapy and is encouraged in the use of sign language. Growth is carefully monitored under the care of a nutritionist on the craniofacial team.

In late childhood and adolescence, speech therapy is maximized, the use of sign language is encouraged as needed, and the child may be a candidate for additional speech surgeries for palatal lengthening/function which may include buccinator flaps, pharyngeal flaps, or sphincter pharyngoplasty. Prior to any speech surgery, a polysomnogram should be performed to ensure that sleep apnea is appropriately managed and not worsened.

By skeletal maturity, speech should be optimized.

For a thorough discussion on this topic, please refer to Chap. 15 under the Treacher Collins section of this book.

Hearing/Microtia

At birth a hearing evaluation is performed. Since the majority of TCS patients have significant bilateral conductive hearing loss, diagnosis and treatment are critical to ensuring appropriate cognitive speech development. Removable BAHA softbands

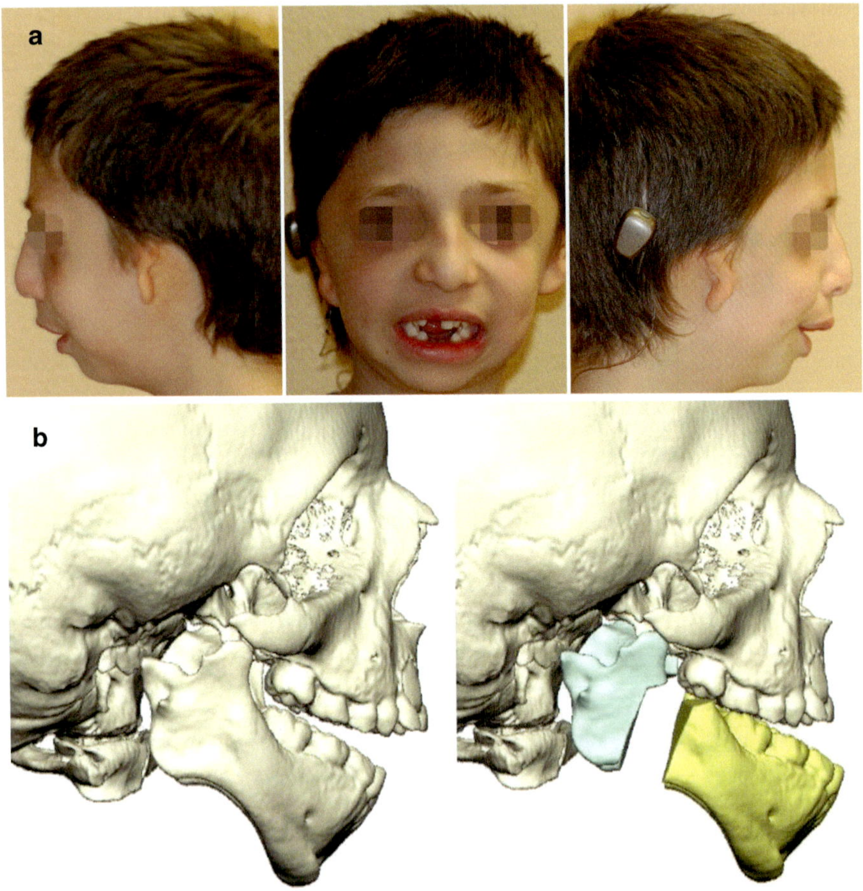

Fig. 26.5 Mandibular Distraction for Worsening Sleep Apnea (**a**) Patient presents with TCS and worsening sleep apnea. No history of mandibular surgery. (**b**) Virtual surgical plan – Kaban IIa mandible – mandibular distraction 20 mm. (**c**) Preop and postop photos of patient before and after mandibular distraction which resulted in resolving of sleep apnea symptoms

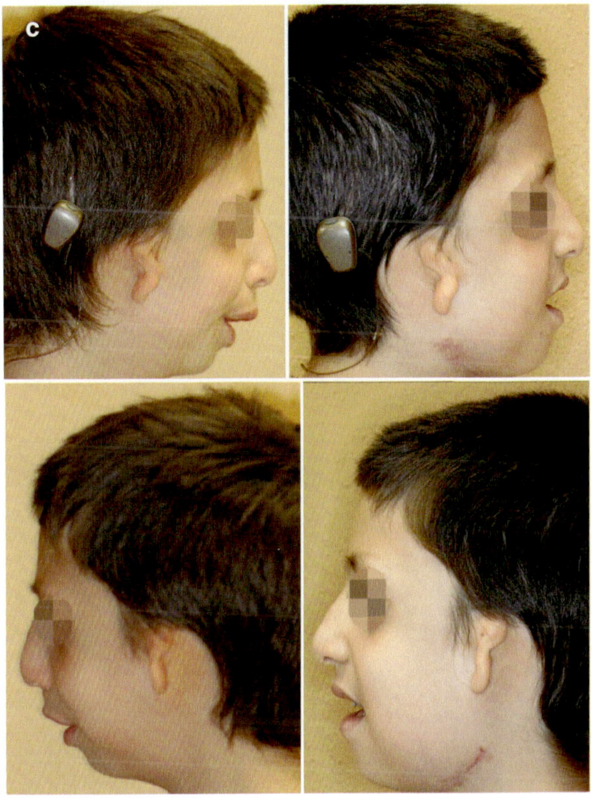

Fig. 26.5 (continued)

may be fitted by 3 months of age, and evaluation by the craniofacial team, audiology, and ENT is critical.

During infancy, it is critical to encourage use of the BAHA headband; yearly audiological testing and excision of ear tags may be considered.

Childhood interventions may include Medpor reconstruction of microtia (3–10 years of age) and surgical placement of a BAHA once temporal bone thickness is adequate. If the family desires autogenous rib reconstruction for microtia, this may be done around 10 years of age and is dependent on the development of the thoracic rib cartilage. Prosthetic ear reconstruction may be performed once temporal bone thickness is adequate for osseointegrated implants (usually 6 years of age to adulthood) (Fig. 26.6a–c). Yearly evaluation by the craniofacial team, audiology, and ENT remains critical.

Once skeletal maturity is obtained, maintenance of ear reconstruction and yearly audiological testing is encouraged. For a thorough discussion on this topic, please refer to Chaps. 23 and 24 under the Treacher Collins section of this book.

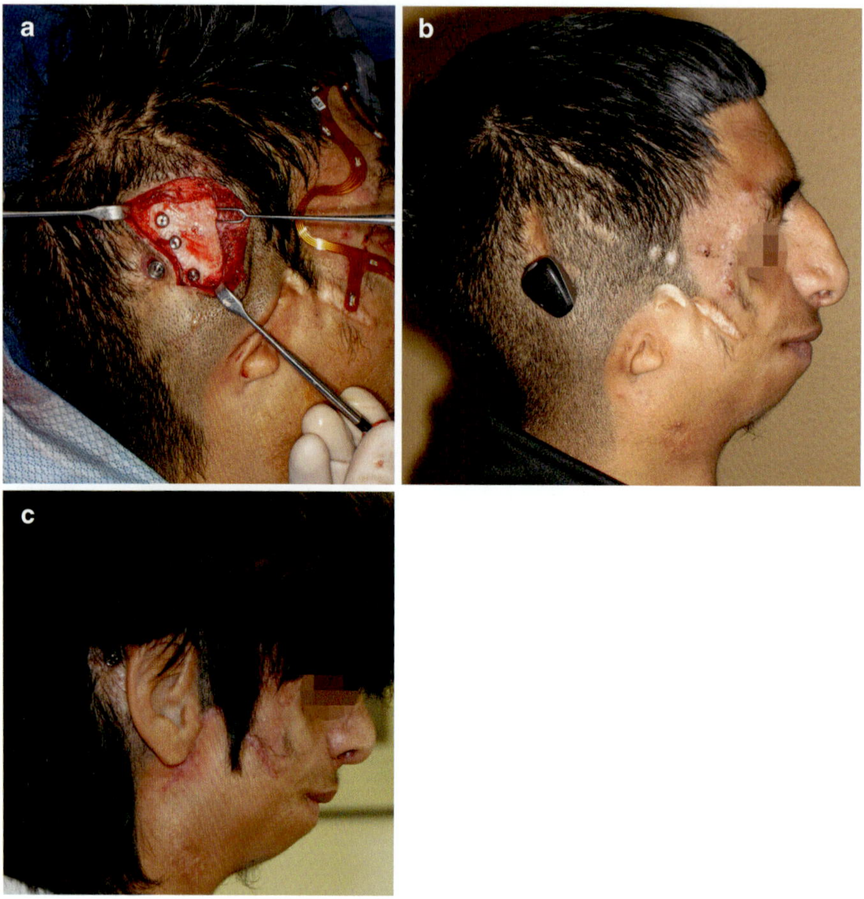

Fig. 26.6 Placement of Implants for Prosthetic Ear Reconstruction (**a**) Placement of implants for prosthetic ear reconstruction – note presence of BAHA posteriorly. Placement of cranial implants can be difficult in this population due to hypoplastic temporal bone. Real-time navigation is recommended. (**b**) Patient before removal of ear tag and placement of cranial implants for prosthetic ear reconstruction. (**c**) Patient after completion and placement of prosthetic ear

Orbito/Ocular

At birth the patient is evaluated to ensure that they are able to achieve appropriate lid closure thus providing sufficient corneal protection. If they are unable to self-protect their cornea due to the presence of a hypoplastic lower lid/coloboma, lubrication and/or a temporary tarsorrhaphy is performed. Pediatric ophthalmology evaluation is performed at birth and yearly.

During infancy (6–9 months), coloboma reconstruction is undertaken for large defects to ensure corneal protection. A lateral canthoplasty may also be undertaken at this time. Visual rehabilitation and, if needed, epibulbar dermoid excision may be performed if the child is symptomatic.

During late infancy (12–24 months), consider strabismus surgery, lacrimal drainage surgery, and continue visual rehabilitation.

Preschool-age children may undergo coloboma reconstruction of small to moderate defects, lateral canthoplasty, and ptosis repair.

In school-age children, one may consider all of the above surgeries and revisions, as well as orbitozygomatic reconstruction – which is generally performed using either malar implants or cranial bone (Figs. 26.7a–d and 26.8a–c).

Once adulthood/skeletal maturity is reached, revisional surgeries may be performed as needed. Fat grafting around the orbits is frequently helpful in softening the appearance of the reconstructed orbitozygomatic complex.

For a thorough discussion on this topic, please refer to Chaps. 17 and 18 under the Treacher Collins section of this book.

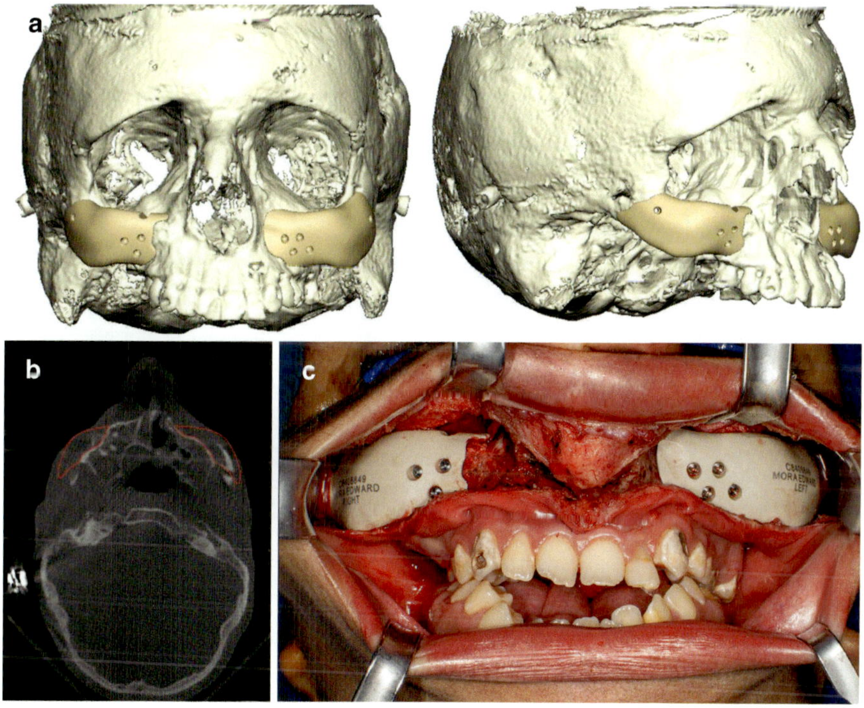

Fig. 26.7 Orbito-Malar-Zygomatic Reconstruction Using PEEK Implants (**a**) Virtual surgical plan – malar (PEEK) implant placement for zygomatic reconstruction. (**b**) Red outline indicates proposed area for placement of malar implants. (**c**) Malar implants being placed through a transoral vestibular incision

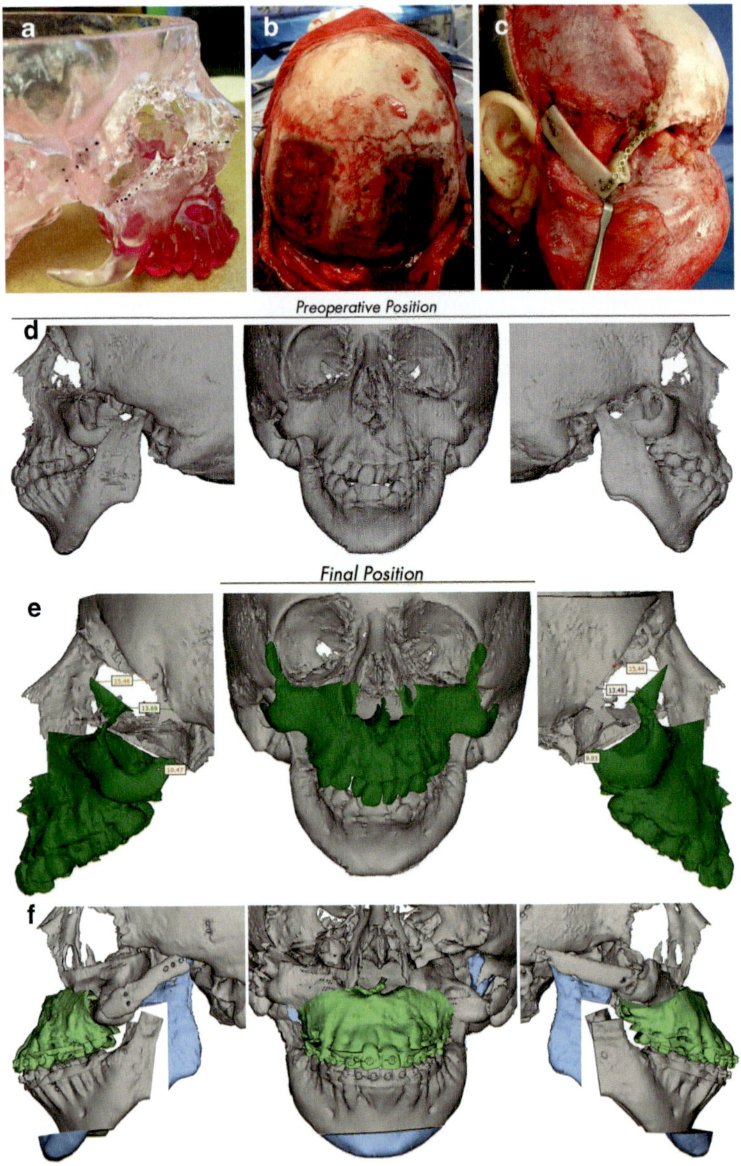

Fig. 26.8 Staged Maxillo-Mandibular Reconstruction (**a**–**c**) Modified LeFort III (Kufner) osteotomy for midface advancement with simultaneous reconstruction of zygomatic complex with cranial bone and fibula allograft. (**d**) Preoperative mature Treacher Collins deformity: note deficient midface and zygomas, clockwise rotation of maxillomandibular complex with steep occlusal and mandibular planes, Kaban IIa mandible (deficient ramus with loss of height, but glenoid fossa and condylar stop present). (**e**) First stage of reconstruction – Kufner osteotomy (modified LeFort III) with advancement of maxilla and inferior orbital rims to aid in reducing scleral show, bone grafting with calvarial bone, and for reconstruction of the zygoma. (**f**) Second stage of reconstruction – LeFort 1 osteotomy and bilateral sagittal split ramus osteotomy (BSSO) with counterclockwise rotation and genioplasty. Pogonion moved anteriorly >33 mm. (**g**) Demonstrating preoperative position as compared to postoperative position – mild relapse noted

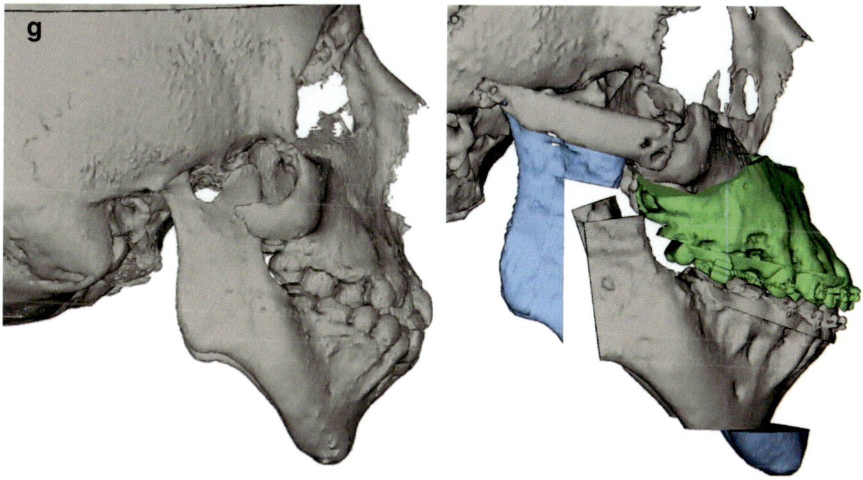

Fig. 26.8 (continued)

Dental/Orthodontic

Children with TCS are at a much higher risk of dental caries secondary to parotid dysgenesis, ectopic eruption, and dental malformations. We recommend regular establishment of a dental home at the eruption of the first primary tooth with regular visits every 3–6 months.

Orthodontic care is established at the first craniofacial team visit, and the patient is regularly followed. During the mixed dentition period, maxillary expansion is frequently needed to correct posterior cross bites and establish compatible arch forms. At this time, a limited phase of orthodontic treatment may be undertaken to facilitate eruption of permanent teeth and correct traumatic occlusions.

Once permanent dentition is in place, comprehensive orthodontic therapy is undertaken – many times in conjunction with orthognathic surgery. Careful planning and combined decision-making are required between the cranio-maxillo-facial surgeon and the orthodontist.

For a thorough discussion on this topic, please refer to Chap. 22 under the Treacher Collins section of this book.

Soft Tissue Concerns

Tessier VII clefting resulting in macrostomia is frequently present in TCS patients. Correction is undertaken less frequently than in patients with CFM, likely due to the bilateral nature of clefting in the TCS patient population and the lack of eye-catching asymmetry.

Fat grafting around the orbits is frequently helpful in softening the appearance of the reconstructed orbito-malar-zygomatic complex.

Maxillomandibular Treatment

Mandibular management is critical in the reconstruction of TCS patients. Treatment protocols vary based upon age and stage of dental development. The specific surgical techniques, methods, and materials vary with the severity of the individual deformity but may involve orthodontic intervention, orthognathic surgical procedures, distraction osteogenesis (DO), and TMJ reconstruction with costochondral grafting, vascularized flaps (e.g., fibula), or alloplastic joint replacement. In general, reducing the number of procedures performed will result in a more cosmetic and functional final outcome.

The first decision is made prenatally. If there is a family history of TCS, the mother should be under the care of a maternal fetal medicine doctor, and during sonographic exams, the inferior facial angle (IFA) is calculated (Fig. 26.3a, b). If the IFA is less than 50 degrees, an EXIT procedure is planned. If greater than 50 degrees, likely the baby will not require an emergency airway – however, an airway specialist is present at delivery ready to intervene if necessary. Likely, conservative measures (i.e., prone positioning, nasal trumpet, oral airway, or a tongue stitch) will be sufficient to maintain the airway.

Upon initial examination, if the patient is unable to maintain their airway and a severe mandibular deformity is present (Kaban IIB or III), consider tracheotomy. If the mandible is a Kaban I or IIa and the patient's airway is unable to be maintained, judicious mandibular distraction may be considered. It is noted that mandibular distraction in Treacher Collins patients is much less reliable than in the straightforward Pierre Robin sequence population. This is likely secondary to the U-shaped mandible often present and the lack of mandibular stop secondary to a hypoplastic cranial base in the region of the glenoid fossa (Fig. 26.4a, b).

During the preschool- and early-school-age years, attention is directed toward maintaining healthy dentition. Due to their deformity and difficulty with oral hygiene, as well as parotid dysgenesis, TCS patients are at a greater risk of dental caries. Occasionally, additional distraction versus tracheostomy is needed as the child continues to grow if struggling with progressive sleep apnea and/or other manifestations of hypoxia.

School-age children (9–14 years) may be candidates for TMJ and mandibular ramus reconstruction. Judicious mandibular distraction may be performed only if airway/sleep apnea demands it. Reconstruction with costochondral grafts or "early" (prior to skeletal maturity) TMJ alloplastic reconstruction may be considered for Kaban/Pruzansky Types IIB and III.

Once skeletal maturity is reached, the maxillomandibular complex may be addressed in its totality. In mild cases, a LeFort I/bilateral sagittal split ramus osteotomy with counterclockwise rotation may be all that is needed for surgical success. In moderate to severe cases, additional considerations need to be taken into account. Key to successful reconstruction is building off a stable temporomandibular joint complex. In severe cases, this may be achieved with successful costochondral grafting bilaterally or with the placement of alloplastic temporomandibular joints. Once TMJ stability has been achieved, significant counterclockwise rotation of the maxillomandibular complex must occur. The midface deformity, steep mandibular plane angle, and severe retrognathia must be addressed (Fig. 26.9). This has been done with the combination of a Kufner osteotomy (Modified LeFort III) followed by a LeFort I in the maxilla and inverted L plus a genioplasty in the mandible (Fig. 26.8d–g). It may also be accomplished with a LeFort III osteotomy/mandibular osteotomies followed by counterclockwise distraction.

The maxilla/mandibular maxillomandibular instead of maxilla/mandibular deformity associated with TCS is among the most difficult issues confronted in their complex care. Key treatment concepts include (1) maintenance of the airway and monitoring of sleep apnea, (2) reducing the number of maxillomandibular surgeries performed which will result in an improved final cosmetic and functional outcome, and (3) successful reconstruction being dependent on building off a stable temporomandibular joint complex.

For a thorough discussion on this topic, please refer to Chaps. 19–21 under the Treacher Collins section of this book.

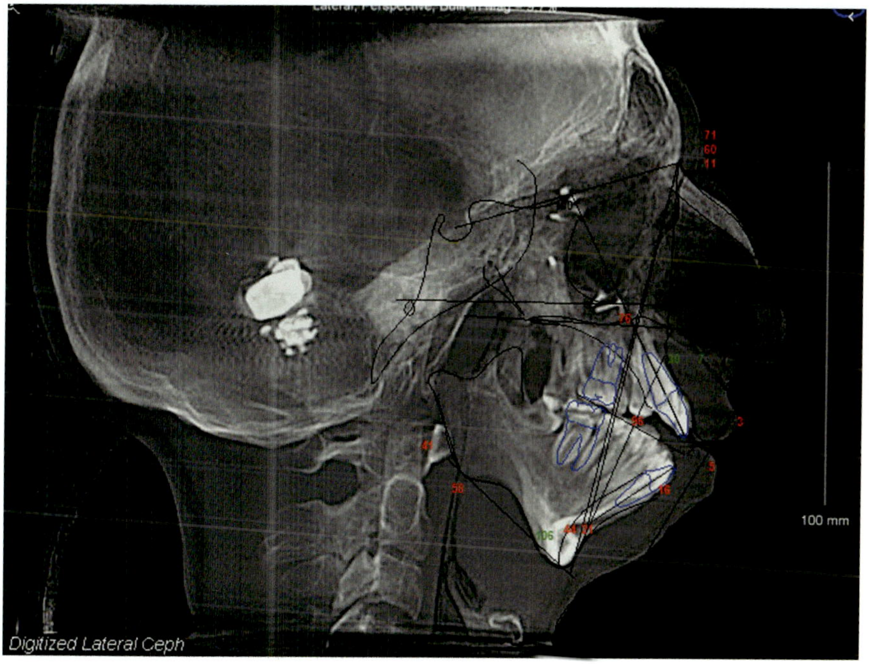

Fig. 26.9 Cephalometric Radiograph Demonstrating Classic Findings in TCS Cephalometric radiograph demonstrating maxillary deficiency, severe mandibular retrognathia, steep occlusal and mandibular plane angle, condylar hypoplasia, generalized clockwise rotation of the maxillomandibular apparatus

Nasal Deformity

TCS characteristically presents with a constricted nasal airway and may present at birth with choanal atresia. Useful exams to determine the extent of the nasal deformity include attempted passage of a 5 French orogastric tube through nasal cavity, nasendoscopy, and CT maxillofacial. If choanal atresia is present, surgical correction is performed.

The typical nasal deformity seen in TCS includes septal deviation, prominent dorsal hump, nasal tip ptosis, bulbous tip, external tip deviation, and a narrowed alar base (Fig. 26.10a, b). Definitive nasoseptorhinoplasty is performed at the cessation

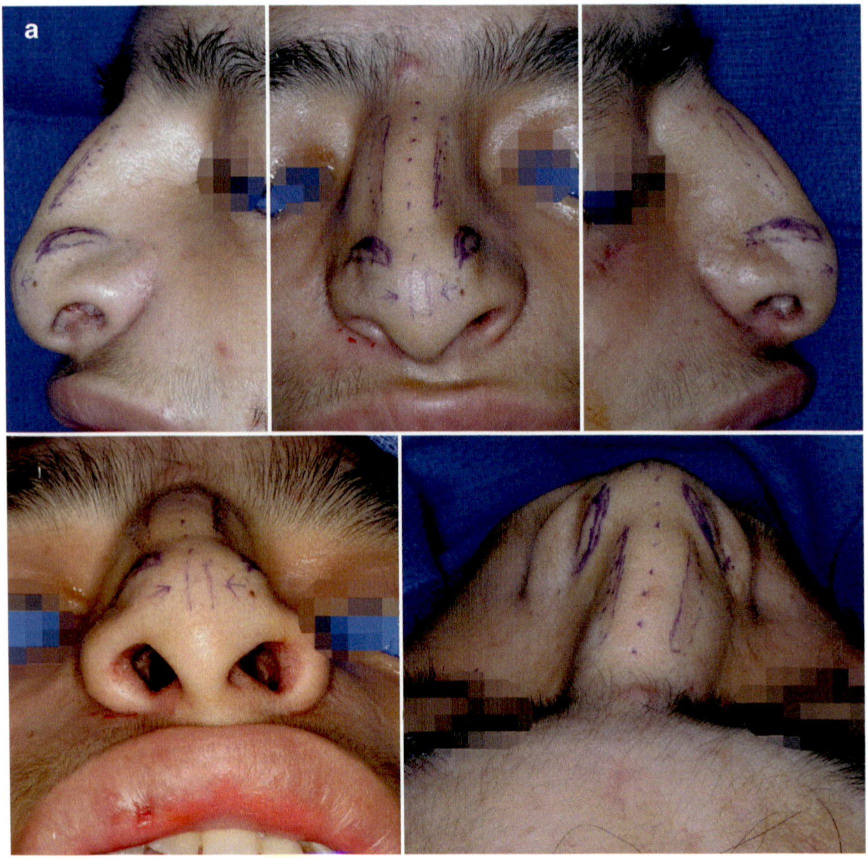

Fig. 26.10 The Treacher Collins Nasal Deformity (**a**) Treacher Collins nasal deformity: deviated dorsum, dorsal hump, deviated nasal septum, bulbous tip, acute nasolabial angle, constricted alar base. (**b**) Procedure performed: nasal osteotomies, dorsal hump reduction, resection and reconstruction of septum using autologous cartilage, spreader grafts using allograft rib, cephalic trim, tip-defining sutures

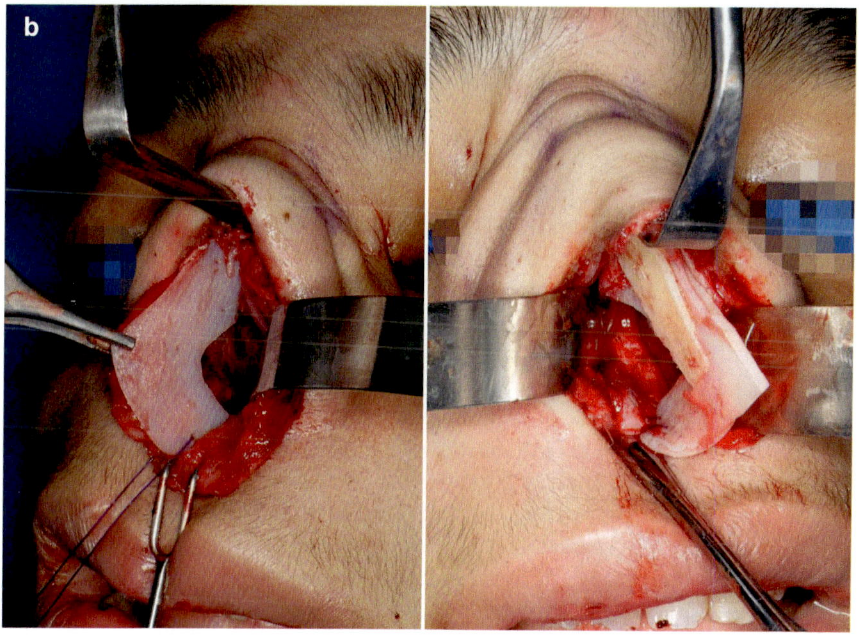

Fig. 26.10 (continued)

of nasal growth and ideally after completion of midface advancement as early as 14 years of age in female patients and 15 years of age in males.

For a thorough discussion on this topic, please refer to Chap. 25 under the Treacher Collins section of this book.

Conclusions

It must be recognized that there is no complete consensus on diagnosis and/or management of TCS. Therefore, evidence-based decisions are difficult; often decisions are based upon the existing low-level evidence and/or the individual practitioner's experience. There is certainly controversy about the preferred treatments and timing. Standardizing treatment algorithms is difficult due to the varying severity of phenotypes present. Individualized treatment planning in the team setting is the most ideal while adhering to certain guiding principles.

Guiding Principles:

1. *Regular craniofacial team evaluation.*
2. *In general, reducing the number of surgeries during active growth will result in better functional and cosmetic outcomes.*

3. *Ensuring that the patient is supported and able to feed, hear, and speak as soon as physically possible is critical to overall success.*
4. *Providing appropriate social and psychological support systems for the child as they develop emotionally and physically.*

Case Studies:

1. This case study importantly illustrates the value of appropriate treatment planning and how it can save lives, prevent unpleasant experiences for patients and their families, and ensure that care is delivered in the correct treatment environment.

   Term infant with prenatal care – not referred for EXIT procedure though inferior facial angle is clearly <50 degrees corresponding to severe mandibular hypoplasia. Patient was born without any planning for an EXIT procedure. Neonatologist present at birth immediately identified the life-threatening airway situation. Due to the extreme micrognathia, visualization of the laryngeal cords was not possible. The neonatologist present was unable to intubate; however the baby was able to be ventilated secondary to supraglottic placement of an ET tube nasally and orally (Fig. 26.11a). The patient was immediately transferred via ambulance to the local children's hospital where a pediatric ENT, pediatric OMFS, neonatologist, pediatric anesthesiologist, and pediatric surgeon were all assembled in the operating room (OR). The patient was brought into the OR, and using a rigid pediatric ventilating bronchoscope, a bougie was used to slide past the vocal cords and an endotracheal tube was slid over the bougie to intubate.

   A CT scan was then obtained to determine if the patient was a candidate for mandibular distraction to assist in avoiding a tracheotomy (Fig. 26.11b). Unfortunately, due to the lack of a condylar stop at the temporal bone and the severe hypoplasia of the mandibular condyle/ramus complex, the patient was not a candidate for neonatal mandibular distraction at that time. The patient underwent a successful tracheotomy.
2. A 2-year-old male presented with Treacher Collins syndrome. The patient was hospitalized every month for the preceding 10 months secondary to multiple bouts of aspiration pneumonia. Born full term, he necessitated a NICU stay secondary to breathing and feeding difficulty x 2 weeks in Peru. Swallow study demonstrated aspiration present. Patient was underweight secondary to chronic malnutrition secondary to feeding difficulties. He presented with severe sleep apnea and frequent aspiration when feeding. The patient at this point did not have a g-tube or tracheostomy present and was an excellent candidate for mandibular distraction secondary to Kaban IIa mandible (glenoid fossa present, mandibular condyle present but diminutive) (Fig. 26.12a). Mandibular distraction was performed, and the mandible was advanced at a rate of 1 mm/day × 20 days (Fig. 26.12b, c). The patient did well after surgery – he gained weight and tolerated feedings without further aspiration, and his sleep apnea significantly improved (Fig. 26.12d, e). Upon team evaluation, the patient was found to be one of the 7% of patients with TCS with sensorineural hearing loss and underwent cochlear implant placement.

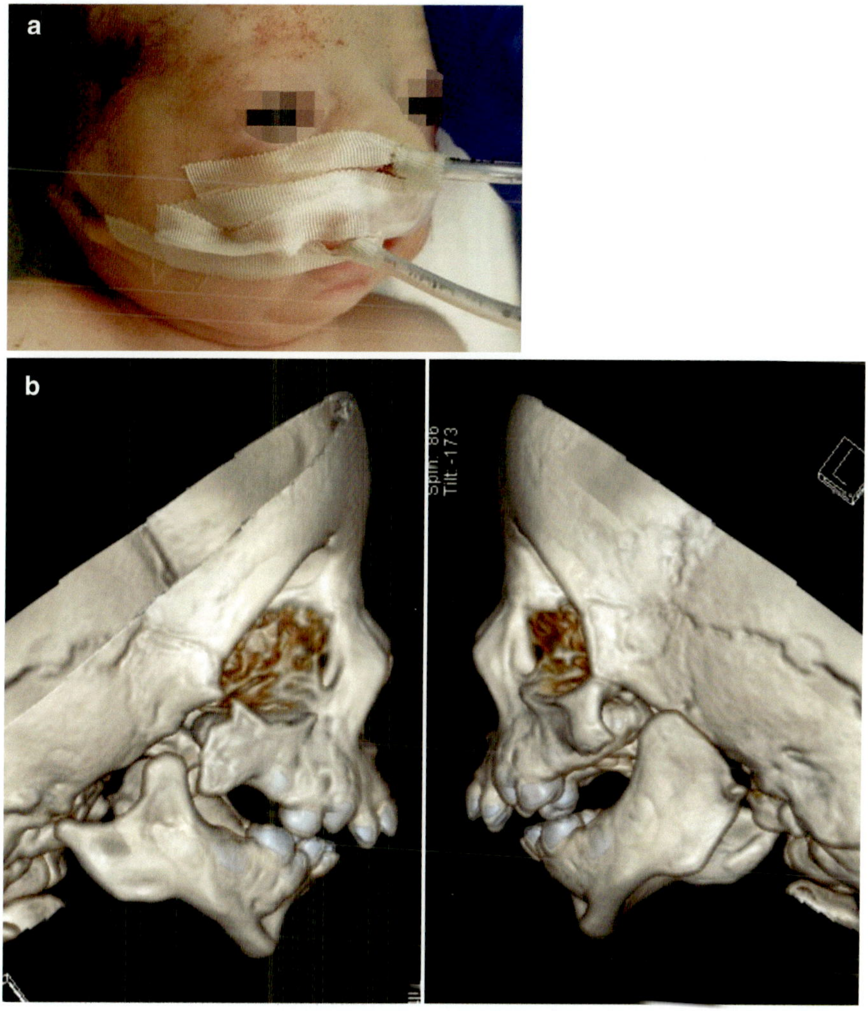

Fig. 26.11 Unexpected Treacher Collins Birth: The Airway (**a**) Baby arrived stable secondary to supraglottic placement of an ET tube nasally and orally. (**b**) Aplasia of glenoid fossa and temporal bone in this region, severe hypoplasia of the mandibular condyle/ramus complex

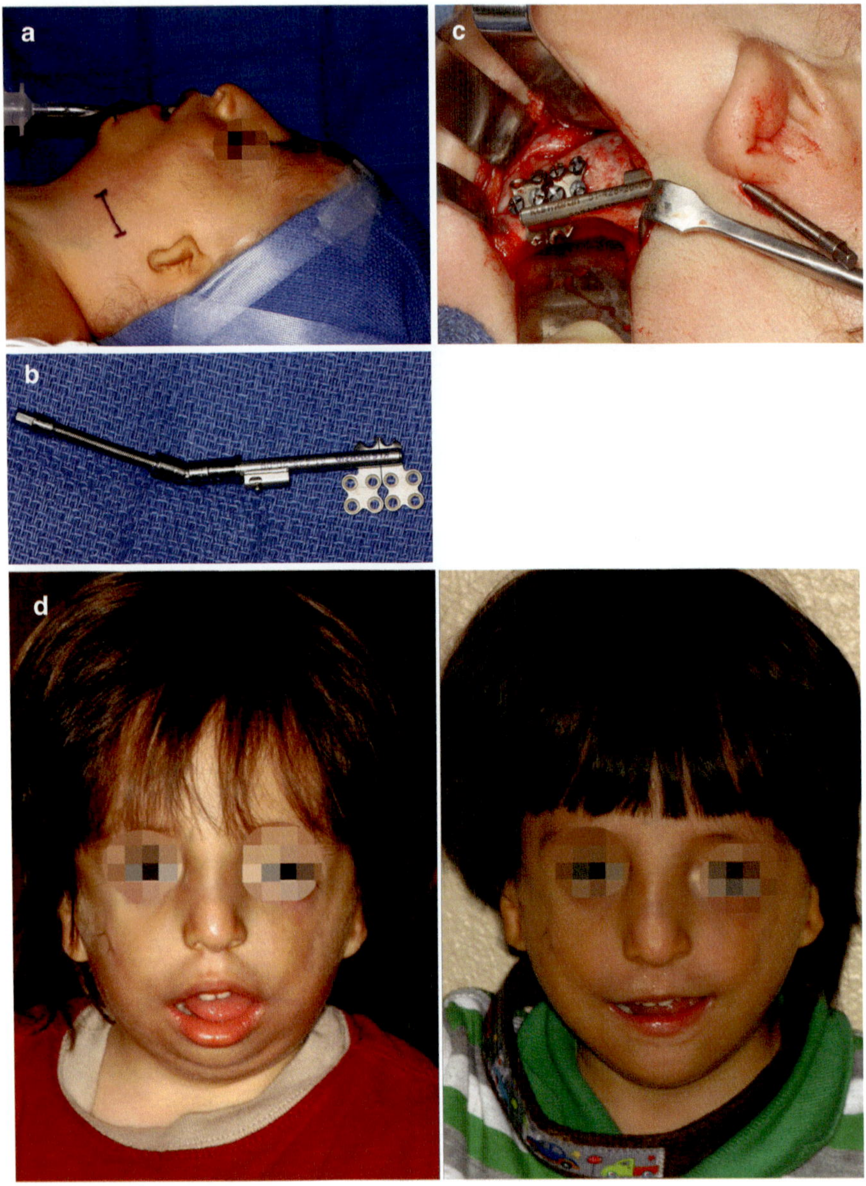

Fig. 26.12 Treacher Collins Syndrome: Failure to Thrive, Multiple Bouts of Aspiration Pneumonia (**a**) Mandibular retrognathia with submandibular incision marked out in the appropriate location 1.5 cm inferior to the inferior border of the mandible. (**b**) Mandibular distraction device (20 mm – KLS Micro Zurich 2). (**c**) Mandibular distraction device in place – may exit anterior or posterior. (**d**) Frontal view: preop and postop 1 year. (**e**) Profile view: preop and postop 1 year

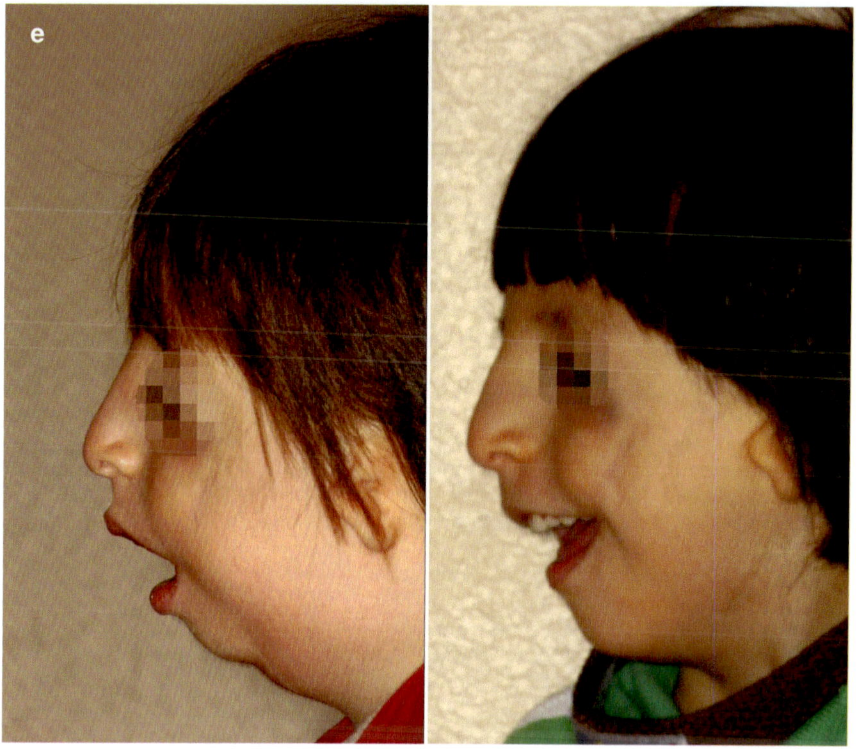

Fig. 26.12 (continued)

References

1. Wieczorek D. Human facial dysostoses. Clin Genet. 2013;83(6):499–510.
2. Posnick JC, Tiwana PS, Costello BJ. Treacher Collins syndrome: comprehensive evaluation and treatment. Oral Maxillofac Surg Clin North Am. 2004;16(4):503–23.
3. Østerhus IN, et al. Salivary gland pathology as a new finding in Treacher Collins syndrome. Am J Med Genet A. 2012;158a(6):1320–5.
4. Cobb AR, et al. The surgical management of Treacher Collins syndrome. Br J Oral Maxillofac Surg. 2014;52(7):581–9.
5. Hertle RW, Ziylan S, Katowitz JA. Ophthalmic features and visual prognosis in the Treacher-Collins syndrome. Br J Ophthalmol. 1993;77(10):642–5.
6. Marsella P, et al. Bone-anchored hearing aid (Baha) in patients with Treacher Collins syndrome: tips and pitfalls. Int J Pediatr Otorhinolaryngol. 2011;75(10):1308–12.
7. Pron G, et al. Ear malformation and hearing loss in patients with Treacher Collins syndrome. Cleft Palate Craniofac J. 1993;30(1):97–103.
8. Marsh JL, et al. The skeletal anatomy of mandibulofacial dysostosis (Treacher Collins syndrome). Plast Reconstr Surg. 1986;78(4):460–70.
9. Buchanan EP, Xue AS, Hollier LH Jr. Craniofacial syndromes. Plast Reconstr Surg. 2014;134(1):128e–53e.
10. Vincent M, et al. Treacher Collins syndrome: a clinical and molecular study based on a large series of patients. Genet Med. 2016;18(1):49–56.

11. Katsanis, S.H. and E.W. Jabs, Treacher Collins Syndrome, in GeneReviews(®), M.P. Adam, et al., 1993, University of Washington, Seattle. Copyright © 1993–2020, University of Washington, Seattle. GeneReviews is a registered trademark of the University of Washington, Seattle. All rights reserved.: Seattle (WA).
12. Teber OA, et al. Genotyping in 46 patients with tentative diagnosis of Treacher Collins syndrome revealed unexpected phenotypic variation. Eur J Hum Genet. 2004;12(11):879–90.
13. Aljerian A, Gilardino MS. Treacher Collins syndrome. Clin Plast Surg. 2019;46(2):197–205.
14. Rosa F, et al. Ear malformations, hearing loss and hearing rehabilitation in children with Treacher Collins syndrome. Acta Otorrinolaringol Esp. 2016;67(3):142–7.
15. Jahrsdoerfer RA, Jacobson JT. Treacher Collins syndrome: otologic and auditory management. J Am Acad Audiol. 1995;6(1):93–102.
16. Plomp RG, et al. Treacher Collins syndrome: a systematic review of evidence-based treatment and recommendations. Plast Reconstr Surg. 2016;137(1):191–204.
17. Takegoshi H, et al. Facial canal anatomy in patients with microtia: evaluation of the temporal bones with thin-section CT. Radiology. 2002;225(3):852–8.
18. Mukari SZ, Tan KY, Abdullah A. A pilot project on hospital-based universal newborn hearing screening: lessons learned. Int J Pediatr Otorhinolaryngol. 2006;70(5):843–51.
19. Amirhassankhani S, Lloyd MS. Accessory auricles: systematic review of definition, associated conditions, and recommendations for clinical practice. J Craniofac Surg. 2018;29(2):372–5.
20. Plomp RG, et al. Nasal sequelae of Treacher Collins syndrome. J Plast Reconstr Aesthet Surg. 2015;68(6):771–81.
21. Akre H, et al. Obstructive sleep apnea in Treacher Collins syndrome. Eur Arch Otorhinolaryngol. 2012;269(1):331–7.
22. Yates, DM, Sinn DP, Chapter 58 Classification, Diagnosis, and Etiology of Craniofacial Deformities; Maxillofacial Surgery, 3rd Edition Authors : Peter Prof. Brennan & Henning Prof Dr Schliephake & G.E. Dr. Ghali & Luke Cascarini 2017.

Correction to: Hearing Loss and Aural Rehabilitation in Patients with Treacher Collins Syndrome

Kevin Chow, Randi Tepper, Jaymee Franknecht, Lauren Kaplan, and Maura Cosetti

Correction to: Chapter "Hearing Loss and Aural Rehabilitation in Patients with Treacher Collins Syndrome" in: D. M. Yates, M. R. Markiewicz (eds.), *Craniofacial Microsomia and Treacher Collins Syndrome*, https://doi.org/10.1007/978-3-030-84733-3_23

This book was inadvertently published with incorrect author name "Jaymee Frankneckt". It has now been updated to correct name "Jaymee Franknecht" in the book.

The updated online version of this chapter can be found at https://doi.org/10.1007/978-3-030-84733-3_23

D. M. Yates, M. R. Markiewicz (eds.), *Craniofacial Microsomia and Treacher Collins Syndrome*, https://doi.org/10.1007/978-3-030-84733-3_27

Index

D. M. Yates, M. R. Markiewicz (eds.), *Craniofacial Microsomia and Treacher Collins Syndrome*, https://doi.org/10.1007/978-3-030-84733-3

T

GPSR Compliance

The European Union's (EU) General Product Safety Regulation (GPSR) is a set of rules that requires consumer products to be safe and our obligations to ensure this.

If you have any concerns about our products, you can contact us on ProductSafety@springernature.com

In case Publisher is established outside the EU, the EU authorized representative is:

Springer Nature Customer Service Center GmbH
Europaplatz 3
69115 Heidelberg, Germany

Batch number: 10756373

Printed by Printforce, the Netherlands